Plastic and Reconstructive Surgery
of the Genital Area

Plastic and Reconstructive Surgery of the Genital Area

EDITOR

CHARLES E. HORTON, M.D.

Professor of Surgery (Plastic), Eastern Virginia Medical School
Chief, Plastic Surgery, Norfolk General Hospital, Norfolk, Virginia

By 76 Contributing Authors

LITTLE, BROWN AND COMPANY
BOSTON

Library of Congress catalog card No. 73-1422

ISBN 0-316-37381

Printed in the United States of America

To my family

Contents

V. Trauma and Infection of the Genital Area

VI. Tumors

X. Unusual Cases

Y EARS AGO when new frontiers were being charted and great advances within various medical specialties were being accomplished, certain limitations and vague restrictions were drawn by men who sincerely believed that their specialty offered all in the treatment of a specific problem. Even though other specialists worked in related areas, they were not expected to delve into what "we know and treat best"—our sacrosanct field. This viewpoint resulted in an undesirable isolation of specialties.

Such isolation existed until recently in the complex field of genitourinary reconstruction. The urologist and gynecologist for anatomical reasons, the plastic surgeon for technical manipulations, the pediatric surgeon for psychological and physical circumstances, and the general surgeon because of his overall dominance, in all honesty felt that those from other disciplines who manipulated and contrived to treat "conditions" they were suspected to know little about were really to be distrusted.

Now, the value of cooperation, mutual respect, and admiration is being realized. Teams of pediatric surgeons, urologists, plastic surgeons, gynecologists, and general surgeons in all combinations are proving that patient care does benefit by sharing knowledge and techniques.

All disciplines have made contributions. In some anatomical areas, certain specialists will perform procedures with greater competence, yet in other areas, the reverse may be true. In these pages are gathered the best of all medical worlds for the use of those who are interested and are properly trained through varying disciplines in surgery of the genital area.

Possessing as it does the basic structures which allow the powerful drive of sexuality to exist, the genital area poses unique psychological and physiological problems. Hushed and repressed for years by even the medical profession, sexuality and all of its attendant problems can now be discussed with a new intellectual freedom. Instead of ignorance and hidden personal anguish for those patients with genital abnormalities, new hope and new horizons are now being offered.

All contributors to this book desire to be a forceful part of a new evolution to produce better care for the mental and physical problems that afflict these patients. Unfortunately, the external genitourinary system presents many difficulties, and not all of the problems inherent in reconstruction are solved. I have attempted to assemble chapters by specialists known over the world for their accomplishments. It is impossible to cover all medical aspects in one volume; however, by selecting what I judge to be major topics, I hope that this book will be a reference for further intensive study.

After opening chapters devoted to the history, embryology, and psychological aspects, the wide area of developmental anomalies is discussed. Of the twenty-three chapters in this section, the one on hypospadias stands out by its length and its format. There are eighteen subdivisions, five of them devoted to one-stage repairs; some duplication was inevitable, but I believe that the importance of the individual author's technique outweighs any objections. The remaining chapters cover trauma and infection, tumors, resurfacing, erectile disorders, and intrascrotal reconstruction. The thirteen unusual cases at the end are included for their interest and for their dramatic illustration of the variety of problems that may occur in the genital area.

My sincere thanks are offered to these experts for their cooperation and to my office staff who indulged my idiosyncrasies and interspaced my writing with necessary patient care and routine.

C. E. H.

Contributing Authors

Jerome E. Adamson, M.D.
Cochairman, Department of Plastic Surgery, Norfolk Medical Center, Norfolk, Virginia
CHAPTERS 25, 27, 35, 37, 42, AND 48

Robin Anderson, M.D.
Chief, Department of Plastic Surgery, Cleveland Clinic Foundation, Cleveland, Ohio
CHAPTER 40

Vinko Arneri, M.D.
Professor of Plastic Surgery and Specialist in General Surgery; Dicertor, Klinika za Plastičnu Hirurgiju VMA, Belgrade, Yugoslavia
CHAPTER 32

Lars Avellán, M.L.
Lecturer in Plastic Surgery, University of Göteborg; Assistant Chief Surgeon, Department of Plastic Surgery, Sahlgrenska sjukhuset, Göteborg, Sweden
CHAPTER 18

Lester A. Ballard, Jr., M.D.
Assistant Clinical Professor in Obstetrics and Gynecology, Case Western Reserve University School of Medicine; Gynecology Staff, Cleveland Clinic Foundation, Cleveland, Ohio
CHAPTER 40

Namik Baran, M.D.
Associate Professor of Plastic Surgery, Military Medical Academy, Ankara, Turkey
CHAPTERS 18 AND 27

Professeur Agrégé J. Barcat, Ph.D.
Membre, Faculté de Médecine de Paris, Chef du Service de Chirurgie Infantile, Hôpital Saint Louis, Paris, France
CHAPTER 18

Hal G. Bingham, M.D.
Professor and Chief of Plastic Surgery, University of Florida College of Medicine, Gainesville, Florida
CHAPTER 12

Thomas Ray Broadbent, M.D.
Associate Professor, University of Utah College of Medicine; Active Staff and Co-director of Resident Training Program, Department of Plastic Surgery, L.D.S. Hospital, Salt Lake City, Utah
CHAPTER 18

Forst E. Brown, M.D.
Clinical Instructor in Plastic Surgery, Dartmouth Medical School; Member, Plastic Surgery Section, Hitchcock Clinic and Hospital, Hanover, New Hampshire
CHAPTERS 41 AND 45

Earl Z. Browne, Jr., M. D.
Assistant Professor, Division, Plastic Surgery, University of Utah College of Medicine, Salt Lake City, Utah
CHAPTER 6

James Carraway, M.D.
Cochairman, Department of Plastic Surgery, Norfolk Medical Center, Norfolk, Virginia
CHAPTERS 25, 35, 37, 42, AND 48

J. Kenneth Chong, M.D.
Associate Professor, Section of Plastic Surgery, Temple University School of Medicine; St. Christopher's Hospital for Children, Philadelphia, Pennsylvania
CHAPTER 46

W. M. Cocke, M.D.
Assistant Clinical Professor of Plastic Surgery, Vanderbilt University School of Medicine, Nashville, Tennessee
CHAPTER 34

Lester M. Cramer, D.M.D., M.D.
Professor and Chairman, Section of Plastic Surgery, Temple University School of Medicine; Chairman, Plastic Surgery, Temple University Hospital and St. Christopher's Hospital for Children, Philadelphia, Pennsylvania
CHAPTER 46

Thomas D. Cronin, M.D.
Clinical Professor of Plastic Surgery, Baylor College of Medicine; Attending Surgeon and Director, Plastic Surgery Residency Program, St. Joseph Hospital, Houston, Texas
CHAPTER 18

Ormond S. Culp, M.D.
Professor of Urology, Mayo Graduate School of Medicine, The University of Minnesota Medical School; Chairman, Department of Urology, Mayo Clinic, Rochester, Minnesota
CHAPTER 18

John D. DesPrez, M.D.
Associate Clinical Professor of Plastic Surgery, Case Western Reserve University School of Medicine; Division of Plastic Surgery, University Hospitals of Cleveland, Cleveland, Ohio
CHAPTER 18

Charles J. Devine, Jr., M.D.
Department of Urology, Norfolk General Hospital and Kings Daughters Childrens Hospital, Norfolk, Virginia
CHAPTERS 2, 18, 19, 20, 21, 22, 23, AND 52

Patrick C. Devine, M.D.
Department of Urology, Norfolk General Hospital and Kings Daughters Childrens Hospital, Norfolk Virginia
CHAPTER 38

John W. Duckett, M.D.
Assistant Professor of Urology, The University of Pennsylvania School of Medicine; Pediatric Urologist, Children's Hospital of Philadelphia, Philadelphia, Pennsylvania
CHAPTER 14

Milton T. Edgerton, Jr., M.D.
Professor and Chairman, Department of Plastic Surgery, University of Virginia School of Medicine; University of Virginia Hospital, Charlottesville, Virginia
CHAPTER 7

A. J. Evans, F.R.C.S.
Consultant Plastic Surgeon, Plastic Surgery and Burns Centre, Queen Mary's Hospital, Roehampton, London, England
CHAPTER 31

Joseph G. Fiveash, Jr., M.D.
Urologic Surgeon, Norfolk Medical Center, Norfolk, Virginia
CHAPTER 26

P. Fogh-Andersen, M.D.
Doctor of Medicine, University of Copenhagen; Plastic Surgeon, Deaconess Hospital, Copenhagen, Denmark
CHAPTER 54

Foster Fuqua, M.D.
Clinical Professor of Urology, The University of Texas Southwestern Medical School at Dallas; Chief of Urology, Baylor University Medical Center; Director of Urology Section, Children's Medical Center, Dallas, Texas
CHAPTER 18

Thomas Gibson, F.R.C.S., D.Sc., M.B.
Visiting Professor, BioEngineering Unit, University of Strathclyde; Regional Director, Plastic Surgery Unit, Canniesburn Hospital, Bearsden, Glasgow, Scotland
CHAPTER 30

Jay Y. Gillenwater, M.D.
Professor and Chairman, Department of Urology, University of Virginia School of Medicine; Urologist and Chief, University of Virginia Hospital, Charlottesville, Virginia
CHAPTER 5

James F. Glenn, M.D.
Professor of Urology, Duke University School of Medicine; Chief of Urology, Duke University Affiliated Hospitals, Durham, North Carolina
CHAPTER 39

Thomas H. Guthrie, M.D.
Clinical Professor of Urology, Baylor College of Medicine; Associate Chief of Urology, St. Luke's Episcopal Hospital and Texas Children's Hospital, Houston, Texas
CHAPTER 18

Donald W. Hastings, M.D.
Professor of Psychiatry, University of Minnesota, Minneapolis Medical School, Minneapolis, Minnesota
CHAPTER 4

Charles E. Horton, M.D.
Professor of Surgery (Plastic), Eastern Virginia Medical School; Chief, Plastic Surgery, Norfolk General Hospital, Norfolk, Virginia
CHAPTERS 18, 19, 20, 21, 22, 23, 25, 27, 35, 37, 41, 42, 48, 52, AND 55

John T. Hueston, M.S., F.R.C.S., F.R.A.C.S.
Chief Plastic Surgeon, Royal Melbourne Hospital, Victoria, Australia
CHAPTER 24

H. B. Jennings, Jr., M.D.
Surgeon General, Department of the Army, Washington, D.C.
FOREWORD TO CHAPTER 33

Bengt Johanson, M.D.
Professor of Plastic Surgery, University of Göteborg; Chief Surgeon, Department of Plastic Surgery, Sahlgrenska sjukhuset, Göteborg, Sweden
CHAPTER 18

M. J. Jurkiewicz, M.D.
Professor and Chief, Division of Plastic and Reconstructive Surgery, Emory University School of Medicine; Chief of Surgery, Grady Hospital, Atlanta, Georgia
CHAPTER 44

Desmond A. Kernahan, F.R.C.S.(C)
Professor of Surgery (Plastic), Northwestern University Medical School; Head, Plastic Surgery, Children's Memorial Hospital, Chicago, Illinois
CHAPTER 9

Wilson J. Kerr, Jr., M.D.
Plastic and Reconstructive Surgeon, Yakima, Washington
CHAPTER 36

Robert A. Loeffler, M.D.
Eden Hospital, Castro Valley, California; Consultant, Plastic Surgery, U.S. Naval Hospital, Oakland, California
CHAPTER 51

Joseph M. Malin, Jr., M.D.

Associate Professor of Urologic Surgery, Wayne State University School of Medicine, Detroit, Michigan
CHAPTER 39

Frank W. Masters, M.D.

Professor of Surgery, The University of Kansas School of Medicine, Kansas City, Kansas
CHAPTER 29

David N. Matthews, M.D., M. Ch., F.R.C.S.

Consultant Plastic Surgeon, Hospital for Sick Children and University College Hospital; Civilian Consultant in Plastic Surgery to the Royal Navy, London, England
CHAPTERS 13 AND 18

Howard B. Mays, M.D.

Assistant Professor of Urology, University of Maryland School of Medicine; Attending Urologist and Chief, Urology Department, Maryland General Hospital, Baltimore, Maryland
CHAPTERS 17 AND 18

Ian A. McDonald, F.R.C.S., F.R.A.C.S., F.R.C.O.G.

Chief Gynaecologist, Royal Melbourne Hospital, Victoria, Australia
CHAPTER 24

Ian A. McGregor, Ch.M., F.R.C.S.

Honorary Clinical Lecturer in Plastic Surgery, University of Glasgow; Consultant Plastic Surgeon, Canniesburn Hospital, Bearsden, Glasgow, Scotland
CHAPTER 47

Jon K. Meyer, M.D.

Assistant Professor of Psychiatry and Assistant Professor of Surgery, The Johns Hopkins University School of Medicine; Psychiatrist, The Johns Hopkins Hospital, Baltimore, Maryland
CHAPTER 7

Richard A. Mladick, M.D.

Cochairman, Department of Plastic Surgery, Norfolk Medical Center, Norfolk, Virginia
CHAPTERS 25, 27, 35, 37, 42, AND 48

B. D. G. Morgan, M.B., F.R.C.S.
Consultant Surgeon, Regional Plastic Surgery Centre, Skotley Bridge General Hospital, Durham, England
CHAPTER 28

I. F. K. Muir, M.S., F.R.C.S.
Lecturer in Clinical Surgery, University of Aberdeen; Consultant Surgeon, Department of Plastic Surgery, Aberdeen General and Special Hospitals, Aberdeen, Scotland
CHAPTER 28

John C. Mustardé, F.R.C.S.
Consultant Plastic Surgery, Glasgow and West of Scotland Regional Plastic and Oral Surgery Service, Canniesburn Hospital; Consultant Plastic Surgeon, Royal Hospital for Sick Children, Glasgow, Scotland
CHAPTER 18

Lester Persky, M.D.
Professor of Urology, Case Western Reserve University School of Medicine; Chief, Division of Urology, University Hospitals of Cleveland, Cleveland, Ohio
CHAPTER 18

Jaime Planas, M.D.
Chief of Plastic and Aesthetic Surgery, Clinica de Cirugía Plástica y Estética, Barcelona, Spain
CHAPTER 18

Eugene F. Poutasse, M.D.
Department of Urology, Norfolk General Hospital and King's Daughters Children's Hospital, Norfolk, Virginia
CHAPTER 49

† Robert J. Prentiss, M.D.
Late Professor of Urological Surgery, University of California, San Diego, School of Medicine, San Diego, California
CHAPTER 53

Peter Randall, M.D.
Senior Surgeon, Division of Plastic Surgery, Children's Hospital of Philadelphia, Philadelphia, Pennsylvania
CHAPTER 18

† *Deceased*

Greer Ricketson, M.D.

Associate Professor of Plastic Surgery, Vanderbilt University School of Medicine, Nashville, Tennessee
CHAPTER 18

Blair O. Rogers, M.D.

Assistant Professor of Clinical Surgery (Plastic Surgery), New York University School of Medicine; Attending Surgeon, Department of Plastic Surgery, Manhattan Eye, Ear and Throat Hospital, New York, New York
CHAPTER 1

Frederic Rueckert, M.D.

Clinical Assistant Professor of Plastic Surgery, Dartmouth Medical School; Member, Hitchcock Clinic, and Chairman, Department of Plastic Surgery Section, Hitchcock Hospital, Hanover, New Hampshire; Consultant in Plastic Surgery, Veterans Administration Hospital, White River Junction, Vermont
CHAPTERS 41 AND 45

Peter L. Scardino, M.D.

Chief of Urology, Memorial Medical Center, Savannah, Georgia
CHAPTER 43

Charles D. Scott, Ph.D.

Assistant Research Professor, University of Utah College of Medicine; Head, Cytogenetics Laboratory, University of Utah Medical Center, Salt Lake City, Utah
CHAPTER 6

Arthur George Ship, M.D., D.M.D.

Assistant Clinical Professor of Surgery, Albert Einstein College of Medicine of Yeshiva University; Associate Attending, Plastic Surgery, Montefiore Hospital and Medical Center, The Bronx, New York
CHAPTER 15

Donald R. Smith, M.D.

Professor and Chairman, Division of Urology, University of California, San Francisco, School of Medicine; Urologist-in-Chief, Herbert C. Moffitt Hospital, San Francisco, California
CHAPTER 18

Clifford C. Snyder, M.D.
Professor of Surgery and Chairman, Division, Plastic Surgery, University of Utah College of Medicine; Chief of Surgery, Salt Lake City Veterans Administration Hospital, Salt Lake City, Utah
CHAPTER 6

Mark B. Sorensen, M.D.
Formerly Resident in Urology, University of California, San Diego, School of Medicine, San Diego, California
CHAPTER 53

Richard B. Stark, M.D.
Associate Clinical Professor of Surgery, Columbia University College of Physicians and Surgeons; Attending Surgeon in Charge of Plastic Surgery, St. Luke's Hospital Center, New York, New York
CHAPTER 3

Edward S. Tank, M.D.
Associate Professor of Surgery, University of Michigan Medical School, Ann Arbor, Michigan
CHAPTERS 10 AND 11

Ian M. Thompson, M.D.
Professor and Chief, Department of Urology, University of Missouri—Columbia School of Medicine, Columbia, Missouri
CHAPTER 12

Esat Toksu, M.D.
Senior Attending Plastic Surgeon, St. Elizaeth Hospital; Chairman, Department of Surgery, St. Luke's Memorial Hospital, Utica, New York
CHAPTER 18

Samuel Torres, M.D.
Chief Resident, Department of Urology, Memorial Medical Center, Savannah, Georgia
CHAPTER 43

William V. Tynes, II, M.D.
Department of Urology, Norfolk General Hospital and King's Daughters Children's Hospital, Norfolk, Virginia
CHAPTER 50

Luis O. Vasconez, M.D.

Assistant Professor, Division of Plastic and Reconstructive Surgery, Emory University School of Medicine; Department of Surgery, Emory University Hospital, Atlanta, Georgia

CHAPTER 44

David Innes Williams, M.D., M.Ch., F.R.C.S.

Dean, Institute of Urology, University of London; Urologist, Hospital for Sick Children, London, England

CHAPTER 16

J. S. P. Wilson, F.R.C.S.

Consultant Plastic Surgeon, University of London, St. George's Hospital; Consultant Plastic Surgeon, Westminister Hospital, London, England

CHAPTER 8

A. Michael Wood, F.R.C.S.

Lecturer, University of East Africa; Consultant Plastic Surgeon, H. H. The Afa Khan Hospital and The Kenyatta National Hospital, Nairobi, Kenya

CHAPTER 36

Robert M. Woolf, M.D.

Associate Clinical Professor, University of Utah College of Medicine; Active Staff, Latter-day Saints Hospital and L. D. S. Primary Children's Hospital, Salt Lake City, Utah

CHAPTER 18

Joseph R. Zbylski, M.D., Lt. Col., M.C., U.S.A.

Clinical Assistant in Surgery (Plastic), University of Colorado Medical Center School of Medicine; Chief, Plastic Surgery Service, Fitzsimons General Hospital, Denver, Colorado

CHAPTER 33

History

I

History of External Genital Surgery

BLAIR O. ROGERS

I

Ye shall circumcise the flesh of your foreskin; and it shall be a token of the covenant betwixt me and you (Gen. 17:11).

Surgical Practices and Medical Knowledge in Ancient Times

IN ORDER to understand ancient man's first attempts at performing genital surgery, we must know something about his early trials with other primitive forms of surgery and about his basic attitudes toward sex itself.

Trepanation, amputation, incision, and circumcision were prehistoric man's first crude attempts at surgery [1]. During the Neolithic age (about 9000 B.C. to about 2000 B.C.), the earliest surgical instruments were sharpened flints or fishes' teeth, by means of which skulls were trepaned, abscesses were emptied [1], blood was let, and tissues were scarified. At a somewhat later period, ritual mutilations such as circumcision were performed [61].

The first example of a skull showing a trepanation wound was found in France in 1843, and the skull was dated as an example of the early Neolithic period [132]. Amputation as a surgical procedure is first depicted in cave paintings of the Aurignacian period [76], which began approximately 40,000 years ago [32].

Incision as a surgical procedure was used for emptying abscesses and letting blood, as well as for piercing ears and ritual tattooing and scarring. The latter is one of the most common ritual mutilations practiced among primitive peoples today. Incision originated in the Late Paleolithic period, which began approximately 70,000 years ago. According to the modern anthropological method of inferring prehistoric practices on the basis of the study of present-day "stone age" primitive tribes, it may be assumed that incision of the external genitalia is probably one of the oldest forms of ritual mutilation [86–88]. Among some of the mountain dwelling primitive tribes of New Guinea, "boys are incised sometime after the first puberty ceremonies, and since in menstruation women are thought to be provided with a natural mechanism for purging themselves of bad blood, the men believe that in order to preserve their health and strength they, too, must similarly purge themselves. At periodic

3

intervals, therefore, they go to a stream where they make light incisions in the glans" [87].

Ceremonial incision of males at puberty initiation rites generally consists of splitting; the foreskin is cut downward for its full length. It also can take the form of making a more or less deep cut only into the glans, which may or may not be periodically repeated [87]. In one section of New Guinea, such periodic incision of the penis is referred to as "men's menstruation." Male novices at puberty rites are told that penile incision "is a way of getting rid of their mothers' blood, so that they will grow strong and handsome" [50]. Ashley-Montagu suggests that men in these primitive societies believe that women rid themselves of "bad blood" by menstruation, and therefore they not only try to imitate the act of bleeding by inflicting a genital wound, but in many cultures they also practiced the art of "subincision," which attempts to make the male genital organ resemble the female's [87].

Subincision is probably the most extraordinary of all genital mutilations practiced by primitive man. It consists of slitting open the penile urethra on its ventral surface, the incision in some instances extending all the way from the urinary meatus to the scrotum. In others, it may be limited to a small incision made into the floor of the urethra at any point along the ventral surface of the penis. Under ordinary conditions, the subincised penis looks perfectly normal on its anterior or dorsal aspects since the ventral urethral aspect is hidden from view, and the mutilation usually escapes the casual observer's eye. Readers are referred to a fascinating book on this subject by Eliade: *Rites and Symbols of Initiation: The Mysteries of Birth and Rebirth* [50].

Excision as a primitive ritual is the removal of either a part or most of the female external genitalia. Excision ranges from the removal of only a part of the clitoral prepuce, as is done among natives in certain parts of Abyssinia and Egypt [116], to the removal of parts of the clitoris, both labia, and the mons, as is done among certain East African tribes [87]. Between these two extremes, every variety of excision operation of intermediate degrees of severity has been described [87]. An Egyptian papyrus attributed to the year 163 B.C. indicates that excision was performed on almost every girl at puberty. It is still widely practiced today in Melanesia, Indonesia, and Africa.

EARLY DEPICTIONS OF GENITALIA

Prehistoric man had no inhibitions when it came to depicting the genitalia of men or animals (Fig. 1-1). Ivory or bone phallus carvings are common, human sex organs were frequently carved on cave walls, and the famous Venus figurines—noted for their stoutness, ample buttocks, and huge dangling breasts—almost always have the genital features emphasized. On the other hand, primitive artistic depictions of humans in the act of sexual intercourse are very rare, but a few exist. In most prehistoric art, male figures are more scarce than female figures, and their male sexual characteristics are seldom emphasized. However, in one of the Pyrenees caves, Le Portel, a bearded man in a wall painting has as an erect penis a three-dimensional stalagmite protruding from the cave wall itself [123]. Of the male figures whose organs are depicted without question, many of the men are shown with the penis in erection. Since late prehistoric art frequently shows warriors in ithyphallic stances, the erect penis may merely be a convention intended by the artist to demonstrate virility [123].

Prehistoric men who existed near the early beginnings of recorded time still lived very close to the natural world, and their reaction to it was certainly more direct. Thus, one should not be surprised to learn that their art indicates that they performed sexual acts

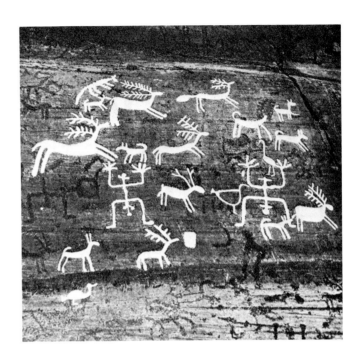

FIG. 1-1. Male figures with obvious penises and scrota among the hundreds of carvings superimposed one upon another on the rock face at Naquanne in the Camonica Valley. (From Bibby [15].)

with animals (Fig. 1-2), although some art historians prefer to believe that such paintings are not literal portrayals but are instead mere "wish fulfillments." Certainly the ancient Greeks and Romans did not hesitate to depict such acts or to display various works of art based on this zoophilic theme in their houses and in their gardens [111]. It was probably not until Judeo-Christian ethics replaced the attitudes of earlier civilizations that the public acceptance of this kind of erotica gradually died out [123].

Since prehistoric times, the erect penis in cave paintings and temple wall friezes and paintings often symbolized fertility, dominance, power, and virility. The Egyptians were often quite realistic in the depiction of this phallic symbolism (Fig. 1-3).

It is not yet known whether prehistoric man was acquainted with congenital genital deformities, nor do we have any depiction of the rituals of incision, subincision,

excision, or circumcision in any of his art. Puberty rites include mutilating forms of genital surgery that primitive man performs with a deadly seriousness, and these ceremonies were almost always religious, involving primitive man and his gods. Thus, any artistic depiction of these operations would probably be forbidden because of the secrecy associated with such rites [50].

Prehistoric art may be concerned merely with eroticism rather than having magical interpretations such as enhancement of fertility. It is felt by some that some African Bushmen have regularly practiced infanticide since a food-gathering and hunting life is much too hard to be able to support too many children. Some writers have suggested that subincision may originally have been introduced as a contraceptive device. In most aboriginal and, by analogy, probably in most prehistoric societies, the approach to such a problem has two much simpler solutions:

custom of circumcising males. There is some evidence that circumcision or excision of the female external genitalia was practiced centuries before Mohammed. In some societies, notably among certain Peruvian tribes, it was performed on all women regardless of their social rank when they became of age to receive their dowries [63]. Even today, circumcision or excision in its simplest form, i.e., in which only a part of the clitoral prepuce is removed, is still found among natives in certain parts of Egypt. The ancient Egyptians were aware of distinctions in the gross anatomy of the female, and in their papyri and hieroglyphic writings, they used different words for the uterus, the vagina, and the external genitals [19].

BLADDER EXSTROPHY

Exstrophy of the bladder has apparently been known since early recorded time. Teratologists have especially been interested in one of the Assyrian tablets in the British Museum that states: "When a woman gives birth to an infant that wants the penis and the umbilicus, there will be ill-will in the house, the wife will have an overbearing eye; but the male descent of the palace will be more extended." Rickham [110] suggests that this is probably a description of a case of ectopia vesicae, or exstrophy of the bladder with a downward displacement of the umbilicus, and if so, this disorder can be said to have been first described in approximately 2000 B.C.

CASTRATION AND OTHER MUTILATIONS

The earliest explicit mention of castration or of eunuchs in recorded history can be found in the code of Hammurabi (about 2000 B.C.), the great Babylonian administrator. Some historians believe there is a suggestion of the presence of eunuchs in the somewhat earlier Minoan civilization of Crete [120]. The Code of Hammurabi forbade a eunuch's adopted children from leaving their foster parent since, quite practically, he would then lack any provision for his old age. The Code of Hammurabi also recommended castration as a punishment for sexual crimes.

When the Vedic people invaded India from approximately 1500 B.C. until 1000 B.C., they brought with them a history of eunuchism, and their Vedas, the hymns of people who preceded the Hindus, mention several forms of castration of animals and men. At the beginning of the Twentieth Dynasty (1200–1085 B.C.), castration or excision of the penis was the punishment for adultery in Egypt, and the same punishment can be found in the Chinese literature of 1122 B.C.

Since castration and eunuchism appeared in Egypt later than in the earlier civilizations of Asia and Asia Minor, one might assume that the Egyptians learned these concepts from their Asian neighbors. Castration was a much more important concept among peoples in the Israelitic lands, and apparently its practice emerged in 1250 B.C. Eunuchs were specifically prohibited by Mosaic law from entering the priesthood or even from entering the "congregation." This is specifically mentioned in Deuteronomy: "He that is wounded in the stones, or hath his privy member cut off, shall not enter into the congregation of the Lord" (Deut. 23:1). Eunuchs are discussed frequently throughout the Old Testament.

Eunuchism occurred only sporadically among the Greeks, and it seems to have been almost nonexistent among the Romans, although in both civilizations castration was used as a form of punishment.

The destruction of the entire male organ either by mutilation or amputation was, in ancient times, a fairly common and distinctive sign of degradation or slavery, or a reli-

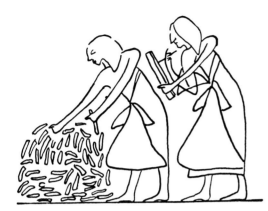

FIG. 1-5. Artist's drawing of a relief at Medinet-Habu showing Egyptian soldiers dismembering their victims after a battle by cutting off either their hands or penises. The tally was kept by a scribe by noting the number of amputated organs. (From Bitschai and Brodny [19].)

gious symbol of the humility of an individual before his god or gods or before his victorious kings. In 1300 B.C., for example, the Egyptian pharaoh Merneptah had inscribed on the walls of the Temple of Karnak the following inventory to commemorate his victory over the Libyan invaders (Fig. 1-5) [37]:

Libyan generals killed, phalluses cut off	6
Libyans killed, phalluses cut off	6359
Sicilians killed, phalluses cut off	222
Etruscans killed, phalluses cut off	542
Greeks killed, phalluses brought to the King	6111

Surgical infibulation, known to the eighteenth century English as "muzzling," consists of the passing of a ring, pin, clamp, leather thong, or similar device through two perforations of the prepuce or the labia majora. In the male, this prevents retraction of the prepuce and hence makes coition or masturbation impossible.

The history of infibulation goes back to at least ancient Greece, but its purpose varied according to the culture in which it was practiced. In Greece, infibulation was used primarily for professional athletes who, following the prevailing code, had to appear in public naked but with their glans covered. The only public exposure which was considered indecent in ancient Greece, Etruria, and Rome was that of the uncovered glans. Among the Greeks, some athletes were said to be infibulated in preparation for Olympic contests, a rather gruesome practice apparently designed to enforce their rigorous rules of sports training [41, 113]. In Greece and Etruria, the device consisted of a leather string or band that either was wound around the tip of the prepuce or was drawn through the perforations of the prepuce and then wound around the loin for purposes of immobilization and protection during the athletic contest (Fig. 1-6). It was referred to as

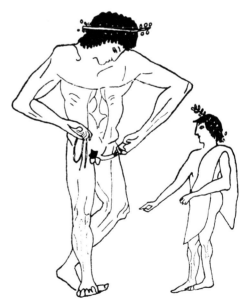

FIG. 1-6. Method of application of the *kynodesme*. Engraving on a Greek kylix-krater now in the Berlin Antiquarium. (From Dingwall [41].)

kynodesme, i.e., "dog chain," and was re-moved after the athletic competition or games were completed. In Rome, athletes passed a pin through the perforations to which a decorative copper sleeve was at-tached to hide the glans. Jewish professional athletes, naturally with more deficient pre-puces because of their circumcised penises, had a greater problem and covered the glans with a clamp. The case has been recorded of Menophilus, a Jewish athlete, who lost his clamp during a fight in the arena, much to his embarrassment [113].

HERMAPHRODITISM

Ombrédanne [95] points out that there were some civilizations prior to the Greeks who worshipped bisexual or hermaphroditic gods. Although Young [139] and Jones and Scott [73] begin their introductory chapters on the historical concepts of hermaphrodit-ism with references made only to the Greeks, Ombrédanne cites the mention of hermaph-rodites in the Asiatic religions of the Chaldeo-Babylonians and the Syro-Phoenicians, both of whom had civilizations that preceded the Greeks by many centuries. In Greek legend, Hermaphroditos was the son of Hermes and Aphrodite [75] and was originally a normal youth. One day at a spring whose waters were said to render those who used them effeminate, the nymph of the spring, Sal-macis, desperately in love with the handsome youth, implored the gods to unite her with him forever. Her wish was fulfilled and the bisexual Greek god, Hermaphroditos, was the result (Fig. 1-7). During these early civiliza-tions, hermaphroditic or androgynous divin-ities had a very high status.

Zarathustra (Zoroaster), who founded the ancient Persian religion in the sixth cen-tury B.C., spoke of the first man as a her-maphrodite. Some medical historians find this same bisexuality or hermaphroditism in

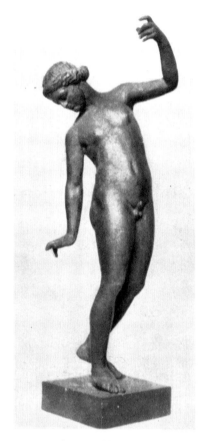

FIG. 1-7. The so-called Hermaphroditos of Mirecourt, now in the Epinal Museum. This bronze statuette is presumably a copy of a work dating from the first or second century B.C. It is interesting to note that this graceful figure is depicted with an erect, hypospadial penis. This realism may be an indication that the sculptor used a live model. (From Ombrédanne, L. *Les hermaphrodites et la chirurgie.* Paris: Mas-son, 1939. By permission of Masson & Cie, Paris.)

the first chapter of Genesis in which Moses is quoted: "So God created man in his *own* image, in the image of God created he him; male and female created he them" (Gen. 1:27).

Aristotle believed that the condition of her-maphroditism was the result of a deviation from natural developmental processes, but his humanism was in sharp contrast to the ideas of later centuries [74]. The Romans exposed deformed children, especially hermaphrodites, on islands in the Tiber, or they executed them [133]. In subsequent centuries, human hermaphrodites were treated with extreme prejudice and general contempt, being regarded as monsters.

THE ANCIENT JEWS

In turning to the Bible for information on the surgical practices of the ancient Jews, the results are disappointing. Guthrie [65] and Castiglioni [25] are among numerous historians who believe that the practice of surgery among the ancient Jews was almost nonexistent. The only surgical operation specifically mentioned in the Bible is circumcision, which was performed by a rabbi as a ritual procedure (see Gen. 17:10–14; Ex. 4:25). Circumcision as a surgical operation was known at least as early as 1300 B.C. by the ancient Jews [16]. Isaiah (Chapter 1, verse 6) speaks of wounds that "have not been closed, neither bound up, neither mollified with ointment" [65], thus indicating that the Jews knew something about first aid.

In the First Book of the Maccabees [82], one of the Apocryphal books of the Old Testament which probably was originally written in Hebrew about the first century B.C., there is a quotation in Chapter 1, verses 15 and 16, of the existence in Jerusalem of certain houses where the prepuce was restored [141]. In Saint Paul's first letter to the Corinthians, the following statement perhaps verifies the Maccabean quotation: "Is any man called being circumcised? let him not become uncircumcised. Is any called in uncircumcision? let him not be circumcised" (1 Cor. 7:18).

Zeis [141], in his exhaustive though occasionally inaccurate bibliography of writings on plastic surgery from ancient times to 1863, cites numerous other references in which allusion is made to the ancient Jewish practice of restoring the prepuce that may have been missing or deficient following too extensive a circumcision or following the removal of tumors in the preputial area.

The Bible, the Apocrypha, the Pseudepigrapha, and the Talmud provide medical historians with some interesting descriptions of genitourinary diseases and deformities [124]. Any man whose penis was cut off was not permitted to marry an Israelite woman. Another rule stated that a man suffering from an abnormal opening in his penis could not marry into the community. This might refer to cases of hypospadias and epispadias [124], as could the Talmudic reference to "one who passes water in two places," although these descriptions could equally apply to the "watering-can" perineum that frequently follows urethral strictures caused by severe cases of gonococcal urethritis.

The ancient Jews were aware of the conditions of unilateral and bilateral cryptorchidism, and this affliction disqualified a priest from temple duties [124]. Two forms of intersex, the androgenes and the tumtom, were recognized. Androgenes probably represented some form of hermaphroditism. Tumtoms were either cryptorchids or some form of intersex whose actual sex was unknown until they were "cut open" [124].

ANCIENT INDIA

The ancient Hindus had a relatively thorough knowledge of male and female anatomy. Sushruta (approximately sixth century B.C.) made no mention of circumcision in his surgical descriptions, but he did refer to the excision of malignant ulcers and necrotic disorders of the penis, the latter resulting from a disease known as *Upadansá* that might have been a very virulent ancient form of gonorrhea or syphilis. Sushruta mentioned the penis by name in some paragraphs and in others referred to it as the "male organ." Simple surgery of the penis is evidenced in Sushruta's description of the treatment of one of the forms of *Upadansá:* "Now hear me discourse on the special treatment of *Tridoshaja Upadansá.* It should be the same as in the case of malignant ulcer.... the putrid portion of the male organ should be cut off and the remaining portion should be fully cauterized [in the incised part] with a *Jambvoshtha* instrument, made red hot in fire" [14]. In another form of *Upadansá,* the veins of the penis were opened for the elimination of "contaminated blood" in a severe case of the disorder, and leeches were applied to the organ in less severe cases.

Apparently, Hindu surgeons—as judged by the writings of Charaka in the sixth century B.C. [38] and Sushruta—knew only the rudiments of urological surgery, but they certainly knew of and probably employed catheters. Catheters were used for urethral dilatation and for the treatment of abdominal swelling caused by urinary retention [38]. One operation was precisely described; it consisted of treating scrotal tumors caused by urinary infiltration in which, if the medical treatment of sweating the patient did not help to draw off the urine, the surgeon resorted to perforating the scrotal raphe on the left and introduced a perforated tube to withdraw the urine. He then placed a ligature in the perforation site.

In the writings of Sushruta, medical historians first encounter ancient man's rather derisive and condescending attitude toward the female in his society and, perhaps even more specifically, a negative attitude toward the female genitalia. A certain sense of naïveté and even prudery pervades the medical literature for the next 2500 years after Sushruta whenever the female genitalia are re-

ferred to. In certain civilizations, this prudery extended to any mention of the male genitalia as well. An example of the attitude of placing blame on the woman can be seen in Sushruta's explanation of the cause of *Upadansá:*

The disease owes its origin to the action of the local Doshas . . . aggravated by promiscuous and excessive intercourse, or by entire abstinence in sexual matters; or by visiting a woman, who had observed a vow of lifelong continence or one who has not long known a man, or one in her menses, or one with an extremely narrow or spacious vulva, or with rough or harsh or large pubic hairs; or by going unto a woman whose parturient canal is studded with hairs along its entire length; or by visiting a woman not amorously disposed towards the visitor and vice versa; or by knowing a woman who washes her private parts with foul water and neglects the cleanliness of those parts; or suffers from any of the vaginal diseases, or one whose vagina is naturally foul; or by going unto a woman in any of the natural fissures of her body other than the organ of copulation (*Vi-yoni*) . . . . The inflammation of the genital thus engendered is called *Upadansá* [14].

ANCIENT GREECE

Only a few records, essentially consisting of artistic depiction, reveal the state of medical practice prior to the Hippocratic period of Greek medicine and surgery. A section of a painting on an antique vase, dating approximately from the period of 510 to 490 B.C., illustrates five patients, four of them, some leaning on crutches with or without bandaged arms and one, most interestingly, a short achondroplastic slave whose nude body and genitalia reveal that he was infibulated, thus providing an example of a practice that was known to exist in Greece in this epoch.

Prior to Hippocrates (approximately 460 to 355 B.C.), there seem to be no medical documents verifying that catheterization and lithotomy were procedures known to the ancient Greeks. Hippocrates, however, defended those who practiced lithotomy, although he stated that it was not performed by him or his pupils [3, 4, 26]. The Hippocratic Oath contains this sentence: "I will not cut persons labouring under the stone, but will leave this to be done by men who are practitioners of this work" [3]. This apparently referred to itinerant lithotomists, who seem to have had no compunctions about operating on and frequently tampering with the penis, the urethra, and the bladder [38]. Thus, one can assume, as did Littré, that lithotomists existed either during or prior to Hippocrates' lifetime in Greece. It is assumed that in Egypt there were specialists for the eyes, the teeth, and the lithotomy operation.

Hippocrates, in his chapter dealing with articulations, described the bladder as anatomically situated together with those parts that were responsible for generation, locating them in the concavity of the sacrum below the fifth lumbar vertebrae. Hippocrates was also familiar with the shape of the urethra [3, 4, 26], but in none of his books is there any mention of hypospadias or other external genital deformities. Urethral abscesses and gangrene of the genitalia, however, were described. Retraction of the genitalia and cases of urinary incontinence were considered "hopeless" [26]. In speaking of the urethra anatomically for the first time in medical literature, Hippocrates describes it as follows:

Calculi do not form so readily in women, for in them the urethra is short and wide, so that in them the urine is easily expelled; nor do they rub the pudendum with their hands, nor handle the passage like males [masturbation]; for the urethra in women opens direct into the pudendum, which is not the case with men, neither in them is the urethra so wide, and they drink more than children do [3].

Although Hippocrates did not write specifically of circumcision, in 460 B.C. Herodotus stated: "The Egyptians ... are the only people who practice circumcision. ... they practice circumcision for cleanliness sake—for they set cleanliness above seemliness" [63].

The Hippocratic school believed that female genitalia were much colder than other abdominal organs [108]; they "should be concealed" and are that "which it is a shame to look upon" [3]. Hippocrates and the Romans were guilty of prudery insofar as the meaning of the word *pudendum* is "that of which one ought to be ashamed," from the Latin verb *pudere,* to be ashamed. Hippocratic gynecology referred to the vaginal orifice and vaginal discharges, but neither the clitoris nor the hymen were described.

Hippocrates was essentially a medical man in the full sense of the word and anything but a surgeon. His avoidance of surgery at almost all costs, with the possible exception of the setting of fractures, is probably due to his conforming to the principle of *"primum non nocere,"* which when translated essentially means "above all, do no harm." The Hippocratic Oath gave Hippocrates and his school a convenient excuse for not taking the knife into their hands. Hippocrates left no outstanding pupils.

Two centuries after Hippocrates, Ammonious of Alexandria (born circa 276 B.C.) perfected a cutting or a breaking up of a calculus by an operation in which he opened the perineum and the neck of the bladder and extracted the sectioned, divided, and broken up calculus with a thin blunt instrument. Ammonious gave the name of lithotomy to this operation [38]. Ammonious might have been an itinerant nomadic lithotomist [38], but he has gained the medical historians' accolade of being the first to describe lithotomy, although it had been performed for centuries before his time.

Roman Medicine and Surgery

Aulus Cornelius Celsus (25 B.C. to A.D. 50) was without doubt the first great Roman physician [93]. His work, *De Medicina* [121], was a vast encyclopedia of medical and surgical knowledge that he had probably acquired both from his Greek and Egyptian predecessors as well as from earlier Roman medicine and surgery, although the last had been somewhat primitive and unremarkable. Unfortunately, Celsus' books did not become widely read texts until the middle of the fifteenth century A.D. [142], and they apparently exerted only a very minor influence on his contemporaries and his immediate successors [108]. Celsus' anatomical knowledge of the details of both male and female external genitalia was the most advanced and most sophisticated of any writer before Galen [108, 121].

Celsus was one of the first to describe catheterization, a techinque that was to be necessary in any of the hypospadias repairs to be performed in the next millennium and thereafter:

Sometimes we are compelled to draw off the urine by hand when it is not passed naturally; either because in an old man the passage has collapsed, or because a stone, or a blood-clot of some sort has formed an obstruction within it; but even a slight inflammation often prevents natural evacuation; and this treatment is needed not only for men but sometimes also for women. For this purpose bronze tubes are made, and the surgeon must have three ready for males and two for females, in order that they may be suitable for every body, large and small: those for males should be the longest, fifteen finger-breadths in length, the medium twelve, the shortest nine; for females, the longer nine, the shorter six. They ought to be a little curved, but more so for men, and they should be very smooth and neither too large nor too small. Then the man must be placed on his back, in the way described for anal treatment, on a low

seat or couch; while the practitioner stands on his right side, and taking the penis of the male patient in his left hand, with his right hand passes the pipe into the urethra; and when it has reached the neck of the bladder, the pipe together with the penis is inclined and pushed on right into the bladder; and when the urine has been evacuated, it is taken out again. The woman's urethra is both shorter and straighter, like a nipple placed between the inner labia over the vagina, and this requires assistance no less often though it is attended by somewhat less difficulty [121].

Another source of objects that gave an accurate picture of the state of urological surgery during the time of Celsus are the votive figures left by gratified patients in the temples of Hygeia or Aesculapius. Many of these ex-votos, which consist of a small cast in either terracotta or other malleable ceramic material, are fashioned in the shape of a penis and the adjacent scrotum and demonstrate such disorders as balanitic ulcerations and swollen prepuces as a result of blennorrhagia. A great number show lesions, indicating the frequency of venereal diseases among the ancients. Some ex-votos demonstrate prepuces of extremely pendulous dimensions, which apparently were rather common in ancient times. Needless to say, some of these little works of art, which also can be traced to the later period of Imperial Rome when everyday morality had relaxed considerably, were fashioned in definitely erotic shapes and dealt with highly arousing subject matter. One must not accuse the ancient Romans purely and simply of eroticism, however, because the phallus was also a symbol of fecundity and phallic symbols were frequently worn as amulets against evil spirits and sorcerers [111].

The Roman reputation for loose sexual morality and degeneracy [111] in later decades and centuries did not seem to affect a certain degree of puritanism in Celsus' writings. He wrote in the introduction to his discussion of diseases of the penis as follows:

Next come subjects relating to the privy parts, for which the terms employed by the Greeks are the more tolerable, and are now accepted for use, since they are met with in almost every medical book and discourse. Not even the common use has commended our coarser words for those who would speak with modesty. Hence it is more difficult to set forth these matters and at the same time to observe both propriety and the precepts of the art. Nevertheless, this ought not to deter me from writing, firstly in order that I may include everything which I have heard of as salutary, secondly because their treatment ought above all things to be generally understood, since every one is most unwilling to show a complaint to another person [121].

In contrast to the "punctures" or "perforations" loosely referred to by the ancient Indian authors, Celsus was probably the first author to describe a specific surgical incision made in the penis:

Sometimes too a stone slips into the urethra itself, and lodges not far from its orifice, because this becomes narrower further down. The stone should if possible be extracted either by an ear-scoop or by the instrument with which a stone is drawn out in the course of lithotomy. If this cannot be done, the foreskin is drawn as far forwards as possible over the glans and tied there by a thread. Then to one side of the penis a longitudinal incision is to be made and the stone taken out, after which the prepuce is released. This is done in this way so that an intact portion of skin covers the incision into the penis and urine flows out naturally [121].

Celsus provides the first detailed description in medical literature of the treatment for a deficient prepuce, an operation that requires a subtle understanding of penile anatomy. Although most modern surgeons and some of those in the eighteenth and nineteenth cen-

turies have been skeptical as to its successful outcome, this operation illustrates the boldness with which Roman surgeons attacked abnormalities in this organ:

For Deficient Prepuce: . . . if the glans is bare and the man wishes for the look of the thing to have it covered, that can be done; but more easily in a boy than in a man; in one in whom the defect is natural, than in one who after the custom of certain races has been circumcised; and in one who has the glans small and the adjacent skin rather ample, while the penis itself is shorter, rather than in one in whom the conditions are contrary.

Now the treatment for those in whom the defect is natural is as follows. [Obviously, Celsus did not consider circumcised cases where too much prepuce was taken away as ideal cases for this rather drastic operation.] The prepuce around the glans is seized, stretched out until it actually covers the glans, and there tied. Next the skin covering the penis just in front of the pubes is cut through in a circle until the penis is bared, but great care is taken not to cut into the urethra, nor into the blood vessels there. This done the prepuce slides forward towards the tie, and a sort of small ring is laid bare in front of the pubes, to which lint is applied in order that flesh may grow and fill it up. It is seen that a large enough part of the penis has been bared, if the skin is distended little or not at all, and if the breadth of the wound above supplies sufficient covering. But until the scar has formed it must remain tied, only a small passage being left in the middle for the urine [121].

Celsus apparently cared little for the procedure known as infibulation:

Some have been accustomed to pin up the prepuce in adolescence either for the sake of the voice, or for health's sake. This is the method: The foreskin covering the glans is stretched forwards and the point for perforation marked on each side with ink. Then the foreskin is let go. If the marks are drawn back over the glans too much has been included, and the marks should be placed further forward. If the glans is clear of them, their position is suitable for the pinning. Then the foreskin is transfixed at the marks by a threaded needle, and the ends of this thread are knotted together. Each day the thread is moved until the edges of the perforation have cicatrized. When this is assured the thread is withdrawn and a fibula inserted, and the lighter this is the better. But this operation is more often superfluous than necessary [121].

Infibulation for the purpose of "locking" the penis and preventing coition or masturbation originally employed a light pin or ring inserted through the foreskin, but in later stages of the Roman Empire the removable pin was replaced by a permanently closed ring, forged together by a silversmith. The motivation was mainly to "preserve the strength of athletes and the voice of singers" [113]. Preservation of the voice was thought to be affected by delaying puberty as long as possible. Although Roman actors were originally infibulated only to preserve their voices, particularly if they were lute players, at a later period in Rome police prefects insisted on the presence of infibulated actors "to prevent lewdness."

Despite Celsus' exhaustive treatment of other disorders of the external genitialia, no mention can be found in his works of either hypospadias or hermaphroditism or their treatment. Celsus did describe, however, surgical correction of phimosis, penile warts, callosities, carbuncles, penile inflamed ulcers and spreading gangrenous ulcers, hydrocele, varicocele, and sarcocele.

Celsus was probably the first to describe imperforate hymen and possibly vaginal aplasia. The following description of an operation to correct the latter sounds familiar to today's surgeons, who find similarities in it to the first stage of reconstruction of the vagina prior to skin graft implants, which, of course, were unknown in Celsus' time:

[There] are also some troubles which are peculiar to females, especially that occasionally their genitals do not allow of coitus, the orifices having coalesced. And this sometimes happens even in the mother's womb; sometimes when ulceration has occurred in those parts, and through bad treatment there the margins have become united during healing. If the condition is congenital a membrane obstructs the vulvar orifice; if due to ulceration flesh has filled the same. The membrane should be incised along two lines crossing one another like the letter X, great care being taken that the urethra is not injured; then the membrane is to be cut away all round. But if flesh has grown there, it must be laid open with a single straight cut; next when the margin has been seized either with a forceps or hook, a fine strip must be cut away from it, after which there is inserted wool rolled lengthwise (the Greeks call it Lemniscus), dipped in vinegar, and over this is bandaged on greasy wool wetted with vinegar; this is changed on the third day and the wound treated like other wounds; and as soon as it begins to heal, a lead tube smeared with a cicatrizing ointment is passed in, and over this the same application applied until the cut surface has cicatrized [121].

Celsus' postoperative use of a lead tube smeared with an ointment and acting as a tamponade to keep the cut vaginal surfaces from reuniting preceded Dupuytren's use of a tampon in a case of vaginal aplasia by approximately 1800 years [97, 104] and McIndoe's use of a skin graft covering an acrylic mould to treat similar vaginal conditions by approximately 1950 years [81].

Alexandrian Surgery

Heliodorus and Antyllus in the first and second centuries A.D. can be given credit for being the first in medical history to describe hypospadias and its surgical correction. In the translation of Bussemaker and Daremberg [19, 24], the description of hypospadias is given in its entirety:

Among certain individuals, the gland [glans], because of a congenital defect, is not pierced according to nature, but the hole is found below the brake (frenum), as it is called in Greek, at the termination of the gland. For this reason, the patient can neither urinate in front, unless the penis is raised sharply toward the pubes, nor procreate children because the sperm cannot be directed in a straight line into the uterus, but forms on the side in the vagina. Some patients develop hypospadias because of an acquired defect: these are the cases where the urinary canal is perforated on the side, although the gland remains in its natural state, the meatus having been corked by callosity [tissue] following an invasive ulceration or some other circumstance. Sometimes the hole is situated far from the frenum, in the middle of the urethra near the base of the gland; these cases are incurable. At other times the hole exists at the level of the brake and then the disturbance can be cured.

The simplest, best, and least dangerous operative procedure is what is called operation by resection. The patient is placed on his back and the gland is fully raised with the left hand. This part is then cut with the edge of the scalpel at the level of the crown. However, the incision should not be slightly oblique but should resemble a delicate circular carving, leaving a projection representing the form of a gland. If a little blood flows, it should be stopped with a bandage and vinegar water; if this does not suffice, medications should be used to stop the bleeding, and if the flow is severe the wound should be cauterized. But the resection must be done in the gland rather than in the penis, for because of its compact structure the gland is less likely to hemorrhage.

If cauterization is used, one should, after the operation, resort to the appropriate treatment for burns; in the other cases the treatment for bleeding wounds should be employed. It is necessary to know why the resection is not an obstacle to reproduction: during coitus the gland does not encounter the orifice of the uterus, but the coupling takes place in the vagina, and the snout of the tench being open, the sperm is directed into the uterus, whether the penis is large or small [19].

Despite the crudeness of this amputation-type operation to correct hypospadias, Alexandrian surgeons at least were concerned about cosmetic results, as is indicated by their emphasis on leaving intact a distal portion of the penis by using an incision which resembled "a delicate circular carving" so that some semblance of a projecting gland (glans) resulted.

Heliodorus and Antyllus also described treatment of rectovesical, rectovaginal, and scrotal fistulas, phimosis, adhesion of the prepuce to the glans, circumcision for preputial gangrene, verrucous papillomas of the glans or prepuce, and preputial fissures. Urethral stenosis, according to Heliodorus, was treated by dilatation, recanalization, and the use of a postoperative indwelling paper-wrapped candle containing in its center a little tin or bronze tube through which the patient urinated during the healing phase.

Galen (circa A.D. 129–200) described such conditions as hermaphroditism and hypospadias. He referred briefly to the surgical correction of hypospadias in a short chapter dealing with such surgery entitled *"De chirurgiae speciebus"* [77]. Leonides of Alexandria, who lived approximately 90 years after Galen, was apparently the first to describe hermaphrodites from a strictly medical standpoint [2, 5].

Following Galen, the Byzantine period (A.D. 476–732) was noted chiefly for its famous medical compilers. Oribasius (A.D. 325–403), Alexander of Tralles (A.D. 525–605), and Paul of Aegina (Paulus Aegineta) (A.D. 625–690) [2] preserved for the future the medical knowledge that otherwise would have disappeared in the Dark Ages which were soon to envelop all of Europe and Asia Minor [118].

Paulus Aegineta lived in Alexandria during the rise of Mohammedan power and the spread of Islam. The city was captured by the Arabs in 640 A.D., and they inherited and preserved the science of the Greeks. The subsequent works of Arab physicians and surgeons reflect their almost total reliance on the recorded works of Paulus Aegineta and his predecessors.

Paulus Aegineta was next, after Leonides, to describe in brief detail the condition of hermaphroditism:

There being four varieties of it, according to Leonides; three of them occur in men and one in women. In men, sometimes about the perineum and sometimes about the middle of the scrotum, there is the appearance of a female pudendum with hair; and in addition to these there is a third variety, in which the discharge of urine takes place at the scrotum as from a female pudendum. In women there is often found above the pudendum and in the situation of the pubes the appearance of a man's privy parts, there being three bodies projecting there, one like a penis, and two like testicles. The third of the male varieties in which the urine is voided through the scrotum is incurable; but the other three may be cured by removing the supernumerary bodies and treating the part like sores [2].

Although Paulus Aegineta was not the first to describe the condition, he is probably the first author whose works come to us first-hand without being interpreted or compiled by a previous author.

Paulus Aegineta's writing on hypospadias is a short description, apparently compiled and drawn from the previous work of Heliodorus and Antyllus.

Paulus Aegineta is perhaps the first to describe castration specifically, although Celsus described removal of the testicle for a condition known as cirsocele, a form of varicocele [121]. Paulus showed his distaste for the operation in the opening lines of his description:

The object of our art being to restore those parts which are in a preternatural state to their natural, the operation of castration professes just the reverse. But since we are sometimes compelled against our will by persons of high rank to perform the operation, we shall briefly describe the mode of doing it. There are two ways of performing it, the one by compression, and the other by excision. That by compression is thus performed: Children, still of a tender age are placed in a vessel of hot water, and then when the parts are softened in the bath, the testicles are to be squeezed with the fingers until they disappear, and, being dissolved, can no longer be felt. The method by excision is as follows: Let the person to be castrated be placed upon a bench, and the scrotum with the testicles grasped by the fingers of the left hand, and stretched; two straight incisions are then to be made with a scalpel, one in each testicle; and when the testicles start up they are to be dissected around and cut out, having merely left the very thin bond of connection between the vessels in their natural state. This method is preferred to that by compression; for those who have had them squeezed sometimes have venereal desires, a certain part, as it would appear, of the testicles having escaped compression [2].

Paulus' operation for an "imperforate pudendum" was undoubtedly derived from the descriptions of Celsus, Aëtius, and Soranus. Of interest to plastic surgeons is his recommendation that following removal of the obstruction, the vaginal surfaces be permitted to heal more naturally by the application of "a priapus-shaped tent covered with some epulotic medicine, in those cases especially in which the operation is performed upon a part not very deep-seated, in order that the parts may not unite again" [2].

With the exception of the Roman surgery described by Celsus, the sixth book of Paulus Aegineta's compilations is the only extant treatise in which surgery was precisely separated from medicine.

The Middle Ages

With the death of Paulus Aegineta in the seventh century, the great period of Greco-Roman medicine came to an end and was replaced by the domination of Islamic medical thought. However, it was not until Albucasis (936–1013) that major references to urological surgery are again found [78]. In addition, Avicenna (980–1036), the most famous of the Arab writers on medicine, actually set back the progress of surgery by his repetition and spreading of the doctrine that the art of surgery was inferior to medicine and only a separate branch of it [93]. The separation of medicine from surgery was a fundamental error of medical science in the Middle Ages [93]. Monastic and scholastic minds gradually became convinced that surgery was a most lowly, undesirable art.

Rhazes (865–925), the astonishingly erudite Persian physician, performed a buttonhole urethrotomy in the perineum when unable to pass a catheter in cases of gonorrheal urethral stenosis [19].

Haly Abbas (930–994), a well-known Persian physician who was often quoted in the literature of the early Renaissance, spoke of castration in the same manner as did Paulus Aegineta. Many sentences from his writings reveal his dislike of the procedure. Haly Abbas also wrote of hermaphroditism:

The cause of hermaphroditism is natural [congenital]; it is a cause of deformity that develops in three different ways among men, and in one way among women. The first type among men is where a formation like a female vulva surrounded by hair appears under the pubis or in the middle of the scrotum [19].

Hot cautery was a characteristic feature of Arabic surgery. Some Arab surgeons completely rejected the Greco-Roman use of the knife, but most apparently did not abandon its use entirely. In fact, Albucasis of Cordoba (936–1013), the greatest and most imaginative of all Arab surgeons, was the first in medical history to describe and illustrate [68] the very delicate bistoury (lance) that was used to make an incision into the glans of a newborn baby to correct an "imperforate urethra." His instructions for postoperative care in such cases were simple and very interesting:

You place in the opening [created by the bistoury] a small lead sound [probe] which you tie in place [with a ligature?] and which you keep in place for three or four days. When he wishes to urinate, you remove the sound and you let him urinate and then you replace it. If indeed you yourself do not replace the sound, it will be possible that the urine which flows on the wound prevents the edges from healing....

There are others in whom the urinary meatus is not situated at its natural location [hypospadias], they are born with the meatus opening laterally on the glans or not situated at the end of the glans. Such is the method of operating: make the patient lie on his back; hold the glans firmly with the left hand; then cut the head of the glans, at the eminence [or the presenting aperture of the meatus] with a knife or a bistoury, as if you were cutting a quill or as if you want to carve a piece of wood, in the manner of reestablishing a natural shape of the glans, and in which the meatus falls into a median position where it should be. Take care during the operation against hemorrhage, which happens frequently, and treat it with hemostatics. You dress it afterward until it heals* [translation by the author].

Albucasis treated urethral narrowness with a lead bougie that was employed long enough to enlarge the canal. He also described castration briefly, mentioning that Moslem laws forbade it, but he suggested that surgeons be familiar with the procedure from a practical standpoint in order to perform it when necessary on "bulls, billy goats, cats" and other animals.

Avicenna (980–1037), the Persian, devotes the third book of his *Canon of Medicine* to urology and urological surgery. This book contains 160 chapters, some of them so long that they could almost be considered monographs. Section 20 of the third book deals with the masculine sexual organs and their pathology and anatomy. The pathological aspects of sexual life, in which normal sexual

---

* Compare this description with a paragraph from Ambroise Paré five centuries later.

---

life and its derangements are dealt with, are covered in approximately 20 chapters [19].

In the eleventh century, Arabic medical doctrine was introduced into the School of Salerno in Italy. The status of medicine was to become greatly elevated in Western Europe during the beginnings of the university systems that were to take hold soon thereafter. Unfortunately, however, the edict of the Council of Tours in 1163 called for the removal of books on surgery and midwifery from libraries, and some universities excluded all those who worked with their hands. Medicine and surgery therefore became totally divorced in this period [93]. In the thirteenth and fourteenth centuries, it was from the hands of lowly and unlettered men that surgery once again began to develop. In this age, the surprisingly skillful barber surgeons came into their own.

In the fifteenth century, Charaf ed-Din (about 1465), a Turkish surgeon, was responsible for a beautifully illustrated surgical text in which numerous drawings revealed the state of Turkish surgery at that time. A

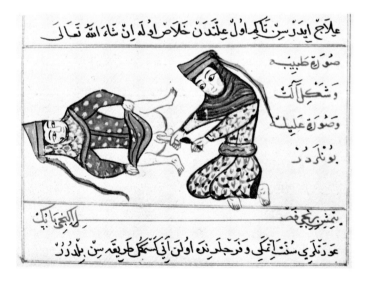

FIG. 1-8. Treatment of hermaphroditism in a woman as depicted in the works of Charaf ed-Din (1465). (From Huard and Grmek [71].)

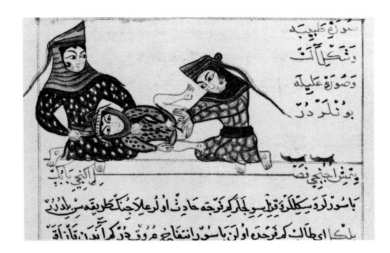

FIG. 1-9. Treatment of imperforation or vaginal atresia, as depicted in the works of Charaf ed-Din (1465). (From Huard and Grmek [71].)

heavy emphasis was placed on the use of cautery [71]; Turkish surgeons had carried on the tradition of the use of cautery from Arab surgeons, and the influence of Arabic medical texts on the Turks was undoubtedly great.

Perhaps for the first time in medical history, actual urological and other surgical operations were depicted in exceptionally colorful illustrations (Figs. 1-8 and 1-9). Specific surgery and other methods for dealing with the following urological disorders were described by Charaf ed-Din: hermaphroditism, imperforate urethra, vaginal atresia, circumcision, emasculation or castration, preputial or glandar warty growths, hydrocele, urinary retention, lithotrity, and bladder lavage [71].

A majority of the operations performed on women's genitalia, both at the time of Albucasis and that of Charaf ed-Din, were done by midwives rather than male surgeons [2]. Among the Moslems and their Semitic cousins, the ancient Hebrews [111], the viewing of a nude female body or a portion of the female body in the nude state by a male was considered shameful and humiliating [2, 71, 111]. In the Charaf ed-Din manuscript, the beautiful illustrations of the surgery of a

female hermaphrodite and of a patient with vaginal atresia reveal the surgeon to be a midwife (see Figs. 1-8 and 1-9).

The Renaissance

The epitome of Renaissance surgery was represented by the work of Ambroise Paré (1510–1590), a provincial barber-surgeon's apprentice, whose perilous life as a Huguenot mirrored this fascinating period in history [98, 101, 102]. Renaissance surgery also benefited from the brilliant discoveries, writings, and teachings of Gaspare Tagliacozzi (1545–1599) [62] and of Pierre Franco (circa 1505–1579), another great Huguenot itinerant barber-surgeon. The latter's operations for hernia and lithotomy did much to put surgery on a dignified basis [58, 59].

Amatus Lusitanus (1511–1561), a Portuguese Jew who studied medicine at Salamanca, described treating a 2-year-old child with an imperforate glans and penoscrotal hypospadias with a silver cannula that he directed from the scrotal hypospadial opening up through the shaft of the penis until it came to the imperforate site, where he used a pointed instrument to perforate the glans [7]. His successful canalization technique was, in 1556, the first major advance in hypospadias surgery since the primitive "carving" and amputation technique of Antyllus, Paulus Aegineta, and Albucasis.

Matteo Realdo Colombo (born 1510) of Cremona, an opponent and the successor of Vesalius in the chair of anatomy of Padua, was probably the first to describe vaginal agenesis in his book, *De re anatomica*, published in 1559. Surgical repair of this deformity, however, was not dealt with by Colombo [31, 122].

Ambroise Paré's exhaustive anatomical and surgical descriptions reflected some rather naïve and bizarre ideas about anatomy, physiology, and pathology. In describing the testes and the penis, which was known as the "yarde" in the English translation, Paré stated:

Those whose testicles are more hot are prompt to venery, and have their privities and the adjacent parts very hairy, and besides their testicles are more large and compact. Those on the contrary that have them cold are slow to venery, neither doe they beget many children, and those they get are rather female than male, their privities have little haire upon them, and their testicles are small, soft and flat.

The action of the testicles is to generate seede, to corroborate all the parts of the body, and by a certaine manly irradiation to breed or encrease a true masculine courage.

Of the yarde.... The yarde is of a ligamented substance because it hath its originall from bones, it is of an indifferent magnitude in all dimensions, yet in some bigger, in some lesse; the figure of it is round, but somewhat flatted above and beneath [102].

His description of the female pudendum is probably in keeping with the thinking of his

time and is almost reminiscent of the Arabic distaste for viewing the female genitalia. Speaking of the pudendum, or "privitie," Paré states that:

[It] is of a middle substance, betweene the flesh and a nerve; the magnitude is sufficiently large, the figure round, hollow, long.... It is one in number, situate above the *Perinaeum*. It hath connexion with the fundament, the necke of the wombe and bladder by both their peculiar orifices.

The latter *Anatomists*, as *Columbus* and *Fallopius*, besides these parts, have made mention of another particle, which stands forth in the upper part of the privities, and also of the urinary passage, which joynes together those wings wee formerly mentioned. *Columbus* calls it *Tentigo*, *Fallopius Cleitoris*, whence proceeds that infamous word *Cleitorizein*, (which signifies impudently to handle that part). But because it is an obscene part, let those which desire to know more of it, read the Authors which I cited [102].

Paré's description of hypospadias is not as sophisticated as that of Paulus Aegineta, considering that the latter at least drew attention to the need for trying to preserve the appearance of a glans in the crude amputation procedure that he recommended. Paré describes the "evil conformation" as follows (note that he was probably the first in medical literature to describe chordee and its surgical correction):

The cure is wholly chirurgicall, and is thus performed. The praepuce is taken hold of and extended with the left hand, but with the right hand, the extremity thereof, with the end of the *Glans*, is cut even to that hole which is underneath. But such as have the bridle or ligament of the yarde too short [chordee?], so that the yarde cannot stand straight, but crooked, and as it were turned downewards; in these also the generation of children is hindred, because the seed cannot be cast directly and plentifully into the wombe. Therefore this ligament must be cut with much dexterity, and the wound cured after the manner of other wounds, having regard to the part.

Children also are sometimes borne into the world with their fundaments unperforated, for a skinne preternaturally covering the part, hinders the passage forth of the excrements; those must have a passage made by art with an instrument, for so at length the excrements will come forth; yet I have found by experience, that such children are not naturally long lived, neither to live many dayes after such section [102].

Paré described hermaphrodites or "scrats" (the latter was apparently an English term) more completely and in more detail than any prior author in medical history. He mentioned that the death penalty was inflicted if the scrats "departed from the sexe they made choice of":

And here also we must speake of Hermaphrodites, because they draw the cause of their generation and conformation from the plenty and abundance of seed, and are called so because they are of both sexes, the woman yeelding as much seed as the man. For hereupon it commeth to passe that the forming faculty (which alwaies endeavours to produce something like it selfe) doth labour both the matters almost with equall force, and is the cause that one body is of both sexes. . . .

[The] lawes command those to chuse the sexe which they will use, and in which they will remaine and live, judging them to death if they be found to have departed from the sexe they made choice of, for some are thought to have abused both, and promiscuously to have had their pleasure with men and women [102].

Two excellent illustrations of hermaphrodites were included in Paré's text, as well as an illustration of the two assistants required

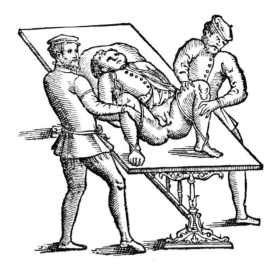

FIG. 1-10. The position of a man on a table prior to removing a stone from the bladder. (From Paré [102].)

to hold a man down on the operating table for a lithotomy (Fig. 1-10).

Paré described and illustrated an artificial penis almost four centuries before the first descriptions of surgically reconstructed penises by Gillies and others. Paré's device consisted chiefly of a pipe or a conduit to draw off the urine:

Those that have their yardes cut off close to their bellies, are greatly troubled in making of urine, so that they are constrained to sit downe like women, for their ease. I have devised this pipe or conduit, having an hole through it as big as ones finger, which may be made of wood, or rather of latin.

A. and C. doe shew the bignesse and length of the pipe. B. sheweth the brink on the broader end. D. sheweth the outside of the brinke. This instrument must be applied to the lower part of the *os pectinis:* on the upper end it is compassed with a brink for the passage of the urine, for thereby it will receive the urine the better, and carry it from the patient, as he standeth upright [102].

Exstrophy of the bladder was probably first described by Schenk in 1595 [47]. Others have assigned a priority for the "first" in describing this deformity to Ruffin in 1637 [46]. Bartolin states that Van Horne published the first case observed in women in 1670 [46].

The Seventeenth Century

Compared with the other branches of medicine, neither general surgery nor urological surgery advanced greatly during the seventeenth century. Among the great names in medicine in this period, Fabricius of Aquapendente (1533–1619) described the restoration of a deficient prepuce in much the same manner as did Celsus and Paulus Aegineta. He drew attention to treatment of an imperforate glans using the technique of Albucasis, cutting away or carving away enough of the glans until the meatus appears [52, 53]. He also described vaginal atresia, imperforate hymen, and hermaphroditism. Fabricius of Aquapendente treated two young women with imperforate vaginas. As described in the colorful eighteenth century English translation of Dionis:

The one...a Servant-Maid which several Scholars could not deflower, and who, after having shock'd all their Vigour against the Ligatures of her *Caruncules,* was forc'd to have recourse to him. The other Example is of a Girl, who, being wholly imperforate, could not discharge her menstruous Terms, they being detained by a Membrane which join'd the *Caruncules,* and intirely lock'd up the Passage, which occasion'd a pressing weight in the *Vagina,* accompanied with insupportable Pains; he made an Incision lengthwise in that Membrane, from whence issued out a great quantity of black and stinking Blood, which gave the Patient ease, and perfectly cured her. There is also an Author who

has written a Treatise in Latin, *de Imperforatis* [42].

Although surgical progress was slow in the seventeenth century, the art of surgical illustration showed great advances and refined techniques, especially in the art of the woodcut.

The Eighteenth Century

Paris was the center of surgical studies in Europe at the beginning of the eighteenth century, and among its most famous surgeons was Pierre Dionis (died 1718). Despite the preeminence of French surgeons, the status of surgery during most of the eighteenth century was quite low, with the exception of the work of Lorenz Heister (1683–1758), the first German surgeon of importance in this century.

Dionis' 1707 book of surgery, *Cours d'opérations,* was a standard work for half a century or more, and in it he described treatment of the imperforate glans, hypospadias, chordee, hermaphroditism, adhesion of the prepuce to the glans, enlarged clitoris and nymphae, imperforate hymen, and imperforate vagina. Dionis taught operative surgery at the Jardin-du-Roi in Paris, a famous training ground for surgeons. Although he described many urological operations in his text, three of them he rejected as "unprofitable." They were circumcision, infibulation (buckling), and *recutili* (surgery for correcting a deficient prepuce). In prefacing his remarks to these three operations, he stated rather derisively: "I shall say no more than what is necessary to give you a sufficient Idea of them, to incline you to be the first in condemning them" [42].

Dionis' operation to correct an imperforate glans in the newborn follows Albucasis' method closely, but he apparently did not pay much attention to reinsertion of a lead sound after each spontaneous urination of the baby as did Albucasis:

I think 'tis not necessary to insert a small leaden Pipe to hinder the re-union of the edges of the Wound, because the frequent Passage of the Urine prevents its closing [42].

Dionis probably wrote the most complete description of surgery of hypospadias in 1707, eleven years before Heister's exhaustive review [66]. Dionis' account is the following:

It frequently happens that the *Glans* is not perforated in the ordinary Place, but below it towards the *Fraenulum;* those affected with this Indisposition, are obliged to raise up their Yard in order to make Water.... This frequently proceeds from a Child's coming into the World without any Aperture of the *Glans,* and the Parent's not discerning it, the Urine which endeavors to pass out, makes its way near the Bridle, which is the thinnest Part of the *Urethra;* ... We must then, with the pointed *Myrtle-Leaf Q,* pierce the *Glans,* and thereby make such an *Aperture* as ought to be there naturally, the Orifice then made, insert in it a small *leaden Pipe S,* long enough to run beyond the lower Aperture in the *Urethra,* and conduct the Urine thro' this new one: Next we must go about the closing the old one, quickening the Edges of it by small Incisions, and procuring its cicatrizing: The Pipe must be left in the urinary Passage, which must be kept fast and tied to it with the String T, 'till the Cure be perfected, that the Urine no longer passing thro' the old Orifice may not hinder its re-union. If we cannot close this Hole, some Authors direct us to make an Incision on the *Glans* from the first Aperture to the second, cutting it like a writing Pen with the small Incision-Knife V, that so the Urine and Seed passing thro' a large Pipe, may be cast to the Places where they ought to go.

I have seen some children whose *Urethra* has been pierc'd two or three Finger's breadth distant from the *Glans:* These were Children subject to piss their Beds, and who to escape Cor-

rection, which frequently fell on them, tied their Yard with a Thread, concluding that an infallible way, and in the interim the Urine pressing its Passage, after violent Pains, made a way near the Ligature, through which that Serosity continually pass'd afterwards. To cure these Patients we must thrust into the *Urethra* a small leaden Pipe, which must be run beyond the Orifice, whose re-union we aim at [42].

Dionis' description of chordee is probably one of the first after Paré's to be found in the surgical literature. Like Paré, he did not give this condition any specific medical name:

There are some who are born with the Bridle of their Yard too short; this *Fraenum* draws the *Glans* downwards, particularly at the Time of Erection: Whence the Aperture being at that Time too low, if the Yard be not rais'd, the Person will piss on his Legs or Feet, and 'twill be impossible for the Seed to be darted directly into the Matrix, whence the generative Work will be obstructed. To remedy this Inconvenience then, by a light *Scissure* of the Incision Knife or Scissars X, we cut the *Bridle* across, in the same manner that we do the String under the Tongue, and so by a very light Operation remedy two Inconveniences which it causes. I have seen some who have been cur'd of this Indisposition by a *Shanker* corroding the *Bridle,* but would not advise any make use of so dangerous a Remedy [42].

Dionis added little or nothing to the literature on hermaphroditism. Also, his operation for correcting adhesion of the prepuce to the glans in the newborn paraphrases the operations previously described by Heliodonus and Antyllus [19], Paulus Aegineta [2], and Albucasis [78].

Perhaps one of the earliest surgical references to lesbian behavior is found in Dionis' explanation of the need for and method of clitoridectomy:

If the *Clitoris* does not extend beyond the Bounds which Nature has prescrib'd it, there is no need of Operation, but sometimes it grows to that degree as to become as big and long as a Man's Yard; this happens frequently to the *Aegyptian* women. The Europeans, who have this Part larger than other Women, are call'd *Fricatrices,* because they may abuse it, and pollute themselves with other Women; which has made way for its Amputation, in order to deprive Women of a continual excitation to Lasciviousness: but there are very few who will submit to this Operation; for if a Woman be chaste she will not abuse it; and if debauch'd, she will not voluntarily lose a Part which contributes to the Pleasure she enjoys in her Debauchery. But if a Chirurgeon is oblig'd to retrench this Part, he must take it in his left Hand in order to cut it off with the curved Knife H, as close to its Root as he can, avoiding the touching the *Urethra* or the *Lacunae* about the *Clitoris* [42].

Dionis described the necessity of operating when the vulva was entirely closed in the newborn:

Of all Indispositions, the most pressing is when a Girl, at her coming into the World, has not her *Vulva* perforated; it must be open'd with utmost expedition; but 'tis not ordinarily perceived before the second or third Day after her Birth, by observing that she is not wet; when the operation is easier than at her Birth, because the Urine being issued out of the Bladder, and stopp'd by the Lips join'd together, pushes them outwards by the Tumour which it there occasions; and also the Skin being extended very tort, we see the Line where the Incision is to be made longways; so that taking the Pen-Knife A, or the Incision-Knife B, we cut the Skin which joins the Lips, and make an Aperture proportion'd according to the Shape and Size which it ought to have naturally [42].

Lorenz Heister (1683–1758), who was the founder of scientific surgery in Germany, published a book in 1718 that was translated into many languages, including English [66]. It included such a wealth of interesting illus-

trations and colorful writing that it is to be recommended to any surgeon interested in the medical history of his specialty [66]. In a manner similar to the descriptions of Dionis, Heister wrote upon the treatment of hypospadias, chordee, imperforate glans, and the enlarged clitoris and nymphae. Some of Heister's methods, however, today seem amusing and apparently useless, such as the following one for treating chordee:

But sometimes the Penis is so incurvated, that it cannot properly be erected, notwithstanding the Fraenulum is sufficiently loose. But that proceeds from a Mis-conformation of the internal Parts of the Penis; and is therefore very difficultly, if at all, curable. If such Men are desirous of entering into a State of Matrimony, and becoming Fathers of Children; and for that End require the Assistance of the Surgeon; he may try what can be done, by the Application of Emollients to the contracted Side of the Penis, and of Astringents to the other Side; assisting both with a proper Bandage, and sometimes by making small Incisions in the Integuments of the contracted Side [66].

Heister was one of the first to discuss the relationship of the site of the hypospadial orifice to the prognosis as far as procreation was concerned. Perineal hypospadiacs were very unlikely to father any children:

[But] those are not so, who have this Perforation about the Middle, or towards the Extremity of their Penis. These last may indeed celebrate the Rites of the Marriage-bed, in all Respects [66].

Heister referred to hermaphrodites only very briefly, and surprisingly in context with the subject of women with enlarged clitori:

In some Women the Clitoris grows to so large a Size, as to equal and resemble the Penis of the male (Instances of which we have in Tulpius, DeGraaf, Platerus, Rhodius, Plazonus, Panarolus,

Paulinus, etc.) upon which Account such Women have been called *Hermaphrodites*, notwithstanding the Clitoris is without any Perforation, and does not discharge either Semen or Urine [66].

Heister, in discussing the amputation of nymphae which were "sometimes so large, as not only to hang without the labia pundendi, but also to prove very troublesome to them walking, sitting, and in their conjugal embraces" [66], was sympathetic enough to be one of the first surgeons to refer to the patient's discomfort in that era of no available anesthesia; he cautioned that the surgeon should "have in readiness styptics for the hemorrhage, and medicines to prevent the patient from fainting" [66].

In the same period, Henri François Le Dran (1685–1770) argued against the appropriateness of trying to bandage the penis in a small child, since, he maintained, "the penis is so short, especially in young children, that no bandage can be applied that will keep on" [79]. In cases following circumcision, he resorted instead to the laying on of lint dressings that were renewed and changed frequently by a nurse every time the child urinated [79].

Chaussier, in the late eighteenth century, was apparently the first to use the word "exstrophy" to describe this condition of the bladder. He was, in 1817, also probably the first or at least one of the earliest to use the word "epispadias." The term "epispadias" was not used in earlier centuries, since both epispadias and hypospadias were described by the word "hypospadias" [46].

The Nineteenth Century

The bold and imaginative innovations of French, German, English, and American surgeons of the early nineteenth century rescued surgery from the doldrums of the seventeenth and eighteenth centuries and charted the way for a succession of rapid developments [25]. Surgeons such as Carpue, von Graefe, Roux, Cooper [33], Warren [134], Dupuytren, Dieffenbach [40], and Mettauer [85], were responsible for a host of new surgical ideas and the development of technical craftsmanship which, in the latter half of the nineteenth century, provided plastic surgery and urological surgery in particular with an unending supply of surgical improvements [11, 13, 20, 21, 27, 34, 35, 69, 83, 89, 106, 107, 115, 119, 126, 127, 138, 140, 141].

John Syng Dorsey (1783–1818) of Philadelphia described in his 1818 textbook of surgery [43] the treatment of imperforate vagina as follows:

When the vagina is closed by a membrane, the operation by which it is to be relieved is extremely simple. A straight incision, or if the membrane be very dense, a crucial incision should be made through it, and the wound kept from uniting by the introduction of a sponge tent, or roll of linen. Cases are recorded in which prodigious quantities of black putrid blood have been discharged by such an operation, and the lives of many patients have been saved by this simple process.

A more difficult operation becomes necessary when instead of a mere membrane to be divided, the surgeon finds an obliteration of the vagina, or a concretion of its size. In this case he must proceed by slow and cautious dissection, guarding with extreme care the bladder, on one side and the rectum on the other. DeHaen related a case in which the bladder was actually opened and death resulted....

Dr. Physick has once been called to dissect a passage to the uterus, in a case where the vagina was entirely closed up to a considerable distance within the os externum. After a cautious dissection through a very considerable thickness of parts, the operation was accomplished, and the vagina was kept open and dilated by the use of tents [43].

Perhaps this patient of Philip Syng Physick (1768–1837) of Philadelphia was the first in medical records to be successfully operated upon for vaginal agenesis [43].

In the early nineteenth century, there was no improvement in the operations intended to repair hypospadias or other genital deformities over what had been practiced in the previous 1800 years, but simple attempts merely to close urethral fistulas showed considerable advancement [33, 126, 127]. European surgeons devoted much attention to the introduction of plastic surgery techniques by Lucas, Carpue, von Graefe, and others, and their notions of the means by which the loss of soft tissue parts in various regions of the body could be surgically corrected greatly advanced. The first attempts to close fistulous openings along the penile shaft probably made use of previous known methods of therapy, including "freshening" of the edges of a fistulous tract with caustics such as nitric acid in order to create enough granulation tissue that could then be brought together. The first purely plastic surgical procedure to close such a urethral fistula was performed by Sir Astley Cooper in 1818 on a 56-year-old patient suffering from urethral stricture and a fistula just anterior to the scrotum. Cooper reported the successful correction of this fistula in 1820 [33]. This was accomplished by the simple maneuver of placing an elastic catheter into the bladder, paring the edges of the fistulous opening, and then dissecting a flap from the scrotal skin. This was merely turned over upon the fistulous wound and fitted exactly, being held in place by interrupted sutures and adhesive plaster. After two months of postoperative catheterization, dressing changes, and control of the inflammation in the operative site, the patient passed urine for the first time "by the natural passage."

Cooper's case was soon followed by another treated by Mr. Earle of Bartholomew's Hospital in London in the year 1819 and reported in the year 1821 [48].

Some early nineteenth century "surgical" attempts were ghastly, especially in an age when anesthesia was unknown. Dupuytren, known as "the Brigand of the Hotel Dieu," thought nothing of striking his patients and abusing them harshly. He treated a young hypospadiac whose urethra opened at the root of the penis by shoving a thin trocar from the urethral opening into the glans to create a new canal [8, 99]. The canal thus formed was then cauterized with a red hot wire, and after the severe inflammation had passed, he kept the new canal open with elastic catheters. These catheters, which were placed through the canal and into the bladder, were used for three months postoperatively, and the original malpositioned urethral opening finally closed after many treatments with silver nitrate.

According to Ricci [109], after DeHaen unsuccessfully operated for an absent vagina in 1761, Dupuytren in 1817 was the next to attempt a plastic surgical correction of this deformity. He, too, was unsuccessful, as was Villaume in 1826, Boyer in 1831, and Debrou in 1851, all of whom used DeHaen's surgical method. This method apparently consisted of attempting to make an artificial vagina by creating an opening between the bladder and the rectum, kept patent by a tampon. Owens pointed out that this fundamentally sound procedure was advocated by Dupuytren in 1817, but it was essentially forgotten· until approximately 1936 when Monod and Iselin "improved Dupuytren's original operation by applying Thiersch grafts over a hard stent and inserting the stent into the newly formed vaginal canal" [97].

John Collins Warren (1778–1856) [134] of Boston probably reported the first successful correction surgically for "non-existence of vagina." His son, Jonathan Mason Warren (1811–1867), also reported surgery of three cases of vaginal atresia in 1851 [135], two of them acquired and one congenital in origin. John Collins Warren wrote in 1833:

The forefinger of the left hand was introduced into the rectum, and a small probe-pointed bistoury employed to make an aperture in front of the rectum as near as might be in the situation of the fossa navicularis.... It was necessary ... to proceed with the same instrument, the convexity being towards the rectum, to dissect from behind forwards. In this way an opening was made sufficient to admit the point of the finger. The dissection being carefully continued in the same manner, a passage was formed about three inches long, and wide enough to admit the finger. The bleeding was considerable; this was arrested by the introduction of a tent.... The wound was carefully dressed by the introduction of a tent daily. The suppuration was considerable; after it had subsided the tent was removed, and the passage exhibited no disposition to close.... Four weeks afterward she was seen by Dr. Hayward; he found the aperture and cavity open and he thought he could distinguish something like an uterus [134].

The first plastic surgical operation following Warren's operation for the reconstruction of an absent vagina in 1833 that proved successful was reported in 1870 by C. L. Heppner in St. Petersburg [109]. He made an H-shaped incision in the rectovaginal septum and lined the walls of this cavity with tongue-shaped flaps of skin that he dissected from the adjacent thigh regions.

In 1831 George Bushe of New York City published his paper "Hypospadias" [23], in which five cases were described, only three of which were congenital in origin. Bushe employed the trocar technique of Amatus Lusitanus [7], though he did not refer to the latter author. He perforated an imperforate glans and an imperforate urethra in two of the patients; in one of the patients, he introduced a silver tube into the urethra thus constructed, and, in the other, he employed a

gum elastic catheter through the cannula of the trochar. Both patients were then repeatedly dilated with bougies, and their original hypospadial orifices were closed with "actual cautery." Cautery served to create granulation tissue which then, with the aid of silver nitrate applications and compression, brought about a scar tissue closure of the openings. The patient with the imperforate glans "afterwards successfully exercised his procreative powers." The other patient, a recruit, also had a successful cure, and within 12 months of the operation, he enlisted in a career with the Army.

Erichsen, writing in 1853, indicates the crudeness of the surgical techniques employed at that time for the repair of an imperforate vagina:

An imperforate vagina is occasionally met with in young children, and occasions a great deal of anxiety to the parents. This condition, however, may always be very readily and speedily removed by tearing up the canal as it were, by dragging upon its walls in opposite directions and breaking through the adhesions, which are little more than epithelial, with the thumbnail, a blunt probe, or the handle of a scalpel, and then introducing a small pledget of greased lint [51].

In the 1830s, many operations utilizing penile or scrotal skin for the repair of urethral fistulas were recorded. French and German surgeons in particular started developing better, less brutal, successful repairs of hypospadias.

Alliott [6] of Montagny in 1833 was completely successful in closing an antescrotal fistula of moderate size by forming a flap from the skin on one side of the fistulous opening.

Dieffenbach recorded his attempts to repair urethral fistulas in several papers and memoirs written between 1829 and 1836 [39, 40, 60]. Many of his earliest experiences were

failures [11], and only after much perse-
verance was he able to obtain success with a
variety of operations (Figs. 1-11 to 1-13). His
operations showed his increasing skill with
the techniques of plastic surgery that were
revolutionizing surgery in early nineteenth
century Europe.

Dieffenbach contrived a method of suturing that gave him more successful results
than any other previously employed, to
which he gave the name of the *schnürnaht*
or the "lace suture" technique (Fig. 1-12). On
the day previous to the operation, the skin
around the fistulous opening and some of the
surrounding normal skin was treated with
tincture of cantharides, which created blistering. The loose epidermis that was raised by
the blistering fluid was then removed by
scraping, a catheter or a sound was introduced into the urethra and passed below the

fistulous opening, and then the lace suture—
which acted like a purse string when
tightened—was introduced into the denuded
tissues around the fistulous tract (see Fig. 1-
12) and then tied. Successful closure of the
fistula resulted if the case proceeded as
planned.

In larger fistulas in which the lace suture
technique was inapplicable, Dieffenbach obtained occasional success by converting the
rounded fistulous opening into a lozenge-
shaped one by removing a small piece of skin
above and below the opening (see Fig. 1-12).

In all of the surgical variations described so
far, none has dealt specifically with the condition of congenital hypospadias. The word
"hypospadias" was misused by surgeons for
many centuries, including those of the early
nineteenth century, to describe any abnormal
position of a urethral opening or a fistula,

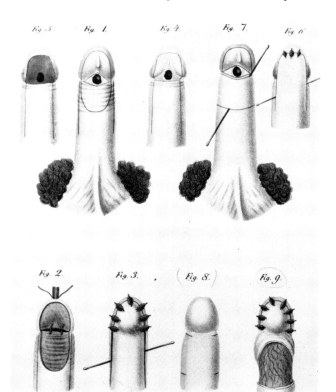

FIG. 1-11. Original plate from
Fritze and Reich [60] demonstrating
various operations performed by
Dieffenbach for the closure of urethral fistulas in the penile frenulum
by use of an outer preputial flap
(*Figs. 1–3*), by an outer and inner
preputial flap (*Figs. 4–6*), and by a
sliding preputial flap (*Figs. 7–9*).

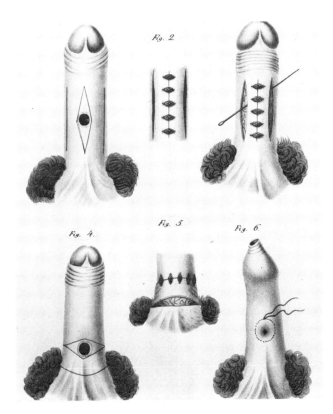

FIG. 1-12. Original plate from Fritze and Reich [60] demonstrating various operations performed by Dieffenbach for the closure of urethral fistulas in the midpenile shaft (*Figs. 1–3*) using a penile "skin bridge" advancement flap closure; in the proximal portion of the penis close to the scrotum (*Figs. 4–5*) using a local scrotal advancement flap; and of a small fistula in the penile shaft using the "lace" or purse-string suture of Dieffenbach (*Fig. 6*).

which quite often was the result of chronic gonorrhea or syphilitic chancres. The first specific case of hypospadias of congenital origin that was described in the surgical literature and for which a specific new operation proved to be successful was reported in 1838 by Liston [80] in London. A similar case was reported four years later by Mettauer [85] of Virginia.

Liston (1794–1847), one of the most dexterous surgeons in Britain in the early nineteenth century, reported in 1838 a variation in the technique of closing the hypospadial malpositioned urethral orifice using a preputial flap. In another case treated by Liston, a 23-year-old patient displayed an epispadias in which approximately 4 inches of urethra were exposed. The patient was completely cured within several days. The operation consisted in paring the edges of the dorsal cleft

thoroughly and joining these edges of penile skin over a catheter by approximating them with a twisted suture.

Although Dieffenbach's works dealt extensively with the repair of urethral fistulas [39, 40, 141], throughout these writings his attitude toward successful repair of hypospadias and epispadias was quite pessimistic. In his 1845 textbook of surgery [40], he describes several operations for simple repair of hypospadias, but he admitted that his experience with more complicated forms of hypospadias was limited. The excellent descriptive work of Mettauer [85] in 1842 and Pancoast [100] in 1844, both Americans, provided the medical world with the first accurately described operations for the repair of several types of hypospadias and epispadias, including good illustrations (Fig. 1-14).

Mettauer should be given the credit for

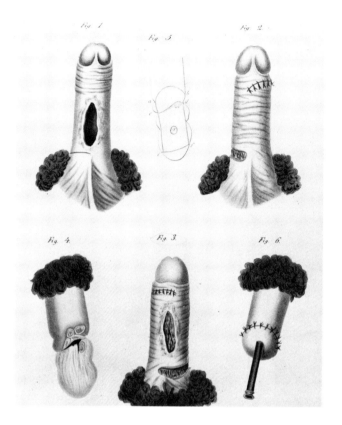

FIG. 1-13. Plate from Fritze and Reich [60] demonstrating various operations performed by Dieffenbach for the closure of a very large urethral fistula (*Fig. 1*) in the penis by a circular displacement of penile skin from the dorsal surface (*Fig. 2*) to cover the ventral surface (*Fig. 3*). A balanoplasty by Dieffenbach is shown (*Figs. 4–6*).

being the first modern surgeon to report a case of the repair of a very intricate and complicated type of hypospadias [131]. In an excellent review [70] of the contributions of John Peter Mettauer, considered by some as America's first plastic surgeon, the authors summarize Mettauer's extensive writing on epispadias and hypospadias:

To repair a distal penile hypospadias, Dr. Mettauer formed a tract with a small trocar and held the passage open by inserting a "...gum elastic tube of proper size and length." The tube was in place "...2 or 3 days or until suppuration was established." Following this a short bougie of proper size was introduced in its depth for half an hour at a time, 3 or 4 times daily until the passage "ceased to matter." Patients were generally confined to bed "...in a state of undress for at least 5 or 6 days after the operation." Dr. Mettauer wrote in 1842: "This mode

of operating has been in our use for over twelve years." This would appear to mean that he had been successfully operating on hypospadias pa-

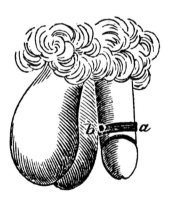

FIG. 1-14. Postoperative appearance of a 2 inch long penis, which when erect became 4½ inches in length, prior to closure of a perineal hypospadial orifice. (From Mettauer [85].)

tients since at least 1830, a time which predates by 44 years the [first] hypospadias repair reported in the French literature [Anger, 1874].

This time is also earlier than the reports of any success by Dieffenbach in the 1830s and 1840s, and his attempts in repairing hypospadias seemed to be more unsuccessful than successful [39, 40]. It is also earlier than the reports of success by Heller [67] in 1834 and by Liston [80] in 1838. Mettauer was probably also the first in medical literature to describe the absence of the corpus spongiosum in hypospadias cases, and he wrote in detail of the pathology of chordee [70].

Mettauer described his operation for proximal penile hypospadias in the following manner:

The same principles of treatment should guide us in cases in which the opening is low down on the penis or in the perineum. In these last however a longer trocar will be required to form the passage. The gum acacia tube should be long enough to enter the bladder and then must fill the passage tightly for the double purpose of rendering it free, and to put an immediate stop to the traumatic bleeding which is sometimes very profuse. The tube should never be left out of the passage long at a time for several days and must invariably be replaced before urination to prevent the painful scalding which would certainly follow as well as to guard against the possibility of infiltration of urine [85].

Mettauer closed the fissure from the previously existing urethral tract by denuding the margins of the fissure by excision and then bringing these together accurately by the use of a uniting bandage or adhesive plasters or by interrupted sutures. He advised:

When the malformation is distinguished by an open cleft or fissure from the termination of the urethra to the extremity of the glans, modifications by no means uncommon, the margins must be carefully denuded with a knife or by touch-

ing them with nitris argenti. The passage corresponding to the tract of the urethra must then be filled with a tube of proper size, and the denuded margins be brought together so as to embrace it and be in exact and close contact throughout their whole extent. The margins are held together with sutures and with bandages [85].

Unless medical history should prove to the contrary, Mettauer was also the next physician to report a successful operation for epispadias following Liston's report in the late 1830s [80]. In treating epispadias, Mettauer suggested:

[Treatment] should be directed by the precepts which have been presented in regard to the several modifications of hypospadias. Generally, however, it will be easier to manage the former than the latter. Complete cures can generally be effected in these malformations in two or three weeks. Should these malformations be complicated with an unsightly and inconvenient curvature on any portion of the penis, the contracted part must be divided by subcutaneous incisions in succession until the organ is liberated. The contractures can be easily distinguished and readily divided as they are generally situated in the subcutaneous cellular tissue which from some cause has lost its soft and yielding qualities. Occasionally the deformity depends on a preternatural shortening of the elastic ligament. In either case the deformity may be easily corrected by division of the contracted tissue, taking care however to employ an exceedingly delicate instrument in the operation. After the contracture is removed the organ may be kept perfectly straight either by using a short tube or by employing delicate splints on the 4 surfaces of the penis [85].

Mettauer, unlike Dieffenbach, was not pessimistic about the treatment of hypospadias, of which he stated: "Many, nay we believe all, of these malformations may be corrected, or greatly relieved by proper treatment, although they have in numerous instances been regarded as irremediable." [70].

Pancoast's superbly illustrated "A Treatise on Operative Surgery . . . ," published in 1844, was one of the first in the medical literature to provide surgeons with an illustration of means by which a hypospadias of the "second variety," or a midpenile shaft hypospadias, was corrected [100].

Simon in 1852 unsuccessfully tried to transplant the ureters into the rectum in a case of ectopic bladder. After this date, numerous attempts of a plastic surgical nature were undertaken but apparently few, if any, were successful [117]. Maydl in 1894 successfully transplanted intraperitoneally the base of the bladder with the attached ureters into the sigmoid colon. His operation was widely practiced before World War I although it carried a mortality rate of approximately 25 percent [110].

Gross, an American surgeon, described in 1864 the then current attitudes toward surgical repair of exstrophy of the bladder, stating that this disorder was more common in males than in females and that of the six cases that came under his attention, all were males. He stated:

Exstrophy of the bladder was, until lately, universally regarded as utterly irremediable. . . . Occasionally an attempt has been made to form a cover for the tumor by autoplasty, by borrowing the integuments from the adjacent parts, and inverting them, in the hope that the cutaneous tissue may ultimately assume the properties of the mucous, and so adapt itself to the presence of the urine. The flaps are united by suture, and are thoroughly protected during the treatment from the contact of the water. . . . This operation, so far as I know, has been performed only twice in this country. In 1858, Professor Pancoast resorted to it at the Clinic of the Jefferson Medical College, but although it was executed with great skill, the edges of the flap only partially united. Soon afterwards, it was repeated by Dr. Ayres, of Brooklyn, upon a woman, 28

years of age, with results, apparently highly gratifying, the cutaneous cover being nearly perfect, and the patient, consequently, much improved in comfort. A full report of the case illustrated by drawings, has been published by the operator [64].

In the third edition of his textbook of surgery, Gross was pessimistic in his attitude about the use of surgical methods for repairing the absence of a vagina. He summarized

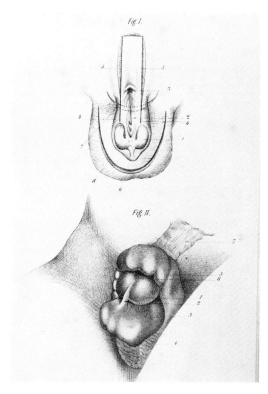

FIG. 1-15. Complete epispadias; the incisions are shown that are necessary for its operative correction according to Nelaton (modification of Dolbeau). (*Fig. I: 1.* glans; *2.* funnel-shaped entrance to the bladder.) (After Dolbeau.) Definitive result of more conservative operations is shown below. (*Fig. II: 1.* glans; *2.* frenulum; *3.* edematous prepuce; *4.* scrotum; *5.* scrotal flap; *6.* new urethra; *7.* scar tissue.) (After Dolbeau, from Thiersch [125].)

FIG. 1-16. Operative correction of epispadias according to Thiersch. (*Fig. I: 1.* glans; *2.* dorsal urethral gutter; *3.* funnel-shaped entrance to bladder; *4.* scrotum; *5.* preputial apron [hood].) Two right-angled skin flaps were created on either side of the dorsal penile urethral gutter (*Fig. IIIa*). Skin flaps were sewn in place off-center so their suture lines were not directly lying superimposed one over the other (*Figs. IIIc* and *d*). (From Thiersch [125].) *Operation* continued on page 36.

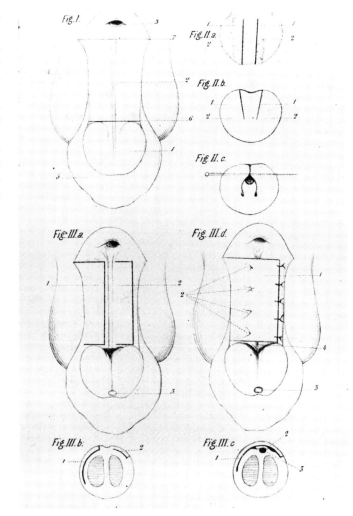

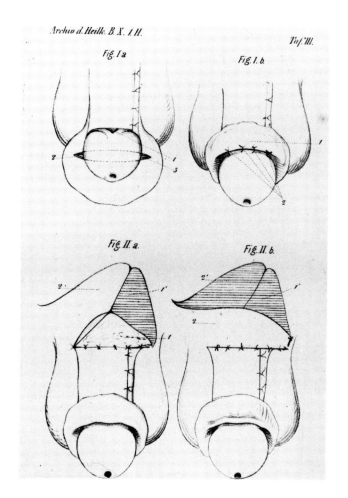

Archiv d. Heilk. B. X. 1 H.   *Taf. III.*

Fig. I a   *Fig. I. b*

Fig. II a.   *Fig. II. b.*

FIG. 1-17. Operative correction of epispadias according to Thiersch (*continued*). Closure of the uncovered area lying between the penis and the glans by transposition of the prepuce (*Figs. Ia* and *b*). Closure of the funnel-shaped opening into the bladder by rotation of an abdominal skin flap (*Figs. IIa* and *b*). (From Thiersch [125].)

bluntly, "nothing is to be done when there is an absence of the vagina, the woman is impotent and therefore, disqualified for marriage" [64]. Some of his bluntness was, however, amusing. In discussing the reasons for amputating an enlarged or hypertrophied clitoris, he stated:

[In] Persia, Turkey, and Egypt, hypertrophy of the clitoris is often immense, the tumor thus formed perhaps equaling the size of an adult's head.... the clitoris has occasionally been removed on account of erotomania, even when it was not materially enlarged. Such an operation is on par with the amputation of the penis for the cure of onanism. Nothing could be more absurd [64].

Despite the descriptions in the literature prior to the nineteenth century of the treatment of hypospadias and the imperforate glans by Albucasis, Paré, Fabricius of Aquapendente, Dionis, Heister, and others, the majority of surgeons in the sixteenth, seventeenth, and eighteenth centuries either neglected or abandoned the treatment of hypospadias and epispadias. Even during the early and middle nineteenth century, some famous surgical luminaries, such as Malgaigne, Boyer, and Berard, believed that operations to correct hypospadias were impractical and had very little chance of success.

Chouet provided an excellent review [28] of the numerous details and variations that were reported, mainly by French authors, about the use of trocars and cannulas to form a new urethral tract in cases of hypospadias prior to the first report of Anger of his new operation in 1874 [9]. Théophile Anger, at a meeting of the Société de Chirurgie in Paris on the 21st of Janurary, 1874, described the successful repair of a penile or penoscrotal hypospadias. The modern era of hypospadias repair began with his report. His technique was based

largely on a method of surgical repair of epispadias described previously by Karl Thiersch (1822–1895) in 1869 [125] (Figs. 1-15 to 1-17). Anger made parallel incisions in the penile skin asymmetrically (Fig. 1-18). The suture lines of the reconstructed urethra and the suture lines of the skin closure were thereby offset so they did not overlap or coincide, and thus there was less chance for fistula formation.

The year 1874 initiated a new era in hypospadias surgery. Duplay, Nové-Josserand, and Ombrédanne were each responsible for what one might call a "school" of hypospadias

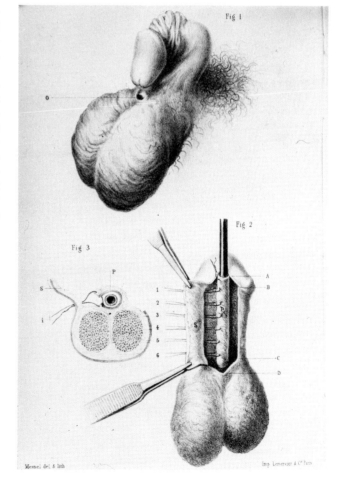

FIG. 1-18. Plate from Anger's original article [10] demonstrating successful closure of penoscrotal hypospadias employing the Thiersch method of closure. The penoscrotal hypospadias orifice (*O*) is shown with the penis base in erection, but the glans is depressed because of the chordee (*Fig. 1*). The penile skin is turned in as a flap to create a skin-lined urethra (*Fig. 2*). A cross section (*Fig. 3*) illustrates the turned-over penile skin flap. The adjacent skin flap (*S*) is to be used to cover the urethral skin tube. (From Anger [10].)

surgery, and the surgeons who came after them often merely modified and refined their basic ideas. Duplay provided the earliest, the more completely described, and perhaps the most significant contributions. Some historians therefore regard him as the "father" of hypospadias surgery.

Duplay, like Anger, used a technique that was similar to the method described by Thiersch to form a glandar urethra for reconstruction of cases of epispadias. Thiersch made two lateral skin incisions and isolated a central skin strip or flap, thereby approximating the edges of the incisions over the skin strip to form a glandar urethra (see Fig. 1-16). This was probably the first recorded instance of the use of a buried skin strip for the reconstruction of the urethra (this method has been utilized by Denis Browne in recent years). Duplay's first stage of hypospadias repair consisted of creating the glandar urethra and correcting the chordee (Fig. 1-19). He created a buried skin strip by making either a single central or two lateral incisions, or two lateral incisions combined with two smaller central incisions, after which he sutured the edges of the central incisions together over the central mucosal strip, leaving a sound in place (Fig. 1-20). In the second stage of the operation, using a technique similar to that described several decades earlier by Dieffenbach, he made parallel incisions on the ventral surface of the penis that extended from the hypospadial opening to the glandar urethra. The central skin flap was then undermined and raised at its periphery bilaterally, and a catheter was inserted into the hypospadial opening up through the glandar urethra. This central skin flap was then wrapped around

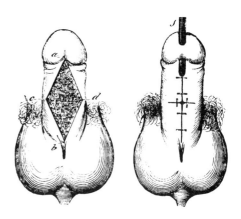

FIG. 1-19. Correction of ventral chordee by a vertically positioned, diamond-shaped excision of tissue, and straightening of the penis by closure of the defect with interrupted sutures. (From Duplay [44].)

the catheter and sutured in a midline closure vertically. Two lateral skin flaps were raised, then advanced medially, and sutured together over the newly formed urethral tube by fine interrupted sutures (Fig. 1-21).

Duplay divided his surgery into three steps. First, correction of the penis deformity or chordee was effected by a transverse diamond-shaped incision of the ventral shaft of the penis distal to the hypospadial orifice and by excision of the first segment of the corpus spongiosum. This was somewhat similar to the operation described by Mettauer in 1842. Duplay then closed the skin using the principle of Heineke-Mikulicz. He constructed a new urethral canal by using skin flaps taken from the penile shaft and sutured to the glandar urethra. This new canal extended from the glans to the hypospadial opening, and the third operation consisted of joining

  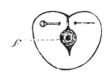

FIG. 1-20. Creation of a glandar urethral meatus. (From Duplay [44].)

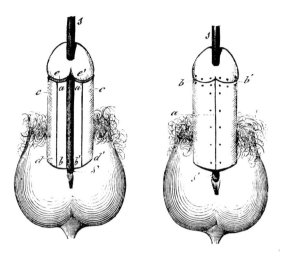

FIG. 1-21. Creation of the new urethral canal by a buried modified Thiersch-type skin flap, which was covered by lateral penile skin advancement flaps sutured in the midline. (From Duplay [44].)

the two parts, the proximal portion of the new urethral canal distally to the old hypospadial orifice proximally. In his earliest report, he described the cure of five cases—four of perineoscrotal and one of penoscrotal hypospadias (Fig. 1-22).

Although Dieffenbach, Thiersch, Anger, Duplay, Rochet (1899), Bucknall (1907), and Ombrédanne (1911) [94] are usually cited chronologically in the history of reconstruction of the urethra with skin flaps in cases of hypospadias [115, 140], the first surgeon to construct a urethra with a free skin graft was apparently Nové-Josserand in 1897 (Fig. 1-23). In principle, his technique consisted of taking a free skin graft from the thigh cut in the manner of Ollier-Thiersch, which was sutured about a trocar and plunged through the glans down through the penile shaft to the abnormal hypospadial meatus [90–92]. This method was subsequently highly favored by McIndoe of England, who devised a special instrument consisting of a trocar that housed a graft-lined catheter and had a detachable tip. The trocar was thrust through the penile shaft, the tip was unscrewed, and the catheter was left in place as the trocar was removed.

Nové-Josserand's case, described in *Lyon Médical* in 1897, was of an 18-year-old young man afflicted with a penoscrotal hypospadias who had previously been operated upon unsuccessfully by the Duplay procedure. Thus, the use of the trocar by Nové-Josserand was in direct continuity and in keeping with the traditional use of such an instrument established centuries previously by Amatus Lusitanus and others.

Ombrédanne in 1911 constructed the urethra in cases of hypospadias with a pedicle flap of skin taken from the ventral penile surface behind the meatus, the posterior edge of which was left unattached (Fig. 1-24). The flap was then turned forward by means of a purse-string suture so its anterior end reached the inferior surface of the glans, where it formed the new meatus. The raw surface thus left was covered by button-holing the preputial hood and bringing it down over the ventral surface of the penis. The two lateral skin pedicles were divided later. Ombrédanne claimed that this operation obviated fistula formation but it left a pouch-like urethra. The dribbling from this pouch-like urethra after urination was likely to be very inconvenient to the patient, especially

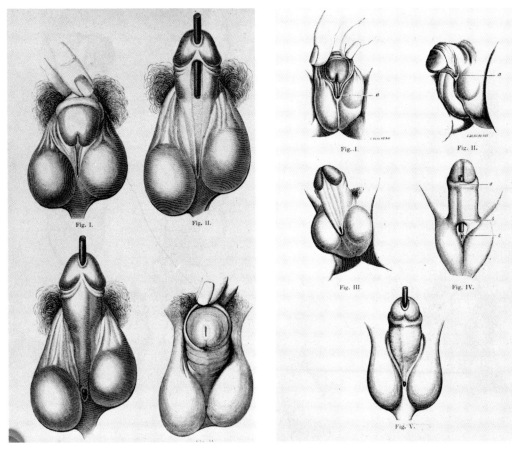

Plate I   Plate II

FIG. 1-22. Original plates from the first article by Duplay [44] on the repair of hypospadias by a modification of Thiersch's technique. *Plate I:* A 21-year-old with perineoscrotal hypospadias (*Fig. I*). Correction of the chordee and creation of a glandar urethral meatus (*Fig. II*). Closure of the penile skin flaps over the newly constructed skin-lined urethra (*Fig. III*). Postoperative result (*Fig. IV*). *Plate II:* A 4-year-old with perineoscrotal hypospadias and ventral chordee (*Figs. I* and *II*). The chordee tended to re-form after its correction (*Fig. III*). Closure of the penile skin flaps over the new urethral canal (*Fig. IV*). Postoperative result (*Fig. V*). (From Duplay [44].)

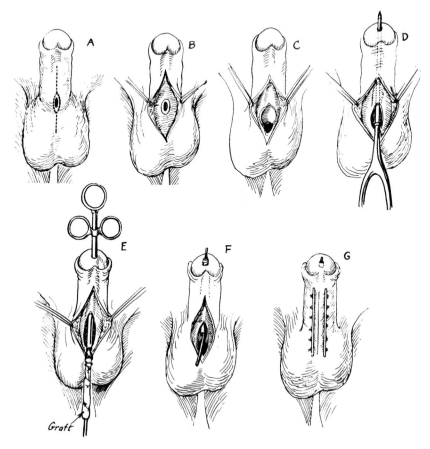

FIG. 1-23.   The method of Nové-Josserand.   *A.* Skin incision is outlined.   *B* and *C.* Skin flaps are raised about the hypospadial opening.   *D.* A cannula is passed to the glans.   *E.* The catheter, wrapped in a split-thickness graft, is drawn through the cannula to exit at the glans.   *F.* The proximal end of the cannula is passed into the posterior urethra.   *G.* The completed procedure. (Redrawn from G. Nové-Josserand; from Wood-Smith [138].)

when several stages were required to bring the urethra to the end of the penis and a series of pouches, each of which being able to retain a little urine, were left [94].

The wealth of endeavors described by our surgical predecessors during the past 2500 years reveals that these were not merely "un-inspiring surgical exercises on the external genitalia," as they were recently described by the English surgeon, J. D. Fergusson [55]. A solid background of technique and theory has been bequeathed to us by our courageous surgical forebearers and by their even more courageous and long-suffering patients.

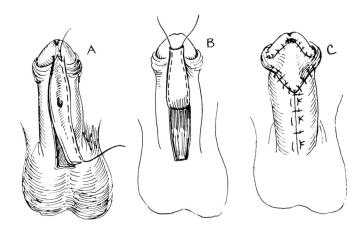

FIG. 1-24.   The method of Ombrédanne.   *A.* Incisions are made parallel to the urethra and its anterior prolongation, and a flap is raised proximally. *B.* The proximal flap is rotated distally, and the skin edges are approximated. *C.* The frenulum is button-holed dorsally, the glans is drawn through, and the frenulum is sutured to the ventral surface of the glans to cover the ventral aspect of the new urethral tube. (Redrawn from Caucci and Caucci; from Wood-Smith [138].)

References

1. Ackerknecht, E. H. Primitive Surgery. In Brothwell, D., and Sandison, A. T. (Eds.), *Diseases in Antiquity: A Survey of the Diseases, Injuries and Surgery of Early Populations* . . . . Springfield, Ill.: Thomas, 1967. P. 635.

2. Adams, F. (Translator). *The Seven Books of Paulus Aegineta.* . . . London: Sydenham Society, 1844.

3. Adams, F. (Translator). *The Genuine Works of Hippocrates.* . . . London: Sydenham Society, Vols. I, II, 1849.

4. Adams, F. (Translator). *The Genuine Works of Hippocrates.* Baltimore: Williams & Wilkins, 1939.

5. Allbutt, T. C. *Greek Medicine in Rome.* London: Macmillan, 1921. Pp. 408–409.

6. Alliott, M. F. Observations cliniques. *Gaz. Med. Paris,* 1834. P. 348.

7. Amati Lusitani [Amatus Lusitanus]. *Curationum medicinalium centuriae quatuor.* . . . [H. Frobenius], Basileae, 1556.

8. Ammon, F. A. *Parallele der französischen und deutschen Chirurgie.* . . . Leipzig: C. H. F. Hartmann, 1823. P. 378.

9. Anger, T. Hypospadias. *Bull. Soc. Chir. Paris,* 1874. P. 32.

10. Anger, T. Hypospadias péno-scrotal, compliqué de coudure de la verge: redressement du pénis et uréthro-plastie par inclusion cutanée: guérison. *Bull. Soc. Chir. Paris,* 1875. P. 179.

11. Backus, L. H., and DeFelice, C. A. Hypospadias: Then and now. *Plast. Reconstr. Surg.* 25:146, 1960.

12. Bandi, H. G., Breuil, H., Berger-Kirchner, L., Lhote, H., Holm, E., and Lommel, A. *The Art of the Stone Age.* New York: Crown, 1961.

13. Bernard, C., and Huette, C. *Précis Iconographique de Médecine Opératoire et d'Anatomie Chirurgicale.* Paris: Méquignon-Marvis, 1855. P. 351.

14. Bhishagratna, K. K. *An English Transla-*

tion of *The Sushruta Samhita Based on Original Sanskrit Text.* Varanasi, India: Chowkhamba Sanskrit Series, 1963.

15. Bibby, G. *Four Thousand Years Ago: A Panorama of Life in the Second Millennium B.C.* Harmondsworth, Middlesex: Penguin Books, 1961.

16. *Bible* in *Encyclopaedia Britannica,* Vol. 3, p. 570. Encyclopaedia Britannica, Inc. Chicago: Wm. Benton, Publ., 1963.

17. Bickers, W. B. John Peter Mettauer of Virginia. *J.A.M.A.* 184:870, 1963.

18. *Bilder-lexikon der Erotik.* Vienna: Institut für Sexualforschung, 1-4, 1928–1931.

19. Bitschai, J., and Brodny, M. L. *A History of Urology in Egypt.* New York: Riverside, 1956.

20. Bouisson, M. F. Remarques sur quelques variétés de l'hypospadias et sur le traitement qui leur convient. *Bull. Ther.* 59:349–362, 1860.

21. Bouisson, M. F. De l'hypospadias et de son traitement chirurgical. *Trib. Chir.* 2:484, 1861.

22. Brothwell, D., and Sandison, A. T. (Eds.). *Diseases in Antiquity: A Survey of the Diseases, Injuries and Surgery of Early Populations.* Springfield, Ill.: Thomas, 1967.

23. Bushe, G. Hypospadias. *New York Medico-chir. Bull.* 2:1, 1831.

24. Bussemaker and Daremberg. *Oeuvres d'Oribase, Texte Grec en Grande Partie Inédit. . . .* Paris: Imprimerie Nationale, 1851–1876. 6 vols.

25. Castiglioni, A. *A History of Medicine* (2nd ed.). New York: Knopf, 1958. P. 720.

26. Chadwick, J., and Mann, W. N. *The Medical Works of Hippocrates.* Springfield, Ill.: Thomas, 1950.

27. Chelius, J. M. In South, J. F. (Ed.), *A System of Surgery.* Philadelphia: Lea & Blanchard, Vol. II, p. 174, Vol. III, p. 87, 1847.

28. Chouet, A. Traitement de l'hypospadius par les greffes de Thiersch (procédé de M. Nové-Josserand). *Thèse de Paris.* Paris: G. Garré and C. Naud, 1899.

29. *Circumcision* in *Encyclopaedia Britannica,* Vol. 5, p. 799. Encyclopaedia Britannica, Inc. Chicago: Wm. Benton, Publ., 1963.

30. Clark, G. *The Stone Age Hunters.* New York: McGraw-Hill, 1967.

31. Columbus, M. R. *De re anatomica. . . .* Venetiis: N. Bevilacquae, 1559.

32. Coon, C. S., and Hunt, E. E., Jr. (Eds.). *Anthropology: A to Z.* New York: Grosset & Dunlap, 1963. P. 182.

33. Cooper, A., and Travers, B. *Surgical Essays* (2nd ed.). London: Cox & Son, 1820. Pp. 222–228.

34. Creevy, C. D. The correction of hypospadias: A review. *Urol. Survey* 8:2, 1958.

35. Creevy, C. D. Surgery of the Penis and Urethra. In Glenn, J. F., and Boyce, W. H. (Eds.), *Urologic Surgery.* New York: Hoeber Med. Div., Harper & Row, 1969.

36. Dawson, W. R. *The Beginnings: Egypt and Assyria.* New York: Clio Medica, Hoeber, 1930. P. 5.

37. Derbes, V. J. The keepers of the bed: Castration and religion. *J.A.M.A.* 212:97, 1970.

38. Desnos, E. *Histoire de l'Urologie.* Paris: Doin, 1914.

39. Dieffenbach, [J. F.]. Mémoire sur quelques nouvelles methodes pour obtenir la guérison des ouvertures contre nature a l'extrémité antérieure libre de l'urétre chez l'homme. *Gaz. Med. Paris,* 1836. P. 802.

40. Dieffenbach, J. F. *Die operative Chirurgie.* Leipzig: Brockhaus, 1845.

41. Dingwall, E. J. *Male Infibulation.* London: Bale & Danielsson, 1925.

42. Dionis, [P.]. *A Course of Chirurgical Operations, Demonstrated in the Royal Garden at Paris.* London: J. Tonson, 1710; 2nd ed., pp. 137–155, 1733.

43. Dorsey, J. S. *Elements of Surgery for the Use of Students.* Philadelphia: Parker and Warner, 1818. Vol. 2, p. 453.

44. Duplay, S. *De l'Hypospadias Périnéo-Scrotal et de Son Traitement Chirurgical.* Paris: Asselin, 1874. (Also in *Arch. Gen. Med.* 1:513; 1:657, 1874, and in *Bull. Soc. Chir. Paris,* 1874. Pp. 49, 157.

45. Duplay, S. Sur le traitement chirurgical de l'hypospadias et de l'epispadias. *Arch. Gen. Med.* 145:257, 1880.

46. Durand, M. *L'Exstrophie Vésicale et l'Epispadias: Étude Pathogénique.* Paris: Ballière, 1894.

47. Durant, W. *The Life of Greece.* New York: Simon and Schuster, 1939. P. 625.

48. Earle, H. On the re-establishment of a canal in the place of a portion of the urethra which has been destroyed. *Phil. Trans.* 4: Part II, 1821. P. 300.

49. Ebbell, B. *The Papyrus Ebers . . . .* Humphrey Milford, London: Oxford University Press, 1937. P. 103.

50. Eliade, M. *Rites and Symbols of Initiation: The Mysteries of Birth and Rebirth.* New York: Harper & Row, 1965.

51. Erichsen, J. *The Science and Art of Surgery . . . .* London: Walton and Maberly, 1853. P. 909.

52. Fabricii ab Aquapendente, H. *Opera chirurgica . . . .* Venetiis: Apud Robertum Megliettum, 1619.

53. Fabricii ab Aquapendente, H. *Opera chirurgica . . . .* Patavii: Franciscum Bolzettam, 1641.

54. Fabricii Hildani, G. *Opera quae extant omnia . . .* (2nd ed.) Francofurti ad Maenum: Sumpt. Ioan. Ludovici Dufour, 1682.

55. Fergusson, J. D. Urological records. *Proc. R. Soc. Med.* 61:417, 1968.

56. Fergusson, W. *A System of Practical Surgery.* Philadelphia: Blanchard and Lea, 1853. P. 566.

57. Flocks, R. H., and Culp, D. *Surgical Urology: A Handbook of Operative Surgery* (2nd ed.). Chicago: Year Book, 1961.

58. Franco, P. *Petit Traité Contenant une des Parties Principalles de Chirurgie.* Lyon: Antoine Vincent, 1556.

59. Franco, P. *Traité des Hernies.* Lyon: Thibauld Payan, 1561.

60. Fritze, H. E., and Reich, O. F. G. *Die platische Chirurgie . . . .* Berlin: Hirschwald, 1845.

61. Garrison, F. H. *An Introduction to the History of Medicine* (4th ed.). Philadelphia: Saunders, 1929. P. 28.

62. Gnudi, M. T., and Webster, J. P. *The Life and Times of Gaspare Tagliacozzi: Surgeon of Bologna: 1545–1599.* New York: Reichner, 1950. Pp. 320–322.

63. Graham, H. *The Story of Surgery.* New York: Doubleday, Doran, 1939. Pp. 25–32.

64. Gross, S. D. *A System of Surgery: Pathological, Diagnostic, Therapeutic, and Operative* (3rd ed.). Philadelphia: Blanchard and Lea, 1864.

65. Guthrie, D. *A History of Medicine.* London: Nelson, 1945. Pp. 29–31.

66. Heister, L. *A General System of Surgery in Three Parts. . . .* London: W. Innys, 1743. Pp. 129–138; 243–250.

67. Heller. Beitrag zur operativen Behandlungsweise der Hypospadia. *Würtemb. Correspbl.* 3:163, 1834.

68. Herrlinger, R. *History of Medical Illustration: From Antiquity to 1600.* New York: Medicina Rara, 1970.

69. Horton, C. E., Devine, C. J., Jr., Crawford, H. H., and Adamson, J. E. Hypospadias. In Gibson, T. (Ed.), *Modern Trends in Plastic Surgery.* London: Butterworths, 1966. P. 268.

70. Horton, C. E., Crawford, H. H., and Adamson, J. E. John Peter Mettauer—America's first plastic surgeon. *Plast. Reconstr. Surg.* 27:268, 1961.

71. Huard, P., and Grmek, M. D. *Le Premier Manuscrit Chirurgical Turc Rédigé par Charaf Ed-Din (1465). . . .* Paris: Dacosta, 1960.

72. Huyghe, R. (Ed.). *Larousse Encyclopedia of Prehistoric and Ancient Art.* New York: Prometheus, 1957.

73. Jones, H. W., Jr., and Scott, W. W. *Hermaphroditism, Genital Anomalies and Related Endocrine Disorders.* Baltimore: Williams & Wilkins, 1958.

74. Keller, R. Historical and cultural aspects of hermaphroditism. *Ciba Symp.* 2:466, 1940.

75. Kiefer, J. H. The hermaphrodite as depicted in art and medical illustration. *Trans. Am. Assoc. Genitourin. Surg.* 58:121, 1966.

76. Krogman, W. M. The medical and surgical practices of pre- and protohistoric man. *Ciba Symp.* 2:444, 1940.

77. Kühn, C. G. (Compiler). *Opera omnia...* (by Galen). Leipzig: Cnobloch, 1821–1833.

78. Leclerc, L. *La Chirurgie d'Abulcasis.* Paris: Baillière, 1861.

79. Le Dran, H. F. *The Operations in Surgery of Mons. Le Dran.* Gataker, T. (Transl.). London: C. Hitch and R. Dodsley, 1749.

80. Liston, R. *Practical Surgery: With One Hundred and Thirty Engravings On Wood.* Philadelphia: Thomas, Cowperthwait, 1838. P. 367.

81. McIndoe, A. The treatment of congenital absence and obliterative conditions of the vagina. *Br. J. Plast. Surg.* 2:254, 1950.

82. *Maccabees, Books of,* in *Encyclopaedia Britannica,* Vol. 14, p. 549. Encyclopaedia Britannica, Inc. Chicago: Wm. Benton, Publ., 1963.

83. Maisonneuve, J. G. T. Une note sur un nouveau procédé opératoire qu'il imaginé pour la guérison de l'hypospadias. *Compt. Rend.* 43:908, 1856.

84. Matthiessen, P. *Under the Mountain Wall: A Chronicle of Two Seasons in the Stone Age.* New York: Ballantine Books, 1969. P. 58.

85. Mettauer, J. P. Practical observations on those malformations of the male urethra and penis, termed hypospadias and epispadias, with an anomalous case. *Am. J. Med. Sci.* 4:43, 1842.

86. Montagu, M. F. A. *Coming into Being among the Australian Aborigines: A Study of the Procreative Beliefs of the Native Tribes of Australia.* New York: Dutton, 1938.

87. Montagu, M. F. A. Ritual mutilation among primitive peoples. *Ciba Symp.* 8:421, 1946.

88. Morrison, J. The origins of the practices of circumcision and subincision among the Australian aborigines. *Med. J. Aust.* 1:125, 1967.

89. Moutet. De l'uréthroplastie dans l'hypospadias scrotal. *Montpellier Méd.* May 1870.

90. Nové-Josserand, G. Traitement de l'hypo-spadias; nouvelle méthode. *Lyon Méd.* 85:198, 1897.

91. Nové-Josserand, G. Hypospadias périnéo scrotal total guéri par le procédé de la greffe autoplastique. *Lyon Méd.* 1906. P. 322.

92. Nové-Josserand, G. Resultates élonginés de l'uréthroplastie par la tunnelisation et la greffe dermo-épidermique dans les formes graves de l'hypospadias et de l'epispadias. *J. Urol. Med. Chir.* 5:393, 1914.

93. Olch, P. D., and Harkins, H. N. A History of Surgery. In Moyer, C. A., et al. (Eds.), *Surgery: Principles and Practice* (3rd ed.). Philadelphia: Lippincott, 1965.

94. Ombrédanne, L. Hypospadias pénien chez l'enfant. *Bull. Soc. Chir. Paris* 37:1076, 1911.

95. Ombrédanne, L. *Les Hermaphrodites et la Chirurgie.* Paris: Masson et Cie, 1939.

96. Oribasius. *Oribasii Sardiani collectorum medicinalium....* Paris: Apud Bernardinum Turrisanum, 1555. P. 298

97. Owens, N. A suggested Pyrex form for support of skin grafts in the construction of an artificial vagina. *Plast. Reconstr. Surg.* 1:350, 1946.

98. Packard, F. R. *Life and Times of Ambroise Paré (1510–1590)....* New York: Hoeber, 1921.

99. Paillard and Marx. Bemerkungen über den unter dem Namen Hypospadia bekannten Bildungsfehler und die dagegen passende Behandlung. *Froriep's Notiz. den Gebiete der Natur-u. Heilk.,* 1834. P. 15.

100. Pancoast, J. *A Treatise on Operative Surgery....* Philadelphia: Carey and Hart, 1844. P. 317.

101. Paré, A. *Les Oeuvres de M. Ambroise Paré.* Paris: Chez Gabriel Buon, 1575.

102. Paré, A. *The Works of That Famous Chirurgion Ambroise Parey, translated out of Latine and compared with the French by Th. Johnson....* London: T. H. Cotes and R. Young, 1634. [Reprint Edition by Milford House, Inc., Boston, Mass., 1968.]

103. Pfeiffer, J. E. *The Search for Early Man.* New York: American Heritage, 1963.

104. Pierce, W. F., Klabunde, E. H., O'Connor,

G. B., and Long, A. H. Changes in skin flap of a constructed vagina due to environment. *Am. J. Surg.* 92:4, 1956.

105. Polk, H. C., Jr. Notes on Galenic urology. *Urol. Survey* 15:2, 1965.

106. Rashad, M. N., and Morton, W. R. M. *Selected Topics on Genital Anomalies and Related Subjects.* Springfield, Ill.: Thomas, 1969.

107. Reybard. Traitement de l'hypospadias par une nouvelle méthode d'autoplastie applicable aux fistules urinaries.... *Gaz. Méd. Paris,* 1857. P. 463.

108. Ricci, J. V. *The Genealogy of Gynaecology: History of the Development of Gynaecology Throughout the Ages: 2000 B.C.–1800 A.D.* ... Philadelphia: Blakiston, 1943.

109. Ricci, J. V. *One Hundred Years of Gynaecology: 1800–1900* (A.D.).... Philadelphia: Blakiston, 1945.

110. Rickham, P. P. The treatment of ectopia vesicae. *Br. J. Plast. Surg.* 10:300, 1958.

111. Sandison, A. T. Sexual Behavior in Ancient Societies. In Brothwell, D., and Sandison, A. T. (Eds.), *Diseases in Antiquity: A Survey of the Diseases, Injuries and Surgery of Early Populations.* Springfield, Ill.: Thomas, 1967. P. 734.

112. Sandison, A. T., and Wells, C. Diseases of the Reproductive System. In Brothwell, D., and Sandison, A. T. (Eds.), *Diseases in Antiquity: A Survey of the Diseases, Injuries and Surgery of Early Populations.* Springfield, Ill.: Thomas, 1967. P. 498.

113. Schwarz, G. S. Infibulation, population control, and the medical profession. *Bull. N. Y. Acad. Med.* 46:964, 1970.

114. Seligman, P. Some notes on the collective significance of circumcision and allied practices. *J. Anal. Psychol.* 10:5, 1965.

115. Serfling, H. J. *Die Hypospadie und ihre Behandlung.* Leipzig: Georg Thieme, 1956.

116. Sigerist, H. E. *A History of Medicine. Vol. 1: Primitive and Archaic Medicine.* New York: Oxford University Press, 1951.

117. Simon. Ectropia Vesicae; (Absence of the anterior walls of the bladder and pubic abdominal parieties); operation.... *Lancet* 2:568, 1852.

118. Singer, S., and Underwood, E. A. *A Short History of Medicine* (2nd ed.). New York: Oxford University Press, 1962.

119. Sorenson, H. R. *Hypospadias with Special Reference to Etiology.* Copenhagen: Munksgaard, 1953.

120. Spencer, R. F. The cultural aspects of eunuchism. *Ciba Symp.* 8:406, 1946.

121. Spencer, W. F. (Translator). *Celsus: De Medicina.* Cambridge: Harvard University Press, 1935–1938.

122. Stark, R. B. Congenital Absence of the Vagina and Other Abnormalities of the External Female Genitalia. In Converse, J. M. (Ed.), *Reconstructive Plastic Surgery.* Philadelphia: Saunders, 1964. P. 2075.

123. Stern, P. V. D. *Prehistoric Europe: From Stone Age Man to Early Greeks* (1st ed.). New York: Norton, 1969.

124. Sussman, M. Diseases in the Bible and the Talmud. In Brothwell, D., and Sandison, A. T. (Eds.), *Diseases in Antiquity: A Survey of the Diseases, Injuries and Surgery of Early Populations.* Springfield, Ill.: Thomas, 1967. P. 209.

125. Thiersch, K. Ueber die Enstehungsweise und operative Behandlung der Epispadie. *Arch. Heilkunde* 10:20, 1869.

126. Thompson, H. Clinical observations on some forms of urinary disease. *Lancet* 2:9, 1856.

127. Thompson, H. The history and practice of urethroplasty. *Lancet* 2:219, 378, and 508, 1856.

128. Thompson, H. The history and practice of urethroplasty. *Lancet* 1:499, 1857.

129. Titiev, M. *The Science of Man: An Introduction to Anthropology.* New York: Henry Holt, 1954.

130. Ucko, P. J., and Rosenfeld, A. *Palaeolithic Cave Art.* New York: McGraw-Hill, 1967.

131. Velpeau, A. A. L. M. In Townsend, P. S. (Ed.), *New Elements of Operative Surgery.*... New York: Langley, 1845. Vol. I, p. 805.

132. Wakefield, E. G., and Dellinger, S. C. Possible reasons for trephining the skull in the past. *Ciba Symp.* 1:166, 1939.

133. Warkany, J. Congenital malformations in the past. *J. Chronic Dis.* 10:84, 1959.

134. Warren, J. C. Non-existence of vagina, remedied by an operation. *Am. J. Med. Sci.* 1833. P. 79.

135. Warren, J. M. Three cases of occlusion of the vagina, accompanied by retention of the catamenia, relieved by an operation. *Am. J. Med. Sci.* 43:13, 1851.

136. Weiss, C. Motives for male circumcision among preliterate and literate peoples. *J. Sex. Res.* 2:69, 1966.

137. Wendt, H. *In Search of Adam.* Boston: Houghton Mifflin, 1956.

138. Wood-Smith, D. Hypospadias: Some Historical Aspects in the Evolution of Methods of Treatment. In Converse, J. M. (Ed.), *Reconstructive Plastic Surgery.* Philadelphia: Saunders, 1964. P. 2010.

139. Young, H. H. *Genital Abnormalities, Hermaphroditism and Related Adrenal Diseases.* Baltimore: Williams & Wilkins, 1937.

140. Young, F., and Benjamin, J. A. Repair of hypospadias with free inlay skin graft. *Surg. Gynecol. Obstet.* 86:439, 1948.

141. Zeis, E. *Die Literatur und Geschichte der plastischen Chirurgie.* Leipzig: Wilhelm Englemann, 1963. Pp. 145–173.

142. Zimmerman, L. M., and Veith, I. *Great Ideas in the History of Surgery.* Baltimore: Williams & Wilkins, 1961.

Embryology

II

Embryology of the Male External Genitalia

CHARLES J. DEVINE, JR.

2

Normal Development

AT THE END of 2 weeks of development, the embryonic disk lying beneath the amnion consists of two cell layers: the ectoderm and the entoderm. A midline groove (the primitive streak) is formed by proliferation of ectodermal cells at the caudal end of the disk. From this groove, a third cell layer (the embryonic mesoderm) forms between the ectoderm and entoderm. These cells proliferate and migrate peripherally, separating the entodermal and ectodermal layers.

Just caudal to the primitive streak before the mesoderm completely separates the ectoderm and entoderm, the latter fuse and form the cloacal membrane. Caudal to this membrane, the allantois develops as an outpouching of the posterior wall of the yolk sac into the connecting body stalk. The embryonic disk grows and elongates due to increasing proliferation and migration of mesodermal cells. This continues through the fourth week, by which time the primitive streak has regressed. The cell layers in the cloacal membrane are inseparable, so the migrating meso-

dermal cells pile up around it and form the cloacal ridge.

Due to rapid and uneven growth, the embryo buckles upward and begins to overgrow its slower growing margins. Head and tail folds form, and the embryo assumes a more or less cylindrical shape. The tail fold has formed by day 21, and the cloacal membrane and the allantois become part of the ventral wall. The entoderm-lined tube at the caudal end formed by this process is called the *hindgut;* this terminates in a blindly ending sac (the cloaca) that terminates at the relocated cloacal membrane.

The external genitalia and anus are formed by developments about the cloacal membrane. The cloacal folds continue to grow as the migrating mesodermal cells continue to be blocked by the fused membrane. As the folds join superiorly, a mound (the genital tubercle) (Fig. 2-1) builds up between the membrane and the allantois. A midline depression (the urethral groove) persists in the genital tubercle and extends to its tip. Here an epithelial tag forms from proliferating ectodermal cells. The tubercle lengthens,

51

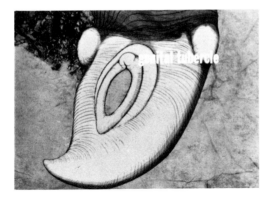

FIG. 2-1. The cloacal membrane surrounded by the cloacal folds with the genital tubercle demonstrating the urethral groove. (Figures 1 through 12 are from the film, *Embryology of the External Male Genitalia,* by Charles Devine, M.D. Reproduced with permission of Eaton Laboratories, Division of the Norwich Pharmaceutical Company, Norwich, New York.)

carrying the groove with it and maintaining the tag at its tip.

Inside the hindgut, cranial to the allantois, an entoderm-lined projection from the infolding abdominal wall grows downward into the cloacal cavity dividing the cloaca into the ventral portion, which becomes the bladder, and the dorsal portion, which becomes the rectum (Fig. 2-2). By 6 to 7 weeks, this uro-

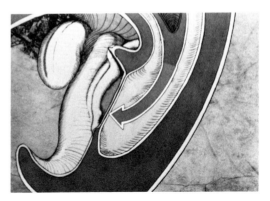

FIG. 2-3. Sagittal section showing the division of the cloaca into the bladder and rectum.

rectal septum meets the cloacal membrane, where lateral tissues have formed a transverse bar dividing it into urogenital and anal membranes (Fig 2-3). The ventral portions of the cloacal folds become the urogenital folds, and the dorsal parts, the anal folds. Then, as the genital tubercle elongates and swells, the urogenital membrane breaks and creates the urogenital ostium (Figs. 2-4 and 5). Mesoderm also piles up around the anal membrane so that it comes to lie in a deep pit (the proctodeum). The anal membrane then ruptures and establishes an outlet for the rectum.

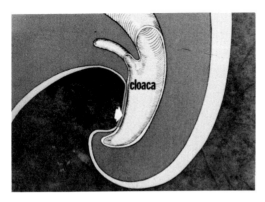

FIG. 2-2. Sagittal section showing the cloaca and the cloacal membrane.

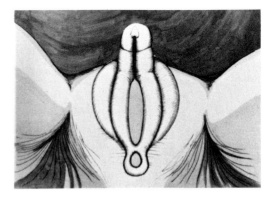

FIG. 2-4. External view showing anteriorly the urogenital membrane, posteriorly the anal membrane.

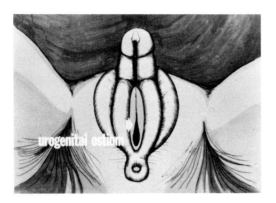

FIG. 2-5. The urogenital membrane has ruptured to form the urogenital ostium.

All this takes place prior to the functional development of the gonads. Although the external genitalia may show hints of sexual differentiation—such as the extent of the urethral groove—this stage is essentially the same for both sexes. If testes did not develop, the external genitalia would grow into a normal female configuration. The genital tubercle would become the clitoris, the urogenital folds would become the labia minora, and the labioscrotal swellings would enlarge to form the labia majora. A hormone from the fetal testis is necessary to direct development into male structures.

Proliferating mesoderm that is lateral to the axis of the embryo differentiates into three parts: the paraxial mesoderm, the lateral plate (which splits to form the lining of the intraembryonic coelomic cavity), and a portion between these called the *intermediate mesoderm*. The caudal end of this structure becomes the nephrogenic cord. In the lower thoracic region at about 5 weeks, the gonadal ridge appears between the midline dorsal mesentery and the nephrogenic cord, which has by this time developed into the mesonephros. Proliferation of the coelomic epithelium and consolidation of the underlying mesenchyme build up this ridge. The primordial germ cells that have formed in the wall of the yolk sac close to the allantois now migrate into the germinal ridge through the dorsal mesentery of the hindgut. This initiates development of the gonads. The coelomic epithelium proliferates and penetrates the underlying mesenchyme, forming the primitive sex structures that surround the germ cells in the mesenchyme.

The sex of the developing embryo is determined by the chromosome content of the spermatozoon that fertilizes the ovum. A sperm containing an X chromosome will yield an XX individual (female) whereas a Y containing spermatozoon will result in an XY (male). In the male subject during the sixth to eighth week, the primitive sex cords continue to proliferate and become separated from the surface epithelium by the tunica albuginea. The interstitial cells of Leydig develop from mesenchyme located between the cords. These are especially notable during the fourth to fifth month of development and have almost disappeared by the eighth month, but they hypertrophy again at puberty. The developing testes secrete a substance that causes the external genitalia to develop a male configuration from the indifferent stage. The genital tubercle grows rapidly and assumes a more cylindrical shape until it is identifiable as a phallus. At its distal end, a definite groove appears, delineating the glans.

The phallus is now perpendicular to the abdominal wall. As it elongates, the urethral groove deepens from the opened urogenital ostium far out onto the shaft. The urethral folds become quite prominent. (Details of this are outlined later in the discussion of chordee without hypospadias, Chap. 19.) At the end of 3 months, the urethral folds begin to close. Mesenchyme coalesces around the deepening groove and in the dorsal portion of the phallus. The original urogenital ostium closes, and as the urethral grooves seam to-

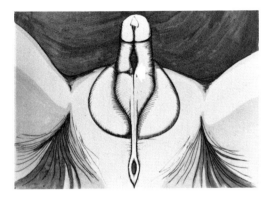

FIG. 2-6. Closure of the urethral groove has progressed. Now the urogenital ostium is on the shaft of the penis.

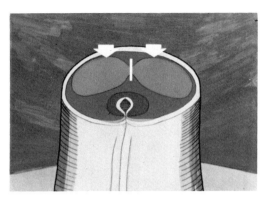

FIG. 2-8. The urethral groove has closed and is being surrounded by mesenchyme. The mesenchyme in the dorsum of the penis is separating to form the two corpora cavernosa.

gether, the tube of the urethra progresses distally with the urogenital ostium advancing before it (Figs. 2-6 and 7). The seam remains as a prominent median raphe that lengthens as the urogenital ostium moves distally.

Later the consolidated mesenchyme in the dorsal portion of the phallus divides in the midline to form the two corpora cavernosa (Fig. 2-8) and the muscular structures that furnish attachments to the bony pelvis.

Proximally, mesenchyme around the developing urethra becomes the corpus spongiosum and its covering muscle that encloses the bulbourethral glands and ducts which form as buds from the urethra (Fig. 2-9). In the shaft of the penis, this mesenchyme forms the corpus spongiosum and the covering fascia.

Closure of the urethra continues to the developing glans penis, and the urogenital ostium is present as a diamond-shaped opening at the corona (Fig. 2-10). The glans en-

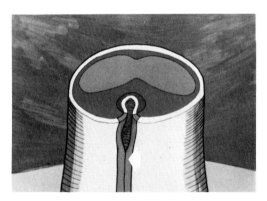

FIG. 2-7. Cross section of the penis. The urethral groove is deepening and closing at the arrow. The mesenchyme is coalescing in the dorsal portion of the penis and around the urethral groove.

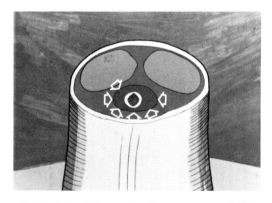

FIG. 2-9. The urethra is now surrounded by mesenchyme that will become the corpus spongiosum and the covering fascias.

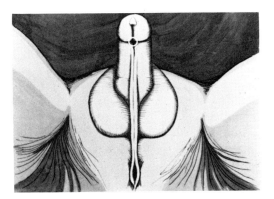

FIG. 2-10. The closure of the urethra has progressed to the glans. The urogenital opening is located within the circle.

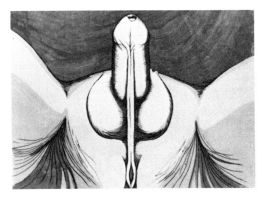

FIG. 2-12. The prepuce has formed and deep to it the glandar urethra has closed. The meatus is now at the tip of the glans. The testes have migrated down to the scrotum, and the development of the external genitalia is complete.

larges, deepening its urethral groove; the glans then closes over the groove but its edges do not fuse at this stage. The deep epithelial-lined tract is still open, filled with desquamated epithelial cells.

At about the third month a roll of skin arises on either side of the urethral opening (Fig. 2-11). Gradually, this ridge extends to encircle the shaft of the penis. Growing out to cover the corona, this skin forms the prepuce, which extends to sheath the glans dur-

ing the next 2 months. As the prepuce grows, the edges of the glans seal the glandar urethra until the urethral meatus reaches its final location at the site of the former epithelial tag. The deep epithelial tract in the glans now forms the navicular fossa of the urethra.

At about 8 weeks, as the genital tubercle elongates, the labioscrotal swellings appear. Sharply separated from the penis by the lateral phallic grooves, they migrate posteriorly and around the phallus. When the swellings meet caudal to the penis, they form the scrotum. The median raphe and septum act as a divider, maintaining two separate compartments. The testes descend into the scrotum by 9 months, completing development of the male external genitalia (Fig. 2-12).

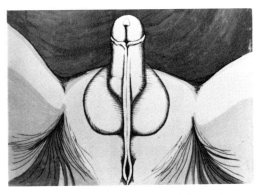

FIG. 2-11. The buds that will form the prepuce have formed laterally to the urogenital opening. The glandar urethra has deepened as the glans hypertrophies.

Abnormalities

HYPOSPADIAS AND CHORDEE

Hypospadias is due to incomplete masculine development of the genitalia. Maximum hypertrophy of interstitial cells of the testis is present over a limited space of time which coincides with the period during which the urethra is formed. The inductor substance is probably generated by these cells. Without this inductor, development will be female. More frequently, we see the result of interruption of androgenic stimulation after normal development has begun. It is my belief that this is due to premature involution of the interstitial cells.

When this occurs, the urethral meatus will remain on the ventral surface of the shaft of the penis, and the penis distal to this will continue to form in a female fashion. The urethral groove will not close but remains as a shallow depression in the skin extending out to the groove in the glans. The glans is flattened and fits ventrally on the end of the penis. The mesenchyme, which would have formed the corpus spongiosum, Buck's fascia, and the dartos fascia, does not differentiate and becomes a layer of fibrous tissue that extends in a fan shape from around the urethral meatus to insert along the ventral aspect of the glans penis, thus causing chordee.

The rolls of skin that develop into the prepuce arise lateral to the normal location; therefore when they encircle the shaft, the prepuce becomes hooded and deficient ventrally. Also, since the outgrowth of the prepuce is involved in closing the glandar urethra, there will be only a groove in the ventrum of the glans. The wide insertion of the fibrous band causing the chordee will extend from one edge of the hooded prepuce to the other.

Chordee can occur without hypospadias. We have encountered three types of this lesion which serve to give additional clues as to the mechanism of formation of the urethra. As the urethral groove deepens, the edges of the skin come together to form the urethra. This tube separates from the skin. If the mesenchyme does not form any of the structures around the urethra, a fibrous band will form and cause chordee. We call this *Type I.*

In what we call *Type II*, the corpus spongiosum forms but Buck's fascia and the dartos fascia do not differentiate. In both Types I and II, fibrous tissue will be found deep to the urethra. In *Type III*, the corpus spongiosum and Buck's fascia form but the dartos fascia does not. In this type, the fibrous tissue causing the chordee will be found lateral to the urethra and superficial to Buck's fascia.

EPISPADIAS AND EXSTROPHY

The defect causing hypospadias occurs late in embryological development, and consequently the more severe forms are less frequently seen. On the other hand, the developmental defect causing exstrophy and epispadias occurs early, being associated with formation of the cloacal membrane. These abnormalities therefore are usually present in their more severe forms.

As the mesodermal layer forms at the primitive streak and migrates outward, it separates the entoderm and the ectoderm. The first cells that move peripherally are the cells which surround the cloacal membrane and form the cloacal ridges. These are extensions of the lateral plate. About 20 days after ovulation, the paraxial mesoderm has formed two broad strips lateral to the notochord and begins to segment into somites. By the end of the fourth week, about 40 pairs of somites have formed, and they begin to differentiate. The cells of the ventromedial part (the sclerotome) migrate toward the midline and form the connective tissue, cartilage, and bone of the axial skeleton. The remainder of the somites divide into a medial (myotome) and a lateral (dermatome) portion. Cells from the dermatome migrate laterally between the ectoderm and the somatic mesoderm to form the deep structures of the skin and subcutaneous tissues. The cells from the myotome penetrate into the already present somatic mesoderm to become the muscles of the body wall. When the layers from both sides have joined in the midline, the abdominal wall is complete. If the cloacal membrane extends too far cranially, it will interfere with penetration of mesodermal cells into the ventral abdominal wall. Thus, when the membrane ruptures, the interior surface of the bladder will be exteriorized and exstrophy of the bladder will be present.

The precise defect in this mechanism that causes exstrophy and epispadias has not been delineated. It can occur because the somatic mesoderm from the lateral plate did not penetrate far enough to open the way for the mesoderm from the myotome to finish the abdominal wall. The cloacal membrane itself could be too large, thus acting as a wedge to hold the two edges apart.

The presence of epispadias indicates that the mesoderm piling up in the cloacal ridge has bridged the cloacal membrane to form a genital tubercle caudal to the urogenital diaphragm. As the diaphragm ruptures, the urethral groove is formed on the dorsal surface of the phallus, resulting in epispadias. Complete exstrophy with epispadias is the most common form of this abnormality. Epispadias alone is seen much less frequently, as are the more severe types of lesions with gastrointestinal involvement and cloaca formation or duplication of the penis or clitoris.

References

1. Barr, M. L. Sex chromatin and phenotype in man. *Science* 130:679, 1959.
2. Boving, B. G. Anatomy of Reproduction. In Greenhill, J. P. (Ed.), *Obstetrics* (13th ed.). Philadelphia: Saunders, 1965.
3. Devine, C. J., Jr. Film: *Embryology of the male external genitalia.* The Film Library of the American Urological Association, Inc., 1970.
4. Devine, C. J., Jr. Film: *Embryology of the male external genitalia. Trans. Am. Assoc. Genitourin. Surg.* 62:123, 1970.
5. Glenister, T. W. The origin and fate of the urethral plate in man. *J. Anat.* 88:413, 1954.
6. Hunter, R. H. Notes on development of prepuce. *J. Anat.* 70:68, 1935.
7. Jost, A. Embryonic Surgical Differentiation. In Jones, H. W., Jr., and Scott, W. W. (Eds.), *Hermaphroditism, Genital Anomalies and Related Endocrine Disorders.* Baltimore: Williams & Wilkins, 1958.
8. Langman, J. *Medical Embryology.* Baltimore: Williams & Wilkins, 1963.
9. Marshall, B. F., and Muecke, E. C. Variations in exstrophy of the bladder. *J. Urol.* 88:766, 1962.
10. Muecke, E. C. The role of the cloacal membrane in exstrophy: The first successful experimental study. *J. Urol.* 92:659, 1964.
11. Patten, B. M., and Barry, A. Genesis of exstrophy of the bladder and epispadias. *Am. J. Anat.* 90:35, 1952.
12. Spaulding, M. H. The development of the external genitalia in the human embryo. In *Contributions to Embryology, No. 61* (Carnegie Institution of Washington, Publication 276). Washington, D.C.: Carnegie Institution, 1921. Vol. 13, p. 67.

Embryology of the Female Genitalia

RICHARD B. STARK

3

THE FEMALE GENITALIA may be said to represent those of the male with arrested development. This is true in view of the fact that the genital development of both sexes is identical until the third month of intrauterine life.

The genital tubercle or eminence until that time is bipotential, capable of becoming the external genitalia of either sex. However, with the development of the testes, the male genitalia undergo changes that move them forward from their previous neutral form. The genital tubercle grows in the male to become the penis. On its ventral or caudal side is a furrow, the urethral groove, flanked on either side by elevations, the urethral folds. These folds are analogous to the palatine shelves of the oral cavity or to the neural plate, which, in the former, close the palate, or, in the latter, produce the neural tube. With tubulation of the urethral groove, the urinary meatus moves from the penoscrotal locus distally to the glans penis. Again, this is analogous to the movement posteriorly of the nasal choanae from their openings into the anterior oral cavity as the palatal shelves fuse, and these two acts of fusion in the penis and in the palate occur at the same time in embryonic development.

Lateral to the genital eminence are the genital swellings which, in the male, will become the scrotal folds that merge in the midline to form the scrotum.

Without pointing out the male-female homologs hereafter, in the female the genital eminence becomes the clitoris. The urethral folds do not meet and fuse to form a urethra located in the clitoris, rather they remain as folds, the labia minora. Thus, the female urethra remains in situ and does not become elongated. The genital swellings become the labia majora (Fig. 3-1 A–C).

As in the case of the external genitalia, the embryo develops with a pair of internal ducts, one of which potentially will produce male ducts (epididymis, vas deferens, seminal vesicles, and ejaculatory duct) and one, female ducts (fallopian tubes, uterus, and vagina). With development, the ducts of the opposite sex become rudimentary. The uterus begins at the second month as paired structures, the müllerian ducts, from which the fallopian tubes, uterus, and vagina arise.

Although the double-barreled uterus may sometimes persist at birth, the usual development consists of the polarization and death of cells of the intervening septum, thus uniting the two cavities into one (Fig. 3-1D–F).

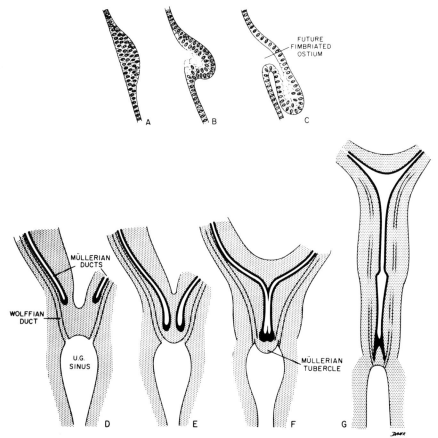

FIG. 3-1. A–C. The müllerian ducts form by cellular proliferation in the urogenital ridges. D–F. At the second month, the paired müllerian ducts form and join. By selective cell death, the intervening septum disappears, thus uniting the two cavities into the uterus. F and G. By the same process, the vaginal canal approaches the external urogenital sinus as the müllerian tubercle disintegrates, leaving behind only a gossamer branchial membrane, the hymen.

The cervix and vagina begin in the solid form initially, then by the process of polarization and cell death, become hollow. As the cavity extends toward the pubic surface, the urogenital sinus—which is well on its way toward becoming the vaginal vestibule—becomes more invaginated until only a cluster of cells, the müllerian tubercle, remains to divide the two approaching tunnels. The müllerian tubercle persists until birth, and it is retained after birth as the hymen (Fig. 3-1G), one of the few branchial membranes, like the tympanic membrane, to remain.

Abnormalities of the müllerian system include a Y-shaped fundic cavity; two cavities; two cavities with a double vagina; Y-shaped bicornuate; bicornuate uterus with two cavities; a double uterus with double vagina (as is the case in marsupials); a bicornuate uterus, one horn of which is rudimentary; atresia of the fallopian tube; cervical atresia; or agenesis of the vagina.

References

1. Conway, H., and Stark, R. B. Construction and reconstruction of the vagina. *Surg. Gynecol. Obstet.* 97:573, 1953.
2. Dmowski, W. P., and Greenblatt, R. B. Ambiguous external genitalia in the newborn and prepubescent child. *J.A.M.A.* 212:308, 1970.
3. Stark, R. B. Congenital Absence of the Vagina and Other Abnormalities of the External Female Genitalia. In Converse, J. M. (Ed.), *Reconstructive Plastic Surgery*. Philadelphia: Saunders, 1964.

Psychological Adjustments to Genital Abnormalities

Counseling in Genital Abnormalities

DONALD W. HASTINGS

4

THERE ARE many sexual problems that require psychological help, but for the purpose of this book the focus will be on two groups of patients:

1. The intersex syndromes, usually genetic in nature, which can present the physician with perplexing problems as to what sex the baby really is and hence whether the child should be raised as a boy or as a girl.
2. Situations wherein genital and psychosexual developments were normal but subsequent disease or trauma rendered sexual intercourse impossible or nearly so.

In this chapter no attempt will be made to deal with symptoms such as impotence, frigidity, and premature ejaculation, although these are the most common types of sexual disorders in adults. Rather, the discussion will be confined to problems of direct urological and surgical interest, problems that would directly involve the reconstructive surgeon either as a consultant or attending physician.

Intersex Syndromes

The path that each human being follows to develop his masculine or her feminine outlook is a complicated one that is by no means fully understood. Only in the past several decades has it become clear just how complex this matter is, and that in the human a great deal depends on how the child is raised, regardless of the chromosome pattern he happens to have. Since the way in which each person regards his make-up, whether masculine or feminine (gender identity), and the role in life this causes him to play (gender role) are central issues in adaptation, since learning seems to occupy the most important position in this process, and since gender identity is largely determined by the first 36 to 40 months of life (never to change), it follows that a physician has a critically important responsibility to determine the correct sex of the baby at the time of birth or shortly thereafter. And, if a mistake has been made, the responsibility to adequately counsel the parents as soon as possible is a great one. Some difficult decisions are often involved regarding the best course to follow.

In simple outline, the steps each person takes in achieving psychosexual maturity are as follows:

1. *Genetic sex.* This is determined by chromosomal composition—XX, XY, or some type of chromosomal abnormality—at the moment of conception.

2. *Anatomical sex.* Under most circumstance, genetics determine bodily architecture, whether male or female. There are some exceptions to this general statement; for example, a new class of drug, the anti-androgens, can cause profound change in body architecture with no relationship to genetic forces.

3. *Sex of assignment.* At the time of birth, the physician inspects the baby's genitalia and decides whether he has delivered a boy or a girl. He conveys this decision to the parents and enters it on the birth certificate. He has assigned a sex to the newborn baby. There may be cases wherein he is not sure (i.e., ambiguous sex) or wherein he makes a mistake, by, for example, deciding that a genetic male is female (i.e., because of abnormalities of genital architecture).

4. *Sex of rearing.* If there is no ambiguity in the sex of assignment, i.e., if the parents have no doubt about the baby's gender, they start the learning and conditioning processes that will establish the child's attitude toward himself: "I am a boy" or "I am a girl." That little boys and girls undergo different learning forces as they grow is evident: the baby girl is dressed in pink and ribbons, the baby boy in masculine things, to give a superficial example. Most importantly, the parents, particularly the mother, convey attitudes about gender to the child both by overt and covert means, verbal and nonverbal. The result of this process is that the child quickly learns that he is a boy or she is a girl. This lesson is learned well and forever. This self-concept is termed:

5. *Gender identity.* This can be defined as the fixed view each person has from childhood (after the age of 36 to 40 months) about his sexual orientation. Based on this identity there follows:

6. *Gender role.* This is the expression each person gives to his sexual identity, i.e., the sexual role he plays in life, masculine or feminine. The sexual role that is played will be determined heavily by the mores and customs of the culture in which he lives, and hence varies widely from one culture to another.

Although it would be grossly misleading to state that genetics and anatomy have little to do with human gender identity and the resultant gender role, it also appears true that they have a much smaller part to play in the total process than does the multitude of psychological forces involved in the "sex of rearing" (such as learning, conditioning, and imprinting). For example, a genetic male baby is born with a bifid scrotum which is interpreted as being vulvae and the penis as an enlarged clitoris. The wrong sex of assignment is made, and the baby is raised as a girl for the first four or five years of life. The gender identity of female comes into being, never to change. Subsequent help for this child cannot consist of trying to reverse the gender identity, since this is impossible. Help must consist of surgery that lets her conform, insofar as this is feasible, with the female gender role. Bing and Rudikoff [1] did a follow-up study of 105 hermaphroditic children and found that the final adoption of gender role was concordant with sex of assignment and rearing in all but five cases. It was not concordant with such physical variables as chromosomal, gonadal, or hormonal sex, or with internal or external genital structures.

The management of intersex problems in infants is primarily the responsibility of pediatricians, but reconstructive surgeons are often consulted. *The rule is that proper sex of assignment must be made early, in the first few months of life at the latest, so that the sex of rearing can be concordant with the sexual role into which the child, when adult, can best fit.* (Usually, but not always, the sex of assignment will be concordant with the genetic sex.) To do otherwise is to create a lifelong tragedy of severe sexual and emotional maladjustment.

From the psychological standpoint, a baby with an intersex syndrome presents a painful and stunning problem to its parents. Their reaction, even if the father is a pediatrician who is expert in these matters, will at first be one of disbelief and shock. It can be likened to a grief reaction, during the early stages of which the parents simply cannot believe, or adequately grasp, that this misfortune has happened. Even the most intelligent and sophisticated of parents conjure up pictures of a child who is a "freak" and who will grow up to become some kind of sexual monstrosity. Both, but especially the mother, often tend to reexamine the events of the pregnancy and to blame themselves for the baby's trouble. Perhaps it was due to the cocktails she had, perhaps she was not as careful of herself as she might have been, and the like; these are the types of thoughts that are apt to occur. Such suffering parents urgently need the help of a physician who well understands intersex problems and who, in equal measure, understands the acute distress such a problem causes. After a few days of inability to cope with the reality of the situation, the majority of parents settle down and are much more accessible for medical explanations of the infant's disorder.

Their methods of coping with the medical facts vary with the parents' education, intelligence, and sociocultural background. The way in which parents adapt represents a broad spectrum. At one end of the scale, the parents are able to quickly visualize the intersex disorder as a quirk of nature, feel relieved by a medical explanation of what is known, consider the treatment possibilities, and cooperate with the physicians; above all, they

accept the child completely and love it. At the other extreme, there are parents who view the disorder as a personal punishment for past sins and who, by the same token, regard the child as an unwanted "thing" they would like to be rid of. The child is rejected by such parents; they are embarrassed by it, cannot mention the problem to relatives or friends, and live with their "secret" in troubled silence. Parents of the latter type often seem to have little interest in seeing that the child gets adequate medical help and may exasperate the physician by their indecision as to whether to follow medical advice. Fortunately such a description is true of only a small number of parents who cannot accept the child's sexual problem, at least at first.

If the newborn has genitals that are ambiguous in nature and the physician cannot, in good conscience and without guessing, determine which sex to assign to the baby, he has a duty to make no sex assignment until further study. Parents should be told something to the effect, "You have a healthy baby except that it was born with external sex organs that make it impossible to tell accurately and without doubt which sex to give the baby. Studies are needed and these will be arranged as quickly as possible so that the correct sex can be assigned and you can give the baby a name. Modern medicine and surgery make it possible for the majority of such babies to develop normally and lead well-adjusted lives. Because of the critical importance for this baby's future in making a correct determination of sex, I will need your cooperation and patience, and I will keep you fully informed as we go along. I know you will feel distressed by the news, but I want to be absolutely frank and open with you on such an important issue. As best you can, try to avoid fixing in your mind whether your baby is a boy or a girl. You will, of course, want to tell your relatives and close friends that you had the baby. I would suggest that you tell them essentially what I have just told you, that by a quirk of Mother Nature your baby has a temporary lack of genital development that makes it impossible to be sure of its sex without further studies and that these will be done as quickly as possible. Also I would hold up sending out birth announcements to more casual friends until the studies have been completed and you can announce whether you have a boy or a girl."

It is obvious that parents need a good deal of support and reassurance as they go through the period of study, and, in large measure, the parents can legitimately be viewed as much as patients during this time as the baby can. It is usually reassuring to both parents if the physician shows the genital defects to them and points out directly on the baby why it is difficult to reach a decision. Parents, upon being told of the condition, often imagine much more bizarre anatomical defects than actually exist and are comforted to see for themselves. The same statement holds for grandparents, particularly grandmothers.

For numerous reasons, it follows that the baby be studied as soon as is feasible, that a logical decision be reached as to the proper sex to be assigned, and that the parents be told this at once and in a clear, unambiguous way. It is difficult for parents, particularly the mother, to regard the baby as an "it" for very long, and in spite of her intellectual understanding, she will begin to regard the baby as either a boy or a girl and treat it accordingly. As mentioned previously, it is thought that the baby soon picks up nonverbal cues from the mother as to her attitudes and thus the "sex of rearing" process begins. If it happens to be in disagreement with the sex that is assigned later, it may cause "confusion" for the infant as he then has to "learn" another sex. Also, the longer the mother makes her own private sex of assignment, the more diffi-

cult it is for her to reverse her attitudes should the studies make this necessary.

If the parents are people of reasonable intelligence and understanding, it is best that they be given the essential facts relating to gender identity and gender role that have composed this chapter so far. It is, I believe, wise to emphasize the reasons for them to accept wholeheartedly the sex of assignment as determined by the studies and to raise the child accordingly. Parents should be told that if they have any doubts about the correctness of the sex assignment (i.e., feel ambiguous), they should voice them so they may be discussed and questions answered. If they harbor doubts and feel ambiguous and uncertain about the gender of the baby, it is a certainty that they will raise him in an ambiguous manner; it is equally certain that the child will develop a confused and uncertain gender identity.

Money [3], one of the foremost experts on intersex problems and gender role, wrote a small and simple book for the layman that explains these matters. It is a very useful volume to have parents read, underlining the parts they would like to discuss or have more information about.

In general, the counseling process for parents who have known of the baby's intersex problem from the time of birth is most intensive during the first several weeks of the baby's life while the studies are being done and the proper sex of assignment determined. Once the sex of assignment is made and the parents informed of this the physician's role in this respect diminishes considerably. However, it is important that follow-up visits be scheduled with the mother about two weeks after and again four weeks after the sex has been assigned. The purpose of these interviews is to discuss her attitudes about the baby's sex and to make certain that she does not have doubts or ambiguous feelings about the baby's gender. If it develops during these interviews that one or both parents have doubtful attitudes, it will be necessary to spend interview time with one or both to try to ascertain what their problems are with regard to acceptance of the baby.

The following case history illustrates the points made above:

At birth the baby appeared normal except for pigmentation of the labial folds which were fused and resembled a scrotum; the clitoris was enlarged and looked somewhat like a small penis. At the base of the clitoris was an orifice through which urine was passed. Buccal smears showed the infant to be chromatin positive. There was no evidence of salt and fluid loss. A diagnosis of adrenogenital syndrome was made. The parents were told that the baby was a girl in spite of the male-appearing genitalia, that cortisone therapy would most likely cause female puberty to appear at the proper time, and that later on surgical correction of the external genitalia would be done.

Because both parents were physicians (although not in specialties that had given them previous contact with the adrenogenital syndrome), the attending pediatrician understandably assumed that they would become acquainted with the syndrome—its causes, its treatment, and the like—by reading the references he had given them. It later turned out that the father did, but the mother did not. The pediatrician scented trouble when the father called him about a month after delivery, saying that they had named the baby "Sally" but that his wife continued to call her "Peter," the name they had originally selected in case the child turned out to be a boy. Further, he said, she made occasional references to her daydreams of *his* becoming a surgeon (the father was a surgeon), and that *he* looked as if he might make a good football player (the baby was quite stocky). The

pediatrician asked her to come in for an interview, and she reported to him that intellectually she knew the child was a girl but that emotionally, "I simply can't accept it." Because she was tearful and depressed as well, the pediatrician suspected a postpartum breakdown and asked for psychiatric consultation.

The consultant psychiatrist substantiated the findings but felt the mother had a neurotic depression with a good outlook and spent 22 hours with her in psychotherapy. In brief, the important events that appeared to produce her difficulties were as follows: Her father was a physician and she was raised as a member of the "upper class" in a small midwestern town. She had two older sisters and a brother two years her junior. She adored her jolly, outgoing father, but he was a busy doctor who had little time for any of the children. What time he had to spare usually was spent with his son building model airplanes and with a large model electric train layout in the basement. The patient said that all the girls were jealous of the young brother and especially she. The father frequently mentioned his dreams that his son would attend medical school, specialize in surgery, and return to the small home town to join him in practice.

When he was 10 years old, the brother was killed in a water skiing accident at their summer home. A neighbor, looking back toward his own child on water skis, ran over her brother, who was in the water after having taken a spill. His body was badly cut by the propeller, and he was dead when his father, who was driving the boat, pulled him from the water. The patient, her two sisters, and the mother did not witness the accident itself, but all helped lift the brother's body onto the dock. The family was totally stunned by this tragedy, and the patient feels that the family was never able to reunite itself after it. She feels that the father never recovered and has been a different person ever since, depressed and lonely instead of jovial. She says to this day (18 years later) the electric train layout is still in the basement of her parents' home just as it was the day the boy died. The father still berates himself for not being more quick-thinking and trying to ram the neighbor's boat, which he knew was going to pass close by his son. The father buried himself in work, and she does not think they saw much of him after that. He received an emergency call at her wedding and was not present for the latter half of it.

The patient had an extremely stormy time through a number of the psychotherapy sessions, particularly those which treated with her highly ambivalent feelings toward her brother. She admitted that shortly after he died, she had conscious feelings that she was glad he was dead. This caused her extreme guilt. She also came to recognize that it was not long after her brother's death that she became fascinated by a medical career, an idea that she had not considered before. Her father did not take her seriously and apparently had no recognition of how desperately this daughter was trying to win his affection. She graduated second in her medical school class, which disappointed her, feeling that her father would be more impressed had she been first.

In her own marriage, she had hoped for a boy to be the first-born. It was a daughter. Her second pregnancy terminated in a stillbirth at term. It was a male child and the patient reports having gone through a severe grief reaction for six or more months after this. Her third pregnancy produced the little girl with adrenogenital syndrome.

As a result of psychotherapy, the patient was able to see and feel why she had so desperately wanted a boy and could not accept the fact that the child was female with an adrenogenital syndrome. The psychiatrist, because she seemed to be recovered and adjust-

ing well and because of the truly difficult emotional experiences she had had, decided against any exploration of the fact that she had married a divorced physician much older than she, i.e., a potential father-figure.

Dewhurst and Gordon [2] suggest several rules about sex assignment in the intersexed baby:

1. Female intersex babies must be raised as females regardless of the status of the external genitalia.
2. Other intersex babies should be raised in the sex that offers them the better chance of normal sexual relations, irrespective of the type of gonad present.

In part, behind both of these rules lies the important fact that it is relatively easy to create a usable artificial vagina by plastic surgery but it is nearly impossible to create a functional artificial penis. Thus, if a genetic male baby has such serious genital deformities, including micropenis, that it appears most unlikely that he will ever be able to function as a male in sexual intercourse, the wise plan of action might be to give him the female sex of assignment and raise him as a girl. When such a decision is taken, it is best to remove any testicular tissue present to prevent later physical manifestations of masculinity at the onset of puberty.

If this were to be considered in a given case, it would require extensive discussion with the parents in order to test their attitudes and to size up their reliability and basic integrity. For what is being asked of them is that they change their thinking from what they know to be a genetic male baby to regarding their baby son as a daughter and raising her accordingly with all of the love and affection that is needed for normal psychosexual development. This is a hard assignment and not all people can do it. If the parents were not able to make this basic switch in thinking but tried to raise the baby as a girl, it is predictable that the child will grow up to have a confused and ambiguous sexual self-concept. Money [4, 5] has this to say:

It is possible, for example, to have four genetic females, each ultimately diagnosed as having the adrenogenital syndrome of female hermaphroditism: one is assigned and reared as a girl, one as a boy, one provisionally as a boy, and one provisionally as a girl. The subsequent medical and social histories differ, relative to the sex of assignment or provisional assignment and rearing. Psychosexual differentiation takes place, respectively, in the four cases as feminine, masculine, ambivalently wanting to be changed to a girl, and ambivalently wanting to be changed to a boy.

The lesson of these four cases does not need to be belabored. They indicate that the outcome in psychosexual differentiation was entirely independent of genetic sex, which was the same in all four and also independent of hormonal sex . . . . The first two cases illustrate also the congruence between sex of assignment and the differentiation of gender identity when the parents and other significant people in the social environment are not ambivalent about the sex to which their child belongs; whereas the second two cases illustrate what may happen when the opposite is true.

All this emphasizes the great importance of settling the sex of assignment as early as possible in the life of the baby and, conversely, not permitting months to go by with the matter remaining unsettled. To do the latter is to court disaster for the future sexual adjustment of the child when he or she becomes an adult. The longer parents do not know what the sex of their baby is, or are raising the baby in the wrong sex of assignment, the greater is the chance for problems in the baby's sexual future.

From what has been said, it follows that if the sex assignment must be changed when the baby is older, say 6 to 18 months of age, a difficult problem lies ahead, particularly for the parents. The child within this age range is not yet particularly verbal and probably can make the gender switch without too much difficulty *if the parents, particularly the mother, can accomplish the difficult feat of now treating him as a girl whereas formerly they treated him as a boy.* When this late a switch in sex assignment must be made, it is imperative that the pediatrician, surgeon, or psychiatrist—whoever is best qualified in knowledge about gender identity and gender role—spend time with the parents and particularly with the mother. Both parents will need a good deal of counsel as they attempt this new adjustment to their baby, and a few hours spent with them at this stage will pay great dividends 20 years later when this child becomes an adult. Parents, even sophisticated ones, will flounder if left alone to solve their doubts and anxieties as best they can. The fact that the physician sees them and talks about their problems and feelings is very important psychotherapy. It offers the hand of support to help them through what can truly be a perplexing and terrifying experience. It is best not to leave an interview up to the parents' initiative, as when one says, "Please call me if you have any questions." Rather, it is preferable to make a definite appointment so there is no chance for an error. It is useful if the mother on occasion brings the baby in to the interview. One can then directly observe how she handles the baby, dresses it, and speaks to it. From this, one can make a reasonably accurate inference as to what gender the child is being raised in.

Acquired Disease and Trauma

Diseases and trauma that injure the genitals (as well as the female breast) are numerous, and there is little purpose served, from a counseling standpoint, in attempting to take them up one by one since little understanding will be gained. Rather, it is more useful to consider if general statements can be made, and what treatment principles and inferences might be drawn from them.

When a person loses someone dear to him or something of high personal value, such as a part of his own body, or his position and status, he enters into a condition that resembles depression but is actually grief. *Grief* is commonly considered to be the phenomenon that surrounds the loss of a loved one by death, but it happens in many other situations of personal loss. The loss of a leg, an eye, or a breast predictably will precipitate a grief reaction. A loss that is castrating, such as loss of the penis or testes, usually initiates a profound grief reaction; the psychological damage and loss pertains to the change in the man's masculine image of himself. He will disparage himself and feel inadequate and inferior with both sexes: with men because he no longer feels equal, with women because he no longer feels capable. Although their genitalia are interior, women go through comparable emotions with the loss of a breast, the uterus, or ovaries. Grief has protean manifestations, and there is no doubt that the loss of one's genitals, in whole or in part, constitutes a most serious insult that is unique. The genitals, as well as the female breast, have tremendously high value and importance. Their loss will plunge the individual into grief just as surely as if someone loved had died.

Grief can be prepared for to a certain extent. One can compare the feelings created by these two situations: First, the death of a loved one suddenly and without warning in an automobile accident; and second, death after many months of suffering with and wasting away from cancer. In the first instance, no preparation is possible and the

shock that hits is hard and severe. In the second instance, much of the emotional work of grieving has been done before death, and when it finally comes, it is often seen as a welcome release from suffering. The point of these examples is that the longer the period of warning about an impending loss (loved one, eye, leg, penis, breast, job, position, and the like), the more opportunity a person has to brace himself against the coming event. Not that he will escape grief—only that it is apt to be less intense and devastating. Specifically, the longer the warning a patient has about the possibility of a surgical sexual mutilation, the better he will be prepared emotionally to meet it. This is a principle that can be followed when the loss is made necessary by disease of the genitals. It cannot be met when mutilation occurs as a result of trauma, such as when a soldier steps on a land-mine and suffers genital loss.

There is no way that a surgeon can prevent the emotional suffering that results from a mutilating operation he must do to save the patient's life or restore his health. Short of an emergency, he can give the patient as much advance notice as possible so some of the work of grieving can be done before surgery. When the cause of the loss is trauma, no preparation is possible, and the surgeon makes such emotional repairs as he can. What is the role of the surgeon as he tries to help his patient work through his grief?

If one considers the classic example of grief caused by the death of a loved one, it is obvious that nothing one can say or do will bring back the dead. Whatever comfort can be given to the grieving survivor is not through words, because rarely will they even be heard. What does matter, and matters beyond measure, is *human contact;* staying with the grieving person fills a great need; the holding of a hand means more than a thousand words.

When a person has lost part of himself,

and especially something connected with his sexual value and worth (genitals and breasts), there is nothing that can be said or done to bring back the part any more than one can bring back the dead. During the period of initial adjustment, what he needs above all is human contact with people he loves or is fond of. He needs to sense from them that their attitude toward him has not changed as a result of his (or her) misfortune. "Am I still loveable?" is the great concern of the mutilated person.

In a loss of this type, the patient will experience many conflicting thoughts about himself and his condition, some of them bordering on the bizarre. At times he will blame himself for what has happened; at other times his mind looks for persons external to himself to blame. (It can be the doctor.) But the overwhelming sensation is that of relative helplessness and dependency. He needs a strong person on whom to lean and he will invariably cast his surgeon in this role. He will look to him for approval and guidance, and it is the wise physician who intuitively recognizes these needs in his patient. It is sometimes difficult for the physician, particularly if he is younger than his patient, to realize adequately that the patient, who might be a captain of industry or a well-known political figure, has strong needs to lean on someone and to be accepted until he has had a chance to work through his grief.

It is important that the surgeon spend sufficient time with his patient who has suffered such a loss so that a firm doctor-patient relationship can be established. This is a time of tenuous adjustment for the patient, and there is one important consideration to be kept in mind: the patient suffering from grief characteristically examines the past—the "might-have-beens," the sins of omission, the sins of commission—and dwells on these. The man who has been a heavy cigarette smoker and who has bron-

chial carcinoma often entertains thoughts such as these: "Why didn't I stop smoking while I still had time?" or "Why didn't someone tell me that I must stop smoking while I still had time?" In the presence of a firm doctor-patient relationship, the thrust of these preoccupations usually will mean that the patient assumes a mature responsibility for his cigarette-related cancer.

In other circumstances, where a good doctor-patient relationship does not exist, this mechanism can take a different turn and be projected outward. What might have been self-blame for smoking can become: "Why didn't you tell me I must stop smoking to preserve my health?" While this is irrational mental behavior, it is common under such stress. Carried a step further, such a projected attitude can become: "The tobacco companies are to blame for my lung cancer and they should settle for the damage *they* have caused me." Another variation on the theme is that unless a trusting doctor-patient relationship exists, the surgeon may be blamed for some of the trouble in a similar manner. The patient, grieving and needing a strong person to lean on in his distress, reaches out for the strongest person he knows, his doctor. If the doctor rejects him, or seems to, by remaining aloof or uninvolved, or if he does not understand the suffering, the dependent need can take this different turn. Instead of being passive, the patient now turns to an aggressive assault (as a defensive measure) and begins to look for areas in which the physician might be blamed for the problem. From an emotional standpoint, these are common reasons for malpractice suits that have no basis in reality.

In summary, when dealing with a patient, man or woman, who has to undergo a surgical procedure that will be regarded as sexually mutilating, there is no way in which the surgeon can prevent emotional responses appropriate to the situation. Rather, by understanding what feelings the patient will encounter and by being willing to support him in adjusting to his predicament, the surgeon will be regarded as friend and valuable ally during this temporary period of acute need. Such an understanding of the feelings and needs of his patient in these trying circumstances constitutes the best of the art of medicine.

References

1. Bing, E., and Rudikoff, E. Divergent ways of parental coping with hermaphrodite children. *Med. Aspects Hum. Sexual.* 4:73, 1970.
2. Dewhurst, C. J., and Gordon, R. R. *The Intersexual Disorders.* London: Baillière, Tindall & Cassell, 1969.
3. Money, J. *Sex Errors of the Body.* Baltimore: Johns Hopkins Press, 1968.
4. Money, J. Sexual dimorphism and homosexual gender identity. *Psychol. Bull.* 74:425, 1970.
5. Money, J., and Ehrhardt, A. A. *Man & Woman, Boy & Girl: Differentiation and Dimorphism of Gender Identity from Conception to Maturity.* Baltimore: Johns Hopkins University Press, 1972.

Developmental Anomalies

IV

Intersex Problems: Diagnostic Aspects

JAY Y. GILLENWATER

5

GENITAL ANOMALIES that require plastic surgical procedures frequently are associated with or are the result of one of the intersex disorders. It is very important to recognize the disorders of abnormal sexual development early because some are life-threatening (congenital adrenogenital syndrome); in some, the sex of rearing will need to be changed to preserve fertility (female pseudohermaphroditism resulting from adrenogenital syndrome); and in some, there is a high incidence of malignancy of the gonad (testicular feminization). It is also important to assign the appropriate sex early to avoid psychological problems.

Criteria of Sex

In evaluating patients with a question of intersexuality, it is helpful to define the five morphological criteria of sex: (1) chromosomal sex, (2) gonadal structure, (3) morphology of internal genitalia, (4) external genital appearance, and (5) hormonal status. The two psychological criteria of sex are: (1) sex of rearing and (2) psychological gender role. Intersexuality usually is defined as one or more contradictions in the five morpho-

logical criteria of sex. The terms "male" or "female pseudohermaphrodite" are assigned according to whether the gonads are testes or overies, and "true hermaphroditism" defines the individual having both gonadal structures.

CHROMOSOMAL SEX

The chromosomal sex can be evaluated by karyotyping (the basic process by which chromosomes are identified and studied) or by studying the nuclear chromatin pattern (Barr bodies). The first accurate count of human chromosomes was made by J. H. Tjio and Albert Levan [10] in 1956. In the succeeding seventeen years, much information has been gathered concerning the chromosomal structure in the various intersex disorders. Karyotyping is done by culturing human cells, usually lymphocytes, and by arresting the division in metaphase using a substance such as colchicine. In metaphase, the chromosomes are discrete and easily visible; when placed in a hypotonic solution, the cell swells, spreading the chromosomes apart. The preparation is fixed, stained, and photographed, and the photograph is cut so that the chromosomes can be arranged in a standardized order. Humans have 46 chromosomes, of which 44 are autosomes and two are sex chromosomes. The normal female has 44 autosomes and two X sex chromosomes (46/XX). The normal male has 44 autosomes and X and Y sex chromosomes (46/XY). Chromosomal mosaicism exists when different cell lines have varying numbers or types of chromosomes in the same individual. Structural abnormalities of individual chromosomes have been described that are caused by translocation or the formation of an isochromosome by an error in meiosis.

In 1949 Barr and Betram [1] noted that it was possible to identify the sex of an individual by a clump of chromatin that is visible in the nuclei of female cells and absent from those of males. The nuclear chromatin, or Barr body, is found in most tissue of the female with the exception of the primary oocyte. It usually is found in 20 percent or more of the nuclei of cells examined from the normal female, and in less than 1 to 2 percent of cells from the normal male. An individual with no chromatin bodies is said to be "chromatin negative"; one having 5 percent or more chromatin bodies is said to be "chromatin positive."

The Y chromosome is believed to be the male organizer that leads to the differentiation of a testis. The testis, through the inducer substance and testosterone secretion, leads to male genital differentiation. There are no true Y-linked disorders. However, there are more than 75 X-linked disorders. the 47/XXX has a decreased IQ, and the 48/XXXX has an even greater reduction in IQ.

GONADAL SEX

Of the various criteria of sex, probably the most important and difficult to obtain is the microscopic identity of the gonad. It is important that the gonadal structure be identified by microscopic examination, since the gross appearance may be deceptive. The iden-

tity of the gonad is necessary to classify the true hermaphrodite and to confirm the diagnosis of male or female pseudohermaphroditism.

MORPHOLOGY OF INTERNAL GENITALIA

The morphology of the internal genitalia may be extremely variable, since every normal embryo has both wolffian and müllerian ducts. The development into male internal genitalia with inhibition of female structures is dependent on the male gonadal inducer substance. The identity of the internal genitalia may influence the choice of sex of rearing, as in the female with adrenogenital syndrome, since fertility may be possible when the individual is reared as a female. The morphology of the internal genitalia may be identified by using appropriate x-ray studies or by laparotomy.

EXTERNAL GENITAL APPEARANCE

The appearance of the external genitalia is the most readily identifiable criterion for sex differentiation but the least reliable. The assignment of sex usually is based on the appearance of the external genitalia; however, ambiguity of external genitalia is often the first suggestion that an intersex problem exists. The external genital development will influence the assignment of sex; if an individual cannot function sexually as a male, the female sex gender will most often be assigned. It is much easier to create surgically a functioning vagina than a functioning phallus.

HORMONAL SEX

The hormonal environment is important in determining the appearance of the external genitalia and is responsible for the secondary sex characteristics. The hormonal state frequently may not correlate with the gonadal tissue, as in cases of testicular feminization or congenital adrenal hyperplasia. The knowledge of hormonal secretions is important in defining and treating intersexuality.

PSYCHOLOGICAL CRITERIA OF SEX

The sex of rearing usually is assigned to the patient by the physician and parents. It has been shown by Money et al. [7] that sexual orientation depends upon assignment of sex and rearing rather than upon genetic determination. Unless there is some contradiction in the five morphological criteria of sex, there is, by definition, no intersexuality. Thus, the individual who sees himself in a contradictory gender role (e.g., a transvestite) does not belong to any of the various hermaphroditic classifications per se. However, the gender role of the individual is an extremely important consideration when deciding the sex of rearing because of the psychological problems that may be caused or prevented by the correct assignment of sex.

Normal Sexual Development*

The undifferentiated gonad appears in the fetus about the fourth week as a genital ridge medial to the mesonephros, and it develops into either an ovary or a testis. The genetic sex is believed to determine gonadal sex by inhibiting one part of the gonad.

The further differentiation of the internal genitalia is delayed until the 25 to 30 mm (eighth to ninth week) stage. According to the work of Jost [5], this differentiation is

* The material in this section first appeared in an article by J. Y. Gillenwater, A. W. Wyker, M. Birdsong, and W. N. Thornton, *J. Urol.* 103:500, 1970. Copyright © 1970, The Williams & Wilkins Co., Baltimore.

dependent upon whether a normally functioning testis is present. In a series of experiments on rabbits (Fig. 5-1), Jost found that if the gonad was removed (either testis or ovary) prior to this stage of differentiation of the internal genitalia, the wolffian duct system was inhibited, and the internal and external genitalia developed toward female organogenesis. If the testis was removed from

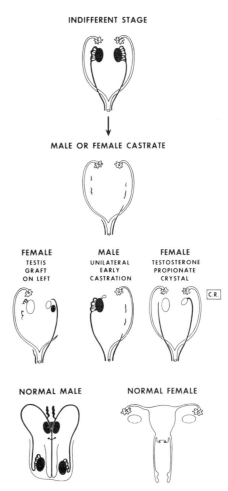

FIG. 5-1. Schematic representation of the development of the internal and external genitalia as proposed by Jost [5].

one side, then only that side developed along female lines with inhibition of that wolffian duct. If a testis was transplanted to one side, that side developed along male lines with development of the wolffian duct and inhibition of the müllerian duct system. He found that no available synthetic androgen could cause these local changes of the fetal internal genitalia; thus, he postulated that the fetal testes have some other masculinizing hormone that causes the local effects of stimulating the wolffian duct and inhibiting the müllerian duct in the fetus. When a crystal of testosterone propionate was implanted unilaterally, there was persistence of the complete wolffian duct system and no inhibition of the müllerian duct. The external genitalia would become masculinized. Jost found that the stage of development at which the testis was removed or implanted was critical. If differentiation was already proceeding along male lines, then the later removal of the testis (or later malfunction of the testis) would produce a wide variety of abnormalities of the müllerian and wolffian duct systems. Thus, any abnormality of the internal duct systems could be explained by the presence or absence of the male inducer substance at various stages of development.

In summary, Jost's classic work shows that the normal testis possesses a locally acting male inducer substance that inhibits the müllerian duct system and stimulates the wolffian duct system. In the absence of this inducer substance, the müllerian structures persist and the wolffian duct structures disappear. If not virilized, the external genitalia also will progress along female lines.

The external genitalia remain in an undifferentiated state until the twelfth fetal week (see Chap. 2).

The human adrenal primordium appears during the sixteenth fetal week and reaches its maximal relative size in the third and fourth fetal months. This is the same period in which androgen stimulus is necessary to masculinize the external genitalia and urogenital sinus in the female fetus to produce a female pseudohermaphrodite.

Effect of Androgen in Fetal Sexual Development*

The age of the fetus is a critical factor in the response of the sex primordia to androgens, since the capacity to stimulate the external genitalia, urogenital sinus, and development of the wolffian duct is limited to a specific period of life. For the development of a complete phallic urethra in the female fetus, the androgenic stimulus must occur before the eleventh fetal week. This concept is supported both by experimental work and by observations in humans. Androgens have been found to be readily transmitted across the placental barrier in humans. They can modify female fetal development of the external genitalia, urogenital sinus, and, rarely, the wolffian duct. Overzier [8] states that the differentiation of the genital ducts is almost complete at the time the fetal adrenal cortex begins to produce androgens, but seminal vesicles and prostatic glands have been found in female patients with noticeable virilism. It is of interest that four cases of masculinization of the female infant have been reported after the mother had received stilbesterol during pregnancy. It was postulated that perhaps this effect was due to adrenal hyperplasia consequent to the administration of estrogens. Conversely, feminization of the male fetus leading to a severe hypospadias has been reported after maternal administration of estrogens and progesterones.

* The material in this section first appeared in an article by J. Y. Gillenwater, A. W. Wyker, M. Birdsong, and W. N. Thornton, *J. Urol.* 103:500, 1970. Copyright © 1970, The Williams & Wilkins Co., Baltimore.

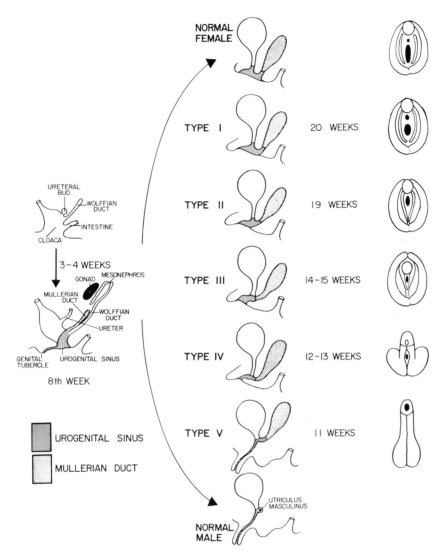

FIG. 5-2. Effect of androgenic hormones on the development of müllerian and wolffian ducts. (Adapted from original description by Prader [9]. From J. Y. Gillenwater et al., *J. Urol.* 103:500, 1970. Copyright © 1970, The Williams & Wilkins Co., Baltimore.)

Prader [9] has divided the different degrees of masculinization of the urogenital sinus into five types (Fig. 5-2):

Type 1: Androgen administration after the twentieth week of fetal life. The vulva has been formed and only clitoral hypertrophy results.

Type 2: Androgen administration after the nineteenth week of fetal life. The vulva gapes but is funnel-shaped, and the clitoris is enlarged. The vagina and urethra open separately.

Type 3: Effect of androgens at about the fourteenth to fifteenth fetal week. The vagina and urethra open into a common urogenital sinus. The clitoris is larger and penis-like.

Type 4: Effects of androgens at about the twelfth to thirteenth fetal week. The perineum is thrust forward, the narrow urogenital sinus is formed, and the labia form a bifid scrotum. The urogenital sinus opens at the base of the penis, corresponding to a hypospadial penis.

Type 5: Effect of androgens at about the eleventh week of fetal life. The external genitalia have a male appearance except for the absence of testes in the scrotum.

Klinefelter's Syndrome

In 1942, Klinefelter, Reifenstein, and Albright [6] described nine men who had small testes, azoospermia, elevated urinary gonadotropins, normal external genitalia, and gynecomastia. Testicular biopsies revealed hypoplastic, sclerotic, and hyalinized tubules. The Leydig cells were clumped in some patients and even appeared hyperplastic. In Klinefelter's syndrome, the internal and external genitalia are as those of the normal male. Gynecomastia is present in some but not all of these patients. The patients with Klinefelter's syndrome have been shown to have a decrease in plasma testosterone. The contradiction in the morphological criteria of sex results from the karyotype abnormality of an extra X chromosome (47/XXY). Thus, these individuals also would be chromatin positive. Other karyotypes of 48/XXXY, 49/XXXXY, 49/XXXYY, and 46/XX have been described. Eighty percent of patients with Klinefelter's syndrome are chromatin positive. The incidence is reported to be 1 in 400 live births and 1 in 100 male mental defectives.

The patients with Klinefelter's syndrome usually are seen by the physician because of gynecomastia or infertility. The diagnosis can be established by obtaining a sperm count, chromatin pattern, or testicular biopsy specimen. The patients usually have a normal male phenotype, but the testes are small and firm. In the patients with small testes resulting from trauma or postinflammatory disease, the testes ordinarily are not as firm as those of the Klinefelter's patients.

Turner's Syndrome (Gonadal Dysgenesis)

Turner's syndrome is a term used synonymously with gonadal dysgenesis. The syndrome includes females of short stature who have congenital anomalies, hypoestrinism, streak gonads, and increased urinary gonadotropins. Other abnormalities encountered in females who have Turner's syndrome include sexual infantilism, primary amenorrhea, webbing of the neck, shield chest, pigmented moles, lymphedema, mental retardation, coarctation of the aorta, deafness, cubitus valgus, retardation of growth, and low-set ears. In the newborn female, the syndrome may present as webbing of the neck and nonpitting edema of hands and feet due to large dilated vascular spaces. A negative chromatin pattern would verify the gonadal dysgenesis. However, 20 to 40 percent of such individuals have positive buccal smears.

In gonadal dysgenesis, it is postulated that there is a defect in the second sex chromosome in some of the patient's cells. The predominant group is 45/XO and chromatin negative. Some patients are mosaics, with the most common combination being XO/XX. Some patients have been reported with 46/XX and are believed to have a structural abnormality of the second X. The internal and external genitalia are those of an immature female. The gonads usually are described as "streak gonads." The hormone studies show hypoestrinism with increased urinary gonadotropins.

Turner's syndrome is believed to represent the human counterpart of the cases in Jost's studies involving rabbits in which the absence of a gonad leads to female differentiation of the internal and external genitalia. The failure of the primitive germ cells to reach the gonad has been postulated as one of the causes of streak gonads.

True Hermaphrodites

The true hermaphrodite is an individual that has both ovarian and testicular tissue. Hermaphrodites usually have been classified according to location and lateralization of the conflicting gonads. The gonads may be combined, such as ovotestes, or there may be an ovary and a testis or an ovary or a testis with or without an ovotestis. The internal and external genital differentiation can vary widely from almost normal female to male with some degree of hypospadias. Most hermaphrodites have been raised as males (70 percent), most develop gynecomastia (75 per-

cent), and half of them menstruate. The predominant karyotype is 46/XX, and the nuclear chromatin test is positive. The hormonal status has been variable. The diagnosis of true hermaphroditism can be made only by microscopic confirmation of the presence of both ovarian and testicular tissue.

The following case history (U.V.H. #57 42 20) has been reported:

An infant was born in The University of Virginia Hospital on February 23, 1967, with ambiguous external genitalia. The mother's pregnancy was normal. No medications had been taken. Examination of the genitalia showed a 3.5 cm phallus with a bifid scrotum and perineal hypospadias as well as cryptorchidism. The karotyping showed 46/XX chromosomes, and the urinary steroid excretion was normal. The parents were told that the child had an intersex problem and that laparotomy and endoscopy should be performed at a later age. It was suggested that the child be reared as a female. At 4 months of age, the child was readmitted and ketosteroids were found to be less than 2 mg per 24 hours, which is normal for that age. Endoscopy showed a female type of urogenital sinus leading to a normal bladder and vagina, with a normal cervix at the apex. A left inguinal hernia was palpable, with a 1 cm gonadal structure. Laparotomy showed a fallopian tube and ovotestis in the left inguinal hernia. The uterus had a suggestion of bicornuate configuration and the right gonad was also an ovotestis. Both gonads and the left fallopian tube were removed. The urogenital sinus was opened and the clitoris partially amputated during another hospitalization at 1 year of age, which provided normal appearing external genitalia.

This case demonstrates the workup of infants with ambiguous genitalia and chromatin-positive nuclear pattern. When the history or hormonal studies do not suggest female pseudohermaphroditism, it is necessary to define the internal genitalia and gonads by endoscopy and laparotomy to make the diagnosis, and to remove contradictory gonadal elements.

Male Pseudohermaphroditism

Male pseudohermaphrodites are individuals with a testis and XY sex chromosomes who have some failure in virilization. The most common condition seen in this group is the testicular feminization syndrome. These patients are phenotypic females whose breasts may be large but the vagina usually is small or obliterated. The gonad is a testis and is usually located in a hernia. Microscopic examination of the testis reveals it to be immature and without spermatogenesis. The internal genitalia are rudimentary and may include a uterus, fallopian tubes, or spermatic ducts. The hormonal studies show normal male urinary 17-ketosteroids and normal male plasma testosterone levels. The pathogenesis of testicular feminization is believed to be a lack of end-organ response to androgen.

Other descriptions of patients with testes and varying degrees of inadequacy of virilization have been reported by Lubs, Gilbert-Dreyfus, and Reifenstein.

Female Pseudohermaphroditism

Female pseudohermaphroditism is seen in patients whose gonads are ovaries and who have various degrees of masculinization. The most common cause of this disorder is the adrenogenital syndrome due to congenital adrenocortical hyperplasia. Masculinization of the female fetus also is seen after maternal administration of androgens, certain progresterones, and even estrogens, as well as with maternal arrhenoblastoma.

The adrenogenital syndrome is caused by adrenal cortical hyperplasia secondary to an inheritable inborn error of metabolism. The incidence suggests that an autosomal recessive genetic factor is responsible. The basic defect is a congenital partial or complete absence of one or several adrenal enzymes necessary for hydrocortisone production, with the resultant accumulation of androgenic steroidal precursors.

Three types of enzymatic defects that cause virilization and three rare enzymatic defects that cause little virilization have been described in congenital adrenal hyperplasia. The most common enzymatic defect is that of the 21-hydroxylase. This defect may be partial, with clinical manifestation of virilism and normal sodium conservation. A complete block in the 21-hydroxylase has been proposed as a cause of salt and water loss as well as virilization. The uncommon 11-hydroxylase enzyme defect produces virilization and hypertension. The rare 3-β-hydroxysteroid dehydrogenase defect causes disturbance in the early stages of hormonal synthesis in both the gonad and adrenal glands. In the male fetus, there are varying degrees of feminization of the external genitalia and urogenital sinus. The female fetus has less virilization than in the two preceding enzymatic defects. Most patients with this disorder have a tendency to lose salt. The rare 17-hydroxylase defects produce sexual infantilism, hypertension, and hypokalemic alkalosis. The 20-hydroxylase defect, which is also rare, prevents the conversion of cholesterol to the active steroids and has been called "congenital lipoid adrenal hyperplasia." This uncommon condition usually involves the gonads as well as the adrenal gland; in most cases, it is fatal. Females show little virilization. Males exhibit varying degrees of male pseudohermaphroditism with female external genitalia because of the absence of androgen.

Adrenal hyperplasia is secondary to increased adrenocorticotropic hormone production by the pituitary because of deficient hydrocortisone production disrupting the adrenal-hypothalmic pituitary feedback mechanisms. The virilization is due to overproduction of adrenal androgens. Thirty percent of these patients have a sufficient decrease in hydrocortisone and aldosterone to be threatened by an addisonian crisis.

The following case history (U.V.H. #35 75 49) is of interest:*

* The material in this section first appeared in an article by J. Y. Gillenwater, A. W. Wyker, M. Birdsong, and W. N. Thornton, *J. Urol.* 103:500, 1970. Copyright © 1970, The Williams & Wilkins Co., Baltimore.

FIG. 5-3. Patient with adrenogenital syndrome at 4 years of age with masculinization and increased growth. (From J. Y. Gillenwater et al., *J. Urol.* 103:500, 1970. Copyright © 1970, The Williams & Wilkins Co., Baltimore.)

This patient, born in 1949, appeared to be a normal, Negro male infant except for poor nutritional development and bilateral cryptorchidism. During his first year, he had repeated respiratory infections and gastroenteritis, weighing only 10 pounds at the age of 10 months. There was a sudden improvement in his health and growth at 1 year of age. At 15 months of age, he weighed 25 pounds and was 30 inches tall. When he was 4 years old, he was much larger than his 8-year-old sister; he weighed 80 pounds and was 50 inches tall. He was noted to have heavy muscular development, a deep voice, a beard, pubic hair, large male genitalia, and mild hypertension (150/90 mm Hg). The patient developed pubic hair at 1 year of age, a deepening voice and large phallus by 1½ years, and at the age of 3½ years he had begun to grow a beard. X-rays of

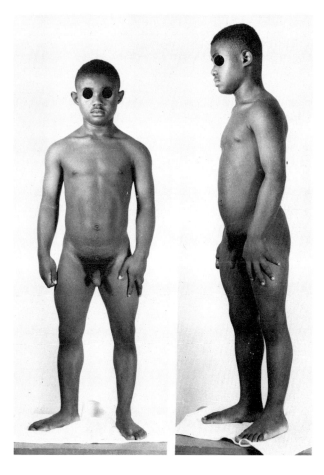

his wrists revealed a bone age of 13 years. The 24-hour urinary 17-ketosteroid secretion was 68 mg per 24 hours. He was referred to The University of Virginia Hospital for evaluation, with a diagnosis of adrenogenital syndrome.

Studies here in 1953 of the 4-year-old patient revealed him to be with facial, pubic, and axillary hair (Fig. 5-3). He had a large penis with a normal urethral opening. The urinary ketosteroid secretion ranged between 56 and 76 mg per 24 hours and suppressed to 4 mg per 24 hours on cortisone. Blood pressure was 150/90 mm Hg. The intravenous urogram and skull X-rays were normal. A skin biopsy specimen was interpreted as chromatin negative with no Barr bodies, and it was compatible with a male pattern. The patient was treated with cortisone.

The patient was readmitted in March of 1956 at the age of 7 years because of intermittent hematuria. Physical examination showed adult male hair distribution, some enlargement of the breasts, bilateral undescended testes, and an adult-sized phallus with the urethral opening at the end of the glans penis (Fig. 5-4). Urinalysis tests confirmed the intermittent hematuria. The intravenous urogram was normal, and the bone age was found to be 14 years. Cystoendoscopy was interpreted as showing a normal bladder and congestion of the "prostatic urethra and verumontanum." The patient was operated upon for the cryptorchidism through a left Gibson incision, and the retroperitoneal area from the bladder to the kidney was explored without locating a vas deferens or testis. The incision was enlarged and the peritoneal cavity opened; enlarged adrenals were found but no testis could be located. The patient continued to have intermittent hematuria.

In August of 1959, the patient was reevaluated. Cystoendoscopy revealed a complete penile urethra and a blood-filled vagina opening into the posterior urethra. This finding was confirmed by urethrograms. With bimanual pelvic examination, a uterus and gonads were palpated. Buccal mucosal smears and review of the patient's old skin biopsy specimen revealed a chromatin positive pattern. The patient was evaluated by the psychiatrists and was found to have a definite male gender role. Abdominal exploration revealed a uterus and two normal ovaries. A hysterectomy and bilateral oophorectomy were performed. The patient has continued

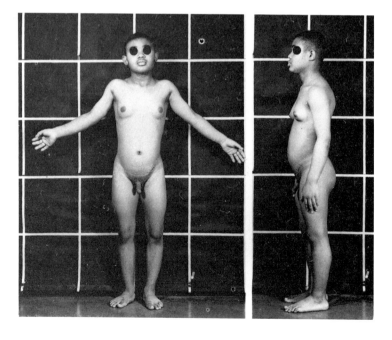

FIG. 5-4. Patient with adrenogenital syndrome at 7 years of age, showing large phallus and prominent breast development. (From J. Y. Gillenwater et al., *J. Urol.* 103:500, 1970. Copyright © 1970, The Williams & Wilkins Co., Baltimore.)

on cortisone treatment and has had some problems with recurrent backache and emotional adjustment.

Differential Diagnosis of Intersexuality

The intersex states usually are suspected when ambiguity of the external genitalia is noted. Hypospadias, a small phallus, cryptorchidism, or the presence of palpable masses in the groin or labia of an infant with female genitalia should suggest a sexual abnormality.

A history of siblings with an intersex state, the phenotype of Turner's syndrome with a short stature or webbed neck, or small testes in an infertile male may be the first clues to an abnormal sexual development.

When the question of intersexuality arises, it can be diagnosed easily by defining the five morphological criteria of sex. Table 5-1 shows a scheme modified from Wilkins [11] and Bunge [2]. The sex chromatin pattern should be determined by the buccal or vaginal smear. This test is obtained easily and should be the first performed, taking care to obtain good staining and fixation in order to

TABLE 5-1. Work-up of Infants with Ambiguous Genitalia

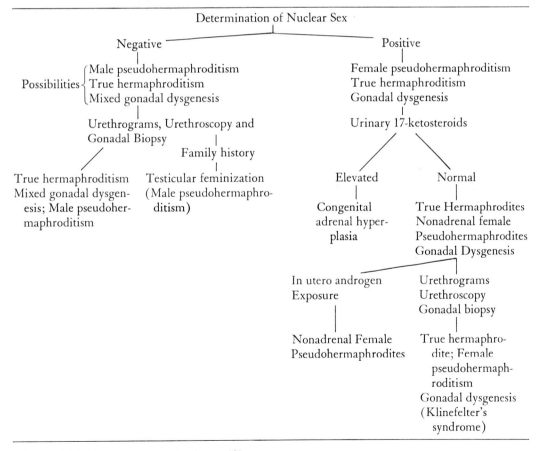

SOURCE: Modified from Wilkins[11] and Bouge[2].

compare the specimen with known controls that are done simultaneously. If the test is interpreted incorrectly, it can certainly result in a misdirected diagnosis, as in our case of adrenogenital syndrome. The newborn female may have lower nuclear chromatin counts during her first several days of life. When there is a positive chromatin nuclear pattern in an individual with a sexual abnormality, the differential diagnosis will be one of the following: (1) female pseudohermaphroditism, (2) true hermaphroditism, (3) Klinefelter's syndrome, or (4) gonadal aplasia.

If there is no history of maternal androgen exposure from drugs or tumor during pregnancy, then the urinary 17-ketosteriod excretion should be determined. In congenital adrenal hyperplasia, there is elevation in the 24-hour excretion of 17-ketosteroids, pregnanetriol, 11-ketopregnanetriol, and 17-ketogenic steroids (the last are elevated because they include pregnanetriol and 11-ketopregnanetriol). Occasionally, the 17-ketosteroids are elevated normally during the first week of life, and it may be necessary to repeat the measurement at two or three weeks of age.

With normal ketosteroids and no history of exposure to androgens, the morphological features of the internal genitalia and gonads must be determined to differentiate true hermaphroditism from nonadrenal female pseudohermaphroditism. Urethrography and urethroscopy should be performed initially to define the internal genitalia. Laparotomy usually is necessary to define the gonadal morphological characteristics and internal genitalia. If cystogenetic study reveals an XX/XY mosaic, the patient should have a laparotomy to rule out true hermaphroditism. All female pseudohermaphrodites are chromatin positive and 46/XX. In the classic case of congenital adrenal hyperplasia with increased 17-ketosteroids, the female sex chromatin 46/XX, and internal female genitalia, surgical exploration is unnecessary and the patient should be reared as a female.

Patients having ambiguous external genitalia with a chromatin-negative nuclear pattern can be true hermaphrodites, male pseudohermaphrodites, or have mixed gonadal dysgenesis. These patients should be given careful urethroscopic and urethrographic examination to rule out a communicating sinus or uterine canal. If bilateral scrotal gonads are palpable, the individual is most likely a male pseudohermaphrodite. In this group, laparotomy usually is necessary to establish the diagnosis.

Management of Intersex States

The management of patients with intersex problems must be individualized. The ideal goal is the achievement of fertility, coital function, and normal psychological adjustment. When an intersex problem is suspected in an infant, it is important that an accurate and orderly examination be accomplished so the correct gender role will be assigned. This procedure can be carried out more effectively at a medical center because of the availability of laboratory facilities and greater clinical experience. It is important that the parents of a child with intersex problems understand that there is a possibility of incomplete sexual development that can usually be completed surgically. Parents should not be told that the child is "half boy and half girl." Money and Hampson [7] have shown that the psychological sex of an individual is not governed by the gonadal or anatomical state, but by many environmental factors. Thus, it is vital that the child receives the complete series of examinations and tests necessary to obtain an accurate diagnosis and a sexual assignment corresponding with the most appropriate sexual function.

Female pseudohermaphrodites are capable

of maturing as fertile women and should be raised as females if the diagnosis is made early. The patients with adrenal hyperplasia usually will need some steroid replacement, since 30 percent will develop adrenal insufficiency. Plastic surgical procedures may be necessary to externalize the vagina.

Male pseudohermaphrodites usually should be reared according to the function of the external genitalia, since all are infertile. The external genitalia may vary from normal male to male with hypospadias. In patients with testicular feminization, most authorities believe that the testes should be removed, since one-third of the reported patients over age 30 had a gonadal tumor. Many physicians allow the testes to remain until puberty to allow a "normal" puberty. When the testes are removed, substitute estrogen therapy is essential to maintain feminization. The female siblings of patients should have nuclear chromatin pattern studies performed, since testicular feminization is familial. In patients

with a male phenotype and hypospadias, the hypospadias can be repaired before school years begin.

The true hermaphrodite should be reared in the gender role most appropriate to the function of the external genitalia. The intraabdominal testes should be removed to prevent malignancy. Certainly, any gonadal element which would conflict with external genitalia should be removed. Since it is not possible to separate surgically most ovotestes, they should be removed. Thus, the only gonadal structure that should not be removed in the true hermaphrodite is a remaining normal unilateral ovary in the phenotypic female.

Infants with bilateral cryptorchidism and hypospadias should have a nuclear chromatin pattern study performed while in the nursery to rule out intersexuality. The high incidence of upper urinary tract abnormalities also warrants an intravenous urogram at this time.

References

1. Barr, M. S., and Betram, E. G. The morphological distinction between neurone of the male and female, and the behavior of the nucleolar satellite during accelerated nucleoprotein synthesis. *Nature* 163:676, 1949.
2. Bunge, R. G. Intersexuality. In Campbell, M. F., and Harrison, J. H. (Eds.), *Urology* (3d Ed.). Philadelphia: Saunders, 1970.
3. Federman, D. D. *Abnormal Sexual Development*. Philadelphia: Saunders, 1968.
4. Gillenwater, J. Y., Wyker, A. W., Birdsong, M., and Thornton, W. N. Adrenogenital syndrome producing female pseudohermaphroditism with a phallic urethra. *J. Urol.* 103:500, 1970.
5. Jost, A. Embryonic Sexual Differentiation. In Jones, H. W., Jr., and Scott, W. W. (Eds.), *Hermaphroditism, Genital Anomalies*

and Related Endocrine Disorders. Baltimore: Williams & Wilkins, 1958.
6. Klinefelter, H. F., Reifenstein, E. C., and Albright, F. Syndrome characterized by gynecomastia, aspermatogenesis without A-Leydigism, and increased excretion of follicle-stimulating hormone. *J. Clin. Endocrinol.* 2:615, 1942.
7. Money, J., Hampson, J. G., and Hampson, J. L. Hermaphroditism: Recommendations concerning assignment of sex, change of sex, and psychologic management. *Bull. Johns Hopkins Hosp.* 97:284, 1955.
8. Overzier, C. Induzierter Pseudohermaphroditism. In Overzier, C. (Ed.), *Die Intersexualität*. Stuttgart: Georg Thieme, 1961. Pp. 394–408.
9. Prader, A. Vollkommen mannliche aubere

Genitalentwicklung und Salzverlustsyndrom bei Madchen mit kongenitalem adrenogenitalem Syndrom. *Helv. Paediatr. Acta* 13:5, 1958.

10. Tjio, J. H., and Levan, A. The chromo-some number of man. *Hereditas* 42:1, 1956.

11. Wilkins, L. *The Diagnosis and Treatment of Endocrine Disorders in Childhood and Adolescence.* Springfield, Ill.: Thomas, 1966.

Intersexuality: Diagnosis and Treatment

CLIFFORD C. SNYDER
CHARLES D. SCOTT
EARL Z. BROWNE, JR.

6

THE ACCURATE diagnosis of intersex variants may be initiated by considering possible hereditary influences, a review of familial predispositions, and a survey of medications and tests that were given during pregnancy. Physical examination of the infant or child must include such factors as (1) the size of the phallus, (2) the urethral orifice position, (3) the scrotal or labial contour and contents, (4) vaginal presence, (5) facies, (6) neck contour, (7) visible hernia, and (8) suspected mental retardation. Laboratory measures of importance are (1) the chromosome pattern, (2) sex chromatin, (3) ketosteroids, (4) gonadotropins, (5) estrogens, and (6) electrolyte patterns. The presence of any body anomaly should be thoroughly investigated. When the patient is of adolescent age or older, further criteria to be recorded are (1) size, shape, and length of the trunk and limbs, (2) breast development, (3) hair distribution, (4) fat distribution, (5) voice, and (6) menstruation.

Because all humans are provided with both male and female hormones, genital complexities are variable. The rapidity of new developments in studying intersex problems is responsible for the changes we observe in the intersex classifications from year to year; current classifications will be tomorrow's controversies. Regardless, a useful clinical classification for surgeons is necessary. There are well-established common intersex syndromes and a number of rare variants. Among the former groups, the surgeon should be acquainted with true hermaphroditism, female and male pseudohermaphroditism, and the gonadal dysgeneses. Of the gonadal dysgenetic types, Turner's syndrome (and mosaic variants thereof) and Klinefelter's syndrome are of particular interest to the surgeon.

Criteria of Sex Identification

CHROMOSOME PATTERNS

Chromosomal sex evaluation is achieved by (1) karyotypic determination and (2) investigation of the nuclear chromatin mass.

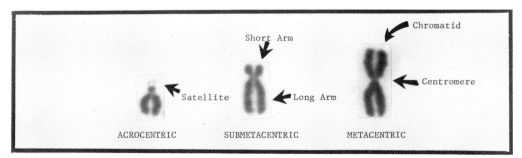

FIG. 6-1. Micrographic study reveals that the centromere may be either exactly centered in the two chromatid arms (metacentric), nearer one end (submetacentric), or almost at the end (acrocentric) of the chromosome. Some chromosomes have antennae or satellites, which appear at the end of the shorter chromatids.

The former is related to chromosome identification, and the current method of determination is to separate white blood cells from a blood sample and incubate them for 3 days, at which time mitoses become accelerated. A hypotonic solution is used to swell the cells for better observation. By careful digital manipulation, they can be flattened out for easier identification.

The textbook pictures of chromosomes which resemble small lobster pincers represent paired chromosomes that have been arrested during mitosis with colchicine. The centromere is the central isthmus that separates the long ends from the short (Fig. 6-1), and when this splits, the pincers become new chromosomes in the daughter cells. Every ovum has a specific chromosome designated as an X chromosome, and every spermatozoon contains an X chromosome or a smaller Y chromosome. Zygotes with XX chromosomes develop into females, whereas XY zygotes become males. Chromosomes become arranged into groups that can be identified and numbered (Figs. 6-2 and 3); in other words, chromosomes have characteristics that fit them into definite patterns. Normally there are 46 chromosomes per cell [5], but there may be only 45 or there may be more, such as 47 chromosomes. If a chromosome is

lost or missing, the condition is known as a monosomy; if an extra chromosome is gained, the variety is a trisomy. An example of a monosomy (X or XO) is found in Turner's syndrome. Trisomy may be illustrated by trisomy-21 or mongolism. Among the interesting chromosomal anomalies known to exist are Klinefelter's syndrome (XXY), Down's syndrome (trisomy-21), and the superfemale XXX. When an individual exhibits valid genital ambiguity and the clinical determination of sex is not absolute, cytological determinations may yield valuable clinical data (see Table 5-1 in Chapter 5).

The second method of chromosomal sex identification is exemplified by inspecting individual cells for a chromatin mass. This test should be done on every patient, without exception, who presents the least suspicion of being other than normal, either mentally or physically. Barr and Bertram in 1949 [2] described a hemispherical satellite of thickened chromatin poised on the inner margin of the nuclear membrane, which was identified as the sex chromatin mass. When it is observed, the subject is designated as *sex chromatin positive;* when it is absent, the subject is *sex chromatin negative.* This so-called Barr body is present in about one-fourth of mucosal cells (Fig. 6-4A), and similar diagnostic

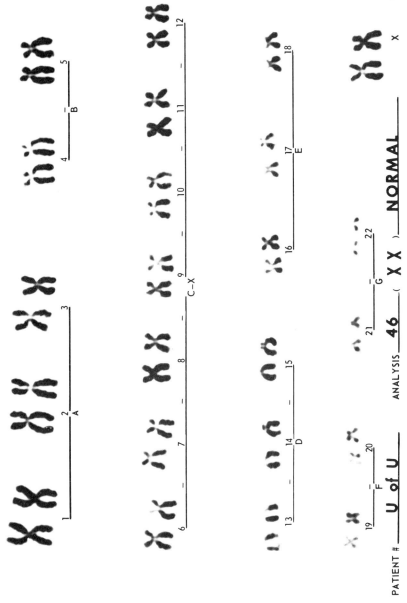

PATIENT # _____ <u>U of U</u> _____ ANALYSIS ___**46**___ (X X) ___**NORMAL**___

FIG. 6-2. Karyotyping consists of arranging chromosomes into pairs and then grouping them. Note that the grouping starts with the longest chromosomes and ends with the shortest.

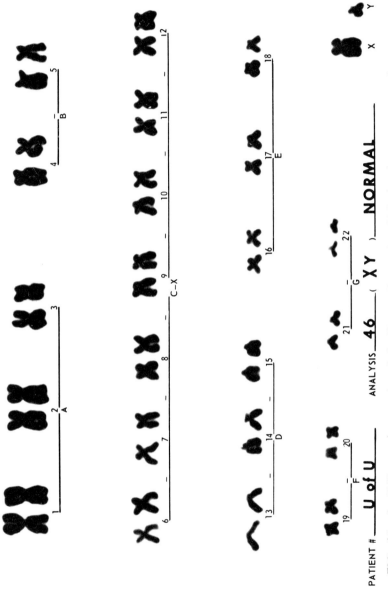

PATIENT # ___U of U___   ANALYSIS ___46___ (X Y) ___NORMAL___

FIG. 6-3. In 1960 a study team issued the Denver Report in which the chromosome complement was segregated into seven groups, designated group 1–3, group 4–5, group 6–12 and X, group 13–15, group 16–18, group 19–20, and group 21–23 and Y. In the same year, Patau proposed the seven groups be labeled by letters instead of numbers (A–G). Both plans are shown in this normal male karyotype.

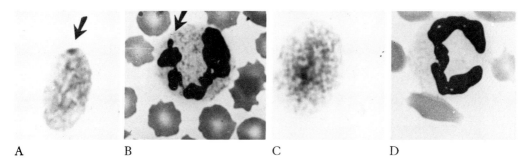

A   B   C   D

FIG. 6-4A–D. Moore and Barr in 1954 provided evidence for the chromatin mass in female cells, which is thought to be formed from one of the two X chromosomes that remain condensed longer than their fellow chromosomes. A. Nucleus from a buccal smear showing a sex chromatin body (chromatin-positive). B. Polymorphonuclear neutrophil leukocyte from a female (XX), showing a drumstick ($\times 2200$). C. Nucleus with no sex chromatin body (chromatin-negative) ($\times 2200$). D. Polymorphonuclear neutrophil leukocyted from a male (XY), ($\times 2200$).

bodies, called "drumsticks," are in one-tenth of the polymorphonuclear leukocytes (Fig. 6-4B) examined in the female.

At the time that Tjio et al. [22] and Ford [4] independently discovered that the normal human had 46 chromosomes, it was thought that anyone with more chromosomes than the normal 46 could not exist. However, three years later Jacobs, Strong, and Ford [10] proved that patients with Klinefelter's syndrome had an additional X chromosome, producing the genotype XXY with a total of 47 chromosomes. As a result of intensive investigations, a variety of chromosomal syndromes were then discovered [8], including gonadal dysgenesis. Gonadal dysgenesis, or Turner's syndrome, is characterized by cells that are mostly chromatin negative with an XO feature and only 45 chromosomes. True hermaphroditism, the sex mosaic with both ovarian and testicular tissue present, was found to exhibit a variety of chromosome patterns such as XX, XXY, XX/XXX, and XO/XY. The kaleidoscope of aberrant sex chromosomes that have been found includes XXX, XXXX, XY, XXXY/XXXY, and the triple genotype XO/XY/XXY. Many patients with these latter abnormalities suffer

from mental deficiency, and have somatic abnormalities as well.

Clinical determination of the genetic sex by chromosome determination provides a reference point from which sexual deviations can be traced. Other identifying factors to be considered are the external and internal gonadal patterns, hormonal patterns, and sex of rearing.

GONADAL PATTERNS

The 1-month-old embryo exhibits primordial germ cells which migrate to the urogenital ridge by the fifth week. The cortex of the genital ridge is the tissue from which the ovary is produced, and from the medulla rises the testis. In the presence of a functioning fetal testis, the müllerian (female) structures involute and the wolffian ducts complete their maturation. It is postulated that the testis secretes a substance that causes regression of the female structures, but this remains to be proved. The testicular inducer apparently is influential only locally, since a true hermaphrodite may have a testis on one side and an ovary on the other.

The external genitalia are undifferentiated

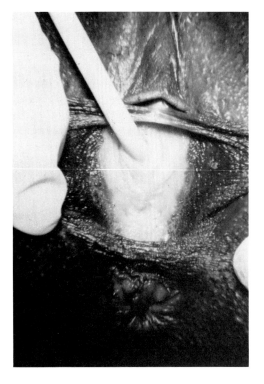

FIG. 6-5. The vesicovaginal septum was completely absent, and this 19-year-old patient with testicular feminization remained incontinent.

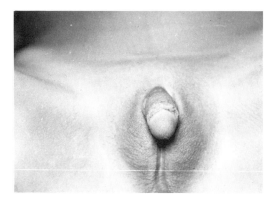

FIG. 6-6. Androgenic excess, endogenous or exogenous, in the female fetus promotes masculinity as manifested by megaloclitoris and labioscrotal fusion in the newborn.

The distinction between a clitoris and penis is based primarily on size and whether the labia minora have fused to form a corpus spongiosum. The morphological characteristics of the internal genitalia are variable, but dependable results can be achieved by roentgenography, cytogenetic investigation, and exploratory laparotomy.

HORMONAL PATTERNS

Hormones are responsible for the secondary sex characteristics that are represented by genital development, breast maturation, fat and hair distribution, voice deepening, bone growth, and body contour.

After the sixth week of embryonic life, the gonad develops either as a testis or ovary [24]. Interstitial cells of Leydig are abundant after the eighth week. Ovarian development begins 2 weeks later and oogonia, primary oocytes, and primordial follicles are identifiable [7]. The hormonal role is a critical factor in testicular and ovarian secretory function; estrogen produces vaginal cornification, nipple and mammary duct development, and uterine growth at puberty. The

at the second fetal month, but androgens are present and they stimulate the genital tubercle to grow, the urethral folds and labioscrotal eminences to become fused, and at the same time inhibit growth of the vesicovaginal septum, preventing a vaginal vault from forming (Fig. 6-5). In the female fetus, an excess of androgen will produce masculine characteristics, such as an enlarged clitoris and the labioscrotal fusion simulating a scrotum that is seen in female pseudohermaphrodites (Fig. 6-6).

The oldest and most common test for determining sex is to examine the external and internal genitalia, and unfortunately this is the least reliable test available to the clinician.

adrenal glands, as well as the gonads of both sexes, secrete androgens and estrogens or their precursors during fetal life. The reticular zone of the adrenal gland enlarges and produces an estrogen precursor for the placenta. At birth, the adrenal involutes and the estrogen and androgen levels decrease, but at puberty the adrenal reticularis thickens again and there is a hormone increase.

The female libido is partly dependent upon adrenal androgen. The female body, including the skeleton, matures faster, and true precocity in the female is more common than in the normally belated adolescent male. Both follicle-stimulating hormone and luteinizing hormone are requisites for normal sexual function in both sexes. The maturation of testicular or ovarian secretory function determines some of the gradients of intersex. If an androgenic hormone is not available before the twelfth fetal week, a vagina will develop. Excess androgen production after this time will afford clitoral hypertrophy but no midline scrotal fusion. Further maturation of testicular secretory function results in voice deepening, penile and prostatic growth, and the development of a male hair pattern.

There is a pseudohermaphroditic state, testicular feminization, in which the testes secrete estrogen, and if these gonads are extirpated, the patient has the symptoms of a surgical menopause. Another intersex condition, congenital adrenocortical hyperplasia, is a common form of hermaphroditism in which there is a virilizing hormone effect in a chromosomal female.

PSYCHOSEXUAL PATTERNS

Psychosexual patterns are inaugurated simultaneously with the sex of rearing [9]. Genitalia, hormones, and chromosomes are not as significant as psychosexual patterns, especially after infancy, in determining the gender role. The gender role is established between 1½ and 3 years of age. If there are medical reasons for the reassignment of gender, this should be achieved not later than the age of 3 years.

Once the gender role has been medically and legally assigned, sex orientation takes precedence over all other therapy. Social indentification and sex mannerisms become a necessary prelude for acceptance into the community. The psychosexual pattern must become consistent with regard to gender activities, sexual attraction, and sexual impulses.

Persons with social aberrations, such as homosexuality, are usually not amenable to sex reassignment. There is an increasing frequency of requests for sex reassignment in adult life by individuals who have been defined as transexuals. Transexualism, which has only recently been recognized, is defined as applying to those individuals who are biologically normal but who have an unalterable mental conviction that they are of the opposite sex and have always regarded themselves as such (see Part IV, Chapter 7). Surgical and endocrinological mutation may be considered favorable if the genitalia can be tailored to accommodate the patient both functionally and socially.

In cases of transexualism, we place male patients on a trial period that is extended or decreased according to patient progress. During this trial, which averages 4 to 6 months, feminization is practiced in reality as well as in pantomime. The individual dresses as a female, including underwear, brassiere, and overgarments; socializes as a female; works as a female; and is administered estrogenic hormones. A monthly physician-patient interview is necessary.

If the decision is made by all concerned that a sex change is indicated, surgical preparations are introduced. We advocate feminization over masculinization, and advise that the middle-age group achieves better results. All the male genital structures are removed

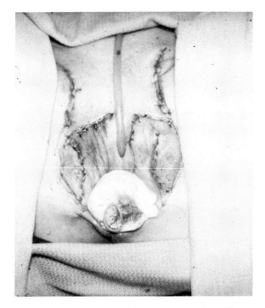

FIG. 6-7. Transexual mutation has been achieved by converting the penile shaft and hood into a clitoris, labia, and the upper one-half of the vaginal vault. The scrotal hamper was converted to the inferior one-half of the vaginal lining.

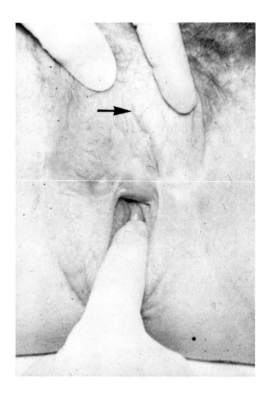

FIG. 6-8. Completion of the genital transformation shown in Figure 7. The arrow indicates the neoclitoris and the index digit is within the vaginal canal. The scrotal integument resembles vaginal rugae.

except the integumentary cloak, which is utilized as one-half of the vaginal vault. The other half is furnished by the scrotal integument (Figs. 6-7 and 8). Augmentation mammoplasty is also performed at the same time. Postoperative hormonal therapy is continued, and examinations are held periodically.

Sex Karyotypes of Surgical Interest

It is astonishing and at times confusing that there are nearly as many different classifications of intersex as there are varieties of intersex, with each geneticist, endocrinologist, obstetrician, urologist, psychiatrist, and surgeon advocating his favorite criteria. Following the classic article published by Tjio and

Levan [22] on discovering the normal human chromosome number of 46, autosomal and sex chromosome syndromes became an authoral sanctuary. Regardless, there are several excellent reviews of classifications [11, 12, 16, 19, 24]. Clinicians are becoming more interested and are intrigued with finding and diagnosing the various sex karyotypes. Among the newborn genital anomalies that have been discovered which are of surgical interest are Turner's syndrome, Klinefelter's syndrome, testicular feminization, male hermaphroditism, gonadal dyscrasias, congenital adrenocortical hyperplasia, and true hermaphroditism.

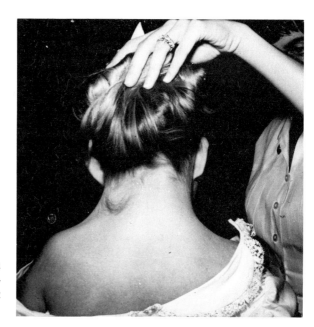

FIG. 6-9. A webbed neck (pterygium colli) is characteristic of Turner's syndrome. This youngster also had a cleft palate and a left ear-lobe deformity.

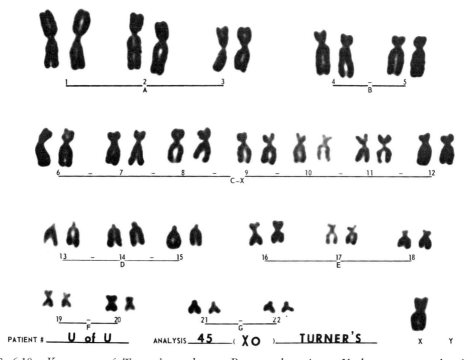

FIG. 6-10. Karyotype of Turner's syndrome. Because there is no Y chromosome and only 45 chromosomes are present, the condition is labeled as an XO chromosomal state.

TURNER'S SYNDROME

It has been estimated that one of 2,000 newborn female infants has Turner's syndrome. Most XO fetuses die during the first 3 months of pregnancy [1], making it a rather uncommon anomaly in newborns. In 1938 Turner [23] reported seven girls with a clinical syndrome of sexual infantilism, webbed neck (Fig. 6-9), short stature, and decubitus valgus. Hamblen [9] thought that the author reported these cases as a variant of hypopituitary dwarfism because Turner prescribed pituitary extract in their therapy. Regardless, Hamblen respected the report enough to name the condition "Turner's syndrome," which has survived the competition of various other terms. Ford and his co-workers [4, 5] found that patients with Turner's syndrome had no Y chromosome, thus having only 45 chromosomes, or one less than normal. Their chromosomal state is therefore designated as XO (Fig. 6-10).

Following the original description by Turner, other somatic anomalies have been

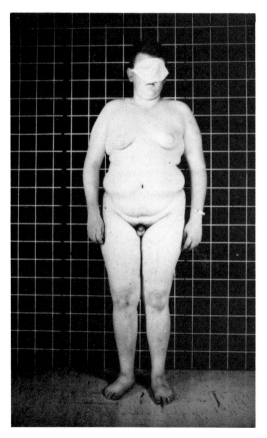

FIG. 6-11. The body adiposity of Turner's syndrome is excessive and is not proportionate as in naturally overweight persons.

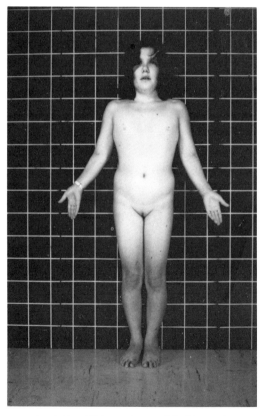

FIG. 6-12. This patient with Turner's syndrome has a shield-shaped chest and widespread nipples. She also has short stature and a lack of body hair for her age.

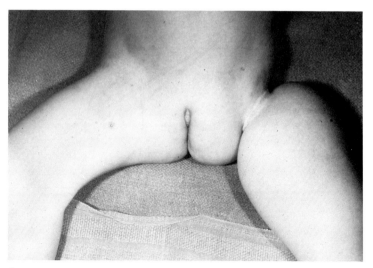

A

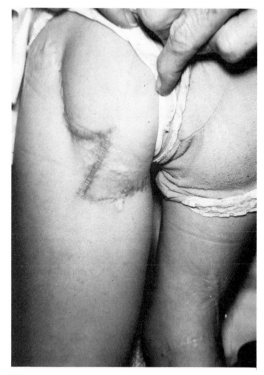

B

FIG. 6-13A and B. The congenital band contracture involving the left upper thigh is relieved by multiple Z-plasties circumferentially; the left popliteal contracture is similarly treated.

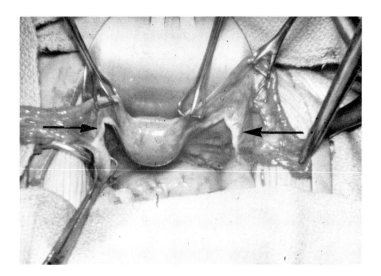

FIG. 6-14. A uterus and oviducts of normal size were found in this patient, but the gonads are atrophic and referred to as "streaks" because of the thin white structures. The gonads are removed after puberty because of possible gonadal neoplastic disease.

added to the syndrome, such as body adiposity (Fig. 6-11), high arched palate, micrognathia, epicanthal folds, misplaced ears, pigmented nevi, peripheral edema, a shield shaped chest and widespread nipples (Fig. 6-12), keloidal tendencies, osteoporosis, and amenorrhea.

The therapeutic approach to this syndrome is to initiate endocrine substitution. Hormone replacement may be instituted at any age, but it seems that a suitable time is during the age of normal puberty so the secondary sex characteristics may develop similarly to those of normal individuals. Estrogen administration stimulates development of the breasts as well as the external and internal genitalia. A suitable drug is Premarin (oral conjugated equine estrogen), which can be given in daily doses of 1.25 to 3.75 mg for 6 months or until the desired breast size is achieved. If breast development has not been satisfactory, Premarin therapy should be substituted on the third week of each month with progesterone (Provera) in 5 to 10 mg daily doses. Usually the girl becomes aware of gradual feminine ascension, thus achieving adolescent body contour and relieving her anxiety.

Many of the symptoms of this syndrome are not corrected by hormonal therapy, and some of these are relieved by plastic surgery. Pterygium colli, pterygium oculi, and edema due to incidental congenital bands are greatly benefitted by Z-plasties (Fig. 6-13). Misplaced ears can be repositioned, micrognathia is corrected by prosthetics, keloids are revised, and pigmented nevi are excised. Because convincing evidence [21] prevails that gonadal neoplasms are to be found in association with Turner's syndrome, it has been suggested that prophylactic gonadal removal be considered after puberty (Fig. 6-14).

KLINEFELTER'S SYNDROME

Klinefelter and his colleagues [13] first reported this anomaly 31 years ago, describing nine males with gynecomastia, small hard testes, azoospermia, and elevated urinary gonadotropins (Fig. 6-15). This XXY chromosomal error is seen once in 500 male births and is therefore recognized as the most common of the sex chromosome errors (Fig. 6-16). There is reasonable indication that the external genitalia may be "decoys" in that

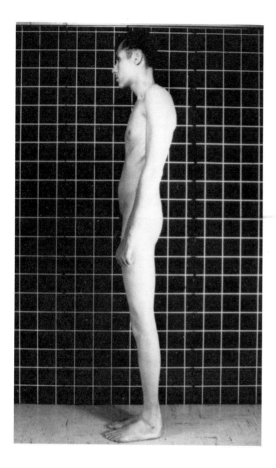

FIG. 6-15. A tall body with a short trunk is characteristic of Klinefelter's syndrome.

they give a boy the appearance of normality who as an adult will be infertile. Those afflicted with this syndrome often shy away from swimming, playing basketball, or taking showers in the presence of other athletes because of the mammary enlargement that occurs in 40 percent of these XXY males. The testicular atrophy is associated with some firmness and tenderness and a decrease in the number of Leydig cells. Regardless, these males may enjoy erections and satisfactory intercourse if treated.

Most patients with Klinefelter's syndrome

search for medical attention either because of their large male breasts (gynecomastia) or because of infertility. Although there is no pharmacological preparation that is specifically effective for infertility, hyalinized testes, or gynecomastia, testosterone substitutional therapy has an important psychological effect. Medicinal and physiotherapy may be harmful when used for breast hypertrophy, whereas plastic surgical reduction is the safest, easiest, and most successful measure. Cryptorchidism has been managed in early stages with chorionic gonadotropins and successfully treated later by surgical advancement. Silicone prostheses are helpful in severe testicular hypoplasia since they tend to relieve psychological problems and improve physical appearance.

TESTICULAR FEMINIZATION

The first known report of this intersexual entity was made by Steglehner in 1817, and very little has been added to the symptomatology since. The term *testicular feminization* was coined by Morris [17] in 1953 when reporting his cases and discussing 82 similar ones in the literature. Clinical features of classic testicular feminization include normal female contours with well-developed feminine breasts but sometimes with juvenile nipples. Body hair is scanty, particularly in the pubic and axillary areas. The patient usually seeks medical advice because of amenorrhea and infantile external female genitalia associated with a shallow vaginal vault (Fig. 6-17). Examinations reveal an absent uterus and no ovaries or oviducts. Further examination reveals intraabdominal, inguinal, or labial testes that produce estrogen. There is a high incidence of inguinal hernia. The family history includes sisters or aunts with identical clinical features. The sex chromatin is negative and there is an XY chromosome constitution (Fig. 6-18). Most

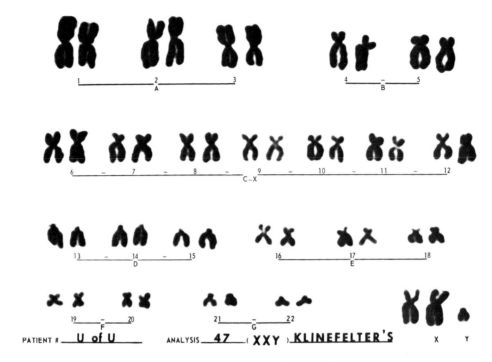

FIG. 6-16. The karyotype of Klinefelter's syndrome exhibits 47 chromosomes.

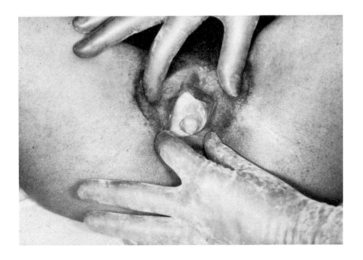

FIG. 6-17. One of the pathognomonic findings in cases of testicular feminization is a shallow vaginal introitus although there is normal hair distribution.

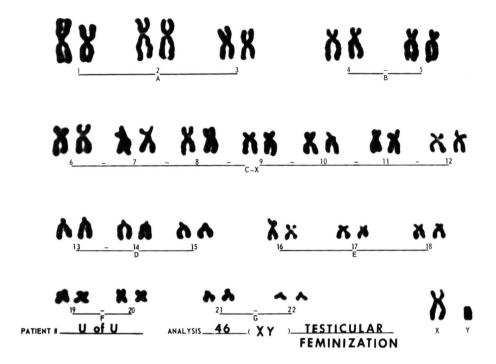

FIG. 6-18. Testicular feminization is associated with a karyotype of 46 chromosomes with an XY constitution.

cases of testicular feminization will demonstrate nearly all of these mentioned features, thus providing a significantly distinct syndrome that can be firmly diagnosed on clinical grounds.

A high familial incidence is typical of this syndrome. Although the exact mechanism for the transmission of testicular feminization is not understood, most of the available data seem to indicate that this syndrome is transmitted as a sex-linked recessive characteristic or a male-limited autosomal dominant characteristic [17].

The first major therapeutic measure to be instituted by the physician is counseling. Although these patients are genetically considered males, they are phenotypically and psychologically females. It is advisable to avoid referring to the masculine aspects of the patient by using the word "testes," for example. This is an instance when "sex glands" is a better reference. The doctor should offer an explanation of the paradoxical function of these sex glands and elicit special concern about the lack of germ cells and sterility. Given supportive psychological help and the needed surgery, these pseudohermaphrodites can lead productive, happy lives.

The next therapeutic measure is directed toward surgical correction of the infantile vaginal vault. Vaginal construction can be done using numerous techniques, but the most popular one is to incise transversely the introital mucosa between the urethral and anal orifices (Fig. 6-19). Digital dissection is carried to the parietal peritoneum or the uterine cervix, if present, in a tissue plane;

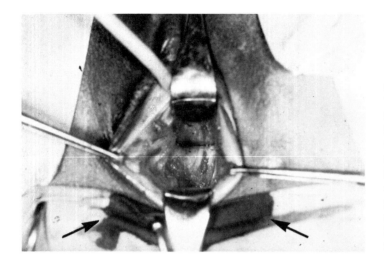

FIG. 6-19. Vaginal construction for patients with testicular feminization is executed by initiating an incision transversely in the introitus and, without further sharp dissection, partitional depth is afforded easily by digital cleavage. When the parietal peritoneum is sounded, vault depth is completed. The total loss of blood is surprisingly small (*arrows*).

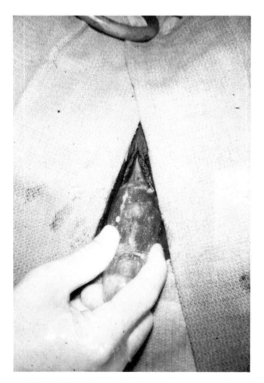

FIG. 6-20. This light-weight, pear-shaped plastic conformer is worn by the patient for 6 months after the operation for vaginal construction.

surprisingly minimal blood loss occurs. A split-thickness skin graft is taken from the buttock and sutured over a conformer like a pillow-case over a pillow. The epidermal side is secured by sutures adjacent to the conformer, which is then inserted into the digitally prepared cavity, and this integumental lining will function as the vaginal wall. The conformer remains in position untampered for 2 weeks. During convalescence, it is removed only for cleansing purposes and is immediately repositioned (Fig. 6-20). The patients wear the conformer for 6 months to prevent vault shrinkage (Fig. 6-21).

The final therapeutic consideration is devoted to the ectopic testes. Opinions differ about the removal of these gonads. Morris [17] reported 15 malignant tumors involving intraabdominal testes and advises removal after adolescence. Hauser et al. oppose prophylactic surgical castration for the presumptive prevention of possible malignant degeneration. Because the existing testes produce estrogen, their excision leads to surgical menopause and therefore substitutional endocrine therapy is indicated. We remove these

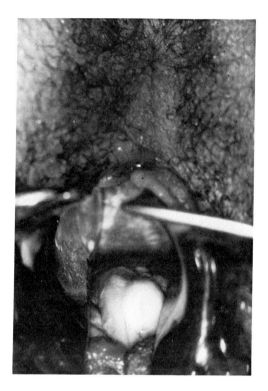

FIG. 6-21. This uncrowded, fabricated vaginal investment is a typical representative of 23 such vaults that were enveloped with split-thickness skin grafts. The urethral meatus is indicated by a metal sound.

gonads during adolescence and use supplemental therapy as necessary.

MALE HERMAPHRODITISM

There are various types of this sex syndrome. Some of the types have been classified as those of gonadal dysgenesis. The patients are chromatin negative with an XY chromosome complement. The hormonal sex pattern exhibits a normal output of 17-ketosteroids. The gonadal sex pattern usually reveals rudimentary müllerian ducts, and the child is thought to be female by the appearance of the external gonads. The phallus is under-

sized, usually hypospadial and with an amazingly small glans, and there is a small vagina, within which lies the urethral orifice (Fig. 6-22). The scrotum is not pendulous, because it is empty of contents. The ectopic testes are found in the inguinal canal or abdomen. Many of the patients develop gynecomastia later in life. This type of sex syndrome is usually referred to the surgeon, tagged with the diagnosis of hypospadias. Many of these hermaphrodites receive excellent treatment for the hypospadias and gynecomastia, but further therapy is rarely instituted.

The three-team therapeutic approach is unequivocally successful. The endocrinologist treats the aspermatogenesis and immature genitalia with testosterone, and may assist the descension of the pelvic gonads with other hormonal treatment. The psychiatrist lends support by adjusting the patient's emotional

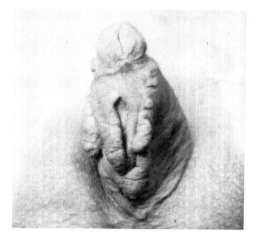

FIG. 6-22. This confusing external gonad of a male hermaphrodite is endowed with a normal-sized vagina, labia majora and minora, and an urethral meatus within the urogenital sinus. However, this feminine architecture developed on a masculine penile shaft consisting of a glans, corona, and prepuce. The labioscrotal fusion resembles an empty miniature cradle; the ectopic testes are in the pelvis.

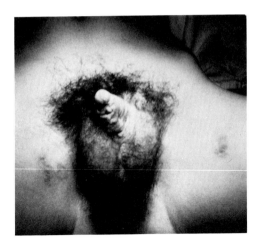

FIG. 6-23. Completed masculinization of a male hermaphrodite. The penile shaft of this 18-year-old patient possesses erectile properties and is a useful urinary organ. The thigh scars are residual from the testicular repositioning procedure.

status. The surgeon reduces the gynecomastia and descends the ectopic testes if they did not respond to hormones. When the first surgical procedure is performed, the pseudovaginal canal is obliterated. The chordee and hypospadias are corrected by a second operation. Because the glans is usually very small, the urethral meatus is constructed proximally at the corona (Fig. 6-23).

FEMALE HERMAPHRODITISM

Female hermaphroditism is an ambisexual development that comprises congenital adrenal hyperplasia as well as other types unrelated to adrenal factors [6, 21]. The former is the most common of all the hermaphroditic conditions, whereas the latter is the rarest form. Female hermaphrodites without adrenal hyperplasia do not secrete androgen and usually do not develop secondary sex characteristics until the age of puberty. They have an enlarged phallus resembling a penis that

may be hypospadial, or they may have have a penile urethra. The remaining anatomy of the genital tract is the same as that found in the adrenal hyperplasia phenotype. Their history usually reveals maternal masculinization during pregnancy or maternal inhibition of androgens.

Females with virilizing adrenal hyperplasia differ from all other hermaphroditic variations because the excessive adrenal androgen produces accelerated and continuous masculinity. The adrenal cortex and the gonads synthesize hydrocortisone, 17-ketosteroids, and other steroids. Adrenocorticotropic hormone (ACTH) accelerates this synthesis. If the adrenal cortex does not produce the needed hormones, then ACTH is hypersecreted, the adrenal cortex becomes hyperplastic, and increased adrenal androgens are secreted. Such a cycle in utero produces female hermaphroditism of the adrenocortical hyperplasia type.

If cortisone is given to the patient with congenital adrenocortical hyperplasia, the pregnanediol values will decrease toward normal (0.8 μg or less). This is a most important diagnostic criterion. Cortisone suppresses the ACTH stimulus of the adrenal reticularis and stops the virilizing hormone secretion.

Congenital adrenocortical hyperplasia is inheritable and familial. It must be suspected in any newborn with abnormal external genitals who is brought to the physician because of persistent vomiting, dehydration, and malnutrition. Early diagnosis and treatment is life-saving, and the moribund infant will recuperate if given sodium and cortisone. Once the child is out of danger, a thorough examination is necessary to confirm the diagnosis. The megaloclitoris has corpora cavernosa but usually no urethra; the urethra is often found at the clitoral base or in the urogenital sinus. The labia are usually partially fused; however, complete fusion may be present, with the labia resembling a male scrotum with a median raphe (Fig. 6-24). There are no scrotal contents. By lateral separation of the labia, a vaginal meatus may be located into which an opaque material is instilled; a vagina is demonstrable by roentgenography (Fig. 6-25).

Children with congenital hyperadrenocorticogenitalism grow rapidly, but bone epiphyses close early and this is responsible for the short, heavy body. Complete growth may be attained before 12 years of age. Mature growth of pubic, axillary, and beard hair appears early. Comedones, acne, and sebaceous cysts are common. Amenorrhea, lack of mammary growth, and wide shoulders are further masculinizing traits.

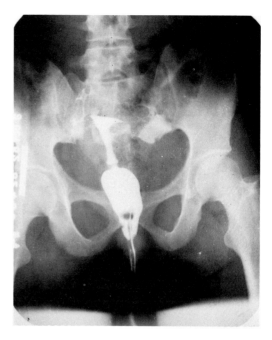

FIG. 6-25. Roentgenographic studies of the vagina reveal the size and shape of the uterine canal and oviducts. Such findings could eliminate the need for a surgical pelvic exploration.

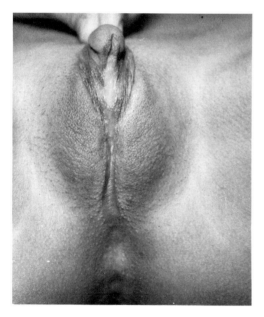

FIG. 6-24. This configuration is found in female hermaphrodites with adrenocortical hyperplasia. The megaloclitoris has corpora but no urethra. The urogenital sinus lodges an urethral orifice and is roofed by a median raphe. There is an abundance of hair, which in the case shown has been shaved preparatory to surgery.

The sex assignment of patients with congenital adrenal hyperplasia is female. The initial and continued treatment should be delegated to a pediatric endocrinologist who is knowledgeable regarding electrolyte balance, bone growth, and maintenance dosages of hormones for lengthy periods. After the 17-ketosteroids have reached the desired level, a maintenance suppressive drug dose schedule is formulated, using repeated urinary determinations as an index. If treatment is started before 2 years of age, precocious virilization is remedied, normal development occurs, and a normal life is enjoyed. If the patient is under 7 years of age and epiphyseal fusion has not occurred, cortisone therapy will prolong bone growth. Cortisone is of no benefit to body growth if the epiphyses are closed. Treatment, however, will inhibit hirsutism and skin blemishes, and it will be beneficial to mammary growth and menstruation.

If surgical treatment is anticipated, hormonal therapy is regulated accordingly. The type of surgical procedure depends upon the existing anomaly, but surgical feminization is definitely required. After positioning a suture through the glans for retraction, a bladder catheter is introduced. If the urethral orifice is concealed by the urogenital sinus, the sinus is incised to the base of the phallus for exposure of the meatus. The megaloclitoris is removed, leaving the prepuce as a skin flap. The corpora cavernosa stump is sutured for hemostasis. Nerve ends are sutured away from the incision to prevent painful neuromas. The remaining clitoral cloak is then divided into equal halves and tailored as labia majora and minora. The inferior portion of the vaginal mucosa is sutured to the integument to form the fourchette. Only absorbable sutures are used. A lubricated tampon is inserted into the vault as a conformer, and the bladder catheter is left in situ for urinary diversion until the wounds are healed. This type of surgical procedure may be modified to accommodate different existing problems.

TRUE HERMAPHRODITISM

The true hermaphrodite, if there were such, would possess the unique distinction of functioning as both sexes. Because this sex syndrome has not yet been accurately defined, it is accepted as a relative concept. Chromosomal and hormonal sex patterns are of little benefit since the diagnosis depends upon the gonadal sex pattern. Ovarian and testicular tissue are found in one or both gonads, which may be labioscrotal, inguinal, or abdominal. One-half of our true hermaphrodites were endowed with a testis in one pelvic floor and an ovary in the contralateral pelvis, one-fourth had ovotestes in both pelves, and about one-fourth had an ovotestis in one

pelvis and either a testis or an ovary in the other pelvis. There may or may not be a uterus. The phallus may be clitoral or penile in form, and the labia may be bifid, as in the female, or fused, forming a scrotum. Some patients with this syndrome develop female breasts and some menstruate.

Successful treatment of this sex syndrome depends on careful interviews with the patient and parents, as well as surgical dexterity and efficient endocrine therapy. The female gender role should be assigned to all such patients whenever possible, especially those under 5 years of age, since a serviceable vagina can be constructed without difficulty. Adolescents who have been reared as males though they are genetically females should be given the option to elect their sex preference. If they choose to be further augmented toward masculinity, then they should be made aware of the time-consuming staged constructive procedures as well as the future consequences to be encountered physiologically with inadequate phallic tissue. Legal problems, such as birth certificate change, name substitution, and parent-doctor concurrence, must be taken care of prior to surgery.

Early surgical feminization is ideal, and if possible it should be performed before the patient is 2 years of age. If clitoral or penile enlargement is of concern, the structure may be partially amputated, or it may be enshrined in a shallow subcutaneous lair to camouflage its size yet permit the exposed glans to serve its purpose as a sensitive erotic organ. Labioscrotal folds that are fused may be surgically separated and repositioned as labia majora. Internal pelvic exploration is necessary for the correct identification of tissues by microscopic survey; all defined, circumscribed testicular tissues in the abdomen are removed with the exception of ovotestes. In the pelvic environment, testicular parenchyma usually becomes atrophic and nonfunctioning. If masculinizing signs, such as

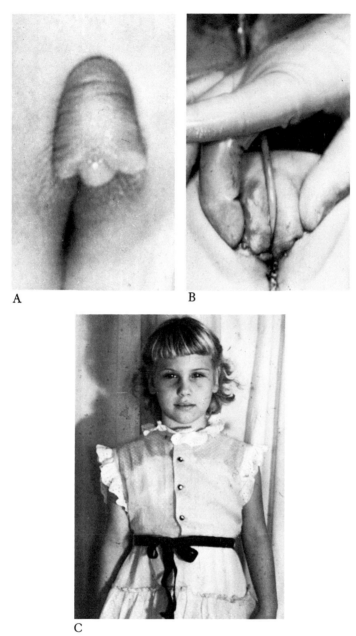

A   B

C

FIG. 6-26. The patient with this external genitalia, despite the masculine appearance, is a hermaphrodite, and the elective surgery was to feminize the subject. B. The integumental cloak has been cleaved from the corpora and utilized for the lining of the vaginal vault. C. The youngster had a definitely feminine appearance when examined 1 year after the operation. Her family environment was of inestimable assistance and was mostly responsible for her successful attainment of her present feminine characteristics.

beard growth, male redistribution of hair, and changes in body proportion, become evident during adolescence, these may be resolved by extirpation of the ovotestes and administration of estrogen therapy. Whether the megaloclitoris is amputated or buried, the integumental hood is dissected free and used as a skin flap to construct the vaginal labia and introitus (Fig. 6-26). Because the flap's innervation is left in continuity, erotic sensation is preserved.

Hormonal substitution is an integral part of continued feminization. Estrogens that are administered too early may stunt growth by causing epiphyseal closure, yet if they are given late, their administration may produce long-legged eunuchoid types. Ideally, the age of puberty (12 to 13 years) is the opportune time. Our drugs of choice are Premarin, 1.25 to 3.75 mg daily for 3 weeks, and Provera, 5 to 10 mg daily for 1 week. This therapy is continued until desired breast proportions are reached, and is utilized at later times whenever necessary.

Surgical masculinization is best adapted to the patient who is fortunately enriched with ample penile and testicular tissue and is personally convinced of his choice of sex assignment. Unfortunately, those desiring virilization are usually deficient in the necessary physical assets. There is the occasional patient for whom there is no other alternative but masculinization (Fig. 6-27A–B). The surgical procedures begin with creating a penile shaft by scalpel that lodges an integumental-lined urethra. The abdominal wall furnishes a de-

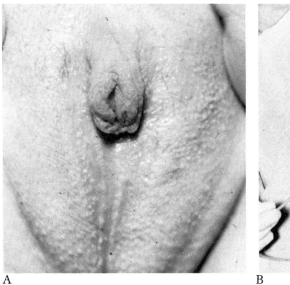 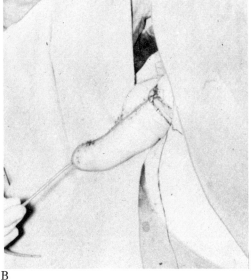

A   B

FIG. 6-27A. Hermaphroditism may be difficult to identify at birth, which may lead to the wrong sex assignment. These external genitalia are those of a 19-year-old who has been reared as a male. Surgical feminization would lead to severe social and psychiatric havoc, and the choice of the patient and parents was to enhance masculinity. B. The phallic shaft is completed; it is an abdominal skin flap with partial rigidity but no erectile properties. The urethral canal provides an excellent guide for the urinary stream. The patient experiences erotic sensation by digital pressure at the penile base. His sexual preference has always been for females.

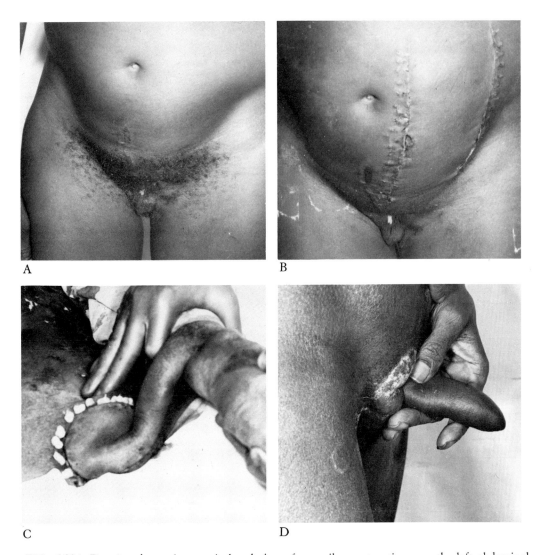

FIG. 6-28A–D. An alternative surgical technique for penile construction uses the left abdominal wall as the donor site for the skin flap, and it is transferred by using the left wrist as a vehicle.

sirable donor site. After "walking" the penile flap into pubic position, the constructed urethra is anastomosed to the bladder urethra (Fig. 6-27B). There are no erectile properties nor innervation present in the shaft; therefore, erotic sensations are usually lacking. The new penis is an excellent guide for micturition. A semblance of the scrotum with contents can be fashioned from thigh tissues. Androgens are administered to the patient seeking masculinization; testosterone in a dosage of 200 mg intramuscularly monthly is given until a semblance of secondary sex characteristics develops. There are alternative surgical means of total phallic construction, one of which is shown in Figure 6-28.

References

1. Barr, M. L. Sex chromosomes of man. *Am. J. Obstet. Gynecol.* 93:608, 1965.
2. Barr, M. L., and Bertram, E. G. A morphological distinction between neurones of the male and female, and the behavior of the nucleolar satellite during accelerated nucleoprotein synthesis. *Nature (London)* 163:676, 1949.
3. Blattner, R. J. Testicular feminization and color blindness. *J. Pediatr.* 56:425, 1960.
4. Ford, C. E. The cytogenetic analysis of some disorders of sex development. *Am. J. Obstet. Gynecol.* 82:1154, 1961.
5. Ford, C. E., and Hamerton, J. L. The chromosomes of man. *Nature (London)* 178:-1020, 1956.
6. Gillenwater, J. T., Wykes, A. W., Birdsong, M., and Thornton, W. N. Adrenogenital syndrome producing female pseudohermaphroditism with phallus urethra. *J. Urol.* 103:500, 1970.
7. Greene, R. R. Embryology of sexual structure and hermaphroditism. *J. Clin. Endocrinol.* 4:355, 1944.
8. Grumbach, M. M., and Barr, M. L. Cytologic tests of chromosomal sex in relation of sexual anomalies in man. *Recent Progr. Horm. Res.* 14:255, 1958.
9. Hamblen, E. C. The assignment of sex to an individual: Some enigmas and some practical clinical criteria. *Am. J. Obstet. Gynecol.* 74:1228, 1957.
10. Jacobs, P. S., Strong, J. A., and Ford, C. E. A case of human intersexuality having a possible XXY sex determining mechanism. *Nature (London)* 183:302, 1959.
11. Jones, H. A., Jr., and Scott, W. W. *Hermaphroditism, Genital Anomalies and Related Endocrine Disorders.* Baltimore: Williams & Wilkins, 1958.
12. Klebs, E. *Hanbuch de pathologischen Anatomie.* Berlin: Hirschwald, 1876.
13. Klinefelter, J. J., Jr., Reifenstein, E. D., Jr., and Albright, F. Syndrome characterized by gynecomastia, aspermatogenesis without aleydigism and increased excretion of follicle-stimulating hormone. *J. Clin. Endocrinol.* 2:615, 1942.
14. Lattimer, J. L. Relocation and recession of enlarged clitoris with preservation of glans: Alternative to amputation. *J. Urol.* 86:113, 1961.
15. Minervini, F., Schwarzenzerg, T. L., Canibus, R., and Natoli, G. The surgical therapy of intersexuality. *Arch. Ital. Pediatr.* 26:275, 1969.
16. Money, J., Hampson, J. G., and Hampson, J. L. Hermaphroditism: Recommendations concerning assignment of sex, change of sex and psychologic management. *Bull. Johns Hopkins Hosp.* 97:284, 1955.
17. Morris, J. M. The syndrome of testicular feminization in male pseudohermaphrodites. *Am. J. Obstet. Gynecol.* 65:1192, 1953.
18. Sandberg, A. A., Koepf, G. F., Crosswhite, L. H., and Hauschke, T. The chromosome constitution of human marrow in various

development and blood disorders. *Am. J. Hum. Genet.* 12:231, 1960.

19. Snyder, C. C. Intersex Problems and Hermaphroditism. In Converse, J. M. (Ed.), *Reconstructive Plastic Surgery*. Philadelphia: Saunders, 1964.
20. Snyder, C. C. Female hermaphroditism. *J. Am. Med. Wom. Assoc.* 22:835, 1967.
21. Taylor, H., Barter, R. H., and Jacobson, C. B. Neoplasms of dysgenetic gonads. *Am. J. Obstet. Gynecol.* 96:816, 1966.
22. Tjio, J. H., and Levan, A. The chromosome number of man. *Hereditas* 42:1, 1956.
23. Turner, H. H. A syndrome of infantilism, congenital webbed neck and cubitus valgus. *Endocrinology* 23:566, 1938.
24. Wilkins, L. *The Diagnosis and Treatment of Endocrine Disorders in Childhood and Adolescence* (3rd ed.). Springfield, Ill.: Thomas, 1966.

Surgical and Psychiatric Aspects of Transexualism

MILTON T. EDGERTON, JR.
JON K. MEYER

7

Attitudes

THE VERY WORD *transexualism* evokes a host of emotional reactions largely because of poorly understood facts about this disorder in the minds of most laymen. The use of surgery to treat transexual patients arouses issues of "morality, medical ethics, the law, psychiatric theory, and the individual patients' right to self-determination" [13]. As a result, patients having this disorder are viewed with aversion by many, and great pressure is placed on surgeons to avoid engaging in sex-conversion operations on such people.

Part of the reason for great caution lies in the fact that transexualism is a dramatic psychiatric syndrome that has only recently been widely recognized. It is characterized by the individual's intense desire for sexual transformation by surgical, hormonal, or other means, based upon his (or her) complete identification with the gender role opposite his (or her) anatomical gender and genital morphology.

It is understandable that doctors and laymen alike would hesitate to undertake or approve surgical treatment of such patients. The majority of these individuals show no evidence of hormonal or chromosomal abnormality. They are not to be confused with pseudohermaphrodites or with other problems of intersex that are associated with incomplete or ambivalent sexual development. The diagnosis must be made entirely on psychiatric criteria, and many of our religious and historical instincts are troubled by the patients' requests. Few long-term studies of such patients are available to give us confidence in the degree of social rehabilitation provided by surgical conversion. The patients are often unreliable historians, and their statements of successful social adjustments must be verified from more objective evidence.

Nevertheless, the existence of thousands of desperate transexuals throughout the world has led to recognition that this extreme form

Dr. Meyer's work was supported in part by Grant No. G68-432 from the Foundation's Fund for Research in Psychiatry.

of psychosexual inversion is not peculiar to any one race, religion, or culture. Each patient gives consistent and eloquent testimony to the loneliness, suffering, and tragedy of the condition, and many turn to self-mutilation, suicide, or crime since they feel both rejected by society and ignored by the medical profession.

Psychiatrists generally agree as to the futility of treatment by psychotherapy, drugs, shock, or hypnosis. It is noteworthy that most transexuals are not psychotic, and the gender identity problem is more appropriately described as an *idée fixe* than a psychosis.

The thousands of individual pleas for help, the needs of society to find ways to make these people productive and law-abiding, the growing community and religious tolerance of sexual attitudes, and the increasing sophistication of plastic surgery have finally combined to produce a medical setting in which scientific and humanitarian studies may be undertaken to clarify the diagnosis, etiology, prognosis, treatment, and (hopefully) prevention of transexualism.

Approximately eight medical centers in the United States have now undertaken careful interdisciplinary medical-team studies directed toward the treatment of transexual patients. There is very limited financial support for such programs, and federal financing of these medical investigations will probably await some measure of public and professional endorsement.

The surgeon who is considering offering his services as a member of a gender identity team must be prepared for criticism from some of his colleagues, for apologies for his activity by his friends, and for numerous disturbing telephone calls from patients concerning their complex social problems. If he can tolerate these pressures, he will be rewarded with the opportunity to learn a great deal about the basic impact of physical deformity (or sexual dissonance) on the human

personality, and he will experience the satisfaction of following the lives of many ever-grateful patients.

Organization of the Medical Team

Many pioneer physicians have made individual contributions to the possible role of surgery in the treatment of transexualism. Outstanding among these were Hamburger [14], Abraham [1], Heppner (1872), Abbe (1898), Gillies [11], Pauly [17], and Benjamin [3].

It is now clear that any in-depth study of gender identity problems requires a multidisciplinary medical team. The programs demand careful selection of patients and detailed postoperative evaluations if meaningful data are to be obtained. In 1964 at The Johns Hopkins Hospital, the senior author, Dr. Edgerton, along with Dr. Howard Jones of the Department of Gynecology, Dr. Eugene Meyer of the Department of Psychiatry, and Dr. John Money, a medical psychologist, organized the first known gender identity medical team dedicated to evaluating the role of surgery in treating the transexual patient. Over the succeeding two years, this team was formalized, and was joined by additional members from the departments of Urology, Endocrinology, Genetics, and Neuro-Psychiatry. The lessons we have learned subsequently from that program and others at several medical centers may be used to arrive at sound principles for the organization of any gender identity clinic.

GUIDELINES FOR A GENDER IDENTITY CLINIC

1. The transexual patient must be thought of as *primarily* a psychiatric patient. Surgery should be viewed as *adjunctive* therapy—if needed. It is desirable to have an informed

and interested psychiatrist acting as "clinic director" whenever one is available. The psychiatric team should be given the right to veto or postpone surgery if they deem it unwise or untimely.

2. The professional team should include psychiatrists, surgeons, clinical psychologists, endocrinologists, a geneticist, a neurophysiologist, a social worker, and a legal consultant. A clinical coordinator and a full-time secretary will usually be needed.

3. The surgical team should include representatives from plastic surgery, gynecology, and urology. The reconstructive procedures are complex and require many skills. Each of these disciplines has proved that it may make special contributions to the surgery of both male and female transexual patients. Usually, at least two of these surgical specialists should be represented at any operation.

4. The team should meet at least monthly and should limit the number of patients accepted to the number they can process and follow with great care. One or two new patients per month may demand much more time than anticipated.

5. Initial evaluation should be undertaken only if the patient understands that such a work-up carries no commitment to offer surgery.

6. Work-up includes many studies (see pp. 125–126 on "Acceptance Criteria for Surgery"), and a careful system of establishing clinical nonoperative controls should be developed. Patients should be matched as to age, economic background, and psychological test results as carefully as possible.

7. Interviews with the spouse or nearest relative are essential in order to assure both accuracy of history and postoperative psychological support.

8. Cost of surgery and aftercare must be carefully outlined since many medical insurance policies have no provision to cover this type of surgery.

9. Police records must be checked to be sure the patient is in no difficulty with the law. Arrangements must be made to assure the reasonable likelihood of long-term follow-up after surgery.

10. Consultations and examinations are best done individually by members of the team, but provision for circulation and review of the resulting recommendations is critical to effective work. When one member of the team arranges a date for later contact with a patient, other members of the team should be notified of this date by the coordinator.

11. When a patient is accepted for surgery, *one member* of the team should be designated as that patient's "responsible physician." From that time onward, he will be responsible for coordinating care, explaining therapy to the patient, contacting relatives, and arranging follow-up. This type of relationship must *not* be left to a group; a one-to-one doctor-patient relationship is imperative to good treatment.

12. If possible, pediatric studies on feminine boys and tomboy girls should be made a part of each gender identity program. The identification, study, and treatment of the transexual patient during the years of early childhood may turn out to be one of the most exciting dividends of these interdisciplinary clinics.

Preliminary Diagnosis of Transexualism

Money and Gaskin [16] have defined transexualism as "a disturbance of gender identity in which the person manifests, with constant and persistent conviction, the desire to live as a member of the opposite sex, and progressively takes steps to live in the opposite sex role, full time." The diagnosis of the condition in some cases may be straightforward, and in others an uncommonly difficult task. The diagnostic criterion most commonly mentioned as a guide to this task is a verbally stated conviction on the part of the patient that the psyche is at odds with soma in such a manner that sexual, personal, and social orientations are fixed at cross purposes to the observable facts of anatomy. Although such a statement of conviction is a necessary component of the transexual picture, in practice its presence alone is not sufficient to establish a diagnosis.

Other disorders, manifested in part through gender identity problems, may lead a patient to seek sex conversion surgery, and to present his belief persuasively that he is at odds with himself as regards psychology and anatomy. Homosexuals, transvestites, adolescents with homosexual impulses or identity problems, schizoid individuals with gender confusion, and psychotics and borderline psychotics among others, as well as transexuals, at one time or another have all applied for sex conversion surgery—almost all of them having an initially stated and often firmly held conviction of a mind-body conflict.

Although in typical cases distinctions may be relatively easy, there is a continuum, rather than discrete states, throughout the gender identity and sexual disorders, so categories often become blurred. For this reason, the work-up of the applicant for sex conversion surgery involves obtaining a detailed history with emphasis on the following areas: family stability and parental orientation toward the child; childhood, adolescent, and adult social adjustment; work and education experience; role assumption at various life stages; physical development and reactions thereto; and sexual practices. The family history may bring to light parental hopes regarding the sex of the unborn child, sexual aberrations in the family, withdrawing from

or particular ties to one parent or the other, or overt encouragement of cross-gender behavior. Features of childhood history, such as the patient's preference for boys' or girls' games, for dolls versus guns and trucks, or for little girls versus boys as playmates, may all help indicate the duration and strength of cross-gender orientation. A normal onset of puberty and associated physiological changes, with the development and the maintenance of secondary sexual characteristics, indicates a normal endocrine status. Inquiry regarding signs or symptoms of seizure disorders (particularly temporal lobe epilepsy), and a readiness to request an EEG will detect those instances of sexual deviancy associated with an epileptic focus [4]. The patient's reaction to pubertal changes, early experience with masturbation and sexual fantasies, and sexual activity and orientation in adolescence are important points of the history. Adult choice of friends, work experience and stability, and the patient's capacity to deal with cross-gender impulses, either constructively or destructively, are important. The sexual history should include the favorite method of sexual encounter, partner choice, arousal and intercourse techniques favored or interdicted by the patient, the subjective experience of, and value placed on, orgasm, and any history of experimentation with cross-gender hormones.

Table 7-1 illustrates the preliminary diagnoses in a series of 31 recent male and female applicants for sex conversion surgery that were seen by the senior author. Out of 31 evaluees, only slightly more than 45 percent were tentatively diagnosed as transexual or transexual/homosexual (the latter category referring to a group of patients intermediate in their behavior and outlook between the homosexuals and transexuals). Although all the diagnoses, and particularly those in the first four categories, are considered tentative and subject to revision upon further evalua-

TABLE 7-1. Tentative Diagnostic Classification of Evaluees

Diagnosis	Males (N = 23)	Females (N = 8)
Transexual	7	2
Transexual/homosexual	3	2
Homosexual	4	3
Transvestite	3	0
Obsessive-compulsive/phobic	2	0
Schizoid personality disorder	1	0
Borderline psychotic	0	1
Psychopath	1	0
Passive-aggressive personality	1	0
Adolescent adjustment reaction	1	0

tion, the table does illustrate the heterogeneity among applicants for sex conversion surgery and should warn surgeons of the need to take great care in processing such patients.

Nontransexual, nonhomosexual, or nontransvestite conditions associated with gender disorders may be identified by history and by observation during the evaluation interview. Psychotic individuals will distort reality in spheres other than the sexual and gender roles. Borderline psychotics will show similar tendencies. Since confusion of sexual identity is a common psychiatric complication of adolescence, a policy of delaying the diagnosis and of not offering conversion surgery to adolescents will allow time for the gender and sexual identity to become more fixed. Psychotherapy in the meantime is essential.

The difficult problems in differential diagnosis are usually presented by transexuals, transvestites, and homosexuals. Schizoid personality disorders may, more rarely, present difficulty. In distinguishing among these clinical entities, some typical historical features are helpful.

A transvestite history will show at least some of the following elements: erotic excitement occasioned by dressing in female clothes; potency in heterosexual intercourse, on some occasions with the adjunct of cross-dressing; erotic fantasies of being forced to assume a passive female role; and exacerbation of the cross-dressing fetish and heightened levels of masturbation as a concomitant of exogenous or endogenous disturbances of emotional equilibrium. As pointed out by Stoller [20], transvestites often nourish a wish to be female, cross dress and pass as female without excitement, and take or apply estrogenic compounds; at other interludes in the history, however, they will show the features outlined above.

The effeminate male homosexual will have a history with some of the following features: a positive desire for erection and ejaculation during homosexual intercourse or with masturbation in the interlude following intercourse with fantasied reenactment of the scene; a relatively infrequent desire to wear women's clothes, usually at parties, with friends "in drag," or at Halloween; pleasure from homosexual male partners and an active seeking of such partners (despite a frequent wish for a "straight" partner); and identification with, and acceptance by, a "gay" crowd. The history of the female homosexual will show identification with and acceptance by a lesbian group; prolonged episodes of living as a masculine ("butch" or "dyke") female rather than a male; and pleasure at having her breasts and genitalia manipulated by a female partner. Sex conversion surgery on homosexuals may be disastrous.

Stoller [20] has commented that he has never seen a female transvestite; certainly none has been seen by the authors.

The schizoid personality will frequently show the following: dissociation and withdrawal from many aspects of life, including sexual functioning; low levels of erotic fan-

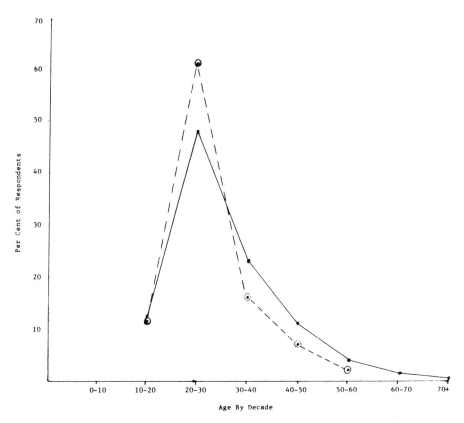

FIG. 7-1. Age distribution of about 600 consecutive respondents who identified themselves as transexual patients seeking operation. Note the predominance of patients in the early twenties age group. Older transexual patients are probably less aggressive in seeking surgery. ●——●, male (436 respondents); •---•, female (163 respondents). (From J. K. Meyer, N. J. Knorr, and D. Blumer, *Arch Sex. Behav.* 1:219, 1971. Copyright © 1971 by Plenum Press, used by permission.)

tasy and activity (a "neutral" approach to sexuality); and only peripheral association or identification with any group.

In contrast to the above, the transexual patient (Fig. 7-1) will typically show the following: absence of, or gradual disassociation from, homosexual contacts; a lack of regard, sense of inappropriateness, or frank repugnance toward his own genitalia to the extent of not wishing the genitalia to be touched or viewed; a decided preference for bisexual or heterosexual partners; absence of erotic

arousal from cross-dressing and a gradual increase in the frequency and extent of cross-dressing (Fig. 7-2); and an attempt to meet and cope with life circumstances in the cross-gender role. The expanded history of the transexual will show the lack of an adequate model in the parent of the same sex, an early lack of aggressiveness and effeminacy (or in the female, "tomboyishness"), preferential association with the opposite sex as peers or friends rather than boyfriends or girlfriends, unhappiness at the development of primary

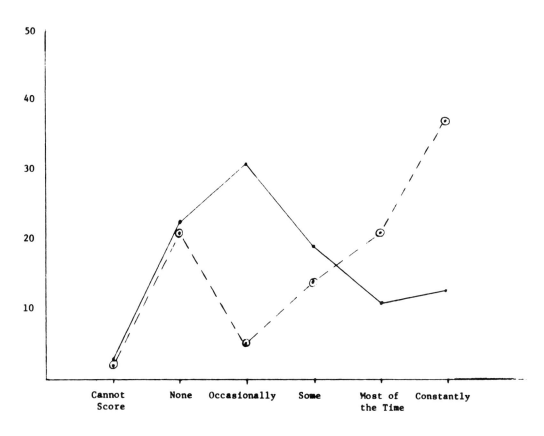

Frequency of Cross Dressing

FIG. 7-2. A study of cross-dressing in patients seeking sex transformation showed that female transexuals are much more likely to cross dress "constantly" than male transexuals. This is undoubtedly due to the present practice of socially accepting a female in male attire but not vice versa. ●——●, male; •----•, female. (From J. K. Meyer, N. J. Knorr, and D. Blumer, *Arch Sex. Behav.* 1:219, 1971. Copyright © 1971 by Plenum Press, used by permission.)

and secondary sexual characteristics, masturbation fantasies in the cross-gender role, lack of satisfaction and sense of belonging in the homosexual role and society, and a gradual seeking of roles and occupations more appropriate to the cross-gender role. (See Benjamin [3], Stoller [20], and Money and Gaskin [16] for more detailed discussions of the diagnosis of transexualism.)

With a compatible psychiatric history and mental status examination, a preliminary diagnosis of transexualism may be established. For several reasons, however, the diagnosis should be considered preliminary and tentative: first, not all patients who request sex conversion surgery are transexual and the distinctions are difficult to make; second, with the increased dissemination of information on transexualism, stereotyped histories may be presented by a patient attempting to put his best foot forward; third, early in the evaluation, supplementary history from family or friends often will not be available; and fourth, orientation and tendency toward cross-gender living is not the same as adaption in reality to the role. Evaluation of desire and capacity to adapt in such a role requires an extended trial period.

The Prediagnostic Trial Period

In view of the variety of conditions that may present with gender identity diffusion or confusion, the often subtle differences among diagnostic categories, and the irreversibility of sex conversion surgery, it is desirable for the patient to have substantial first-hand experience in the cross-gender role and for the physician to have the benefit of observing behavioral adaptation before the final diagnosis is made and surgery is offered.

Although the preliminary psychiatric evaluation should not be underemphasized, perhaps the single and most important phase of the evaluation is the trial period during which the patient lives and works in the cross-gender role and experiences the physiological changes brought about by iatrogenically altered hormonal status [16]. The trial period requires the complete assumption of the feminine or masculine role with the safeguard that, provided the hormone dosage remains within prescribed limits, there will be no irreversible physiological or physical changes. It is true that breast development in the male and beard development in the female do not totally regress with the cessation of hormone administration, but the former may be reduced surgically and the latter by means of electrolysis. Clinical experience indicates that, at recommended hormone levels, menses and spermatogenesis will return following cessation of hormone therapy, should the patient decide to accept his anatomical sex after this trial period.

To live and work in the desired gender role requires sufficient motivation to develop those skills of self-presentation—dressing, speech, and gestures—that will allow the patient to be accepted in the feminine (or masculine) role. Reality issues must be faced during this serious trial period; for example, separation from family, friends, and community and the problems of seeking new employment. In some cases, these changes are in progress or have been completed at the time of preliminary evaluation; in others, the patient must start from the beginning. Although many patients have a tendency to urge the doctors to bypass the trial period as time consuming or unnecessarily rigorous, similar upheavals and problems must be faced following surgery, and it is in the best interest of the patient to have faced those issues in a real sense and to have either adjusted to or decided against such a life style prior to permanent surgical change.

The physiological experience of cross-gender status is accomplished by administration of the appropriate hormones. In the case of the male evaluee, feminization is achieved by what would be maintenance doses of estrogens in the normal female; for example, diethylstilbestrol, 0.25 to 0.50 mg daily. For some possible additional breast development, progesterones may be used in combination with estrogens; for example, Provera (methoxyprogesterone acetate) in doses of 2.5 to 5.0 mg daily. If insufficient feminization is achieved after several months, dosages may be doubled as the upper limit. In the female, masculinization is achieved by the administration of 100 mg of intermuscular testosterone enanthate weekly.* Precautions in the case of estrogen administration involve alertness to signs and symptoms of increased clotting, blood pressure elevation, or neoplasm. Hor-

---

* Hormone levels are those recommended by Claude Migeon, M.D., Associate Professor of Pediatrics, The Johns Hopkins University School of Medicine.

monal dosages should be kept within the limits prescribed in order to ensure that gonadal changes are reversible should the patient desire to return to the sexual role in keeping with his or her anatomy. The physician will often come under pressure from the patient to increase hormone dosage in order to accomplish more striking or more rapid masculinization or feminization, but the development of cross-sexual characteristics, though dose related, seems to be largely idiosyncratic; i.e., larger doses increase risks without necessarily improving the results.

In the female, testosterone administration will result in increased growth of beard and body hair, possible loss of hair from the scalp, increased muscle tone, some masculinization of body contour, and, in some cases, cessation of menstruation. Libido will be increased, and the patient will become more sexually responsive to visual stimuli. Estrogen administration to the male transexual will result in slowed growth, but not elimination, of facial and body hair, increased breast development, rounding of contours, suppression of libido, inhibition of spermatogenesis, and partial or total impotence. Some male patients report a change in the nature of orgasm, i.e., a warm glow in contrast to acute release. All these changes should be experienced and be acceptable to the patient prior to surgical intervention.

In particular, the patient's reaction to a reduction in libido and potency will be helpful in identifying those male applicants for sex conversion surgery who are predominently homosexual or transvestite in orientation. Since the major purpose of the transvestite's fetish is to preserve potency [20] and since the homosexual has a basically masculine identity, over a prolonged trial period these groups will not tolerate well a loss of their potency. These changes will be less helpful in identifying the schizoid individual who may welcome a chance to withdraw

from troublesome sexual feelings. In this situation, the patient's approach to life and his general adjustment will have to guide the physician. Hormonal masculinization will also be helpful in distinguishing the female homosexual who basically considers herself a woman while preferring other women as sexual partners.

A trial period is considered successful when the patient is able to make the adjustment to living and working in the cross-gender role with physiological reversal, and, as a positive consequence, finds this role more satisfactory in terms of personal peace of mind, social adjustment, and the ability to love and to work. When this is not the case, the patient will either drop out of the program or remain in an ambivalent limbo somewhere between the two sexes. Following the successful completion of the trial period, the patient must be reevaluated to establish a definite diagnosis prior to the offering of sex conversion surgery.

Acceptance Criteria for Surgery

When the final diagnosis of transexualism and the decision regarding surgery are to be made, the criteria for diagnosis and acceptance into the surgical program are in many ways pragmatic. The patient has been tentatively diagnosed as transexual prior to entering the trial period, and the trial period itself has served as an important screening device. Those patients who are less serious or more ambivalent about conversion will often become discouraged by the rigors of cross-gender role assumption and will not request further consideration for sex conversion surgery.

Nonetheless, review is indicated in those patients who complete the trial period and request surgery. Positive and negative physiological, psychological, personal, and social consequences of the trial period must be scrutinized. Evidence of incomplete role assumption, adverse reactions to physiological changes, and emergence of other psychiatric disorders or increased anxiety or depression rather than psychosocial stabilization are contraindications to surgery. Inability to complete the trial period should be looked upon with utmost seriousness. Completion should be insisted upon before final evaluation is undertaken and certainly before surgery is offered.

To be accepted into the surgical program, the requirements are as follows:

1. Based on longer observation and more detailed history, the patient's psychiatric diagnosis must be that of transexualism.

2. The patient must have demonstrated psychosocial adaptation during the trial period.

3. The patient must be over 21 years of age. The patient must be of sufficient maturity, as well as being legally entitled, to make the decision for himself. In instances in which the patient is not considered sufficiently mature at the age of 21, there should be no hesitation about requiring an extended trial of cross-gender living.

4. The patient must be nonpsychotic and without significant depression. Psychotic individuals, of course, would not be considered as candidates to begin the trial period. We have never known a patient to become psychotic during the trial period, but such an event would be an indication for psychotherapy rather than surgical conversion. Serious depression manifested during the trial period is a contraindication to surgery.

5. The patient must be supported in his request for sexual conversion by at least one close relative. The family, or part of it, is requested to accompany the patient during the final evaluation in order to provide supplementary history. Obviously, a strong point in favor of surgery would be family recognition that the cross-gender role is appropriate for the patient. Perhaps the most important reason for family involvement, however, is that the patient will be able to count upon at least some emotional and even financial support from his family in the postoperative period.

6. The patient must supply documentation of his police record. This requirement serves as some check on intentions to deceive or defraud as a motivating factor in the patient's request for conversion. Furthermore, it has been our experience that serious antisocial behavior is not significantly modified by sex conversion surgery.

7. The team must have the written permission of any spouse or common-law partner for the sterilization.

8. The patient's general body features should be reasonably acceptable for the chosen gender.

9. There should be reasonable evidence that the patient is sufficiently reliable for good follow-up studies.

10. A history of heavy use of drugs or alcohol must be taken into consideration, since this makes rehabilitation after surgery extremely difficult.

Although psychiatric, psychological, and social evaluations will play a major role in establishing the diagnosis, the final decision about acceptance into the surgical program must remain a team decision in which all the disciplines have an equal voice.

Surgical Techniques

CONVERSION OF MALE TRANSEXUALS

It is critically important that all patients seeking sex conversion know the current limitations of surgery and hormones. Hormone therapy will not completely remove the unwanted beard nor raise the voice pitch to feminine levels, but electrolysis and training in voice modulation will certainly help with these problems.

Excellent and dependable surgical breast augmentation is now available, but hormone therapy alone will produce modest breast enlargement that will satisfy some patients.

The male larynx is often large, but these cartilages may be reduced in size and sculptured to female proportions if the patient wishes to eliminate the embarrassing "Adam's apple." This must be done with great care, or the pitch of the voice will be lowered by the operation.

Body contours gradually become more feminine with estrogens. Rounding-out of the hips and thighs by surgical implants, however, produces excessive scarring, and the dangers of fluid migration make silicone liquid injections unwise for these complaints.

Removal of the male genitalia and surgical construction of a vagina is now quite practical, but the patient must realize that occasionally contracture, stenosis, fistulas, scars, and tenderness may occur with even the most advanced techniques. If this happens, additional unexpected surgery may be required. The patient should be psychologically and financially prepared for such possibilities before starting a surgical conversion.

The male transexual must understand that there is, as yet, no possibility of pregnancy or transplantation of reproductive organs. Some patients may even experience difficulty in achieving orgasm after vaginal construction. Others report complete satisfaction.

Once the drawbacks of surgery are understood, the patient and surgical team may consider the possible approaches. Typically, an anatomically male patient will have lived for one or more years completely in the role of a female—dressing, working, and relating in this role—without reversion to the male role. This patient will be assisted during the

trial period by modest doses of supportive estrogen therapy and an identification card that he carries so legal authorities will know the patient is under medical care. Some patients with heavy beards require electrolytic removal of facial hair before satisfactory life in the role of a female is practical.

If the patient, the psychiatrist, or the surgeon feels the slightest ambivalence at the end of this period, it may be wise to limit the initial surgery to an augmentation mammoplasty. This operation on the breasts produces an intensification of feminine identity and is relatively reversible if the patient should have a change of heart.

Six months after breast surgery (if that constitutes the first step), the patient may enter the hospital for sterilization and amputation of the male genitalia and construction of a vagina. Although vaginal construction by means of free split-thickness skin grafts has been used for many years (Dupuytren [7], Counsellar [6], and McIndoe [15]) to correct congenital absence of the vagina in the female, this method does not take advantage of the valuable elastic tissue available in the phallus and scrotum of the male transexual. The results of vaginal construction by split-thickness graft techniques are often satisfactory, but they are definitely more inclined to develop contracture and to produce additional donor site scarring than the newer operations designed especially for the male transexual.

One of the most obvious of the new techniques involves the removal of the testes and penis, shortening of the urethra, creating a surgical pocket for the vagina in the male perineum just posterior to the prostate, and lining this new cavity with a full-thickness skin graft that is taken from the non-hair-bearing surface of the shaft of the penis [8]. This thin, elastic skin makes an excellent lining for the vagina, but two drawbacks remain: (1) The use of a free graft of any

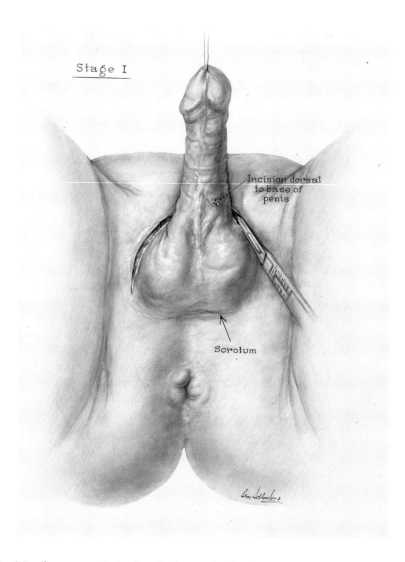

Stage I

Incision dorsal
to base of
penis

Scrotum

FIG. 7-3.   The first stage of the "penile inverted-tube flap technique" for reconstruction of the vagina is started with a U-shaped incision extending just anterior to the base of the penis. (From M. T. Edgerton and J. Bull, *Plast. Reconstr. Surg.* 46:529, 1970. Copyright © 1970, The Williams & Wilkins Co., Baltimore.)

type requires the patient to wear a mold or form almost constantly for several months after surgery to avoid contracture and (2) the junction of the skin graft with the perineum may produce a circular stricture unless some type of Z-plasty or interdigitating graft or flap is used to interrupt the circular scar.

The most satisfactory vaginal constructions (Figs. 7-3 to 7-18) have involved the use of the entire cutaneous and subcutaneous thickness of the male penis by inverting this structure as a pedicle flap to line the new vagina. This method does not require the prolonged use of a form or stent, and the tendency to contracture is greatly reduced. In addition, some sensation is retained in the wall of the new vagina, and the scrotal tissues may be used to construct the labia. The patients having this type of construction have been extremely pleased [8]. A minor disadvantage of the method is that a two-stage operation is required, with a 3-week period between steps. This is necessary in order to retain a scrotal pedicle with needed blood supply until the new vagina develops its own independent circulation from the pelvic pocket.

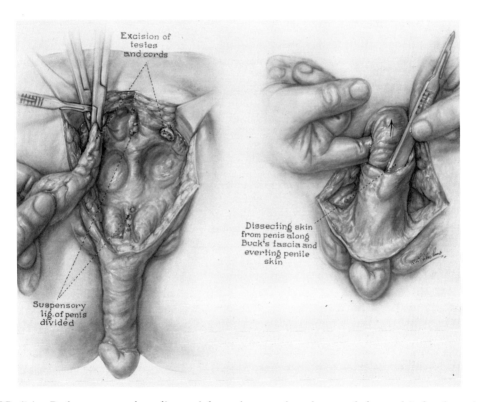

FIG. 7-4. Both testes are then dissected from the scrotal pockets, and the cord is freed on either side up to a point above the pubis. Here the vessels and vas are ligated on either side. The shaft of the penis is then elevated with the finger, and a combination of sharp and blunt dissection along Buck's fascia will free the penile skin in a tubular fashion. (From M. T. Edgerton and J. Bull, *Plast. Reconstr. Surg.* 46:529, 1970. Copyright © 1970, The Williams & Wilkins Co., Baltimore.)

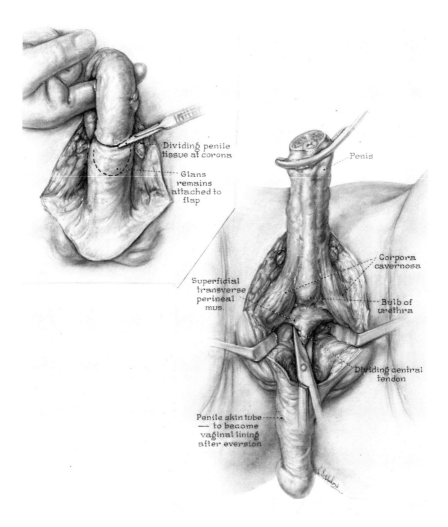

FIG. 7-5. When the tip of the penis is reached, it is transected so as to leave some of the deep glans attached to the skin. This tissue may later simulate a small cervix at the vault of the new vagina. The central tendon of the perineum is divided in order to begin dissection along a plane between the prostate and the rectum. This pocket is at least 2¼ inches posterior to the base of the shaft of the penis. (From M. T. Edgerton and J. Bull, *Plast. Reconstr. Surg.* 46:529, 1970. Copyright © 1970, The Williams & Wilkins Co., Baltimore.)

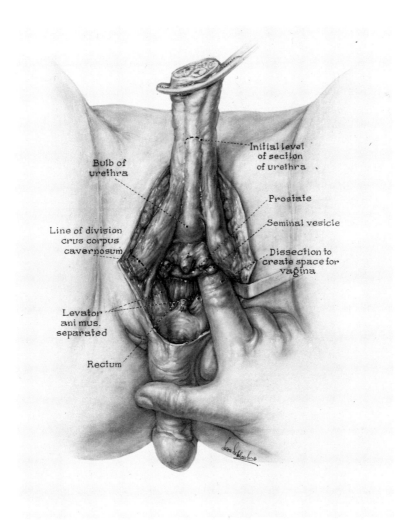

FIG. 7-6. The dissection is carried out between the central fibers of the levator ani muscles and close to the posterior capsule of the small prostate. The seminal vesicles are identified, and the dissection is carried up to the reflection of the pelvic peritoneum. (From M. T. Edgerton and J. Bull, *Plast. Reconstr. Surg.* 46:529, 1970. Copyright © 1970, The Williams & Wilkins Co., Baltimore.)

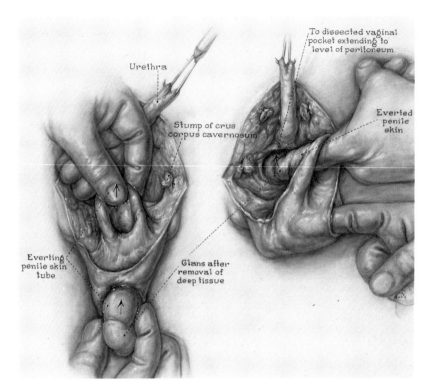

FIG. 7-7.   Once the pocket has been established, the skin flap of penile skin is turned inside out and fitted up to the floor of the pelvis. The urethra has intentionally been left long at this stage of the operation. (From M. T. Edgerton and J. Bull, *Plast. Reconstr. Surg.* 46:529, 1970. Copyright © 1970, The Williams & Wilkins Co., Baltimore.)

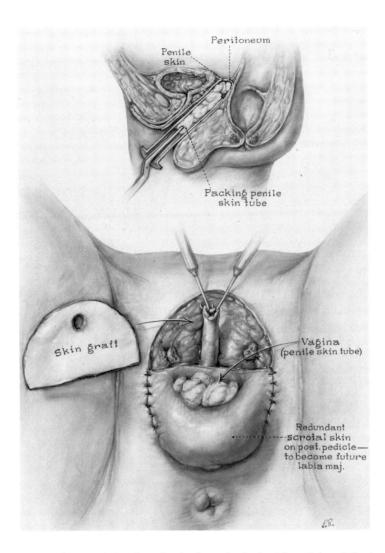

FIG. 7-8. The circulation of the skin flap is then checked with a light while the flap is in the new position of the vagina, and packing is then inserted gently with an anoscope to maintain the full length and diameter of the vagina. Redundant scrotal tissue forming the pedicle is left posteriorly, and a simple split-thickness skin graft is dressed anteriorly to cover the urethral stump and soft tissue defect. This completes the first stage. (From M. T. Edgerton and J. Bull, *Plast. Reconstr. Surg.* 46:529, 1970. Copyright © 1970, The Williams & Wilkins Co., Baltimore.)

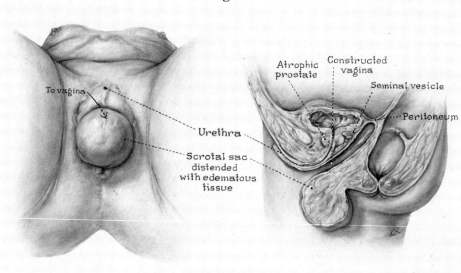

FIG. 7-9. Stage two is carried out about 3 weeks later, and the scrotal pedicle is usually still edematous if the patient has been ambulatory during that interval. The depth and diameter of the vagina are first checked. (From M. T. Edgerton and J. Bull, *Plast. Reconstr. Surg.* 46:529, 1970. Copyright © 1970, The Williams & Wilkins Co., Baltimore.)

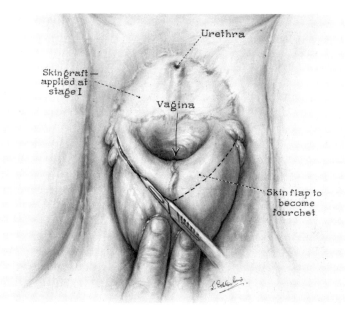

FIG. 7-10. A triangular posterior skin flap of scrotal tissue is then left attached to the rim of the vagina by the V-shaped incision. This prevents later constriction of the introitus. (From M. T. Edgerton and J. Bull, *Plast. Reconstr. Surg.* 46:529, 1970. Copyright © 1970, The Williams & Wilkins Co., Baltimore.)

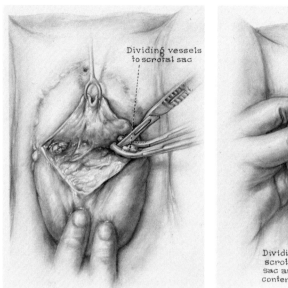
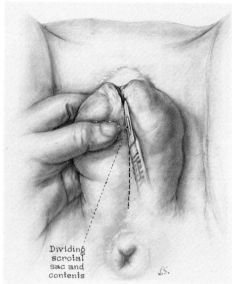

FIG. 7-11. The superficial perineal arteries are divided on either side and ligated, and the remainder of the scrotal pedicle is divided in the midline back to a point 1 inch anterior to the anal canal. (From M. T. Edgerton and J. Bull, *Plast. Reconstr. Surg.* 46:529, 1970. Copyright © 1970, The Williams & Wilkins Co., Baltimore.)

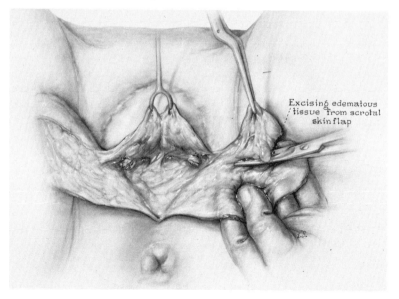

FIG. 7-12. The scrotal flaps are then reflected laterally, and the edematous tissue is removed from the undersurface. If desired, some of the tissue may be left in place and used in the construction of the labia. (From M. T. Edgerton and J. Bull, *Plast. Reconstr. Surg.* 46:529, 1970. Copyright © 1970, The Williams & Wilkins Co., Baltimore.)

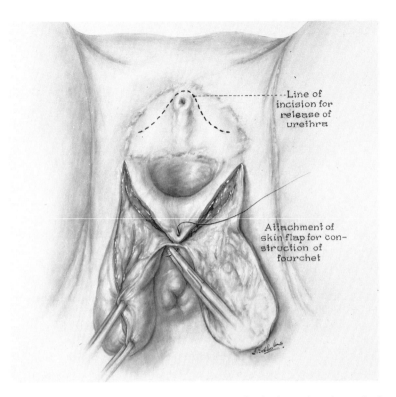

FIG. 7-13. The posterior margin of the vagina is brought backward and attached appropriately to the midline anterior to the rectum, and the urethra is released anteriorly by a bell-shaped incision in the healed skin graft. (From M. T. Edgerton and J. Bull, *Plast. Rconstr. Surg.* 46:529, 1970. Copyright © 1970, The Williams & Wilkins Co., Baltimore.)

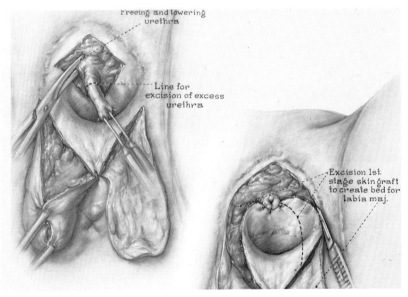

FIG. 7-14. The overly long urethral stump is freed so that all erectile tissue can be removed, and the urethra is shortened to the level of the pubic rami. At this point, it is attached to the anterior vaginal wall, and the scrotal flaps are then fitted on either side of the vagina to create labia. (From M. T. Edgerton and J. Bull, *Plast. Reconstr. Surg.* 46:529, 1970. Copyright © 1970, The Williams & Wilkins Co., Baltimore.)

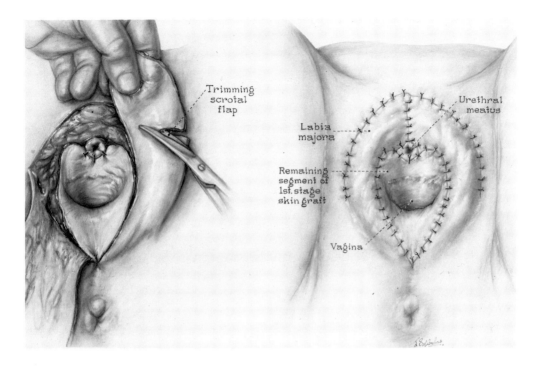

FIG. 7-15. Final trimming and fitting of the scrotal flap is carried out so that, if desired, a small clitoral-like structure may be formed anteriorly, or simple folds on either side of the vagina may be created. These patients are not required to wear the vaginal forms that are needed with techniques involving split-thickness skin graft reconstructions of the vagina. (From M. T. Edgerton and J. Bull, *Plast. Reconstr. Surg.* 46:529, 1970. Copyright © 1970, The Williams & Wilkins Co., Baltimore.)

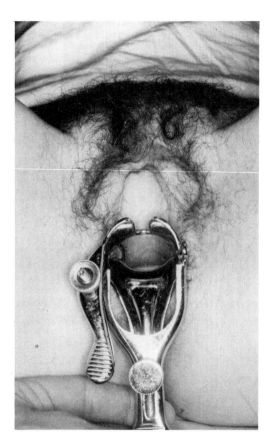

FIG. 7-16. Several weeks postoperatively a speculum may be inserted to full depth. Patient now states that she perceives definite sensation when the wall of the vagina is touched. (From M. T. Edgerton and J. Bull, *Plast. Reconstr. Surg.* 46:529, 1970. Copyright © 1970, The Williams & Wilkins Co., Baltimore.)

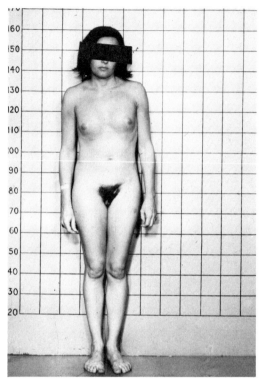

FIG. 7-17. Postoperative appearance of the first patient treated by the penile-flap technique for construction of the vagina. Estrogens have been used to produce this degree of breast enlargement. Reasonably feminine body habitus is apparent. (From M. T. Edgerton and J. Bull, *Plast. Reconstr. Surg.* 46:529, 1970. Copyright © 1970, The Williams & Wilkins Co., Baltimore.)

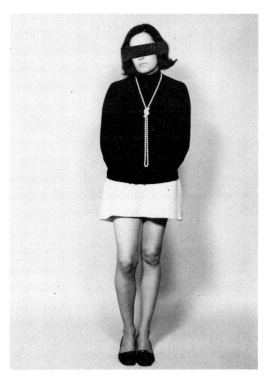

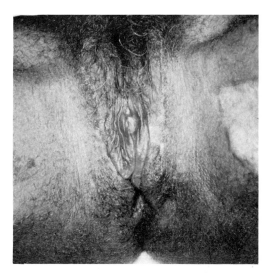

FIG. 7-19. This shows another patient 4 months after operation by the "penile inverted-tube flap tehnique." There has been no tendency to contracture and the appearance of the perineum very much resembles that of a normal female. The donor site on the left thigh was used for the temporary skin graft in the pubic region between stages one and two.

FIG. 7-18. When dressed, the patient is an attractive woman. She has a good job and a significant increase in salary since surgery. She reports quite normal social activities for a female of her age. She is currently anticipating marriage and the adoption of children.

Male transexuals having penile pedicle-flap construction of the vagina have reported "normal" orgasms in sexual intercourse, and at least two have been known to pass military medical examinations permitting them to join women's branches of the armed services. Thus, if the psychiatric and social indications justify the surgery, the male transexual may usually obtain a satisfactory surgical conversion (Figs. 7-19 and 7-20).

CONVERSION OF FEMALE TRANSEXUALS

A totally different set of problems confronts the surgeon who contemplates surgical conversion of the patient from female to male anatomy. The selection of patients requires even greater care, and the doctor must explain the reservations and drawbacks, since these are even more considerable than in the case of a male transexual.

The patient's voice will gradually deepen with continued use of testosterone and the menses will cease, but breast size will *not* appreciably diminish. Some degree of male-pattern hirsutism will appear, but troublesome acne may also develop, and the body contours become only slightly more masculine. Clitoral size does increase with testosterones (Fig. 7-21), but a satisfactory phallus has not been known to develop. Libido may increase and cause social problems and tension.

The construction of the male genitalia has been completed in only a few patients (the

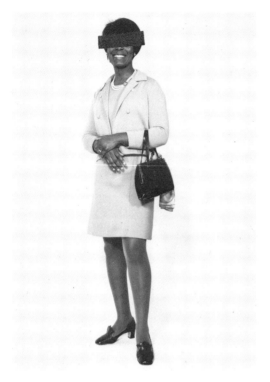

FIG. 7-20. Externally, the patient has a very natural feminine appearance and manner in her work and dress. She has changed her birth certificate and is now married.

authors' total operative experience includes only six female transexuals), and this limited experience has shown the need for faster and better techniques if surgery is to become a practical solution for the treatment of any significant number of female transexuals.

At the present time, however, the female transexual may reasonably aspire to construction of a phallus and scrotum of reasonable appearance that will allow him to stimulate a female partner in intercourse. He must realize that the new penile tissue will not be erectile, that he will remain sterile and without ejaculatory ability, and that usually four to six operations are required to complete the surgery. In an effort to simplify the surgical program, some patients have been asked to choose between the construction of a urethra throughout the length of the new phallus (so they will have the ability to stand and void from the tip of the phallus in normal male fashion) and the surgical insertion of an implant of sufficient rigidity within the phallus (to permit adequate stimulation of a female partner in intercourse). The incorporation of both a urethra and an implant within a phallus constructed from pedicle flap tissue

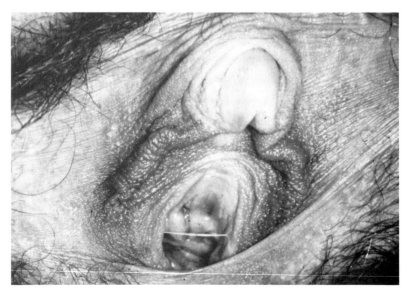

FIG. 7-21. Typical appearance of the vagina and the enlarged clitoris in a female transexual after several years of testosterone therapy. This represents about the maximum hypertrophy that we have seen in the clitoris.

can be accomplished, but the surgical techniques are considerably more complex. Some patients express an interest only in achieving the ability to function sexually like a male, whereas others are more concerned with obtaining patterns of voiding like the male.

In general, the construction of male genitalia involves use of abdominal skin and fat to provide the body of the phallus. Stiffeners of autogenous cartilage, acrylic, Dacron-coated silicone, or metallic mesh may be added (see Figs. 7-41 and 7-42). The cartilage or implants have a tendency to erode or extrude if improperly located or fixed. These implantation techniques have improved greatly in recent years.

The construction of the urethra involves two distinct segments: (1) the normal termination of the female urethra must be elongated about 1¾ inches in a forward direction to bring it near the pubic symphysis where it may enter the base of the constructed phallus in a normal male anatomical location; (2) from this point the urethra must be extended throughout the full length of the phallus to the tip of the new glans. The choice of tissue for building these epithelial-lined urethral segments deserves some comment. Free split-thickness or full-thickness skin grafts have been tried repeatedly within the abdominal tubes. Although the urethra may be readily repaired by this method (the Denis Browne technique) in patients with hypospadias, the reduced blood supply (about one-tenth the capillary clearance rate of normal abdominal skin) in the pedicle flaps used for phallus construction makes "takes" of these grafts unreliable.

Gillies [11] used a second pedicle flap inside the first to make the urethra. We have used secondary reversed flaps, elevated from the non-hair-bearing female labia minora, to create a urethra (Fig. 7-22). These are technically limiting procedures. Ideally, we would

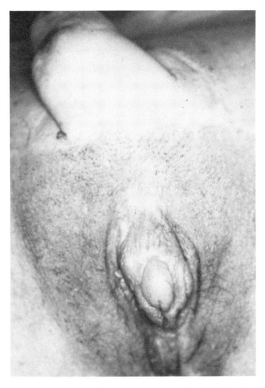

FIG. 7-22. The construction of a phallus has been started in this patient and is attached superiorly at the pubic region. The horizontal portion of the perineum between the base of the phallus and the female opening of the urethra constitutes an important area of urethral construction if the patient is to void like a normal male.

like the urethra to be lined with mucous membrane rather than skin. Such a mucosal tube should be long enough to provide both phallic and perineal segments of the urethra; we would like the new urethra to provide its own blood supply during the critical early days of its residence within the relatively avascular abdominal tube flap. Finally, the urethral construction should not rquire additional operative steps other than those required for construction of the phallus and scrotum.

In an effort to meet the above criteria, we designed a procedure using an isolated segment of ileum on a vascular pedicle to provide the entire urethral segment (Figs. 7-23 to 7-40). This technique was only partly successful, since the patient developed a silk abscess at one point along the midshaft of the phallus with resulting stricture at that point (see Fig. 7-38). However, the resulting urethra was healthy and viable, and the method has interesting possibilities. The steps could be easily streamlined by incorporating the ileal segment within the abdominal tube at the first stage and by leaving the mucosal tube 2 inches longer than the phallus to furnish the perineal section of the urethra. This is done at the time of dividing the mesenteric neurovascular pedicle. The division of nerve supply to the mucosa resulted in elimination of the major part of troublesome mucus production. The patient illustrated has been very pleased with his physical conversion to the male sex, and subsequently has had silicone implants to provide artificial testes and a scrotum (see Figs. 7-39 and 7-40). Present efforts are in progress to develop a rapid two-stage construction of the male genitalia using the wall of the vagina as a new urethra.

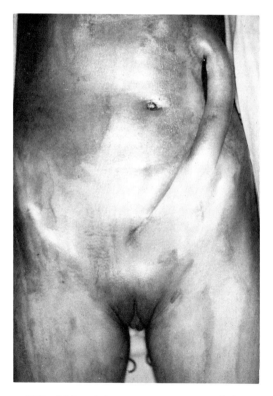

FIG. 7-23. A hysterectomy was carried out through a left rectus incision, and, at the same time, the abdominal tube flap was constructed for construction of the phallus.

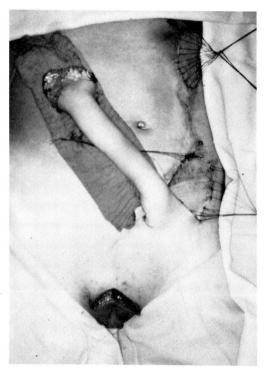

FIG. 7-24. After 3 weeks, the upper edge of the pedicle flap is divided, and the epidermis only is removed over a 1 inch segment. Split-thickness skin grafts are applied to the abdominal defect.

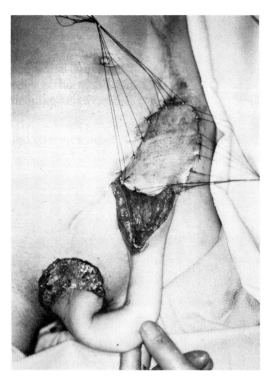

FIG. 7-25. One end of the tube flap has been inserted so that the dermis lies beneath the skin of the pubic region to form a secure attachment.

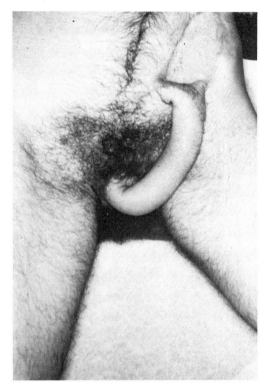

FIG. 7-26. After 3 weeks, the patient returned to the hospital for construction of a urethra throughout the length of the new penile tube flap.

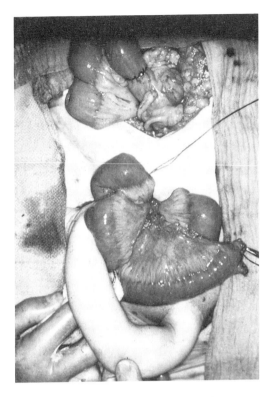

FIG. 7-27. A 10 inch segment of ileum was isolated on a vascular pedicle, and the remainder of the bowel was closed by an end-to-end anastomosis (shown in the upper incision). The isolated segment of ileum has been brought out through a second small incision just above the pubis.

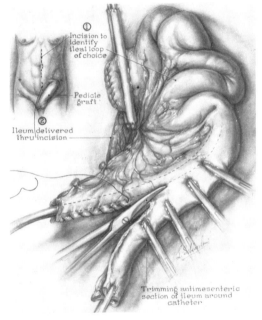

FIG. 7-28. The exess of bowel in the ileum was next removed along the antimesenteric border in order to reduce the diameter of the new urethra. The penile tube was then opened along its former incision and the ileal tube was ready for insertion.

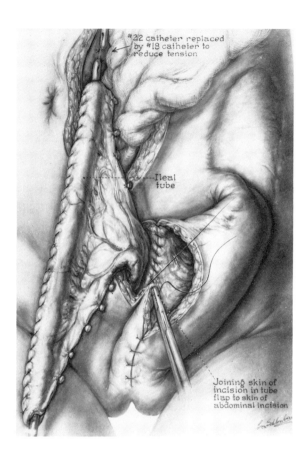

FIG. 7-29. The reduced ileal segment is then transferred into the abdominal tube flap in such a manner as to maintain the pedicle of mesenteric vessels through the incision in the lower abdomen. By closing the skin margins of that incision to the opening created in the tube flap, a completely closed wound may be maintained around the mesenteric vascular pedicle.

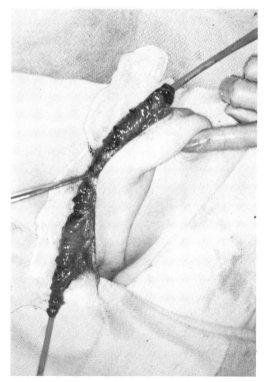

FIG. 7-30. The ileal urethra is gently laid into the abdominal tube; just sufficient fat is removed to avoid tension on closure.

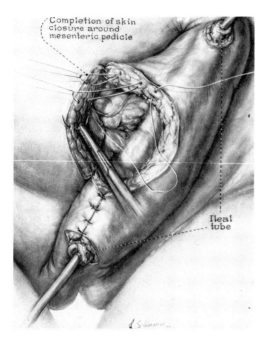

FIG. 7-31.   The tube flap is then carefully closed around the abdominal incision to protect the still intact mesenteric pedicle. Each end of the ileal tube is brought to the skin surface.

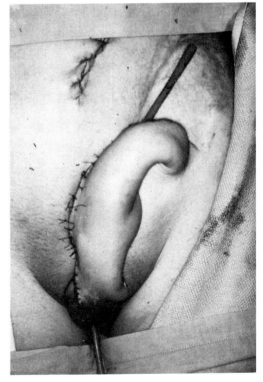

FIG. 7-32.   At the conclusion of this stage, a small catheter is passed through the ileal tube as a stent.

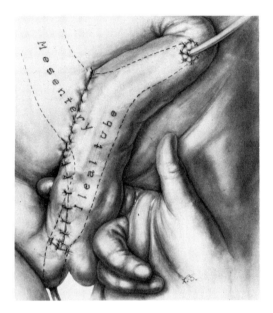

FIG. 7-33. After a 3 week interval, the patient returns to the hospital for division of the mesenteric pedicle.

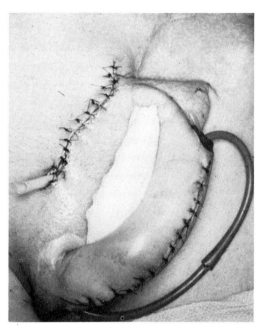

FIG. 7-35. The abdominal wound is closed with drainage, and the pedicle flap making up the new phallus is also sutured.

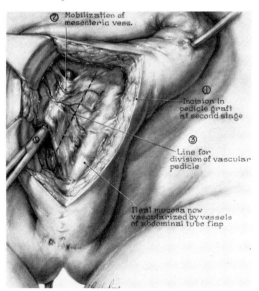

FIG. 7-34. The mesenteric vessels are identified, clamped, and divided along with the accompanying sympathetic nerves. The division of these nerves greatly reduces the mucous discharge within the new urethra.

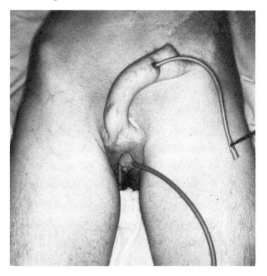

FIG. 7-36. After 2 additional weeks, the patient returns for division of the remaining abdominal attachment of the new phallus and connection between the penile and perineal portions of the urethra.

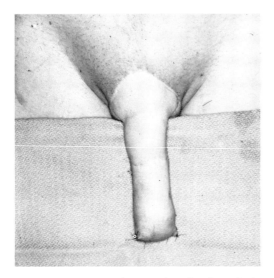

FIG. 7-37. An adequate length of penis is produced by this technique, and often the fibrosis within the tube provides such sufficient rigidity that later implants may not be required.

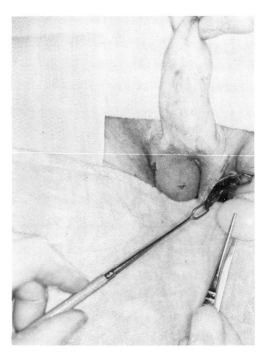

FIG. 7-39. Later, this patient returned and requested silicone implants to simulate testes.

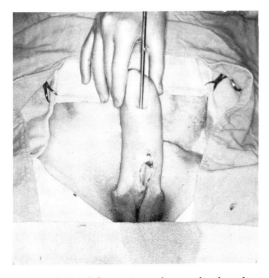

FIG. 7-38. The patient shown developed a silk abscess at one point along the ileal urethra and this fistula developed, necessitating a secondary procedure for closure.

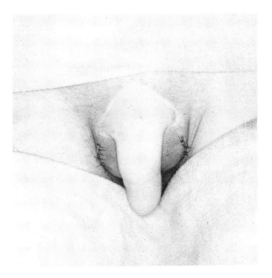

FIG. 7-40. The implants were inserted into the elastic tissue and have caused no subsequent difficulty over the past $1\frac{1}{2}$ years.

Many times, the stiffness that is imparted to the new phallus by the fibrous tissue along its seam will make an implant unnecessary for satisfactory intercourse. This was the case in the patient illustrated in Figure 7-40. At other times, cartilage or silicone may be inserted. To reduce the danger of extrusion, smooth-surfaced implants may be covered with a Dacron mesh to increase tissue fixation (Figs. 7-41 and 7-42).

Other surgical measures to aid conversion of the female transexual include the use of subcutaneous mastectomies to remove unwanted breast tissue. When the breast development has been modest, these operations are identical to those long used for gynecomastia and should always utilize circumareolar incisions in order to avoid the tell-tale branding that results with bilateral submammary incisions (Fig. 7-43).

In certain instances, careful injections of liquid silicone into the vocal cords will lower the pitch of the voice and improve the patient's social confidence. Most patients achieve adequate voice control by training.

Complications of Surgical Treatment

SURGICAL COMPLICATIONS

Surgeons operating on transexual patients will encounter a number of complications. Some of these will be produced by poor techniques undertaken by a previous surgeon, some will have resulted from the patients' desperate acts of self-mutilation or their lack of dependability in following instructions for postoperative care, and some will result from the surgeon's own failure to predict the va-

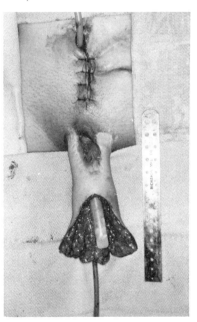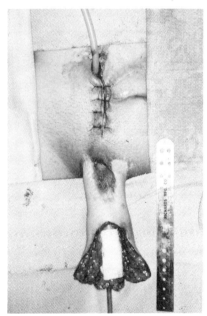

FIG. 7-41. This female transexual had a phallus constructed by a slightly different technique. The original clitoris was allowed to present on the dorsum of the phallus at the base. This was done in order to provide additional erogenous tissue for sexual intercourse. This patient returned for a silicone implant to provide rigidity, and it was placed dorsal to the reconstructed urethra. It was wrapped with dacron mesh to provide better attachment.

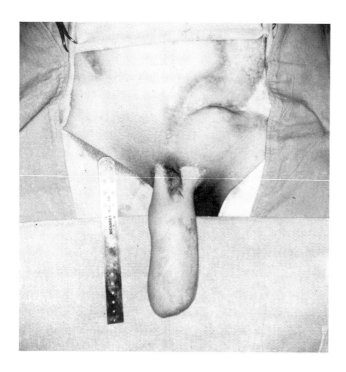

FIG. 7-42. The rigidity obtained by this patient made it possible for him to have satisfactory coitus with his wife, and he has not sought construction of the scrotum or testes.

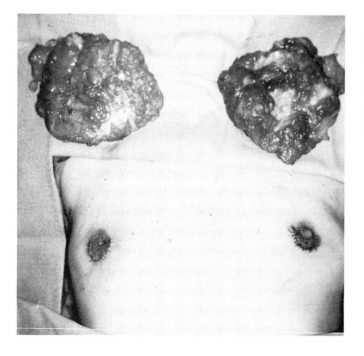

FIG. 7-43. Many female transexuals first seek surgery to remove the undesired breast tissue. The circumareolar incisions suggested by Webster allow the removal of all the breast tissue with no distressing scars on the skin of the chest wall.

garies of wound healing. Many of these complications may be avoided by anticipation.
There are several special problems that may
arise:

1. *A vagina that is too small or stenosed.*
This is usually due to construction with a
free graft technique in which there was im-
complete "take" of the graft, to failure of the
patient to wear her form conscientiously in
the postoperative period, or to inadequate
depth of dissection of the pocket. Secondary
surgery is usually required (Figs. 7-44 and 7-
45).

2. *Urethrovaginal fistulas.* These may be
caused by injury to the posterior wall of the
urethra during the dissection, but more commonly they result from pressure necrosis of
the urethral wall at the point where a tight
pack or form in the new vagina presses anteriorly against a rubber postoperative indwelling Foley catheter. This complication may be
prevented by the use of a suprapubic cystostomy for postoperative emptying of the bladder or the use of a vaginal form that is
grooved to avoid pressure on the urethra.

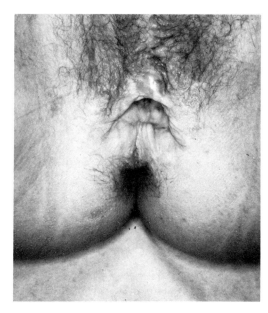

FIG. 7-45. This result was obtained with
the patient shown in Figure 7-44, which was
adequate but certainly not as esthetically satisfactory as a primary construction of the vagina
would have been.

FIG. 7-44. Complications following surgery include contracted and
stenosed vaginas, such as shown in
this patient. Secondary correction
with a free skin graft technique over
a soft foam-rubber form will often
be successful. One must be careful
that the form does not press against
the indwelling catheter in the urethra to produce a fistula.

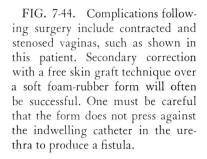

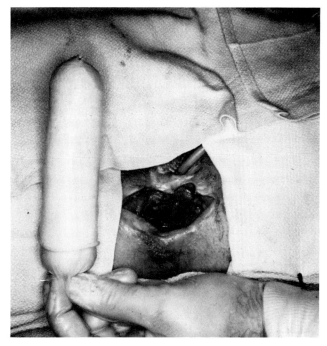

3. *Pubic or perineal pain on intercourse.* Unless the male urethra is carefully shortened so as to lie beneath the level of the pubic rami, the patient will experience engorgement and pain of the erectile tissue in this stump when sexually stimulated. Shortening and repositioning the urethra will relieve the symptoms.

4. *Urinary incontinence.* We have not seen patients with this problem, provided the internal sphincter has not been injured and no urethrovaginal fistula has developed.

5. *Excessive perineal scarring.* Very little scarring is produced by the penile flap-inversion technique (see Fig. 7-16). Any scars in the region of the labia are covered by the regrowth of hair (see Fig. 7-19). However, dark-skinned patients may have a history of keloid formation, and the pubic region is notorious for such scars. If these are encountered, prednisolone injections will help reduce them and prevent recurrence.

6. *Extrusion or erosion of penile implants in the female transexual.* This is likely to occur if the implants are too large, too long, embedded too near the skin surface, too highly polished (preventing tissue ingrowth), or mistreated by an irresponsible patient. Autogenous cartilage or steel mesh seems to be tolerated better than the synthetic materials.

7. *Flap necrosis of the distal phallus.* In *any* part of the body, a dependent and relatively anesthetic skin flap will have reduced microcirculation within the dermis, making it vulnerable to injury. Once ulceration occurs with exposure of fat, it may be necessary to shorten the phallus surgically in order to obtain healing. If the original flap was moved without vascular complication, this type of breakdown is not likely to occur.

8. *Penile urethrocutaneous fistulas.* These are most likely to develop if the reconstructed urethra is near the longitudinal scar on the tube flap or if a suture abscess develops at the site of junction of two segments of urethra. These are minimized if the perineal and penile portions of the urethra are made of a single structure and if the urethra is placed deeply within the phallic flap.

9. *Urethral stricture.* We have seen this only once. It developed at the site of a suture abscess in a patient whose penile urethra was constructed from an ileal segment of bowel (see Fig. 7-38). Reoperation with resection of the stricture was required.

SOCIAL AND PSYCHIATRIC COMPLICATIONS

To date, no serious psychiatric sequelae have been observed among the group of 26 males and 6 females who were treated surgically at The Johns Hopkins and University of Virginia Hospitals. Certainly no "latent psychoses" were uncovered as the result of surgical procedures. In general, the patients seemed relieved and happy to have achieved what, for many, had been a life-long goal; namely, of having an anatomical sex in harmony with the psychological gender.

This is not to say that serious sequelae do not occur. We have seen several difficult problems in patients who had initial surgical efforts at other hospitals before we saw them at the Gender Identity Clinic. It is to be stressed that these patients did not have the original careful screening and testing procedures that we advocate. At least one patient, seen after surgery elsewhere, had been chronically depressed prior to surgery, remained chronically depressed following surgery, and eventually committed suicide. Furthermore, it has generally been observed that those patients who had character problems or showed dissocial behavior prior to surgery continue to have similar problems in the postsurgical period. In none of these instances, however, was the problem engendered by surgery.

A common finding in the postsurgical period is an episode of anxiety and tension induced by a problem situation facing the patient as her confidence expands and brings her more into contact with life in the new cross-gender role. For example, in the case of an originally female transexual who, after operation, had adopted a little girl, how does this transexual father behave when he takes his daughter swimming and must go into the men's locker room in order to change clothes? Such anxiety states respond to supportive therapy and counseling in the cross-gender role. Anxiety or tension states and episodic depressions are usually ameliorated in the postsurgical period as well as in the trial period.

PSYCHIATRIC COMPLICATIONS
OF THE TRANSEXUAL'S
HOSPITALIZATION FOR SURGERY

The psychiatric and milieu complications attending the transexual's hospitalization for surgical conversion were well outlined by Wolf et al. [21], who reported their experiences with a group of eight male transexual patients who underwent sex reassignment surgery.

For the purposes of predicting and dealing with subsequent problems, these authors found that the patients could profitably be divided into two groups, the first more theatrical, and the second more reserved. Hospital nurses and personnel react to the anxiety-provoking and unfamiliar situation of having patients undergoing sexual conversion by the use of denial and suppression. In view of this tendency, the more hysterical patients presented special problems. Their exhibitionism weakened the staff's ability to use denial, with resulting anger, withdrawal, and reduc-

tion in the quality of care. The more reserved group was looked upon by the staff as "better patients" and consequently received more emotional support and care. In counteracting staff tendencies to withdraw from anxiety-provoking and often demanding and hostile patients, the primary physician must take particular care to make himself available to the staff to answer questions and deal with anxieties. Group meetings with the staff have been found to be helpful in dealing with uncertainties and anxieties and in encouraging the feeling of shared responsibility.

As pointed out by Wolf et al., the reaction of the patient to hospitalization can be divided along a time frame into several periods. In the preoperative phase, he is obviously concerned with the upcoming surgery, a significant moment in his life. At this time, anxiety levels may be moderate to high. In this regard, transexual patients are indistinguishable from others about to undergo major surgery. In the early postoperative period, the patients report relief at the accomplishment of a long-sought goal. This immediate postoperative euphoria is rapidly replaced by concern about the functional and cosmetic success of the procedure. "Throughout this period, the patient's level of anxiety, general behavior, and focus of attention correlate with the stages of the physical healing process in the perineal area" [21]. Anxiety and irritability are in evidence from approximately the second to the tenth postoperative day, particularly in the more hysterical group. When the patient is first able to view the perineal area (sometime after the tenth postoperative day), there is usually a shock at seeing the residual evidence of tissue trauma. Whatever the degree of preoperative preparation and postoperative reassurances that the appearance will substantially improve, the patient may succumb to previously denied fears of becoming a "freak," rather than an anatomically acceptable female or male. In the late postoperative period, there is a gradual decrease in concerns about uncomfortable feelings and appearance and about the possible adequacy of the genitals, such misgivings being replaced with the real concerns of facing the new gender role. Obviously, these concerns are greatly reduced if adequate care has been taken in the prediagnostic trial.

When the ward milieu has been adequately managed, the staff will have a sense of achievement at having helped a troubled individual through a difficult period. In achieving this goal, it is critical that the appropriate tone be set when the first transexual patient is admitted to the ward. Perhaps the best means of accomplishing this task is for the primary physician to be available in some routine manner to those who come in contact with the patient in order to provide adequate exchange of information. Candor will clarify areas of potential misunderstanding among the members of the ward staff and between the staff and the physician. The physician's acceptance of, and frank dealings with, the patient will serve as a model for the ward staff. Availability and openness on the part of the physician when the early patients are admitted in a transexual program will be repaid by better nursing care, a smoother hospital course, and better physical, emotional, and social rehabilitation.

SOCIAL COMPLICATIONS

Nothing less is required of the transexual than the establishment of a completely new identity with as little reference as possible to the previous one. Seen in this light, it is apparent that whenever the change of gender role is attempted, whether during evaluation or postsurgically, social complications are legion.

Those to whom the transexual has affectionate ties—spouse, children, family, and friends—may not initially be understanding of his desire for sex conversion. Over time, however, they are often persuaded of the wisdom of his choice. When legal obligations pertain, for example toward a wife or children, specific arrangements must be made. (A wide variety of legal implications and complications of cross-gender living and surgical conversion will be discussed separately; see pp. 155–156.)

A community or neighborhood which the transexual might not otherwise wish to leave may become inhospitable when confronted by an individual who wishes to change his sex. The transexual may be forced to leave his home, neighborhood, or community in order to prevent potential embarrassment—or even harassment—to himself, family, or friends. In developing a new circle of acquaintances, particularly if intimacy develops, the patient may be faced with the agonizing decision of how much to reveal about his previous life and the changes he has undergone.

The transexual's specific job or position in one role often must be abandoned at the time of gender change. Finding new employment may be difficult under any circumstances, but for the transexual to take advantage of previous training or experience, he must request transcripts, letters of reference, and records of previous employment that will refer to him by a different name and a different sex.

For the patient who has already taken the major steps in role conversion, expanding confidence and activity will bring him into new problem situations. For example, how does a female transexual behave at a stag party, or how does a male transexual behave when hostessing the bridge club?

Minor episodes of anxiety and depression that occur as the transexual attempts to cope in the new role usually respond quickly to support and counseling. A short course in grooming, make-up, movements, and voice control will aid many patients.

Legal Implications and Complications

The legal implications of gender change and sex conversion surgery are myriad, both before and after the surgical procedures.

Prior to surgery, the male or female who appears in public in the attire of the opposite sex is subject to prosecution, most commonly under a variety of disturbing-the-peace or public nuisance statutes that punish the "commission of any act which unreasonably disturbs or alarms the public" [9]. The particular statute depends upon the specific jurisdiction. Such prosecution disregards the basic difference between the potential criminal who may masquerade or impersonate in order to cause a disturbance, commit a fraud, or escape identification, and the transexual who dresses to express gender orientation. To add to the hazard of pursuing his gender goal, the preoperative transexual, by virtue of his gender orientation, may seek sexual relief through contact with a member of the same anatomical sex. By definition, this behavior is "homosexual," and the transexual may then be arrested under statutes pertaining to homosexuals. In some cases, the situation becomes bizarre; for example, a preoperative female transexual known to the junior author was recently arrested while in female attire and charged with impersonation. Following a trip to the precinct station, examination by a matron confirmed the patient's anatomical femininity. The arresting officers apologized profusely, but the patient had already suffered the embarrassment and damage to character involved in public arrest. There had been no question of her sexual status over the many years she had dressed as male.

The transexual has difficulty, both social and legal, in severing ties with the past. When a transexual prior to surgery has been married—or to make matters more complex, has children—divorce proceedings, which are difficult under the best of circumstances, become even more sensitive out of the necessity to protect the patient, his spouse, and his children from embarrassment and stigma. Such things as visitation privileges for the father (soon to become a female) must be handled with tact. Support provisions in the divorce also present difficulties, since the husband may, as a female, find difficulty in employing his skills and have to accept a lower paying position. An individual's inheritance in one sex may be contested when that sex is changed. Wills of transexuals may be contested on the grounds that anyone undergoing such a procedure could not be "of sound mind and body."

Assuming that ties with the past can be cut with delicacy and discretion, creating a new life for the transexual still presents serious problems. As Sherwin [19] states, "One does not realize how often one is required to prove one's identity until one disowns the past." One device that transexuals have attempted to use in creating a new identity has been to change their birth certificate. However, in a few places where the matter has been litigated in the courts, they have held in effect that a birth certificate is precisely that, i.e., it is a certification of a set of facts that were held true at the time of a person's birth [19]. Another course has been to seek a name change by court decree, the certified copy of the decree serving as legal proof of identification. This may be useful in many cases, but it has the disadvantage of carrying a reference to the previous name and sexual status.

A series of affidavits may be used to begin the process of altering the significant records that the patient must use in identification and in sustaining claims of past training or experience. Such affidavits may be required from the lawyer, the physician (particularly the surgeon who accomplished the sex conversion procedure), and the transexual himself. (For further discussion, see Sherwin [19].)

The surgeons, psychiatrists, and other treating physicians who deal with the transexual may make themselves liable. The finality of the operation renders the operating physician vulnerable should the patient later claim that surgery should not have been performed in the first place and that, for example, the physician should have recognized that he was homosexual and not transexual. The psychiatrist who initially diagnoses the case as transexual, or who certifies the case as transexual for the surgeon, may also be liable.

In general, it is impossible to cover all legal contingencies facing the transexual and the physician who treats him. Common sense requires discretion and tact on the part of the transexual with regard to family, friends, associates, and the law. On the part of the physician, openness and frankness about what he is attempting to do, as well as the potential hazards to the patient, are important.

Results of Surgical Treatment

EARLY SURGICAL RESULTS

Certain observations may be made regarding 25 patients who have received a total of over 70 operations by members of the Gender Identity team. There has been a steady evolution in the quality of surgical repair. Some of the first patients were operated on by simple split-thickness skin graft constructions of the vagina. In later patients, a technique was attempted that utilized pedicle flap tissue from the scrotum to construct the vagina. The earlier patients tended to have contractions of the split-thickness grafts, and the patients with scrotal-flap operations were troubled by a lack of depth of the vaginal vault and by hair-bearing tissue within the vagina. At the present time, neither of these techniques would be recommended for vaginal construction in the previously unoperated male transexual. We now prefer to construct the vagina either with a free full-thickness skin graft removed from the circumference of the phallus or to use this same source of donor tissue as a pedicle flap, basing its blood supply on a posterior scrotal pedicle (see Figs. 7-3 to 7-19). These techniques have eliminated many of the problems of the early surgical constructions.

Interestingly, even with a number of somewhat mediocre technical results in the first half of the series, no patient indicated that he wished he had not undergone the attempt at surgical conversion. Several patients have accepted what would appear to be less than ideal physical result rather than undergo the additional expense of another operation to improve the effects. All of the first eight patients that were treated surgically had genuine evidence of some deficiency in the repair of the vagina or phallus. These problems included a vagina that was too small and pain in the residual urethra; there was one patient with a urethrovaginal fistula; one patient had keloids of the abdominal wall; two patients complained of hair-bearing scrotal-flap tissue within the vagina; and one patient suffered from persistent neuralgic pain in the labial region (this patient had received her initial vaginal surgery in another hospital). In contrast, of the last seven patients, who were all treated with improved techniques, the surgeon and the patient concurred that excellent functional results were obtained. The use of an improved type of grooved vaginal form and the use of a suprapubic postoperative cystostomy drainage have added to the safety of these more recent procedures.

In summary, if one judges the potential for vaginal construction by the most recent patients treated, the surgical results for the conversion of the male transexual have been quite satisfactory.

The surgical results of treatment of the female transexual have been less satisfactory, but surgery was still justified in the judgments of the six patients who were treated by the author. The principal drawback to these surgical results has been the multiple-staged procedures necessary to achieve a reasonable result. Before widespread use of these techniques could be recommended, plastic and urological surgeons should develop an accelerated two- or three-stage technique for construction of the male genitalia. There is encouraging evidence that such rapid methods of repair may indeed be practical. Even with multiple-staged methods, all six of the surgically treated female transexuals continue to reaffirm the personal benefits that they have experienced as a result of the surgical procedures. One female transexual was seen after conversion surgery had been initiated by another surgeon. He was only 22 years of age and obviously had some ambivalence about his gender. This patient soon thereafter developed a lesbian-like relationship with another female and decided not to complete the surgical program for phallic construction. Such a patient would clearly not meet the current criteria for selection by the Gender Identity Clinic, and obviously would not be accepted for operation under the present program.

We have also had the incidental opportunity to observe a number of patients coming to the clinic with surgical or psychiatric complications following surgical treatment that they had obtained overseas or in Mexico. Most reported little or no psychiatric work-up prior to the surgery, and they returned to the United States with results ranging from rather extensive mutilation to very satisfactory constructions. A few of these perigrinating patients were homosexual and had clearly been misdiagnosed as transexuals. The psychiatric repercussions of such an error will usually be violent and tragic.

It is important that the surgeon establish a good working relationship with any transexual patient on whom he undertakes treatment. In order to do this, it is essential that he deal with the patient as a member of the psychological sex chosen by the patient. To think of a male transexual as a "male" is to defeat completely the working doctor-patient relationship. In general, we have found the properly selected and carefully oriented transexual patient to be a most cooperative and helpful individual.

EARLY PSYCHIATRIC RESULTS

Benjamin [3], in reporting his experience with 51 male patients who had undergone sex conversion surgery, estimated "good" results in 33 percent (successful life situation with integration into the world of women and acceptance by the family), "satisfactory" in 53 percent (less successful social adjustment; inability to experience orgasm), and "doubtful" in 10 percent (appearance and sexual function unsatisfactory despite relief from unhappiness in the male role). One patient was deemed as having an unsatisfactory result. Randall [18], in summarizing his experiences with 29 male and 6 female transexuals both preoperatively and postoperatively, maintained that "the majority of males and females undergoing operation for sex reassignment are subjectively and objectively improved both in their adjustment to their environment and in their own feelings of well-being and satisfaction in their gender role."

Early psychosocial follow-up on the first 13 male transexual patients to undergo sex conversion surgery at The Johns Hopkins Hospital was summarized for us by Blumer [5]. These patients, who ranged from 21 to 46 years of age and from 1½ to 3½ years postsurgery, were evaluated by questionnaire and by psychiatric interview of those patients who returned for personal follow-up evaluation. All reported "no regrets" concerning their initial requests, evaluations, and subsequent surgery. In each case, the patient claimed that she "would do it again" and regretted only the inability to obtain surgery earlier. Although these reports undoubtedly show bias in view of the patients' irreversible anatomical commitment to femininity, the reports came in the face of partial dissatisfaction with the physical results of their transformation on the part of 12 of the 13 patients.

All patients claimed to feel a relief of tension following surgery, in part due to no longer feeling apprehensive about public dressing in female clothing. One patient later reported increased tension and depression at learning that her new husband was in fact dating other women, a revelation that led to several threats and one attempt at suicide. One patient experienced a mild postoperative depressive reaction, seemingly related to unfulfilled expectations of a whirlwind courtship and marriage immediately after surgery. Her depression was relieved after a few weeks, without using medication or psychotherapy. One patient related feeling moody when she focused on the poor physical result. Three other patients reported tending to be intermittently moody or irritable from nonspecific causes, but none required treatment.

Socially, one of the four patients who had been previously involved with "gay" groups gave this up to lead a more conventional life. Six of the 13 patients married, and each claimed "happiness and fulfillment" following the marriage. Three of the six, however, separated or divorced some 6 months to 2 years after marriage. The economic status of the patients remained relatively constant, with only one reporting a decrease in pay as the result of a necessary change of occupation following sexual reassignment.

Nine of the 13 patients reported adequate adjustment in their relationships with their family prior to surgery; three of the four remaining found their relationships with parents improved following surgery.

Some of the patients avoided sexual intercourse, either because of the unsatisfactory physical results of the operation or because of a preference for other methods of sexual release. Some patients found themselves frigid, but eight reported achieving orgasm.

In summary, the psychosocial outcome for the 13 patients, including seven with serious character and social problems, who underwent surgical conversion in the early part of the experimental treatment program showed the following results. With the exception of one patient who made a suicidal gesture, none experienced gross emotional disorders after surgery. No "latent psychoses" were mobilized. All patients claimed relief from anxiety associated with illegal, presurgical cross-dressing. Social gains were made except by those patients who were considered to have significant character disorders. More attempts to achieve social adjustment and to undertake greater social responsibility were made in the postsurgical period, and sexual adjustment was mixed.

Six of the 13 patients in this group were categorized by psychiatric examiners as reliable informants and without serious character impairment. Seven of the patients were noted to have character problems and past social or legal problems, and they were considered relatively unreliable for both the investigation of initial history and the postoperative evaluation of psychosocial outcome. In general, it was seen that those patients who had antisocial backgrounds did not make the social gains of those who did not demonstrate this history. This difference between the two groups of patients emphasizes the importance of evaluating their adjustment during the trial period. Although more follow-up is obviously required, some caution is advocated in accepting patients with serious character disorders as candidates for sex conversion surgery.

Future Use of Surgery for Transexualism

Plastic surgeons have altered body deformities for many years and have observed the lasting benefits on human behavior. Individual sexual organs, such as the breast and genitalia, have been augmented, reduced, constructed, or removed when the indications were appropriate.

The anatomical validity of the "deformity" is much less important to the plastic surgeon or the patient than the "patient's body imagery" of that feature. Thus plastic surgery is designed to improve the patient's body imagery of himself (and only incidentally, the actual anatomy).

The transexual patient may thus be viewed as one with a fixed gender identity of one sex and a "body image" of the opposite sex. Since this body image conflicts with anatomical reality, it is at least possible for surgeons to alter the genital anatomy as one means of resolving the primary conflict. Whether or not this constitutes the *best* treatment for

transexual patients will be decided by comparison with the alternative methods of management that are offered and by the long-term social, economic, and personal productiveness of the patients who receive sex conversion surgery.

Dr. Howard Baker has recently summarized his investigations of the possible role of surgery in the treatment of transexualism:

I have attempted to show that theoretical bias as well as what appear to be purely subjective negative attitudes have created a climate of misunderstanding and confusion that has resulted in promoting and prolonging the suffering of fellow human beings. I have been unable to find evidence in the literature to support the forebodings of Ostow, Gutheil, Lukianowicz, Stafford-Clark, Meerloo, and others against the conversion operation or for the continued application of an insight-oriented approach with the exception of children.

While I wish to emphasize that I am in no way calling for the mass indiscriminate application of sex-conversion surgery, I do feel that the opposition to such procedures is predominantly emotional and that there is an indication for such an approach in those rare individuals who are afflicted with transsexualism. The unfortunate consequence of our unwillingness to be objective in our dealings with these people has been to drive the problem underground, only to have it emerge in some other country, often in the hands of an unscrupulous operator. There, in desperation, transsexuals submit to major surgery with general anesthesia often without the benefit of a physical examination or a blood count.*

There is almost no limit to the possible sophistication of future sex conversion sur-

* Reprinted from *The American Journal of Psychiatry*, volume 125, pages 1412–1418, 1969. Copyright 1969, by the American Psychiatric Association.

gery. Some methods to make the constructed phallus erectile are being tested. Even uterine and ovarian transplants may follow. But at present, the focus must be on the psychodynamics of transsexualism and on producing simple, reliable, inexpensive methods of surgery for a very carefully selected group of patients.

In the meantime, several clinical and basic specialists are reaping the benefits of true team collaboration, and basic research in several areas of human behavior will progress. The recognition and study of the transsexual patient in early childhood should prove especially fruitful.

References

1. Abraham, F. Z. *Sexualwiss.* 18:223, 1931–32.
2. Baker, H. J. Transsexualism: Problems in treatment. *Am. J. Psychiatry* 125:123, 1969.
3. Benjamin, H. *The Transsexual Phenomenon.* New York: Julian Press, 1966.
4. Blumer, D. Transsexualism, Sexual Dysfunction, and Temporal Lobe Disorder. In Green, R., and Money, J. (Eds.), *Transsexualism and Sex Reassignment.* Baltimore: Johns Hopkins Press, 1969. Pp. 213–220.
5. Blumer, D., Knorr, N., Meyer, J., and Chapanis, N. Evaluation of Surgically Reassigned Transsexuals. Paper presented at the 123rd Annual Meeting of the American Psychiatric Association, San Francisco, California, May 11–15, 1970.
6. Counseller, V. S., and Sluder, F. S., Jr., Treatment for congenital absence of the vagina. *Surg. Clin. North Am.* 24:938, 1944.
7. Dupuytren, W. (1817). Cited by Paurez, A. Formation of an artificial vagina to remedy a congenital defect. *Zentralbl. Gynaekol.* 47:883, 1923.
8. Edgerton, M. T., and Bull, J. Surgical construction of the vagina and labia in male transsexuals. *Plast. Reconstr. Surg.* 46:529, 1970.
9. Enelow, M. Public Nuisance Offenses: Exhibitionism, Voyeurism and Transvestism. Slovenko, R. (Ed.), *Sexual Behaviour and*

the Law. Springfield, Ill.: Thomas, 1965. Pp. 478–486.
10. Fogh-Anderson, P. Transvestism and transsexualism: Surgical treatment in a case of auto-castration. *Acta Med. Leg. Soc.* 9:1, 1956.
11. Gillies, H., and Millard, D. R. *The Principles and Art of Plastic Surgery.* Boston: Little, Brown, 1957. P. 387.
12. Green, R. Sex reassignment surgery. *Am. J. Psychiatry* 124:997, 1968.
13. Green, R. Persons seeking sex change: Psychiatric management of special problems. *Am. J. Psychiatry* 126:1596, 1970.
14. Hamburger, C., Sturrup, G., and Dahl-Iverson, E. Transvestism. *J.A.M.A.* 152:391, 1953.
15. McIndoe, A. Treatment of congenital absence and obliterative conditions of the vagina. *Br. J. Plast. Surg.* 2:254, 1950.
16. Money, J., and Gaskin, R. Sex reassignment. *Int. J. Psychiatry* 9:249, 1970–71
17. Pauly, I. B. The current status of the change of sex operation. *J. Nerv. Ment. Dis.* 147:460, 1968.
18. Randall, J. Preoperative and Postoperative Status of Male and Female Transsexuals. In Green, R., and Money, J. (Eds.), *Transsexualism and Sex Reassignment.* Baltimore: Johns Hopkins Press, 1969. Pp. 355–381.
19. Sherwin, R. V. Legal Aspects of Male

Transsexualism. In Green, R., and Money, J. (Eds.), *Transsexualism and Sex Reassignment*. Baltimore: Johns Hopkins Press, 1969. Pp. 417–430.

20. Stoller, R. J. *Sex and Gender*. New York: Science House, 1968.

21. Wolf, S., Knorr, N., Hoopes, J., and Meyer, E. Psychiatric aspects of transsexual surgery management. *J. Nerv. Ment. Dis.* 147:525, 1968.

Diphallus

J. S. P. WILSON

8

THE CLASSIC definition of *diphallic* is having two more or less well-formed penes. However, one must exclude cases in which in addition to a double penis, there is a supernumerary lower extremity. The most celebrated of all such cases was that of Jean Baptista dos Santos (Fig. 8-1), who had two distinct penes with a third lower extremity consisting of two fused limbs pedicled between the scrotum and anus [24]. The incidence of true diphallus in the United States was given by Adair and Lewis [1] as one in 5½ million births. Diphallus, however, is often associated with anomalies of the urogenital and other systems that may well be incompatible with survival; consequently many cases may not have been recorded.

J. J. Wecker in 1609 first described a case of double penis, which he saw on a cadaver in Bologna (Fig. 8-2); cited in Schenkius [57]. Historical reviews giving clinical details of the then known cases were published by Ballantyne and Scot-Skirving in 1895 [2], Neugebauer in 1898 [48], and Nesbit and Bromme in 1933 [47]. Reviews of additional cases without clinical details were published by Villanova and Raventos in 1954, [70] and Adair and Lewis in 1960 [1]. In the last paper, the authors stated that to the best of their knowledge there were 70 authenticated cases in the literature. A review of the case reports of the last decade, together with previously unpublished personal communications and two personally observed cases, provided a total of 108 case reports on diphallus that are available for study.

Double penis occurs naturally in snakes and lizards and occasionally in animals such as rats and calves. It has been produced artificially by teratogenic agents in rats. Little is known of the cause of diphallus in man. Theories of atavism, teratogenic structure (Taruffi, cited in Ballantyne and Scot-Skirving [2]), or minor degree of duplication as in polydactyly (Ballantyne and Scot-Skirving [2]) have been abandoned. Diphallus is not inherited but arises spontaneously in whites and Negroes alike.

Anatomy and Embryology

The mechanism of the failure in development giving rise to double penis is not well recognized. The penis normally develops from bilateral phallic rudiments derived from mesodermal extensions from the caudal ends of the primitive streak, skirting around the margins of the cloacal membrane. The mesoderm passes forward between the ectodermal and the entodermal layers to raise up the phallic rudiments, and then extends on up to

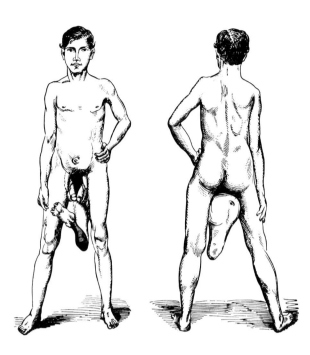

FIG. 8-1. Jean Baptista dos Santos.

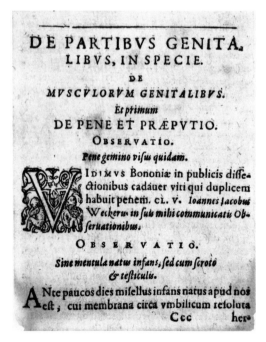

FIG. 8-2. Schenkius's account of Wecker's description in 1609 of the first case of diphallus.

the umbilical cord to form the lower part of the abdominal wall. These bilateral mesodermal extensions meet in the midline, and the two phallic rudiments are brought together to form a single midline penis. Failure of the lateral plate mesoderm to fuse into a single genital tubercle results in the condition of diphallus.

It follows from the above description of the development of the penis from bilateral analogs that any degree of division of the penis may occur. The condition of diphallus may range from a mere fissure or split of the glans to two well-developed penes placed widely apart. In one bizarre case, the glans was united but there were two bodies which were separate but covered by a single sheath of skin [19].

In Figure 8-3 a classification of diphallus is presented. In general, the penes may be symmetrical or asymmetrical and equal or unequal in size. They may lie side by side, or one above the other. Occasionally, they may

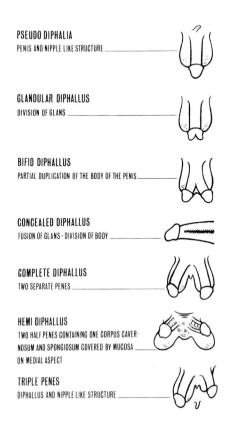

PSEUDO DIPHALIA
PENIS AND NIPPLE LIKE STRUCTURE _____

GLANDULAR DIPHALLUS
DIVISION OF GLANS _____

BIFID DIPHALLUS
PARTIAL DUPLICATION OF THE BODY OF THE PENIS _____

CONCEALED DIPHALLUS
FUSION OF GLANS - DIVISION OF BODY _____

COMPLETE DIPHALLUS
TWO SEPARATE PENES _____

HEMI DIPHALLUS
TWO HALF PENES CONTAINING ONE CORPUS CAVER-
NOSUM AND SPONGIOSUM COVERED BY MUCOSA _____
ON MEDIAL ASPECT

TRIPLE PENES
DIPHALLUS AND NIPPLE LIKE STRUCTURE _____

FIG. 8-3. Classification of Diphallus.

be ectopic and based in the thigh or perineum.

Small nipple-like structures containing erectile tissue are sometimes found and these were termed *pseudodiphallia* by Villanova and Raventos [70]. If this condition is associated with a true double penis, it may be regarded as one of triple penes [15].

Hemipenes is a term coined by Kindred [36] to describe a condition in which there are two small penes, each containing a single corpus cavernosum, surrounded by skin on three sides with transitional epithelium medially which, followed caudally, leads to a small pit. It is usually found in association with

major defects of the developing cloaca (see Chapter 10).

Numerous variations in the anatomy of the genitalia have been described in association with diphallus. The penes usually have a prepuce, but this may be absent in one or both organs. The glans may be perforate or imperforate; in the latter case, hypospadias often occurs. The urethra may be absent or present in one or both penes. If it is duplicated, it commonly drains a septate or double bladder; sometimes, however, the double urethras unite to enter a single bladder. Cases have been described in which one urethra drained the bladder and the other drained the seminal vesicles or the colon.

The scrotal sac is often duplicated, but it may be normal or bifid and found in the usual position or ectopic. When a double scrotum is present, it usually contains a single testis, but cases of polyorchidism and ectopic testis have been reported. The testis itself may be normal or atrophic, descended or undescended.

As would be expected, the upper urinary tract often exhibits numerous forms of anomalies. A knowledge of the various abnormalities and an understanding of their significance is essential in planning the treatment of a patient with diphallus. The urinary bladder may be single, septate, bifid, or even double. In one of the cases of double bladder described, the bladders were connected by a thin duct (Sangalli, cited in Ballantyne and Scot-Skirving [2]). One to four ureters may be present and drain a supernumerary kidney, a kidney with a double pelvis, or a horseshoe kidney.

It is not uncommon to find abnormalities of the anus associated with double penis. The anal impression may be duplicated, and one or the other, or even both, may be imperforate. The possibility of duplication of the bowel, although uncommon, deserves consideration.

Numerous cases of diphallus have now been reported in association with an ectopic bladder. On occasions the entire cloaca may be ectopic; this condition is known as *vesico-intestinal fissure,* and in its most severe forms, it presents an eventration of the gut below the level of the ileocecal valve. In the lower abdomen and perineum, the exstrophy presents medially as an intestinal field that is flanked by hemibladder pads, each with their typical mucosa. Lying below and laterally are commonly found the hemipenes, although they are often concealed by an associated exomphalos. This merely represents a major defect of the lateral plate mesoderm that failed to fuse into a single genital tubercle, thus giving rise to diphallus. The extension of the lateral plate mesoderm stops short of the midline in the body wall, the ectoderm remaining in contact with the entoderm centrally. This leads to a breakdown and a defect in the abdominal wall, which thus provides communication with the urogenital sinus and results in ectopia vesicae, or exstrophy of the bladder. If there is complete dehiscence of the cloacal membrane and its infraumbilical extension, ectopia vesicae and vesicointestinal fissure result.

The picture is somewhat confused clinically, since various degrees of the deformity are found. It may, however, be helpful to have a simple classification (Fig. 8-4):

Group I. Diphallus and ectopia vesicae.
Group II. Double penis or hemipenes with ectopia vesicae and sequestrated rectal mucosa in the perineum.
Group III. Hemipenes, hemibladder pads, and eventration of the bowel.

As with all major congenital abnormalities, the child with diphallus may have anomalies of other systems. Commonly, there may be defects of the lower vertebral column, usually spina bifida or spina cystica, but bizarre defects, such as duplication of the lower spine, have been reported. Associated congenital abnormalities of the heart, hands, and feet have been described.

Surgical Management

The patient with diphallus may require no surgical intervention. Indeed, it may be unwise if the organs drain reduplicated bladders. However, a man so endowed may request removal of one of the organs, either because it interferes with sexual intercourse or because he considers himself to be an anatomical curiosity. Many, but by no means all, of these patients are sterile.

The surgical problem should be considered from several aspects, depending on the exact anatomy of the genitalia and the associated defects of the urinary tract. In all cases, urethral patency must be established or maintained. Therefore, a full urological investigation is mandatory. Intravenous pyelography will demonstrate the function of the kidneys and any abnormalities of the ureters and bladder. If anomalies are found, cystoscopy and urethroscopy may be helpful, and the lower urinary tract may be further visualized by urethrography and cystography. Urinary analysis and culture allow the treatment of an accompanying urinary infection preoperatively. A straight x-ray examination of the pelvis will reveal any separation of the os pubis, and a contrast enema will confirm continuity of the lower intestine and the position of the rectum and sigmoid colon.

Relatively few cases of diphallus have undergone surgical treatment. The first recorded surgical procedure was by Englisch in 1895, as cited in Ballantyne and Scot-Skirving [2]. He united the two halves of a bifid glans and successfully repaired the asso-

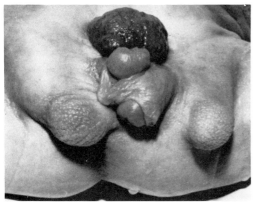

A

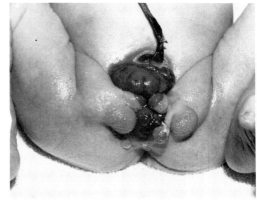

B

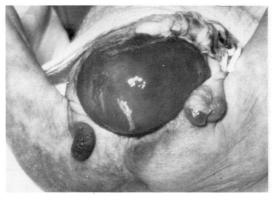

C

FIG. 8-4. Major defects of the developing cloaca. A. Group I. Diphallus and ectopia vesicae. B. Group II. Hemipenes with ectopia vesicae and sequestrated rectal mucosa in the perineum. C. Group III. Hemipenes, hemibladder pads, and eventration of the bowel.

ciated hypospadias. Following this report, several accounts of treatment have been described, and recently, major defects of the developing cloaca associated with double penis have been repaired. However, no one surgeon has had sufficient experience with the condition to permit dogmatism.

The principles of treatment depend on the degree and type of the deformity. The small swelling that may contain erectile tissue but is without a urethra, such as pseudodiphallia, presents no difficulties and can be dealt with by simple excision. With various degrees of

split glans and bifid penis, the parts can be united if they are symmetrical. However, if they are asymmetrical, amputation of the nonfunctioning smaller organ is preferable.

Where there are two distinct organs (Fig. 8-5A), investigation usually reveals only one patent urethra. Surgery is then confined to the amputation of the other penis. Should both penes contain a urethral canal draining either a single, septate, or double bladder or the seminal vesicles, continuity must be established by transplanting a ureter or by uniting a double bladder. The integrity of the lower

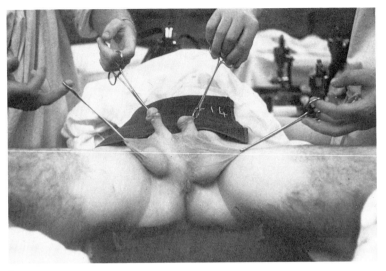

A

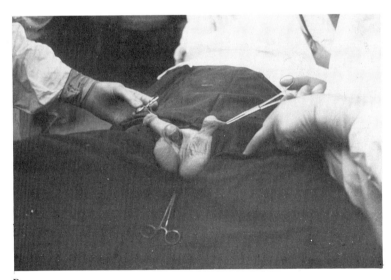

B

urinary tract having been established, an elliptical incision is made around the base of the nonfunctioning penis (Fig. 8-5B), and the crura and bulb of the corpora are mobilized and amputated (Fig. 8-5C). The scrota are then brought together and the wound is closed in two layers (Fig. 8-5D).

The management of a patient with hemi-penes is dominated by the necessity to treat the associated major anomalies. Hemipenes are found only in association with ectopic vesicae, and it is noteworthy that there is a true skin shortage that requires the introduction of a pedicle skin flap to avoid tension in the repair.

The bladder may be reconstructed, but be-

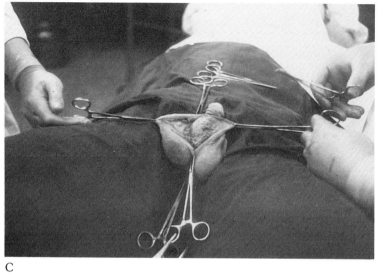

C

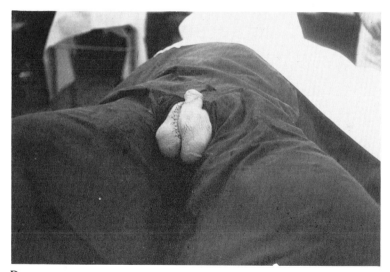

D

FIG. 8-5A–D. Treatment of a case of complete diphallus. (From Hughes [30]).

cause of the complication of the repair (with doubtful primary wound healing and subsequent incompetence of the reconstructed sphincter) and because of the possibility of vesicoureteral reflux developing, a simpler procedure is preferred. It is better to perform a preliminary transplantation of the ureters into an ileal conduit, after which the bladder mucosa can be excised and the abdominal wall repaired in a dry field. Occasionally a perineal hernia is present, and the opportunity should be taken to repair this at the same time.

In Group II cases of hemipenes, the sequestrated rectal mucosa should be excised; the resultant defect in the perineum can be closed by the same pedicle flap that is used to repair the lower abdomen. Attention is then directed to uniting the hemipenes, which are covered by mucous membrane, not skin, on their medial aspect. The paired scrota and penes are first transposed by a double Z-plasty technique (Fig. 8-6). The corpus cavernosum of the smaller organ is amputated, allowing its skin to be donated to resurface the medial defect on the other penis and to cover a central strip of mucosa that has been preserved for the reconstruction of the urethra.

Surgical procedures are illustrated for a case of hemipenes with ectopia vesicae and rectal mucosa in the perineum (see Fig. 8-4B). The staged procedure begins with a laparotomy and the transplanation of the ureters into an ileal conduit (Fig. 8-7A). Following a suitable convalescence, a long flap based on the left inguinal region is delayed (Fig. 8-7B). At the next stage, the ectopic bladder mucosa is excised by blunt dissection with scissors. The resultant defect in the lower abdominal (Fig. 8-7C) wall is closed by advancement caudally of the fibrous remnant of the rectus sheath, which is then sutured to the fibrous bar that is always found in the pubic region. A finger placed per rectum guides the depth of excision while the sequestered bowel mucosa is excised from the perineum. This maneuver results in a large defect of the lower abdomen and perineum, where adequate hemostasis must be secured before the defect is closed by the transposition of the delayed flap. The apex of the flap is drawn downward between the scrota to close the triangular defect in the perineum and the lower abdomen, and the

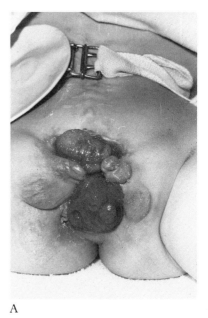

A

FIG. 8-7A–F. Treatment of a case of hemipenes.

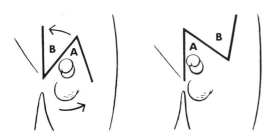

FIG. 8-6. Centralization of hemipenes by Z-plasty.

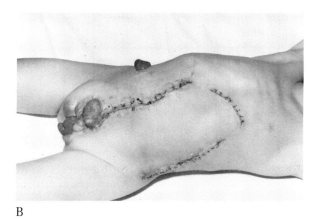

B

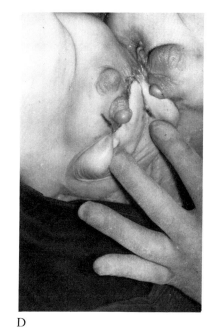

D

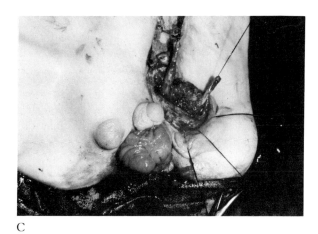

C

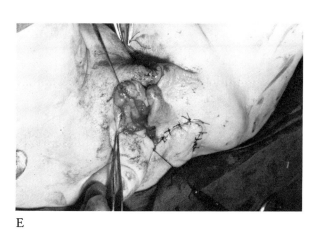

E

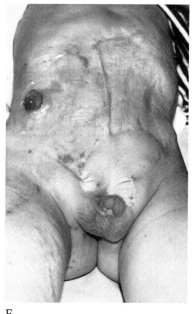

F

donor area of the flap is covered by a split-thickness skin graft.

When the abdominal flap has softened, the penes are transposed to the midline. A large "Z" is planned, based on the lower edge of the flap. The medial limb consists of half the apex of the abdominal flap, and the lateral limb contains the penis and scrotum (Fig. 8-7D). Simple transposition of these flaps will move these structures to the midline once the corpus cavernosum of the penis is mobilized and its shortened suspensory ligament is divided. A similar procedure is performed on the opposite side after a short interval. At this stage the two penes should be united. It is not usually possible to unite the corpus cavernosum to its fellow; it is therefore removed from its sheath and then mobilized from its origin on the ischiopubic ramus, where it is transfixed and divided.

Attention is now directed to the other penis. A narrow Denis Browne-type strip of mucosa is outlined, and the rest of the mucous membrane is excised (Fig. 8-7E). This strip of mucosa will fold in to form the new urethra; although it will not conduct urine, it may form a channel from the entrance of the ejaculation ducts that lie in a pit at its origin and thus allow the passage of seminal fluid. The inner limb of a second "Z" is now moved outward, and the skin and scrota of the other penis are moved in to the midline. The contiguous surfaces of the scrota are united. Finally, the penile skin flap supplies abundant tissue to be draped over the raw area of the penis, completing its skin sheath and prepuce (Fig. 8-7F).

In the case of an infant with a Group III deformity, the hemipenes are only a minor factor in the condition of vesicointestinal fissure. The abnormalities may be so gross that they are incompatible with life, and therefore, therapeutically, surgical procedures are not justified. Recently, successful attempts have been made to salvage some of these infants, especially if there are no associated major neurological or cardiac anomalies [56, 63].

The principle of treatment involves bilateral sacroiliac osteotomies to approximate the os publis. This maneuver aids in the closure of the abdominal wall, especially if an associated omphalocele is treated, and moves the hemipenes toward the midline. Next, mobilization and closure of the medial intestinal field by longitudinal sutures reestablishes intestinal continuity. The blind end of the colon is then pulled down into the perineum to form a perineal proctostomy, or, alternatively, an abdominal colostomy is constructed. Finally, the medial free edges of the hemibladder pads are sutured together.

The infant now has the appearance of a child with a Group I defect. At a second stage, reconstruction of the bladder or cystectomy may be performed, and transplantation of the ureters into an ileal conduit is undertaken.

References

1. Adair, E. L., and Lewis, E. L. Ectopic scrotum and diphallia. *J. Urol.* 84:115, 1960.
2. Ballantyne, J. W., and Scot-Skirving, A. A. Diphallic terata with notes of an infant with a double penis. *Teratologica,* 92–95, 184–209, 225–268, 1895.
3. Bartels, M. Ueber die Bauchblasengenitalspalte, einen bestimaten Grad ehr Sogenannten Inversion der Harnblase. *Arch. Anat. Physiol.* 165, 1868.
4. Bauza, J. A. Malformación genital (bifallia parcial) con extrofia y malformaciónes multi-

ples de las maños y pies. *Arch. Pediatr. Urug.* 3:354, 1932.

5. Beck, C. A case of double penis, combined with extrophy of the bladder and showing four urethral orifices. *Med. News* 79:541, 1901.

6. Blanco, S. Diphallus (double penis). *J. Urol.* 53:786, 1945.

7. Bockenheimer, P. Zur Kasuistik der Bauchblasengenitalspalte. *Arch. Klin. Chir.* 69:669, 1903.

8. Bokay, J. von. Ueber Diphallie. *Jahrl. J. Kinderheilk. Phys. Ersich.* 127:432, 1930.

9. Bruni, C. Seltene Anomalie de Urogenitalorgane droppelter Penis. *Z. Urol.* 21:193, 1927.

10. Campbell, M. F. *Pediatric Urology.* New York: Macmillan, 1937. P. 324.

11. Cochrane, W. J., and Saunders, R. L. de C. H. A rare anomaly of the penis associated with imperforate anus. *J. Urol.* 47:810, 1942.

12. Cohen, S. J. Diphallus with duplication of colon and bladder. *Proc. R. Soc. Med.* 61:305, 1968.

13. Cole, J. D. A case of double penis and imperforate anus. *Nashville J. Med. Surg.* 77:159, 1894.

14. Coutino, A. P. Difalia completa. *Arch. Esp. Urol.* 13:10, 1957.

15. Davis, D. M. A case of double, triple or quadruple penis associated with dermoid of the perineum. *J. Urol.* 61:111, 1949.

16. De Gaetani, G. Diphallus bitious asymmetrious. *Genesis* 12:101, 1932.

17. Donald, C. A case of human diphallus. *J. Anat.* 64:523, 1930.

18. Ferulano, O., and Alfono, C. Su di un raro caso di difallia associata a poliorchidismo. *Riforma Med.* 71:1145, 1957.

19. Fowler, F. Double penis: Report of a case with surgical management. *Am. Surg.* 29:555, 1963.

20. Not used.

21. Ghelani, L. L., and Kodwavala, N. Y. Personal communication, 1969.

22. Glenister, T. W. A correlation of the normal development of the penile urethra and of the infra-umbilical abdominal wall. *Br. J. Urol.* 30:117, 1958.

23. Goligorskii, S. D., and Bardier, L. G. A case of plastic repair of bladder sphincter in congenital bifurcation at penis with incontinence. *Urologiia (Moskva)* 21:70, 1957.

24. Gould, G. M., and Pyle, W. L. *Anomalies and Curiosities of Medicine.* London: Saunders, 1901. P. 196.

25. Green, J. A. S. Personal communication, 1968.

26. Hall, E. G., McCandless, A. E., and Rickhan, P. P. Vesico-intestinal fissure with diphallus. *Br. J. Urol.* 25:219, 1953.

27. Harrenstein, R. J. Ein Fall von droppelter Entwicklung des Penis und Skrotums. *Beitr. Klin. Chir.* 154:308, 1931.

28. Heller, J. Zwei seltene Missbildungen des Penis. *Z. Urol.* 2:612, 1908.

29. Hofmokl, J. Mittheilungen aus der chirurgischen Casuistik und kleinere Mittheilungen. *Arch. Klin. Chir.* 54:220, 1897.

30. Hughes, N. C. Personal communication, 1969.

31. Johnstone, J. H., and Penn, I. A. Exstrophy of the cloaca. *Br. J. Urol.* 38:302, 1966.

32. Keith, A. Three demonstrations on malformations of the hind end of the body. *Br. Med. J.* 2:1857, 1908.

33. Keppel, J. W. A double penis. *New York J. Med.* 68:710, 1898.

34. Kermaunner, F. Ueber Missbildungen mit Stoerungen des Korperverschlusses. *Arch. Gynäk.* 78:221, 1906.

35. Kimura, H. On double penis and its complications. *Jap. Med. World* 10:63, 1930.

36. Kindred, J. E. Eventration of the abdominal viscera associated with umbilical hernia, hemipenes, and hydromyelomeningocele in a newborn infant. *Anat. Rec.* 128:379, 1957.

37. Kirsch, E. von. Totale Diphallie: Ein Beitrag zur Kasuistik der Fehlbildungen der Harnorgane. *Z. Urol.* 48:711, 1955.

38. Kuttner, H. Ueber angeborene Verdoppelung des Penis. *Beitr. Klin. Chir.* 15:364, 1896.

39. Lanman, T. H., and Mahoney, P. J. Intravenous urography in infants and in children. *J. Dis. Child.* 42:611, 1931.

40. Liaschutz, A. A note on a case of bifid penis. *J. Anat. Physiol. Paris* 58:254, 1924.

41. Lionti, G. Ein Fall von Penisverdoppelung. *Dtsch. Med. Wochenschr.* 40:393, 1912.

42. Lorthioir, J. Un cas teratologique rare. *Soc. belge de Chir.* 1:82, 1901.

43. MacLennan, A. Double penis and double vulva. *Glasgow Med. J.* 101:287, 1924.

44. Messler, B., and Gagnon, R. Complete diphallus in a rat. *Rev. Can. Biol.* 26:317, 1967.

45. Mingazzini, E. A case of double penis. *Urol. Int.* 1:188, 1955.

46. Mogg, R. A. A case of diphallus with vesica duplex and rectal agenesis. *Acta Urol. Belg.* 30:533, 1962.

47. Nesbit, R. M., and Bromme, W. Double penis and double bladder. *Am. J. Roentgenol.* 30:497, 1933.

48. Neugebauer, F. L. Fälle van Verdoppelung der ausseren Geschlechteile. *Mschr. Geburtsh. Gynäkol.* 7:550, 1898.

49. Pagano, F. Su un caso eccezionale di doppio pene. *Urol. Int.* 13:362, 1962.

50. Palieri, D. Anomali degli organi esterni maschili (scrotaschisi-o biscsctismo) con ambo i te testicoli. Penepalmato-etiologia. *Gazz. Osp. Clin.* 53:1476, 1932.

51. Pawlukiewicz, S. Zdwojenie pracia i olbrzyim moczowod. (Double penis and megaloureter.) *Pol. Przegl. Chir.* 31:1227, 1959.

52. Pendino, J. A. Diphallus (double penis). *J. Urol.* 64:156, 1950.

53. Phillps, J. R. Diphallus and gastroschisis. *J. Indian State Med. Assoc.* 25:372, 1932.

54. Pires de Lima, J. A. Note on a case of bifid penis with penial hypospadia. *J. Anat. Physiol.* 49:85, 1915.

55. Rickham, P. P. Vesico-intestinal fissure. *Arch. Dis. Child.* 35:97, 1960.

56. Rickham, P. P. Personal communication, 1969.

57. Schenkius, J. Observationum medicarum rararum novarum admirabilium et monstrosarum volumen. *Monst. hist. Francofurti.* Lib IV, 1609, p. 577.

58. Schnieder, G. *Lichtenberg's Handbuch der Urologie.* Berlin: Springer, 1928. P. 160.

59. Seth, R. E., and Peacock, A. H. Double penis. *Urol. Cutan. Rev.* 36:590, 1932.

60. Sloboziano, H., Georgesco, M., and Floru, E. Contribution à l'étude de la diphallie. *J. Urol.* 36:556, 1933.

61. Smith, A. P. Report on 52 successful cases of lithotomy. *Trans. Med. Chir. Faco. of Maryland* 1891. Pp. 86–93.

62. Solomon, A. A., Rosenthal, I., and Linker, M. H. Double penis associated with supernumerary kidney. 64:705, 1950.

63. Sopor, R. T., and Kilger, K. Vesico-Intestinal fissure. *J. Urol.* 92:490, 1964.

64. Thompson, D. P., and Lynn, H. B. Genital anomalies associated with solitary kidney. *Mayo Clin. Proc.* 41:538, 1966.

65. Thompson, R. A case of diphallus. *Proc. Anat. Soc. G. B.* 64:121, 1929.

66. Trenkler, R. Ueber einen Fall vorkommener angeborener Penisspaltung (doppelpenis). *Wien. Med. Wochenschr.* 64:1079, 1914.

67. Tschmarke, G. Beitrag zur Kasuistik der Diphallie. *Beitr. Klin. Chir.* 151:631, 1931.

68. Vaudescal, M. Présentation d'un cas de malformation rare des organes externes Diphallus. *Bull. Soc. Obstet. Gynecol. Paris* 10:271, 1921.

69. Veen, P. J., and Misdorp, W. Penis duplex in a grass-fed calf. *Tijdschr. Diergeneesk* 89:160, 1964.

70. Villanova, X., and Raventos, A. Pseudodiphallia, a rare anomaly. *J. Urol.* 71:338, 1954.

71. Volpe, M. Dell'asta doppia. *Policlinico [Chir.]* 10:46, 1903.

72. von Geldern, C. E. The aetiology of exstrophy of the bladder. *Arch. Surg.* 8:61, 1924.

73. Williams, D. *Paediatric Urology.* London: Butterworth, 1968. P. 319.

74. Wojewski, A., and Kossowski, W. Total diphallia: A case of plastic repair. *J. Urol.* 91:84, 1964.

75. Zischka-Konorsa, W. von, and Bibus, B. Uber ein partiell in de Harnblase hineinragenden Diphallus bifidus. *Zentralbl. Allg. Pathol.* 107:166, 1965.

Congenital Abnormalities of the Scrotum

DESMOND A. KERNAHAN

9

Function of the Scrotum

THE SCROTUM is a structure found only in mammalian species and serves as a temperature-regulating mechanism for the testis. In contrast to lower species, maturation of spermatozoa will not occur if the testis is at intraabdominal temperature. In mammals with intermittent periods of sexual activity, the testes are only periodically present in the scrotum, retracting during the infertile periods through the open inguinal canal. In the human, however, there is no such retraction and the testis is normally constantly present in the scrotum; the inguinal canal above it is closed.

Development of the Scrotum

Development of the scrotum [10] begins with the appearance of the genital swellings that may be seen in the 6-week-old embryo lying to either side and posterior to the genital tubercle. Internally and opposite to these swellings lies the peritoneum of the processus vaginalis with the fibrous tissue known as the scrotal ligament extending between them. The genital swellings increase in size and develop into the labioscrotal folds. At this stage there is no discernible sexual differentiation in the appearance of the external genitalia. In the male, considerable increase in size of the scrotal folds occurs to form the scrotal pouch, and it is into this that the testis subsequently descends. The majority of the growth of the scrotal pouch occurs caudal to the root of the developing penis, where finally the scrotal sacs on either side fuse to form the definitive scrotum with its central raphe. That this more extensive process of development in the male is stimulated by the secretion of androgens is shown by the excessive growth of the labial folds that occurs in the adrenogenital syndrome. These patients, though always genetically and chromosomally female, may resemble a hypospadiac male with a bifid scrotum or even show fusion of the folds to give the appearance of a comparatively normal "scrotum" (Fig. 9-1).

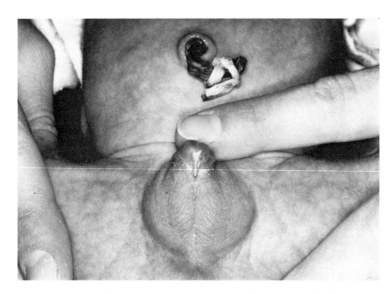

FIG. 9-1. Adrenogenital syndrome with labial fusion and an enlarged clitoris.

Abnormalities of the Scrotum

Abnormalities of the scrotum are comparatively rare, and often they are only part of a more extensive and functionally important deformity of the genitalia, such as the bifid scrotum associated with perineal hypospadias.

The three deformities most commonly reported on are all nevertheless extremely rare: prepenile scrotum, webbed scrotum, and ectopic scrotum.

PREPENILE SCROTUM

Thirteen cases are described in the literature on this condition. The clinical appearances are those of a penis of greater or lesser degree of normal development lying behind an essentially well-formed and normal scrotum.

In the majority of these cases there are associated abnormalities of the genital tract such as hypospadias [3, 12], absence of the

urinary tract [7], polycystic kidney [13], or imperforate anus [8]. Hinman [11] described the condition in a stillborn child whose genitourinary tract was otherwise normal. Campbell [4] and McGuire [14] reported living cases that were normal in other respects, one being that of a 40-year-old African who had married and had one child. Remzi [18] reported a patient in which the right testis lay in the inguinal canal but no gonad could be detected on the left. Another case is listed in the references [17], and two further cases are added herewith.

In a case of prepenile scrotum (Fig. 9-2), the scrotum was fully developed and lying in the anterior position almost over the pubic symphysis. No true penis was present but a longitudinal mass of erectile tissue, adherent to the perineum, was situated behind the scrotum (Fig. 9-3). This mass was covered by ectopic scrotal skin. No urethra or meatal dimple was identifiable. Intravenous pyelography carried out within a few hours after birth showed two functioning kidneys with

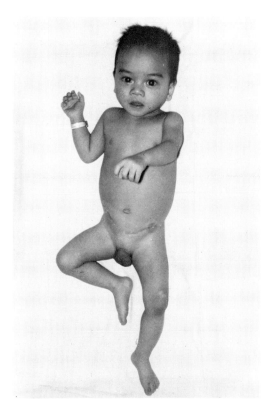

FIG. 9-2. Absence of a penis anterior to the scrotum.

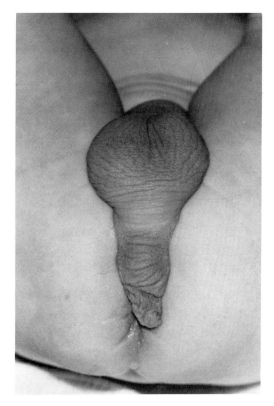

FIG. 9-3. Mass of erectile tissue posterior to the penis is covered with ectopic scrotal skin.

ureters ending blindly. At laparotomy, no bladder was found to be present, and a bilateral cutaneous ureterostomy was carried out. An attempt to bring the mass of erectile tissue through the scrotum to form some semblance of a penis was a failure, and in view of the impossibility of creating a functioning penis, a change of sex was suggested. This was refused by the parents.

The second case (Fig. 9-4) is interesting because it appears to show an intermediate stage between a scrotum in normal position and one in prepenile position. It can be seen that although the majority of the scrotum is fused and lies behind the penis, there is con-

siderable extension of scrotal skin anterior to the penis and extending almost to the midline so the penis appears to come through the center of the scrotum.

It may be noted that in marsupials it is normal for the penis to be situated posterior to the scrotum. McGuire [14] showed this condition to exist in the wallaby.

It has been suggested [20] that the embryological explanation of the condition is that there is retardation in the development of the pars phallica of the urogenital sinus associated with retardation in the development of the genital tubercle. This in turn influences the development of the labioscrotal swellings

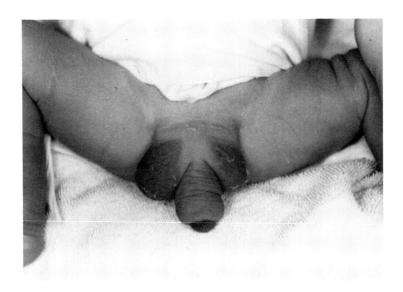

FIG. 9-4. Case showing the penis emerging from the center of the scrotum.

anterior to the genital tubercle, where they continue to grow and fuse to form the pre-penile scrotum.

Treatment involves correction of the abnormalities if they are not such as to be incompatible with life. The penis is generally brought through the scrotum by means of a suitable through-and-through incision, and the scrotum is reconstituted in the normal position behind the penis.

WEBBED SCROTUM

This term is applied to the condition in which a web extends between the penis and scrotum [10] (Fig. 9-5); the condition is seen most commonly in cases of intersex and perineal hypospadias. Generally the penis is small and poorly developed, and it would appear that sufficient growth of the genital tubercle has not occurred to bring the penis away from the developing scrotal folds. Such a case is shown in Figure 9-6. Treatment consists of resection and Z-plasty to the web, which are carried out at the same time as correction of chordee (in cases associated with

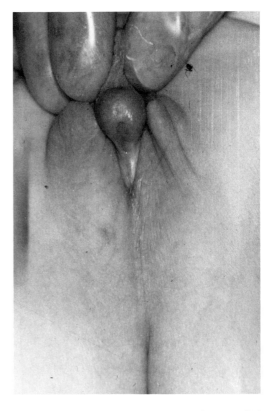

FIG. 9-5. Webbing between a hypospadial penis and bifid scrotum.

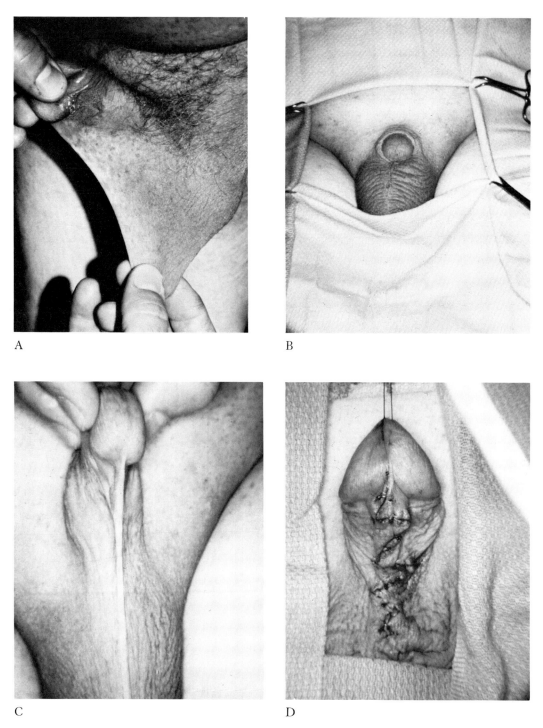

FIG. 9-6.   A.   Webbed scrotum extending to old circumcision scar at frenum. Patient had pain on coitus because the scrotum pulled on the scar. This case was treated by Z-plasties.   B.   A short penis partially retracted into scrotum may be noted.   C.   Congenital web, anterior view. This fibrous band causes pain with erection.   D.   Same case immediately postoperatively after Z-plasties have been performed.

hypospadias) or of clitoridectomy and labial reduction (in cases of adrenogenital syndrome). In cases of perineal hypospadias, the associated bifid scrotum must also be dealt with.

ECTOPIC SCROTUM

This condition has been described even less frequently than prepenile scrotum, seven cases having been reported in the literature. Adair and Lewis [1] reported a case in which the ectopic scrotum lay on the anterior abdominal wall and in which there was associated diphallia, the seventieth such case reported in the literature. Flanagan et al. [5] described a case in which the left half of the scrotum was located cranially and the right half caudally to the penis. Both halves of the scrotum contained testes and the penis appeared normal. The right renal pelvis was reduplicated, and the left kidney and ureter were absent. In addition, multiple orthopedic abnormalities were present. Bajaj and Bailey [2] have reported a case in which the right half of the scrotum was situated on the medial aspect of the right thigh, and Milroy [16] described a case of an adult West Indian in whom the left half of the scrotum was absent and a small patch of ectopic scrotal tissue in the left inguinal region contained an atrophic testis.

Most of the cases reported showed the presence of a testis within the ectopic scrotal tissue, and in all but three cases the kidney was absent on the affected side. A case seen by the author (Fig. 9-7) shows an ectopic scrotum lying behind the penis, which was found on excision to contain a teratomatous mass extending deep into the perineum.

Treatment has consisted of excision of the ectopic scrotal tissue together with the atrophic testis if it is lying too far away from the normal half of the scrotum to be reconstructed with the normal side by transposition of the ectopic scrotum and testis. A full investigation of the upper renal tract should certainly be undertaken in such a case, and it would seem probable that most of the testes present in the ectopic tissue would be functionless and best removed. No reports of testicular biopsy results were found in the cases reviewed.

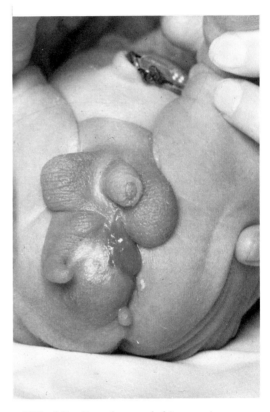

FIG. 9-7. Ectopic scrotal skin covering a teratomatous mass in the perineum.

References

1. Adair, E. L., and Lewis, E. L. Ectopic scrotum and diphallia. *J. Urol.* 84:115, 1960.
2. Bajaj, P. S., and Bailey, B. Ectopic scrotum: A review of the literature and report of a further case. *Br. J. Plast. Surg.* 22:87, 1969.
3. Bergmann, J. F. *Normale und abnormale Entwicklung des Menschen.* Weisbaden, 1911.
4. Campbell, M. F. Transposition of Penis and Scrotum. In Campbell, M. F. (Ed.), *Urology,* vol. 2. Philadelphia: Saunders, 1970, Pp. 1576–1577.
5. Flanagan, M. J., McDonald, J. H., and Krifer, J. H. Ectopic scrotum. *J. Urol.* 86:273, 1961.
6. Forshall, I., and Rickham, P. P. Transposition of the penis and scrotum. *Br. J. Urol.* 28:250, 1956.
7. Francis, C. L. Prepenile scrotum. *Anat. Rec.* 76:303, 1940.
8. Gross, R. E. *Abdominal Surgery of Infancy and Childhood.* Philadelphia: Saunders, 1953.
9. Gualatieri, T., and Segal, A. D. Prepenile scrotum in a double monster. *J. Urol.* 71:488, 1954.
10. Hamilton, W. J., Boyd, J. D., and Mossman, H. W. *Human Embryology.* Cambridge, England: Heffer, 1962.
11. Hinman, F. *Principles and Practice of Urology.* Philadelphia: Saunders, 1935.
12. Hontan, E. S. *Paediatr. Esp.* 24:344, 1935.
13. Huffman, L. F. Prepenile scrotum. *J. Urol.* 65:141, 1951.
14. McGuire, N. G. Prepenile scrotum. *Br. J. Surg.* 42:203, 1954.
15. McIlvoy, D. B., and Harris, H. S. Transposition of penis and scrotum. *J. Urol.* 73:540, 1955.
16. Milroy, E. Ectopic scrotum. *Br. J. Urol.* 41:235, 1969.
17. Nagata, M. Case of transposition of the penis and scrotum. *Jap. J. Urol.* 57:305, 1966.
18. Remzi, D. Transposition of the penis and scrotum. *J. Urol.* 95:555, 1966.
19. Slikodny, A. Congenital accretion of the penis to the scrotum. *Urol. Nefrol. (Moskva)* 31:55, 1966.
20. Spalding, M. H. *Contributions to Embryology.* Washington, D.C.: Carnegie Institute, 1921.

Exstrophy
of the Cloaca

EDWARD S. TANK

I O

FORTUNATELY, the complex anomaly termed *exstrophy of the cloaca* occurs only once in 200,000 live births. During the past 100 years, 94 cases of exstrophy of the cloaca have been recorded in the world literature [2, 3, 4]. The first successful reconstruction was reported by Rickham [2] in 1960. Three subsequent survivors have been documented.

The anomaly primarily involves the intestinal and genitourinary tracts. The major presenting defect is exstrophy of the cecum lying between two exstrophied halves of the bladder (Fig. 10-1). Two of the four orifices may be found on the central colonic plate. The most cephalad aperture is that of the terminal ileum, which is frequently prolapsed. The caudal opening leads into a pouch of colon of variable length that usually ends blindly in the pelvis. The anus is imperforate. One or two appendices may open on the everted cecum. The ureters open onto the exstrophied halves of the bladder.

An omphalocele is part of the complex in 90 percent of the recorded cases (Fig. 10-2). Vertebral anomalies occur in 75 percent of these newborns, and meningoceles have been recorded in 40 percent of the patients. Lower extremity deformities, especially talipes equinovarus, are frequent. Upper urinary

tract anomalies occur in 60 percent of the cases. These defects range from total absence of the kidneys to simple ptosis of the kidneys. Sex distribution is equal. Failure of complete fusion of the müllerian system almost always results in complete or partial uterine duplication and frequently results in a duplicated vagina. The vagina is absent in 25 percent of the female patients. In 50 percent of the males, the penis is small and bifid, and it is absent in another 30 percent.

Significant anomalies in other major systems are rare. Central nervous system aberrations, aside from meningocele, are uncommon, and survivors are reported to be of normal intelligence. Consequential cardiovascular defects are infrequent. Many infants who survive past the first few weeks of life will manifest a "short-bowel syndrome" that eventually causes their death. Subsequent necropsy usually reveals a small intestine of normal length, so it is presumed that the rapid transit time is due to physiological rather than anatomical factors.

Embryology

Patten and Barry [1] have proposed a generally accepted embryological basis for epi-

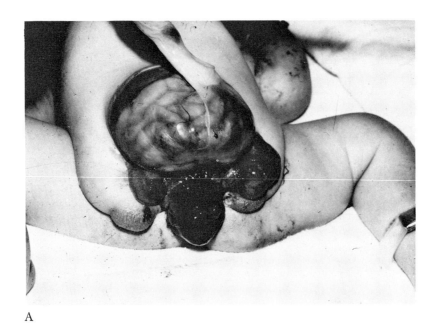

A

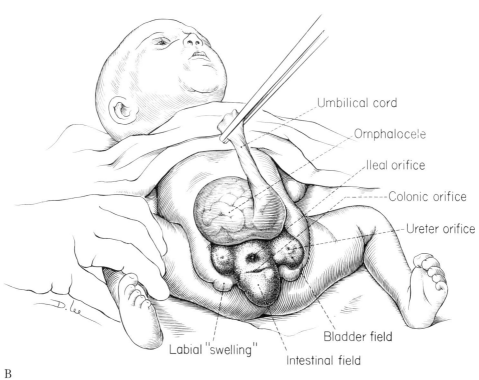

Umbilical cord

Omphalocele

Ileal orifice

Colonic orifice

Ureter orifice

Bladder field

Labial "swelling"

Intestinal field

B

FIG. 10-1. A and B. External anatomy of exstrophy of the cloaca.

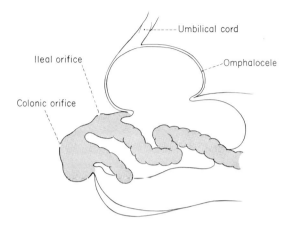

FIG. 10-2. Internal anatomy of exstrophy of the cloaca. (From Tank and Lindenauer [5].)

spadias and exstrophy of the bladder. This concept has been extended by Rickham [2] as an explanation for exstrophy of the cloaca. Anyone wishing to understand this concept clearly must read their original articles carefully.

Normally, the primordia of the genital tubercles (which are apparent at 2 weeks of gestation) are located anterolateral to the margins of the cloacal membrane. During the fifth week of life, the urorectal fold descends to divide the cloaca into an anterior urogenital sinus and posterior rectum. At this time, the genital tubercles migrate to the midline and fuse cranial to the cloacal membrane. The same convergent growth process also brings mesoderm into place, which is essential to the formation of the infraumbilical portion of the abdominal wall. The solitary median genital tubercle then differentiates into the penis and scrotum or the clitoris and labia. The cloacal membrane subsequently ruptures, and the urethral, vaginal, and anal orifices open onto the perineum.

Patten and Barry [1] hypothesize that anomalous development results when the paired genital tubercles arise caudally to their normal anterolateral location in relation to the cloacal membrane. Location of the genital tubercle primordia at the midportion of the cloacal membrane, where the urorectal fold completes partition of the cloaca into the urogenital sinus and rectum, causes incomplete fusion of the tubercles and produces epispadias. Incomplete migration of accompanying mesoderm leaves the lower abdominal wall ectoderm and bladder entoderm unsupported. This results in the rupture of these lamina and extroversion of the bladder.

A further caudal locus of these primordia prohibits any tubercular fusion and eventuates in either completely absent or bifid, undeveloped external genitalia. The absence of essential supportive connective tissue prohibits development of the urorectal fold. This results in arrest at the cloacal stage, with the occurrence of atresia of the distal colon and imperforate anus. Extroversion of the proximal colon and bladder also occurs when the infraumbilical abdominal wall ruptures because of the lack of critical connective tissue. Associated failure of development or fusion of the müllerian system causes vaginal and uterine atresia or duplication.

Preoperative Evaluation

Complete and critical preoperative evaluation is the most fundamental step in the management of these children. In spite of the initial dismay over the multiplicity of defects, careful analysis frequently confirms that the anomalies are primarily structural and do not compromise the essential physiological functions of the infant. These children seldom present surgical emergencies, and time is available for careful and complete consideration of all aspects of the problem.

It is my opinion that these infants should be given the opportunity to survive if certain anatomical and physiological criteria are met.

Urogenital Sinus Outlet Obstruction

EDWARD S. TANK

11

A FEMALE child born with a persistent urogenital sinus will usually require a corrective surgical procedure some time during her early life. Newborn infants with imperforate urogenital sinus outlet present with urinary tract obstruction and need immediate decompression by removal of the obstructing membrane. Infants and children with outlet stenosis may manifest recurrent urinary tract infections or urinary incontinence which may necessitate early surgical correction. Girls with asymptomatic urogenital sinuses will at some time require plastic revision to create an adequate vaginal introitus in order to ensure proper sexual function [3].

Embryology

An understanding of the embryology of the female lower genitourinary tract is essential. During the fifth week of intrauterine life, the cloaca divides into the dorsal rectum and ventral urogenital sinus by ingrowth of the urorectal folds into the cephalic portion of the cloaca where the allantois and midgut meet (Fig. 11-1). Completion of this septation divides the distal cloacal membrane into the anterior urogenital sinus and posterior proctodeal membranes. These membranes rupture at the seventh week of intrauterine life, and the urogenital sinus and anus open separately onto the perineum. The allantois then dilates and becomes the urinary bladder. At this time, the müllerian ducts have fused and meet the urogenital sinus at the müllerian tubercle. This area of junction is excavated and the vaginal lumen is separated from the urogenital sinus by a thin membrane which will become the hymen. The urogenital sinus exphiates, and the urethral meatus and vaginal introitus open separately onto the perineum. The urethra is formed entirely from the urogenital sinus. The vaginal introitus usually is partially occluded by the posterior portion of the urogenital sinus membrane that later becomes the hymen. If this final stage of development is arrested, a urogenital sinus results. If the outlet membrane persists, complete obstruction of the passage of urine to the outside occurs.

Complete Urogenital Sinus Outlet Obstruction

Three newborn infants with complete membranous outlet obstruction have been

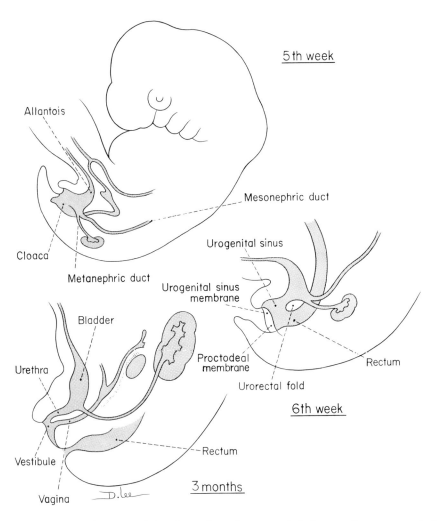

FIG. 11-1.   Initial partitioning of the cloaca into the urogenital sinus and rectum, and the subsequent division of the urogenital sinus into the urethra and distal vagina.

treated at the University of Michigan Hospital. All three presented with anuria and a lower abdominal mass. On careful examination of the perineum, a membrane of varying thickness completely obstructing the urogenital sinus was found.

Since the production of urine commences during the seventh week of intrauterine life, other routes of passage of urine beyond the bladder must be developed in utero to prevent damage to the urinary collecting system. In the infant with complete urogenital sinus outlet obstruction, voided urine reflects off the obstructing membrane and flows into the vagina, uterus, and fallopian tubes, which gradually enlarge and may reach phenomenal size. The ability of the genital tract to accommodate this large volume of urine usually protects the urinary collecting system. The urine reaches the perineal cavity through the uterus and fallopian tubes and is reabsorbed and eliminated by way of the peritoneum. The handling of waste products by way of the maternal circulation is precipitously interrupted at birth, and decompression of the urogenital sinus becomes urgent before azotemia develops.

A recent case illustrates these points. A child, who was first examined here at 48 hours of age, had absence of urine, elevated blood urea nitrogen, and a lower abdominal mass. Intravenous pyelography had been performed at an outside hospital 24 hours before the child was transferred to the University of Michigan Hospital. This study revealed right hydronephrosis and hydroureter, and there was nonvisualization of the left kidney and ureter. Films taken 24 hours later revealed a

lower abdominal mass filled with contrast material (Fig. 11-2). The diagnosis was made at this time, and the membrane was excised. Injection into the urogenital sinus confirmed the presence of a capacious but completely decompressed vagina, and spilling of the contrast media into the peritoneal cavity by way of the uterus and a solitary right fallopian tube was noted (Fig. 11-3). Direct catheterization of the urethra demonstrated anterior displacement of the bladder (Fig. 11-4). Subsequent peylograms taken 1 month later revealed a normal collecting system on the right. Persistent nonvisualization of the urinary collecting system on the left was believed to be due to agenesis of the left kidney. Excision of the obstructing membrane led to a prompt return of the urinary collecting

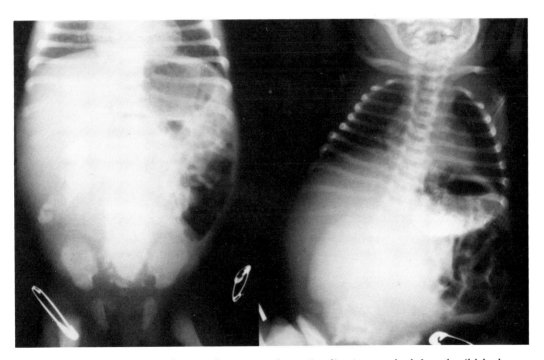

FIG. 11-2. Intravenous pyelogram demonstrated nonvisualization on the left and mild hydroureteronephrosis on the right. Twenty-four hours later, contrast medium was pooled in a large pelvic structure.

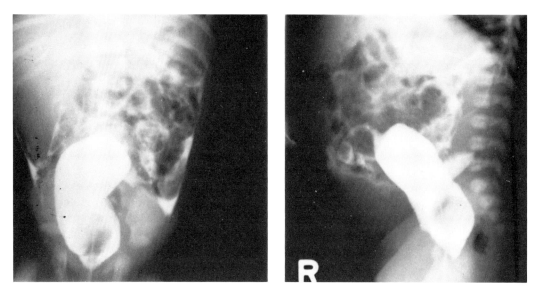

FIG. 11-3. Injection of the urogenital sinus demonstrated a capacious vagina, a uterus, and a solitary fallopian tube as well as spillage into the peritoneal cavity.

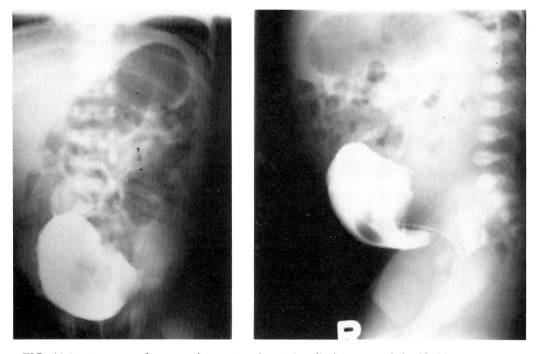

FIG. 11-4. A cystourethrogram demonstrated anterior displacement of the bladder.

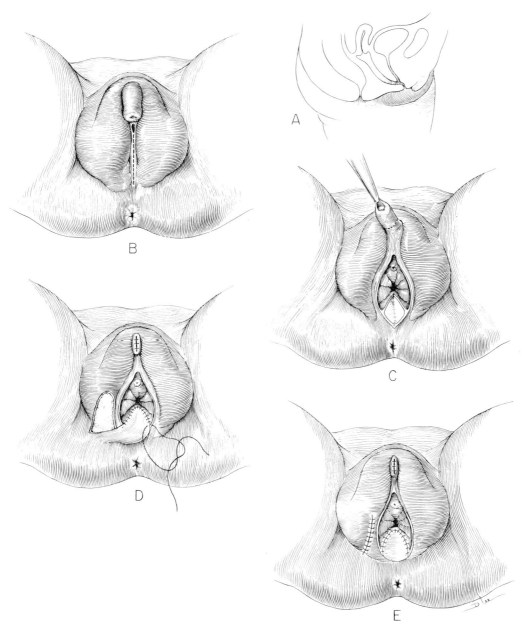

FIG. 11-5. Complete clitoridectomy is performed. Vaginoplasty is accomplished by posterior incision into the urogenital sinus with insertion of a labial skin flap.

system and genital organs to almost normal size.

Urogenital Sinus Outlet Stenosis

These children usually present with recurrent urinary tract infections secondary to pooling of urine in the dilated vagina and urogenital sinus. Another frequent manifestation of this condition is incontinence of urine. On voiding, urine flows into the capacious vagina, rather than through the narrow outlet passage, and then dribbles slowly out through the stenotic sinus. A membrane that partially occludes the outlet or actual narrowing of the distal portion of the sinus is apparent on perineal examination. The urethral meatus is at the cephalad end of the urogenital sinus and usually cannot be seen without instrumentation. The most effective form of surgical correction consists of posterior incision of the stenotic outlet and interposition of a lateral, labial skin flap (Fig. 11-5). It is not necessary to alter the location of the urethral meatus.

Slightly less than half of the female patients with adrenogenital syndrome will have a persistent urogenital sinus. A large phallus will almost always be present. If the family desires clitoridectomy in the newborn period, a vaginoplasty should not be attempted at this time. Only two of the 20 vaginoplasties performed on female patients with persistent urogenital sinus secondary to adrenogenital syndrome have required revision. In both cases, plastic revision of the sinus was attempted at the time of clitoridectomy, which was performed within the first 2 months of age. Vaginoplasty should not be considered until the child reaches such a size that technical success will be assured; two years of age is the youngest that this should be done on an elective basis [1].

Simple labia minora fusion that partly occludes the vaginal introitus may mimic urogenital sinus outlet obstruction or stenosis. The urethral meatus, however, is normally placed and is readily seen on careful examination. Simple separation or incision of the labial adhesion is definitive if care is taken to ensure separation until healing and reepithelialization [4].

References

1. Fortunoff, S., Lattimer, J. K., and Edson, M. Vaginoplasty technique for female pseudohermaphrodites. *Surg. Gynecol. Obstet.* 118:545, 1964.
2. Harrison, R. G. *Textbook of Human Embryology.* Philadelphia: F. A. Davis, 1963. Pp. 157–174.
3. Jones, H. W., and Scott, W. W. (Eds.) *Hermaphroditism, Genital Anomalies and Related Endocrine Disorders* (2d. ed.). Baltimore: Williams & Wilkins, 1971.
4. Lodi, A. Contributo clinico statistico sulle malformazione della vagina osservate nella Clinica Obstetrica e Ginecologia di Milano del 1906 al 1950. *Ann. Ostet. Ginecol.* 73:1246, 1951.
5. Patten, B. M. *Foundations of Embryology.* New York: McGraw-Hill, 1958. Pp. 449–483.
6. Stephens, F. D. Urethro-vaginal malformations. *Aust. N. Z. J. Obstet. Gynaecol.* 6:64, 1966.
7. Tank, E. S., Konnak, J. W., and Lapides, J. Urogenital sinus outlet obstruction. *J. Urol.* 104:769, 1970.

Exstrophy of the Urinary Bladder

IAN M. THOMPSON
HAL G. BINGHAM

12

Historical Background

UNTIL THE FIRST urinary diversion procedure was attempted for exstrophy of the urinary bladder in 1852 by Syme [16], the management of this socially appalling defect was concluded to be hopeless. Although a great number of surgical procedures to ameliorate the condition have been carried out since that time, the problem remains as difficult a clinical situation as ever. From the time of Syme's ureterosigmoid anastomosis in a patient with exstrophy, implantation of the ureters into the colon for continent storage of urine was the major goal, and excision of the bladder with reconstruction of the abdominal wall was of secondary priority.

When Maydl [11] in 1894 transplanted the bladder trigone into the rectum, he acknowledged that ureteral anastomosis to the intact colon had serious inherent deficiencies with regard to ascending infection and electrolyte disturbances. Unfortunately, his attempt to protect the upper tracts with the sphincteric mechanism of the trigone was unsuccessful. Despite the deficiencies of this form of urinary diversion, Coffey's [3] standardization of ureterosigmoidostomy in the early 1900s perpetuated it as the best solution for exstrophy until the gradual accumulation of data regarding the hazards inherent in the operation culminated in the report of Harvard and Thompson [6]. This report showed that even for benign disease, there was not only considerable morbidity but substantial mortality resulting primarily from renal failure. The increasing popularity of a conduit form of diversion—the ileal segment of Bricker [2], which appeared about the time of this report—brought about the rejection of ureteral anastomosis to the intact bowel and the substitution of a controllable form of incontinence for the unmanageable incontinence of exstrophy.

A great number and variety of surgical procedures were devised and sporadically utilized after the early 1900s in an attempt to retain the benefits of continence of urine and yet avoid the hazards posed by renal infection and electrolyte absorption. Of these ingenious and technically complicated assortments of anastomoses of the small to large bowel and reversals of intestinal loops with intussusceptions into intact large bowel, none had the desired effect and gradually most were abandoned. Surgeons in Britain still prefer in many instances to implant the ureters into the distal large bowel and sacrifice fecal control by performing proximal colostomy. Indeed, throughout the years, the options have not been considerable, since the only sphincter that is available in the area is the anorectal sphincter, and the sporadic early attempts at forming a sphincter surgically from the everted bladder neck area had not been promising.

In the 1950s, a resurgence of interest in the possibility of utilizing the exstrophic bladder as a reservoir for urine was stimulated by an occasional report of a successful outcome of bladder inversion with reconstruction of the bladder neck and posterior urethra in a form similar to the normal tubular disposition of the vesical outlet. A number of medical centers then embarked on series of cases of bladder reconstructions.

Orthopedic surgeons had periodically attacked the abnormal pelvic girdle of the child with bladder exstrophy in an attempt to change the characteristic waddling gait to an ostensibly more normal one, and many osteotomies to approximate the widely separated pubes were done for this purpose. They were almost universally abandoned when it became apparent that no orthopedic benefit resulted from these procedures. When urologists began their most recent attempts to invert the bladder and reconstruct the posterior urethra, osteotomy was again performed in a large number of patients to permit approximation of the pubes and the performance of an allegedly easier tubularization of the residual muscular structures of the posterior urethra. Lattimer and others [9] indicated that with posterior osteotomy, the pubes could be brought much closer together and the bladder and urethra could be more readily invaginated, but when wire was used

to provide for more permanent fixation of the pubes, it very frequently cut across and through the newly formed urethra as the pelvis splayed out again.

In most instances, it has been difficult to maintain the approximation of the pubes that is provided by posterior osteotomy, and this engendered attempts to divide the pubic rami near the arch and approximate them in this fashion. Leslie and Cook, who utilized this form of advancement of the pubes, found that approximation could be maintained more permanently than with posterior osteotomy. Although the invagination of the bladder and tubularized posterior urethra into the pelvis is somewhat easier when an osteotomy is performed, its effect on subsequent urinary continence does not seem to be pronounced. Approximation of the posterior urethral musculature that is available is just as easily performed without osteotomy, and osteotomy has never appeared to us to be the limiting factor in securing either tubularization of these structures or of urinary continence.

Although surgeons had utilized the bladder in a number of ways in the management of the child with exstrophy, Hepburn [7] was the first to retain the bladder musculature, after denudation of its mucosa, to support and give substance to the anterior abdominal wall in the midline. However, Culp's histopathological studies [5] indicated that the bladder in the patient with exstrophy might be a dysgenetic structure that perhaps should be removed to avoid complications, such as the development of the carcinoma that is known to ensue in the exstrophic bladder that remains everted. Although this has been a deterrent to vesical reconstruction, it has never been documented that exstrophic bladders are truly dysgenetic. It has been difficult to determine whether the changes described by Culp are really precursors of cancer or whether early inversion of the bladder might not obviate his histopathological findings by removing the constant irritation to which the everted bladder is subjected.

Muecke [12] and Marshall in their experimental studies have shown that the placement of a small foreign body on the developing anterior abdominal wall of the chick embryo reproduces forms of exstrophy seen in the human. They have postulated that the various types of exstrophy in the human can be explained on the basis of such a local deterrence to mesenchymal formation of the abdominal wall. Even though a precise mechanism for this deterrence has not been delineated, the theory is compatible with the various forms of exstrophy that have been reported.

Surgical Management

The most severe form of exstrophy occurs in association with omphalocele, and the least severe is epispadias without exstrophy. The most common type is, unfortunately, complete vesical exstrophy with eversion of the entire urethra. *Superior fissure* refers to an opening of the bladder into the abdominal wall in its cephalad portion only; *inferior fissure* consists of varying degrees of eversion of the bladder neck or posterior urethra that can, in less severe forms, be compatible with socially acceptable urinary control.

The selection of a course of action in the patient with exstrophy is governed by the nature and extent of the defect. There is no great difficulty in managing situations such as the superior fissure, where the upper portion of the bladder simply needs to be freed from the anterior abdominal wall and dropped back into the abdominal cavity. Similarly, the patient with a relatively well-apposed bladder neck or posterior urethral musculature may be successfully managed by

simple imbrication of these muscles. The child with epispadias alone will have continence of urine, and the creation of a distal urethral channel can be done quite readily with a number of standard techniques for urethroplasty.

The more severe forms of inferior fissure will require mobilization of the bladder, bladder base, vesical neck, and posterior urethral muscles, but tubularization of these structures will often result in satisfactory degrees of urinary control.

The omphalocele-exstrophy group may have such an assortment of anomalies that it is difficult to categorize the surgical approaches that may be needed, but a sorting out of exposed bowel and the performance of intestinal and cutaneous urinary diversions are usually the only feasible measures.

We have attempted almost every basic surgical alternative for classic exstrophy, and 20 years of experience has made us less than hopeful about the possibility of achieving a satisfactory bladder reservoir or a competent urethral sphincteric mechanism.

We believe that if the patient has a bladder with a small surface area, any attempt at inversion and reconstruction is doomed to failure. These bladders are composed more of fibrous tissue than muscle, and even if loops or patches of bowel are used in an attempt to enlarge the vesical capacity, considerable morbidity can result. Massive vesicoureteral reflux can be incurred by enclosing the ureteral orifices in such an unresilient cavity, even when urethral reconstruction has not produced any semblance of urinary continence. Since urethral muscle tubularization in these circumstances adds the hazard of producing stricture and further elevating intravesical pressure, we believe that the bladder should be removed and a compatible form of urinary diversion be instituted. We believe that if the anal sphincter has been shown to be competent and the upper urinary tracts are relatively normal, ureterosigmoidostomy should be done (see Fig. 12-7).

It is at times difficult to determine whether the anal sphincter is competent in the first few months of life, and we prefer, when the upper tracts are normal, to delay abdominal wall closure and ureterosigmoidostomy until we are certain of its competence. Surgery is usually feasible between 6 months and 1 year of age.

The reason why we feel ureterosigmoidostomy is the preferred diversion is that there is increasing evidence that a long submucosal tunnel (3 to 4 cm) provides sufficient periureteral muscularization to minimize, if not prevent, ascending infection. With currently available antibiotics and antibacterial agents, pyelonephritis can be readily treated should it occur, and with prophylactic medication, it may be avoided entirely. Under these circumstances, the patient with ureterosigmoidostomy can be continent of urine and probably also look forward to a relatively uncomplicated normal span of life.

If, after ureterosigmoidostomy, the patient does have difficulty with regard to pyelonephritis or electrolyte disturbances that pose a threat to renal reserve, then, without taking down the ureterointestinal anastomosis, the segment of the sigmoid in which the ureters are implanted can be brought out as a conduit, with reanastomosis of the large bowel. The sigmoid is equally as suitable as the ileum for urinary conduit diversion, and the operation is far simpler than the preparation of an ureteroileostomy.

Unfortunately there is a fairly high incidence of less-than-normal competence of the anal sphincter in children with exstrophy, and here—as in instances in which there is hydronephrosis, ureterectasis, or renal function depletion—ureterosigmoidostomy should best be avoided. Ureteroileostomy can be

done under these circumstances, or if the ureters are dilated and well-vascularized, any of the variations of nonintubated, skin-flap interposition cutaneous ureterostomy may be performed. In accord with the current lack of conclusive information as to the potential hazards of retaining a possibly dysgenetic bladder wall, bladders should probably be removed, leaving the prostatic and membranous urethra or vagina in place.

The type of bladder that we believe may warrant an attempt at closure with urethral reconstruction is one that is obviously capacious, that is easily inverted into the abdomen by digital pressure, and that seems to have muscular compliance similar to the normal bladder. There are, unfortunately, very few of these, and even under these circumstances, closure should be contemplated only if the child can be followed closely throughout the subsequent years to make certain that upper-tract form and function do not deteriorate.

In closing the bladder, dissection is begun at the top, encircling the upper portion of the vesical circumference with an incision down to the peritoneum. In this manner, the bladder may be peeled from the peritoneum and dissected downward on each side so that prior to the more tedious dissection and tubularization of the bladder neck and urethral areas, an assessment of the potential capacity and compliance of the bladder and its muscle can be made. It may become apparent that the muscularity and potential size of the vesical cavity have been inaccurately or too optimistically assessed, and the attempt at inversion can then be abandoned.

If closure appears to be feasible, dissection is continued down to where the inferior vascular pedicle becomes apparent at the bladder neck area. Here, dissection must preserve blood supply in order for the posterior urethral muscle to be adequately nourished. At the vesical neck and posterior urethral areas, the incisions should be carried out laterally to the visible musculature in the area where the fibrous bands have their attachments to the interpubertal fascia. These fascial handles can then be used to roll the vesical neck and posterior urethral musculature inward to permit their tubularization without putting tension upon the muscles themselves.

The muscle margins should be skirted widely, and only the fibrous tissue structures overlying the pubes are undermined and turned in to be sutured to each other. This will permit apposition of the vesicourethral outlet musculature and its imbrication with fine sutures without tension, since the fibrous tissue handles from each side will hold the heavier sutures and permit coaptation of the outlet muscle around a small catheter with preservation of its vascularity. The posterior urethral tubularization should extend up through the vesical neck area to a point just below the ureteral orifices, and transverse incisions into the bladder muscle at this juncture will permit the formation of a longer muscular tube to serve as a urethral sphincter. We no longer employ osteotomy in any form, but rely on careful dissection lateral to the vesicourethral outlet musculature in order to provide coaptation and tubularization in the sphincteric area. With the technique that has been developed by one of us (Dr. Bingham) to close the abdominal wall defect in the patient with exstrophy, osteotomy has also been unnecessary. Since the rectus muscles are widely separated at their insertion in the cleft pubic rami, either removal or reconstruction of the urinary bladder requires reconstitution of the abdominal wall to provide coverage of the defect between the divergent recti. Several procedures have been utilized in which fascia is brought in to cover the midline defect. Rectus fascial autografts have been employed, and lateral thigh fascia lata has been woven back and forth between the rectus muscles to buffer the defect in the infraumbilical wall.

In the majority of instances, iliac osteotomy has been necessary to approximate the rectus muscles and lateral fascia when grafts have not been employed, and often the abdominal closure has been disrupted or compromised as fixation of the osteotomy has been lost.

The closure that we rely on provides a sound abdominal wall without osteotomy and without fascial grafts. It consists of a rotation-advancement of rectus muscle and fascia in the following manner. The paired rectus muscles are divided about halfway between their pubic and costal attachments, and the cephalad portion is allowed to retract (Fig. 12-1). The caudal segments of rectus muscle are then dissected from the rectus fascia to their lateral borders, where an attempt is made not to disrupt the segmented innervation (Fig. 12-2). The nerves to the distal segments of rectus muscle are preserved so the flaps remain dynamic (Fig. 12-3). The muscles then provide a "continuous force," or midline pull, on the pubic rami after they are united by imbrication (Fig. 12-4). The posterior rectus sheath is left undisturbed, but the anterior rectus sheath is divided at the same level of the rectus muscle. The anterior sheath is then incised laterally, allowing for rotation and advancement, so that it can be approximated to its fellow in the midline to form a double-layer closure with the rectus muscle (Fig. 12-5).

The technique utilizes the rotation-advancement principle and provides an opportunity for a subsequent spontaneous closure of the cleft between the pubic rami. This is somewhat analogous to a cleft lip repair that reconstitutes the orbicularis oris muscle and, in many cases, forces the malaligned and separated maxillary segments into proper position by a continuous dynamic force.

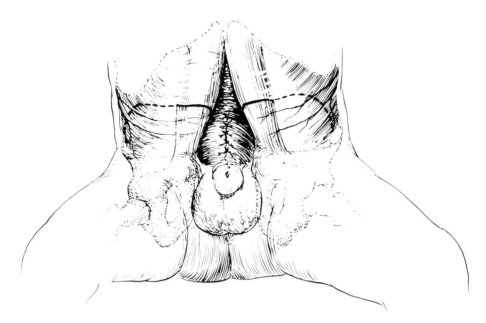

FIG. 12-1. Incision through the rectus muscle.

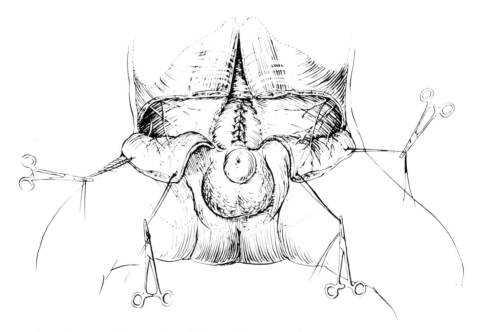

FIG. 12-2. Segmental innervation of the recti is preserved.

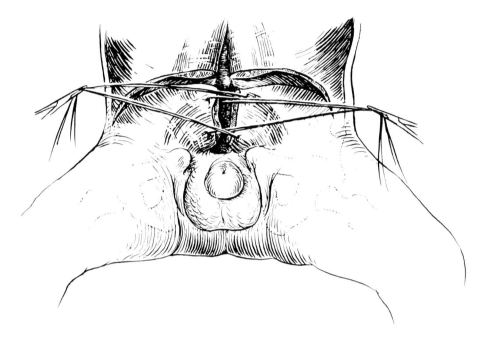

FIG. 12-3. The flaps remain dynamic.

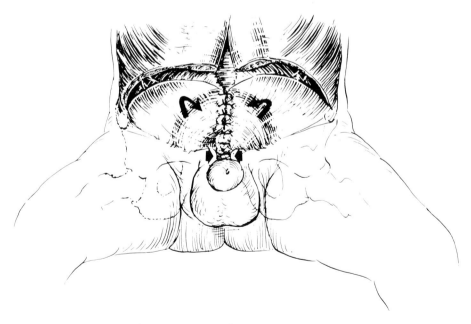

FIG. 12-4. Continuous midline pull is provided by the recti.

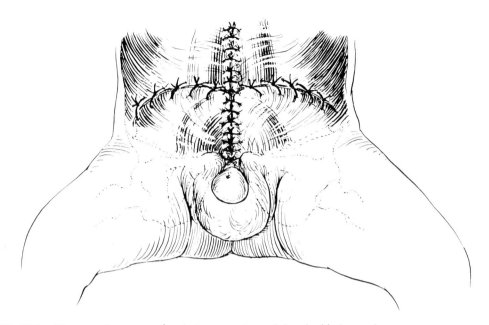

FIG. 12-5. The anterior rectus sheath is approximated for double-layer closure.

FIG. 12-6. Cutaneous closure is obtained with French rotation flaps.

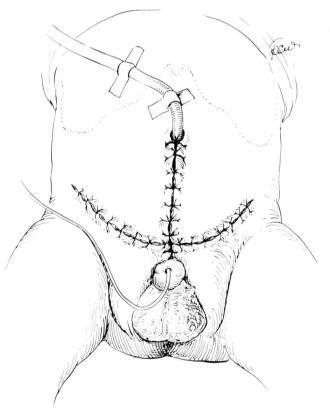

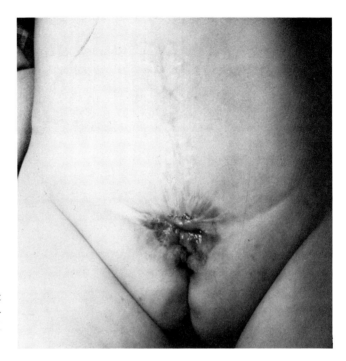

FIG. 12-7. Postoperative patient with rectus muscle and fascia rotation flap closure. Urine was diverted by ureterosigmoidostomy.

The cutaneous closure over the exstrophied bladder is accomplished by a French rotation flap technique, with the incisions being made in the skin just above the level of the pubic rami (Figs. 12-6 and 7).

In summary, management of the patient with exstrophy must be tailored to the type and extent of the abdominal wall and vesicourethral defects. Superior and inferior fissure forms of the condition and the infrequently observed large exstrophic bladder are amenable to vesical closure and sphincteric reconstruction. Small exstrophic bladders should not be closed, but should be removed and an appropriate diversion of the urine carried out. Closure of the abdominal wall does not require osteotomy when the rectus fan-type reconstruction that we employ is performed.

References

1. Baret, A. C., DeMuth, E. E., Murphy, J. J., and Muri, M. W. Experimental repair of exstrophy of the bladder without cystectomy by using a free fascial graft. *Surg. Gynecol. Obstet.* 97:633, 1953.
2. Bricker, E. Substitution for urinary bladder by use of isolated ileal segments. *Surg. Clin. North Am.* 36:503, 1956.
3. Coffey, R. C. Transplantation of the ureters into large intestine. *Surg. Gynecol. Obstet.* 47:593, 1928.
4. Cook, F. E., Jr., Leslie, J. T., and Brannon, E. W. Preliminary report: A new concept of abdominal closure in infants with exstrophy of the bladder. *J. Urol.* 87:823, 1962.
5. Culp, D. A. The histology of the exstrophied bladder. *J. Urol.* 91:538, 1964.
6. Harvard, B. M., and Thompson, G. J. Con-

genital exstrophy of the bladder: Late results. *J. Urol.* 55:225, 1951.

7. Hepburn, T. N.   Repair of exstrophy of the bladder. *J. Urol.* 65:389, 1951.

8. Hinman, F., and Weyrauch, H. M. J.   A clinical study of different principles of surgery used in uretero-intestinal implantation. *Trans. Am. Assoc. Genitourin. Surg.* 29:15, 1936.

9. Lattimer, J. K., and Smith, M. J. V.   Exstrophy closure: A followup on 70 cases. *J. Urol.* 95:356, 1966.

10. Longacre, J. J., DeStefano, G. A., and Davidson, D. A.   Plastic repair of congenital defects of the ventral body wall. *Plast. Reconstr. Surg.* 23:260, 1959.

11. Maydl, K.   Ueber die Radikaltherapie der Blaseneftopie. *Wien. Med. Wochenschr.* 44:25, 1894.

12. Muecke, E. C.   The role of the cloacal membrane in exstrophy. *J. Urol.* 92:659, 1964.

13. O'Phelan, E. H.   Iliac osteotomy in exstrophy of the bladder. *J. Bone Joint Surg.* [*Am.*] 45:1409, 1963.

14. Shultz, W. G.   Plastic repair of exstrophy of the bladder combined with bilateral osteotomy of the ilea. *J. Urol.* 79:453, 1958.

15. Sweetser, T. H.   Exstrophy of urinary bladder. *Arch. Surg.* 68:525, 1954.

16. Syme, J.   Ectopia vesicae. *Lancet* 2:568, 1852.

17. Thompson, I. M.   Management of exstrophy of the urinary bladder by primary closure. *South. Med. J.* 54:1069, 1961.

18. Young, H. H.   Exstrophy of the bladder. *Surg. Gynecol. Obstet.* 74:729, 1942.

Ectopia Vesicae
and Epispadias

DAVID N. MATTHEWS

13

THESE CONDITIONS are both manifestations of the same congenital malformation, varying only in degree. Ectopia vesicae, or exstrophy of the bladder, is almost invariably accompanied by epispadias. The majority of patients in whom the deformity is limited to epispadias are incontinent, although occasionally a child is partially or even wholly continent.

Embryology

Initially, the cloacal membrane extends forward onto the ventral surface of the embryo as far as the allantois (Fig. 13-1A). This ectodermal-covered and entodermal-lined membrane should receive mesodermal ingrowths to separate its layers and form the musculature of the anterior abdominal wall as far as the allantoic stalk at the umbilicus, as well as to form the pelvic bones, genital tubercles, and the musculature of the anterior bladder wall. Thus, only the posterior part of the cloacal membrane should persist in its original form and subsequently rupture. Similarly, a mesodermal downgrowth should take place between the hindgut and the allantois; in

cases of epispadias and ectopia vesicae, some downgrowth does occur but in varying degree (Fig. 13-1B and C). This downgrowth is responsible for the musculature of the perineal floor and the rectal and bladder sphincters. This muscle mass can be demonstrated histologically, and the fibers responsible for the sphincters can be identified at the level of the bladder neck, although their arrangement is haphazard and their number very much less than normal (Fig. 13-2). Excellent papers on the embryology of this region have been published by Wyburn [6] and Davies [3].

The condition of epispadias and ectopia vesicae is essentially brought about, therefore, by failure in the development of and penetration by the mesodermal masses. This leaves the pubic symphysis and genital tubercles unfused, the anterior abdominal wall deficient, and the posterior bladder wall filling the gap. For the same reason, the crura and corpora are widely separated, being only fused at their dorsal extremities, with the urethral channel lying open upon them. From the foregoing, it will also be appreciated why the rectal as well as the vesical sphincter is often defective.

Restoration of normality in the face of such gross failures of development is a formidable

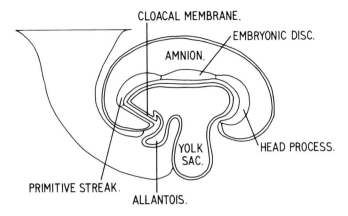

A

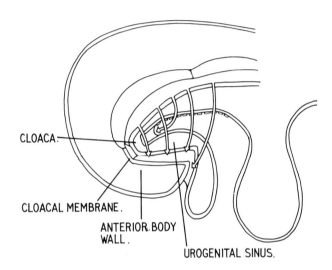

B

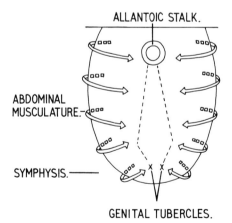

C

FIG. 13-1. A. Cloacal membrane extending forward to allantois. B. Mesodermal masses growing round the embryo to the anterior abdominal wall and down to separate the hindgut from the urogenital sinus. C. Mesodermal mass encircling the developing embryo. (From D. N. Matthews, *Br. J. Plast. Surg.* 11:188, 1959.)

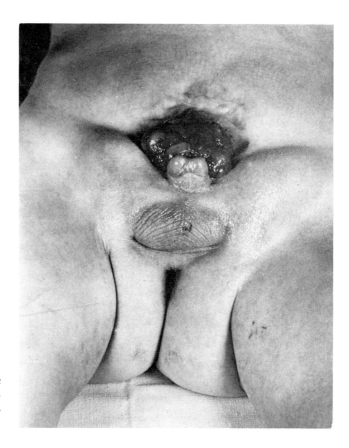

FIG. 13-2. Case in which the small amount of bladder tissue available makes reconstruction impossible.

undertaking, and the recognition that it is impossible in some circumstances is essential for the proper management of these unfortunate children. Ill-conceived operations that have no chance of success must be avoided by carefully assessing each individual. Only too often, repeated attempts are made when better judgment would save the child much suffering and the parents much anguish before the situation is finally rationalized and a tolerable solution is attained, for example, by a diversionary operation. Overriding and obvious facts, such as the absence of sufficient bladder mucosa and musculature to make a contractile bladder of useful size, are often overlooked (Fig. 13-3).

Epispadias

The most favorable case is one of epispadias with a bladder of normal size and little or no symphyseal separation. Some of these may be continent, in which case all that is required is simple closure of the urethra. The operation of Denis Browne [2] for fistula is as applicable to these as it is to hypospadias and is equally successful. It should also be employed preliminarily to a bladder neck resection in those patients with a bladder of normal size but without adequate control. The resection is aimed at tightening the sphincter by narrowing the outlet, and this may be combined with a suspensory sling if

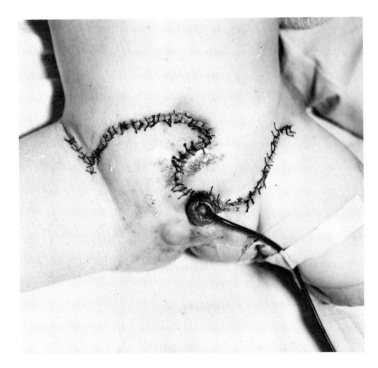

FIG. 13-3. Reconstructed bladder covered with double rotation flaps. (From D. N. Matthews, *Br. J. Plast. Surg.* 11:188, 1959.)

the neck of the bladder is initially very wide. This sling can be fashioned from a strip of the rectus sheath that is left attached to the symphysis and passed behind the vesicourethral junction immediately above the ejaculatory ducts.

If the symphyseal gap is wide, the operation of bilateral transiliac osteotomy to bring it together is indicated since the chances of obtaining a successful sphincteroplasty are thus improved. The immediate closure of the gap is always obtainable with this operation, but there is a tendency toward relapse no matter how firmly the symphysis is lashed together or whatever material is used to hold it. The operation is not difficult. With the child prone, a vertical incision is made over each buttock, and the outer table of the ilium is cut with an osteotome from the crest to the iliac notch behind the hip joint, taking care not to damage the superior gluteal artery in the notch. When both have been divided, the surgeon lifts the child and fractures the inner tables by manual compression. The child is then turned and the symphysis exposed for transfixion with fascia or wire. Any hopes that this operation will lengthen the penis by approximating the crura are disappointed because the backward rotation of the pubic bones, which accompanies symphyseal approximation, retracts the crura and draws the penile tip further upward and backward.

Ectopia Vesicae

Efforts to restore normality in the majority of these cases fail, but occasionally one presents in which the quantity of good bladder wall is large enough to justify the attempt. In the author's opinion, a transiliac osteotomy with symphyseal fusion is then an essential preliminary. This is followed by dissection of sufficient bladder wall to permit restoration of its anterior wall by infolding it, and by closure of the accompanying epispadias by the Denis Browne technique [2]. The reconstructed bladder is covered by double rotation flaps, which can easily be obtained from the abdominal skin, and the bladder is drained by a catheter. No attempt is made to narrow the bladder neck until the wound is well healed, however wide it may be. Occasionally, the sphincter proves strong enough to permit normal distensibility of the bladder and success is achieved. More often it is not, and incontinence results. Bladder neck resection, with or without a suspensory sling, is undertaken in these circumstances.

If a bladder is reconstructed in this way using rotation flaps for cover, it is not necessary to strengthen the hiatus between the rectus abdominis muscles; the skin flaps are adequate.

Cases of ectopia vesicae in which there is insufficient bladder mucosa, or in which it is of such poor quality that there is no chance of making a functioning bladder, must be treated by a diversionary operation without hesitation. There are several choices as to the type of diversion. If the rectal sphincter is strong enough, the time-honored method of implanting the ureters into the sigmoid colon can be very successful. With proper attention to details of technique, the risks of ascending ureteral infection are not prohibitive. Many patients treated in this way lead useful and comparatively trouble-free lives of average span. Only too often, however, inadequacy of the rectal sphincter makes the operation impossible.

The best alternative under these circumstances is to use an isolated ileal loop as a urinary reservoir into which both ureters drain and a closely sealed abdominal bag to collect the urine. Obviously, this is a great handicap to a child as well as to an adult, but it is infinitely preferable to struggling through life incontinent and infected. The operation was introduced by Bricker in 1950 [1] and is the natural successor to the abdominal reservoir fitted over the exposed trigonum vesicae, which was advocated by Holmes [4] in 1868. The author has no experience with the technique using the isolated rectum as a urinary reservoir and creating of a new anal opening behind it.

If a diversionary operation is needed, all bladder mucosa should be excised, no matter whether it is still on the surface or whether it is buried as the result of an attempted reconstruction that has failed. If allowed to remain, it becomes excoriated and infected and may lead to malignancy. In many such cases, the amount of mucosa is small and the area can be satisfactorily resurfaced with a free skin graft. If it is large, however, the resultant weakness of the abdominal wall should be strengthened either by a fascial graft or by suturing together the inwardly rotated anterior sheaths of the divaricated rectus abdominis muscles; the latter is the better method. If this or a fascial graft is required, the skin defect should be closed with rotation flaps instead of skin grafts.

In all male cases in which a diversionary operation is performed, the urethra should be closed by the Denis Browne technique up to and including the openings of the ejaculatory ducts.

References

1. Bricker, E. M. Bladder substitution after pelvic evisceration. *Surg. Clin. North Am.* 30:1511, 1950.

2. Browne, D. Hypospadias. *Postgrad. Med. J.* 25:367, 1949.
3. Davies, D. V. Ectopia vesicae. *Br. J. Urol.* 14:1, 1942.

4. Holmes, T. *Surgical Treatment of the Diseases of Infancy and Childhood* (2d ed.). London: Longmans, Green, Reader & Dyer, 1868.

5. Matthews, D. N.   Ectopia vesicae. *Br. J. Plast. Surg.* 11:188, 1958.

6. Wyburn, G. M.   The development of the infra-umbilical portion of the abdominal wall, with remarks on the aetiology of ectopia vesicae. *J. Anat. Lond.* 71:201, 1936.

Urinary Diversion in Exstrophy of the Bladder

JOHN W. DUCKETT

14

SINCE ONLY a small portion of exstrophied bladders are large and flexible enough to justify an attempt at reconstruction, some permanent form of urinary diversion will eventually be required in nearly all cases. Although the ileal conduit of Bricker [2] has the disadvantage of an abdominal stoma, it is certainly the safest diversion available today. Of the other possible diversions, ureterosigmoidostomy is generally favored as an acceptable compromise for the particular deformity of exstrophy. Spence [23] has reported an acceptable long-term result with this diversion in exstrophy, and the recent long-term evaluation at the Boston Children's Hospital [1] of 94 children with exstrophy of the bladder who were treated by ureterosigmoidostomy is indeed impressive.

Ureterosigmoidostomy should be undertaken only with the awareness and apprehension of the potentially devastating results. Only those patients with normal upper urinary tracts and normal caliber ureters are selected, and only then provided that the parents are fully aware of the long-term, specialized care required. Anal sphincter tone should be good, with no previous problem of

rectal prolapse. Postponement of diversion until the latter half of the first year of age allows a reasonable assessment of these considerations and an opportunity to know the family.

Ureterosigmoidostomy

SURGICAL TECHNIQUE

The infant's bowels are prepared for surgery with a clear liquid diet for 48 hours, and neomycin sulfate is given orally for 24 hours preoperatively. Cleansing enemas are given until clear, and a neomycin enema (1 g in 100 ml) is administered with the premedications of surgery.

The midline abdominal incision should not violate the bladder muscle. The ureters are then divided near the posterior bladder wall. A reflux-preventing implantation of the ureter into the sigmoid is accomplished with a mucosa-to-mucosa anastomosis in either of two techniques. With the Leadbetter [13, 14] combined technique, a tunnel is created on the side of the bowel by incising the seromuscular layer for a length of 3 to 4 cm between two vertically placed holding silks. Then the edges are dissected free from the underlying mucosa with blunt dissection for a width of 1 cm on each side. The mucosa is incised at the distal angle, and the end of the ureter is anastomosed to the mucosa with fine catgut using six interrupted sutures. The end of the ureter may need slight spatulating. The flaps of bowel muscle are then reapproximated over the ureter lying in the trough, making certain that no tension compresses the ureter and that the ureter is fixed to the seromuscular layer proximally. If the incision in the bowel muscle is made over the tenia, the seromuscular layers seem to separate easier from the mucosa, but there is probably no

other advantage for using the tenia. The posterior peritoneal incisions are then closed, covering the anastomotic sites. The uretero-colic anastomosis should be put into the rectosigmoid approximately 4 to 5 cm above the peritoneal reflection (Fig. 14-1).

The other commonly used technique for ureterosigmoidostomy is that described by Goodwin [7, 8]. He advocates a transcolonic exposure with a long vertical incision on the anterior bowel wall. The ureters are divided and the retroperitoneal posterior rectal wall is tented up into the anterior exposure. A mucosal incision is made, and, using a sharp-pointed curved clamp, the mucosa is separated from the seromuscular layer in a manner similar to a transvesical tunnelling proce-

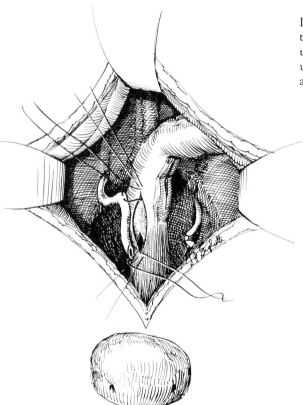

FIG. 14-1. Ureterosigmoidostomy; Leadbetter technique. A seromuscular trough is closed over 3.5 cm of ureter with a ureteral-to-mucosal anastomosis. The other ureter is placed in the bowel wall 3 cm above.

dure. Goodwin maintains that a 1 to 1.5 cm tunnel is adequate; it is difficult to obtain more length without tearing the mucosa or muscle. The curved clamp is turned to penetrate the bowel muscle wall posteriorly, and the ureter is then pulled through this newly created submucosal tunnel. The excess ureteral length is brought into the lumen of the rectum and excised obliquely so a mucosa-to-ureter anastomosis can be accomplished. After both ureters are transplanted, the anterior rectal wall is closed in two layers and the posterior peritoneal rents are closed. A drain can be left retroperitoneally and brought out through a side stab wound. The Goodwin technique requires an elaborate 4-day bowel preparation to clear and sterilize the colon and this, as well as the difficulty in establishing a long seromuscular tunnel, makes it less attractive (Fig. 14-2).

POSTOPERATIVE CARE

Immediately after ureterosigmoidostomy, the rectum should be drained with a large bore catheter with several holes until the child has begun stooling and is resuming oral intake. Even a mild atelectasis or pneumonia will cause pronounced hyperchloremic acidosis since the prime buffer mechanism of respiration is inefficient; thus, good pulmonary toilet is essential. Much that is useful to the surgeon has been written concerning the cause, management, and effects of chronic hyperchloremic acidosis and total body potassium deficiency [6, 16, 17, 27, 28]. To maintain an acceptable status, salt restriction and the use of Schol's solution (5 parts sodium citrate and 3 parts citric acid) as an oral buffer are helpful. Most important in the daily care is establishing a routine trip every 2 hours to the toilet to evacuate the rectum. A 3:00 A.M. alarm clock call is necessary if the patient prefers not to use a rectal tube at night.

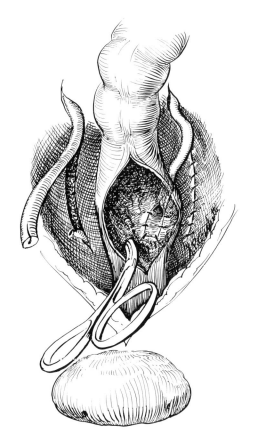

FIG. 14-2. Ureterosigmoidostomy; Goodwin technique. A submucosal tunnel is created from within the lumen of the rectosigmoid.

COMPLICATIONS

Failure of a ureterosigmoidostomy may be expected in one of five patients [1, 23] and should be apparent within the first 2 years. Urography every 3 to 6 months during that time will detect obstruction, parenchymal scarring, or stone formation sufficiently early before much damage is done. Recurrent attacks of pyelonephritis strongly indicate that obstruction or a refluxing state exists and that failure is imminent. Further surgical attempts at salvaging this arrangement, once failing, are discouraging. Conversion to another form of diversion separated from the fecal stream is then mandatory. The segment of colon into which the ureters are already implanted can be isolated and diverted through a left-sided stoma and the bowel continuity reestablished. This technique is more popular in Britain, with Mogg being the chief advocate. For American physicians, the next step is usually an ileal conduit.

Ileal Diversion

SURGICAL TECHNIQUE

Creation of a separate ileal segment with reanastomosis of the ureters to the small bowel provides a conduit of urine into an abdominal collection appliance. The left ureter is brought under the sigmoid mesentery and through the retroperitoneum with the right ureter just at the right pelvic brim. A segment of ileum is resected from the terminal 2 feet. Selection of a good vascular pedicle for the segment is aided by a cross-the-table spotlight transillumination of the mesentery [18]. It is preferable to choose a two-vessel arcade, being sure to keep the segment as short as possible. A 4 to 5 inch conduit is usually sufficient for a child. Normal bowel continuity is reestablished with a two-layer closure, and the appendix is removed.

Isoperistalsis must be maintained so the bowel will function as a conduit. A suture tag at one end or the other will help prevent the mishap of reversal. Bringing the ureters parallel as described by Wallace [26], with the spatulated ends overlapping slightly, provides a conjoined unit to which the proximal end of the ileum will be sutured. The edges of the ureters should be joined with a continuous fine catgut suture. Both ureters can be stented with the end of a T-tube, bringing the tail of the T out the segment. A fixing stitch will prevent this from pulling out. A

watertight closure is achieved by suturing the proximal bowel end circumference to the edges of the ureteral base with continuous fine catgut in three sections. The posterior peritoneum is closed around the anastomosis, and a drain left in the retroperitoneum is brought out the left side. The bowel segment is brought transperitoneally to the stoma site in the right lower quadrant, which has been previously selected and marked with a skin scratch. A standard Turnbull-type stoma is created with a 1 cm bud [25]. A permanent collecting device is attached to the stoma, with the stent lying freely within at the close of surgery so the child will remain dry.

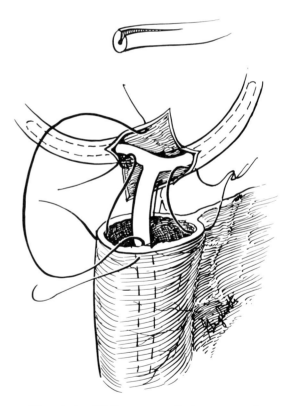

FIG. 14-3. Wallace ureteroileal anastomosis. The spatulated ureters are fixed beside one another and sutured into the end of the ileal segment with a T-tube stent.

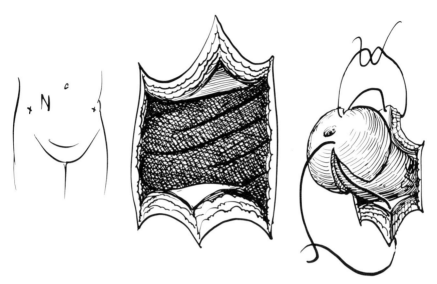

FIG. 14-4. Smith stomatoplasty. An N-shaped incision preserves a flap of skin to be placed into the superior and inferior sides of the bud of the ileum, creating an increased mucocutaneous junction.

COMPLICATIONS

The late complications of ileal segment diversion in children are primarily related to stenosis of the stoma at the skin level. The mucocutaneous junction seems to stricture more readily in children and can be expected to need surgical revision in 25 to 35 percent of the cases [20]. Smith [21] reports much less difficulty with the stoma when an N-type skin incision is made, using the X skin flaps to increase the mucocutaneous junction. More than 15 to 20 ml residual urine in the conduit is considered stasis and indicates the segment is redundant or that stenosis of the outlet exists [20]. Shortening of the conduit or revision of the stoma is then necessary. Hydronephrosis is usually caused by stricture at the ureteroileal anastomosis, which then requires revision. This may be a "silent" occurrence that only routine urography will detect. It is anticipated that the Wallace-type conjoined end anastomosis will diminish this problem. Certainly the complication rate with ileal conduit diversion is significant, and therefore close surveillance is required. Although several revisions may be required, a constant attempt to maintain a urine that is free of infection is rewarded with good results (Figs. 14-3 and 14-4).

Other Forms of Urinary Diversion

End cutaneous ureterostomies have very little use as permanent diversion except in instances where the renal function is so greatly diminished as to contraindicate the use of a bowel segment [5]. Bringing a grossly dilated obstructed ureter to the skin can sometimes temporize, but fluoroscopic evidence of effective peristalsis should exist. Normal or slightly dilated ureters brought to the skin will invariably stricture and require intubation, and therefore this technique should not be attempted.

Attempts to create a urinary reservoir that utilizes the anal sphincter for control of both bowel and urine have, in general, been disappointing. Lowsley and Johnston [12, 15] revived interest in the Gersuny procedure (1898) in which a closed rectal pouch for urine is created and the proximal sigmoid anterior to the rectum is brought through the anal sphincter. Fecal continence, however, may be difficult with this arrangement. Powell and Hays [19] modified the colonic diversion by interposing a segment of ileum between the reconstructed bladder and rectum in order to separate the fecal and urinary contents, but their long-term follow-up report is discouraging [9]. The Heitz-Boyer operation (1912) [10], revived and modified by Culp and Flocks [4], brings the sigmoid down posteriorly to the rectal pouch and makes a Duhamel-type anastomosis to the rectal ampulla. Snyder [22] modified the Heitz-Boyer technique slightly by connecting the rectal pouch to the turned-in exstrophied bladder and by bringing the sigmoid posteriorly to the skin. The complications resulting from these more elaborate arrangements to attempt to utilize the anal sphincter are less than satisfactory, but with renewed interest and modifications, some better form of diversion may evolve. Until that time, the safest—though by no means perfect—form of diversion remains the ileal conduit (Bricker [3]). However, the condition of exstrophic bladder with normal ureters lends itself optimally to a ureterosigmoidostomy diversion, thus avoiding the use of an abdominal stoma and appliance.

References

1. Bennett, A. H., and Eraklis, A. J. Long-term evaluation of ninety-four children with exstrophy of the bladder treated by ureterosigmoidostomies. In press.
2. Bricker, E. M. Bladder substitution after pelvic exenteration. *Surg. Clin. North Am.* 30:1511, 1950.
3. Bricker, E. M. Ileal Segment Urinary Diversion. In Cooper, P. (Ed.), *The Craft of Surgery* (2d ed.). Boston: Little, Brown, 1971. Pp. 1551–1567.
4. Culp, D. A., and Flocks, R. H. The diversion of urine by the Heitz-Boyer procedure. *Trans. Am. Assoc. Genitourin. Surg.* 57:25, 1965.
5. Eckstein, H. B., and Kapila, L. Cutaneous ureterostomy. *Br. J. Urol.* 42:306, 1970.
6. Ferris, D. O., and Odel, H. M. Electrolyte pattern of the blood after bilateral sigmoidostomy. *J.A.M.A.* 142:634, 1950.
7. Goodwin, W. E., Harris, A. P., Kaufman, J. J., and Bell, J. M. Open transcolonic uretero-intestinal anastomosis: A new approach. *Surg. Gynecol. Obstet.* 97:295, 1953.
8. Goodwin, W. E. Ureterosigmoidostomy (Open Transcolonic Uretero-intestinal Anastomosis). In Cooper, P. (Ed.), *The Craft of Surgery* (2d ed.). Boston: Little, Brown, 1971. Pp. 1514–1520.
9. Hays, D. M., Powell, T. O., and Strauss, J. Vesico-ileosigmoidostomy in the treatment of exstrophy: Re-evaluation. *Surgery* 66:1103, 1969.
10. Heitz-Boyer, M., and Hovelaque, A. Création d'une nouvelle vessie d'un nouvel urétre. *J. Urol. Nephrol.* 1:237, 1912.
11. Hinman, F., and Weyrauch, H. M., Jr. A critical study of the different principles of surgery which have been used in uretero-intestinal implantation. *Trans. Am. Assoc. Genitourin. Surg.* 29:15, 1936.
12. Johnston, T. H. Further experiences with a new operation for urinary diversion. *J. Urol.* 76:380, 1956.
13. Leadbetter, W. F. Considerations of problems incident to performance of ureteroenterostomy: Report of a technique. *J. Urol.* 65:818, 1951.

14. Leadbetter, W. F., and Clark, B. G. Five years experience with uretero-enterostomy by the combined technique. *J. Urol.* 73:67, 1955.

15. Lowsley, O. S., and Johnston, T. H. A new operation for creation of an artificial bladder with voluntary control of urine and feces. *J. Urol.* 73:83, 1955.

16. Madsen, P. O. The etiology of hyperchloremic acidosis following uretero-intestinal anastomosis: An experimental study. *J. Urol.* 92:448, 1964.

17. Nesbit, R. M. Another hopeful look at ureterosigmoid anastomosis. *J. Urol.* 84:691, 1960.

18. Peters, P. C. Personal communications.

19. Powell, T. O., and Hays, D. M. An improved surgical procedure for exstrophy of the bladder: A preliminary report. *West. J. Surg.* 68:282, 1960.

20. Retik, A. B., Perlmutter, A. D., and Gross, R. E. Cutaneous uretero-ileostomy in children. *N. Engl. J. Med.* 277:217, 1967.

21. Smith, E. D. Ileocutaneous ureterostomy. II. Operative technique. *Aust. N. Z. J. Surg.* 34:89, 1964.

22. Snyder, C. C. A new therapeutic concept of the exstrophied bladder. *Plast. Reconstr. Surg.* 22:1, 1958.

23. Spence, H. M. Ureterosigmoidostomy for exstrophy of the bladder. *Br. J. Urol.* 38:36, 1966.

24. Stamey, T. A. Pathogenesis and implications of electrolyte imbalance in ureterosigmoidostomy. *Surg. Gynecol. Obstet.* 103:736, 1956.

25. Turnbull, R. B., Jr. Intestinal stomas. *Surg. Clin. North Am.* 38:1361, 1958.

26. Wallace, D. M. Ileal conduit. *Br. J. Urol.* 39:681, 1967.

27. Williams, D. I. Uretero-sigmoidostomy in children. *Urol. Int.* 23:35, 1968.

28. Williams, R. E., Davenport, T. J., Burkinshaw, L., and Hughes, D. Changes in whole body potassium associated with uretero-intestinal anastomosis. *Br. J. Urol.* 39:676, 1967.

Reconstruction of the Female Escutcheon in Exstrophy of the Bladder

ARTHUR GEORGE SHIP

15

EXSTROPHY of the bladder is a rare congenital anomaly that is said to occur approximately once in 30,000 births [1]. It is usually accompanied by varying degrees of separation of the pubic rami and associated diastasis of the rectus muscles and attached perineal muscles. If present, the vaginal introitus lies immediately below the bladder, facing anteriorly. The clitoris is divided into two separate bodies on either side of the vaginal introitus.

It has been demonstrated by Wyburn [9] that the infraumbilical portion of the anterior abdominal wall, the genital tubercle, the symphysis pubis, and the muscular coat of the bladder are all formed from a well-defined band of mesoderm in the embryo. Thus, the association of deformities—exstrophy of the bladder, diastasis recti and absence of the symphysis pubis, cleft clitoris, and widely separated labia minora—can be readily understood. Snyder [8] has characterized the deformity as a cleft or failure of fusion, rather than a deficiency, as has been commonly considered. He notes no less than

55 different operations that have been described for bladder exstrophy.

Bilateral ureterosigmoidostomy has been one of the most widely used methods of treatment. This has usually been performed [4, 7] as a two-stage procedure, the right ureter being transplanted at the first operation, the left ureter approximately 10 days later. Removal of the bladder mucosa was occasionally performed at the time of the second operation, but was frequently deferred until a later time. Gross [3] believed that it was not necessary to remove all of the bladder tissue, although Kickham and Keegan [6] recommended removal of "left behind" bladder tissue.

Repair during childhood of exstrophy of the bladder by bilateral ureterosigmoidostomy results in a characteristic deformity in the adult, who may present for cosmetic repair of the extensive deformity of the lower abdominal wall and absent mons veneris. The patient may be referred for vaginal reconstruction, since the vagina, which is usually present, may be obscured by the ventral displacement of the perineum and the proximity of apparent fistulas. If the vagina is present, it is accompanied by a bifid clitoris and remnants of the labia minora.

The deformity results at least in part from a prominent diastasis of the pubic bones. The lower part of the anterior abdominal wall is depressed, with wide separation of the rectus abdominus muscles. The lower abdominal wall seems to continue straight downward to a forward facing anus. The depression in the area of absence of the symphysis pubis is accentuated by the absence of a mons veneris. Pubic hair is displaced and occurs in triangular patches in each groin (Fig. 15-1A).

The lower abdominal wall is extensively scarred, with several sinus tracts that represent bladder or ureteric remnants. These occur low down and are adjacent to the vaginal introitus, which may therefore be obscured upon casual examination (Fig. 15-2A).

These patients exhibit a characteristic waddling gait, not unlike that of a pregnant

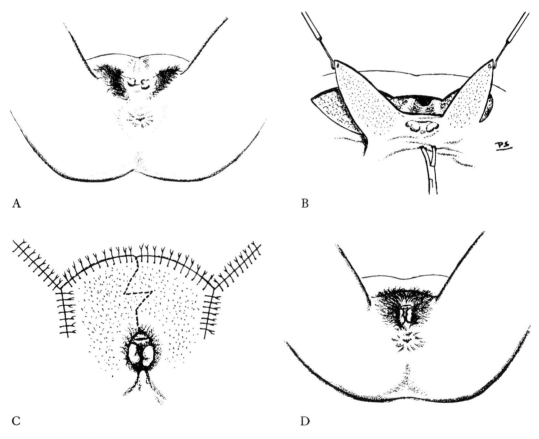

A

B

C

D

FIG. 15-1. A. Deformity of perineum and lower abdominal wall with displacement of pubic hair and diastasis recti. B. Operative stage after removal of scarred lower abdominal wall and elevation of hair-bearing flaps. C. Operative stage after transposition of hair-bearing flaps to construct escutcheon. D. Restored escutcheon simulating normal appearing perineum.

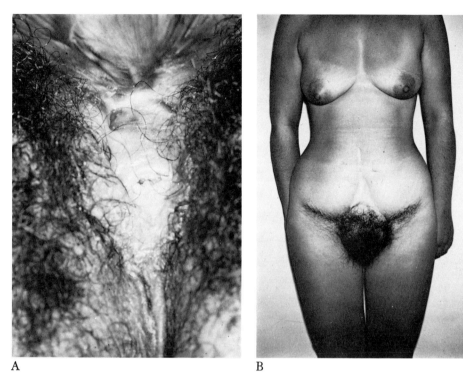

A   B

FIG. 15-2. A. Deformed lower abdominal wall with sinus tracts adjacent to vaginal introitus. Note lateral displacement of inguinal hair. B. Postoperative appearance of mons veneris after transposition of hair-bearing flaps. Note persistence of diastasis recti.

woman shortly before delivery. This is presumably related to the wide diastasis of the pubic bones and outward rotation of the femurs.

Roentgenography confirms the absence of a symphysis pubis. Work-up of these patients should also include intravenous pyelography, which may show upper tract dilatation. Barium enema may be done cautiously with water-soluble radiopaque dye in the well-prepared patient, and it may demonstrate reflux into one or both ureters. Serum electrolyte studies frequently reveal mild hyperchloremic acidosis, and blood urea nitrogen measurements are usually normal. The presence and location of the vagina can be con-

firmed by observing the menstrual flow. Its size and shape can then be delineated by injection of radiopaque dye.

Surgical Reconstruction

The goal of surgical reconstruction is the formation of a normal female escutcheon with labia majora and a mons veneris.

Historically, there are few references to the "third-stage procedure" in which bladder and ureteric remnants are excised and reconstruction is attempted. Gross [3] and Lower [7] make passing references to reconstruction procedures. Hoffman and Spence [5] and

Erich [2] illustrate methods of repair that are basically similar to the technique outlined below.

The scarred tissue of the lower abdominal wall is excised along with the remnants of bladder tissue and the defunctionalized distal ureters that were the cause of the sinus tracts. The diastasis of the rectus muscles is noted—simple approximation is usually impossible (see Fig. 15-1B). Two inferiorly based pedicle flaps of hair-bearing inguinal skin are outlined in the groins. These are elevated and rotated medially around the remnants of the clitoris, labia majora, and the vaginal introitus. They are then approximated in the midline (a Z-plasty will provide additional height in the reconstruction of the lower abdominal wall) (Fig. 15-1C). The donor defects are closed primarily; adequate drainage is important (Figs. 15-1D and 15-2B).

The final result provides an escutcheon that appears normal, with a mons veneris of relatively normal contour and appearance.

References

1. Chisholm, T. C. Exstrophy of the urinary bladder. *Am. J. Surg.* 101:649, 1961.
2. Erich J. B. Plastic repair of the female perineum in a case of exstrophy of the bladder. *Proc. Mayo Clin.* 34:235, 1959.
3. Gross, R. E., and Cresson, S. L. Exstrophy of bladder. *J.A.M.A.* 149:1640, 1952.
4. Higgins, C. C. Transplantation of the ureters into the rectosigmoid for exstrophy of the bladder: Review of 41 cases. *J. Urol.* 57:693, 1947.
5. Hoffman, W. W., and Spence, H. M. Management of exstrophy of the bladder. *South. Med. J.* 58:436, 1965.
6. Kickham, C. J. E., and Keegan, J. J. The bladder "left behind." *J. Urol.* 89:689, 1963.
7. Lower, W. E. Transplantation of the ureters into the rectosigmoid in young children and infants. *J. Mount Sinai Hosp. N.Y.* 4:650, 1938.
8. Snyder, C. C. A new therapeutic concept of the exstrophied bladder. *Plast. Reconstr. Surg.* 22:1, 1958.
9. Wyburn, C. M. The development of the infra-umbilical portion of the abdominal wall, with remarks on the etiology. *J. Anat.* 71:201, 1937.

Epispadias—I

DAVID INNES WILLIAMS

16

EPISPADIAS is not simply an anomaly of the penis, it is a part of a generalized disturbance of the lower urinary tract that can be present in both males and females. It involves the pelvic ring, which is incomplete anteriorly; the abdominal wall, which is weak in the midline and often associated with a low umbilicus; the bladder neck, which is incompetent; and the ureters, which enter the bladder at right angles and are not, therefore, usually capable of preventing reflux. In the female, the urethra is very short and wide, and the clitoris is separated into two separate portions by a strip of mucosa leading anteriorly to a flattened mons veneris. In the male, the corpora cavernosa arise from separated ischiopubic rami and are loosely joined to one another ventral to the urethral strip; the urethra itself is short and wide, opening at the base of the penis or farther up on the dorsal surface.

Operative correction is therefore usually required both for the control of urinary incontinence and for the achievement of a normal external appearance with effective sexual function. These two objectives demand separate approaches and are usually better undertaken on separate occasions. In the female, the external correction is perhaps unimportant and need only be very simple, but in the male a staged procedure of external operation is usually appropriate.

Operation for Incontinence

A small proportion of male epispadiacs have normal or near normal control, so no operation on the sphincter mechanism is required for them. However, the majority of patients of both sexes have severe stress incontinence at least, and most have a continuous dribble from an empty bladder. Assessment of the degree of control should be postponed until the child is at least 3 years old. Operation should not be considered before this age and may even be delayed a year or two longer with profit.

Incontinence is due to a failure of the formation of the bladder neck—the bladder cavity extends down to the verumontanum—and to a failure of the external sphincteric muscle to encircle the urethra, which is displaced anteriorly. Most operations are aimed at constructing a bladder neck from the tissue at the base of the bladder or at constricting this region by an encircling sling of muscle or tendon. Operations aimed at reconstruction of the external sphincteric system have been less successful, and in all reported series, some children have failed to gain urinary control by any reconstructive procedure and have required urinary diversion. These diversionary procedures are not considered in this article, nor are methods depending upon the implantation of muscle stimulators, although the latter do appear to offer some chance of success in failed operative cases.

I am accustomed to employing either a procedure based on the operations described by Young and by Dees [1, 2] or a sling operation. The two procedures can, if necessary, be combined, and a decision regarding this can be made at the time of exploration.

Preliminary investigation should include intravenous pyelography and cystography; the latter is particularly important for giving an indication of bladder capacity and the presence or absence of reflux. The chances of successful treatment are greater with a bladder of large capacity, and reflux must be corrected at the time of bladder neck revision.

The operation is performed by a transverse incision a little above the pubes: the rectus sheath and external oblique aponeurosis are incised transversely and dissected free from the rectus muscles, which are then parted in the midline. The pubes are united only by fibrous tissue and, if necessary, this can be cut through to give better exposure.

The bladder is defined and the urethra is freed from its anterior attachments, where there is often a considerable plexus of veins.

The bladder is opened by a vertical midline incision, and a self-retaining retractor is inserted. The ureteral orifices are identified and the state of the bladder outflow is assessed. In some cases, there is an identifiable, though widely relaxed, bladder neck; in others, there is no such formation but the verumontanum is found located at the base of the bladder.

The object of the operation is to construct a tubular urethra of at least 3 cm in length above the verumontanum, with a bladder neck area supported by the best muscle tissue that is available. If the ureteral orifices allow reflux or are placed very low down, they must first be reimplanted at a higher level. This requires extravesical mobilization, since the ureters at their lower ends make wide lateral loops. Reimplantation must be performed with a submucous course of at least 2 to 3 cm, and this tunnel can be made either from inside the bladder, or from outside.

The area at the bladder base which is to be formed into a tube and the bladder neck are then defined, and incisions are made laterally from the midline opening in the bladder at the appropriate level (Fig. 16-1), thus mobilizing lateral flaps of muscle and mucosa.

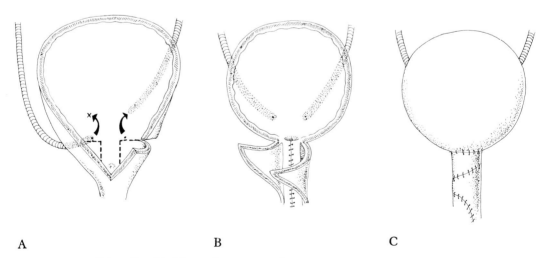

A   B   C

FIG. 16-1. Epispadias; bladder neck reconstruction.

The mucosa is then freed and trimmed so that an epithelial tube can be formed around an 8 Ch. catheter. This tube should not be tight; rather, it should allow a redundancy of mucosal folds that can interdigitate when closed by the muscular coats. The muscle flaps are then brought across, one on top of the other, to form a snug ring around the newly formed bladder neck. The flaps are then supplemented by such adventitial tissue as is locally available. The bladder is closed with a cystostomy drain, which should be maintained for 10 days.

The sling operation is suitable when a bladder neck is already present though relaxed and unsupported. The approach is similar to that already described, but if a sling procedure is chosen, the aponeurosis of the external oblique muscle is cleared of its fat above and below the line of the transverse incision. Slings about 1 cm broad are cut from the aponeurosis above and below, one based on the left and one on the right, the base consisting of the external oblique muscle. Each sling is then led into the abdomen lateral to the rectus muscle.

The plane immediately behind the bladder neck is opened up, a procedure that requires considerable care in patients of both sexes to avoid damage to the bladder or posterior structures. The slings are crossed over in front of the urethra, brought around behind the bladder neck, and sutured to one another in front. They should be fixed with a nonabsorbable suture, and they should be under only slight tension when the abdominal wall is relaxed but still capable of tightening up with the contraction of the external oblique muscle. Complete closure of the anterior rectus sheath after formation of the slings is not usually possible, but incomplete closure does not appear to result in any serious weakness of the abdominal wall provided the fibrae intercrurales (Scarpa's fascia) are closed.

After either operation, a period of some months is required before continence can be expected.

Correction of Chordee

Upward chordee that is sufficient to render intercourse difficult or impossible is present in a high proportion of male epispadiacs, and correction of this deformity is required prior to urethral construction in this group.

Chordee is maintained by the shortness of the urethral strip that cuts the corner between the base of the bladder and the dorsum of the penis, as well as by tethering bands that bind the corpora cavernosa upward to the region of the pubic tubercles. In a few cases, there is a very diminutive penis for which a full correction is impossible. However, in most cases, although the penis appears short during childhood, after puberty it is entirely adequate for sexual intercourse provided chordee has been corrected.

This operation clearly requires severance of the tethering bands, elongation of the urethral strip, and the movement of skin onto the dorsal surface of the penis. Several methods are available for this. Basically, the urethra is cut across and dissected free from the corpora cavernosa so that it retracts upward, allowing the penis to lengthen. This dissection may be carried up almost as far as the verumontanum, although care must be taken to avoid damage to the ejaculatory ducts. Laterally, dissection proceeds upward on the surface of the corpora cavernosa until no upward tethering can be palpated. Both these dissections involve a good deal of hemorrhage from vessels that are hard to identify, but bleeding ceases spontaneously on wound closure.

Skin cover for the denuded dorsum of the penis is best obtained from the prepuce,

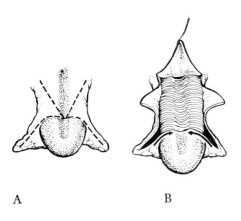

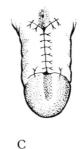

A   B   C

FIG. 16-2. Chordee correction. The urethral strip is allowed to drop back, and skin cover on the dorsum of the penis is obtained by shifting the preputial skin.

which is usually redundant on the ventral aspect of the penis. The simplest operation is shown in Figure 16-2. An initial V-shaped incision on the dorsum of the penis allows the urethra to retract upward; lateral incisions from the apex of the V into the redundant skin of the prepuce allow this skin to be brought around onto the dorsum and sutured in a Y-shaped manner. Alternatively, the prepuce can be entirely separated at the coronal sulcus and unfolded; it can then be buttonholed and a part brought onto the dorsal surface of the penis, reversing the procedure customary in Ombrédanne operation for hypospadias. With this method, however, care should be taken not to leave the redundant skin on the dorsum, since it will render later urethral reconstruction more difficult.

In cases in which the prepuce itself is lacking, a circumferential incision can be made around the base of the penis, and chordee release can be performed as described above. The consequent defect in skin cover on the dorsum of the penis can then be repaired by displacing the shaft under the skin in front of the scrotum and bringing the tip out through the button-hole low down, as shown in Figure 16-3. This scrotal skin is not very satisfactory for the formation of a urethra, but it is adequate if preputial skin is not available. A subsequent operation releases the penis with full skin cover prior to urethral closure.

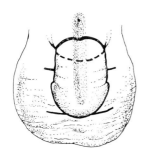

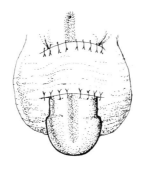

A   B

FIG. 16-3. Chordee correction (continued). Skin cover on the dorsum of the penis is obtained by displacing the shaft under the skin of the anterior scrotum.

Reconstruction of the Urethra

Although many of the methods used for correction of hypospadias can be adapted for epispadias, the simple formation of a urethral tube from the skin or urethral remnants on the dorsum of the penis gives satisfactory results, provided the preliminary chordee correction has been adequate. It is important to note, however, that the glans penis is not the same in cases of epispadias as in those of hypospadias: in the condition now under consideration, the glans is broad and unrolled. It can be rolled up again to enclose a terminal urethra of good caliber without tendency to stenosis, and the process of rolling up restores a normal appearance to the tip of the penis.

The penis is held extended and the strip designed to form the urethra is defined and isolated by the longitudinal incisions (Fig. 16-4). In a child of 3 to 5 years of age, this strip should be 12 to 15 mm broad, which is sufficient to wrap loosely around an 8 Ch. catheter. The lateral flaps should be freely mobilized, undermining close to the corpora cavernosa. Proximally, the incisions should join anteriorly where the urethra disappears under the pubic arch. Distally, they should turn laterally for a short distance at the coronal sulcus. Flaps of tissue cannot be raised on the glans, but beyond the coronal sulcus the two areas on the dorsum of the glans on each side of the urethral groove should be denuded of epithelium, leaving an inner epithelial edge continuous with the edge of the urethral strip (see Fig. 16-4B). This strip, which should not be mobilized at all, can now be closed as a tube by a continuous 4-0 chromic catgut suture that is so placed as to invert the skin edge. The suture line continues up through the glans to the tip of the penis, where the new meatus is to be formed. A second suture, which can also be of catgut, is placed in the subcutaneous tissues, bringing the penile fascia together to cover the urethral tube; this suture stops short at the coronal sulcus area. Finally, the skin is closed and the glans is rolled up; the two bared areas are brought together by an external row of sutures (see Fig. 16-4C). It may at times be necessary to make a small relieving incision on the under surface of the penis if the suture line is tight. The indwelling catheter is allowed to remain for 7 or 8 days.

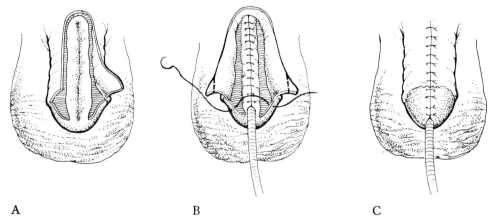

A   B   C

FIG. 16-4. Closure of urethral strip.

References

1. Dees, J. E.   Congenital epispadias with incontinence. *J. Urol.* 62:513, 1949.

2. Young, H. H.   *Genital Abnormalities*. Baltimore: Williams & Wilkins, 1937.

Epispadias—II

HOWARD B. MAYS

17

THE SELECTION of a plan of treatment for the epispadias patient requires careful consideration of the basic problems involved and a well-planned program if the eventual result is to be as close to normal as possible. The great variation of abnormal circumstances found in association with the degrees of epispadias encountered clearly indicates the necessity for differing methods and plans of treatment [3]. Epispadias is never present as a normal embryological development, and, unlike hypospadias, the most frequently encountered varieties of epispadias present the most significant associated anatomical and functional problems. Because primary attention must be directed to the related factors, their correction will significantly influence the planning of epispadias correction.

The simple spadic penis is the rarest form of epispadias encountered; the balanic and simple penile deformities are less rare. The next most frequently encountered form is penopubic epispadias, which may occur with or without incontinence. A most important characteristic of this group is the possibility of borderline or transitional continence that might not be readily apparent. Epispadias with associated vesical exstrophy is the most commonly encountered variety. Because of the relative rarity of the least distorting forms of epispadias requiring comparatively simple

corrective measures, attention is directed to the more significant and challenging problems of complete epispadias. The frequent occurrence of total epispadias with involvement of the bladder neck area suggests the need for treatment planning and procedures that are somewhat at variance with long-established concepts.

The problem of epispadias without exstrophy requires critical attention to the possible existence of a functioning sphincter or the conceivable existence of transitional or borderline continence. The decisions involved may depend on prolonged observation, and premature corrective efforts may prevent a good functional and cosmetic result. Any degree of exstrophy requires evaluation of the status and size of the bladder and estimation of the amount and effect of eventration accompanying the more significant deformities. The status of the upper urinary tract requires early attention, although the ureters and kidneys are usually quite satisfactory. Some form of urinary diversion may subsequently be necessary, but even the presence of a very small bladder does not necessarily indicate the need for early diversion. The existence of incontinence is not significant, since an infant will in any event be incontinent during the early months. Generally, the ureterovesical junctures require no immediate attention.

The apron of preputial tissue that is always associated with epispadias is left untouched until its eventual use as a valuable aid to plastic reconstruction. Definitive penile plastic surgery at a very early age is contraindicated in any degree of epispadias [4].

Inguinal hernia occurs frequently with epispadias, and it may be sufficiently severe to require very early and probably separate surgical correction. Concurrent rearrangement of the existing abdominal wall components with approximation of otherwise normal rectus muscles and fascia may be accomplished effectively. Experience has shown, however, that large hernia defects require very early correction. The best abdominal wall revision may be attained by a separate surgical endeavor. Revision and closure of the abdominal defect to the level of the intersymphyseal deficiency, including closure of the bladder whether large or small, provides a measure of protection of the bladder epithelium and trigone. Closure of a larger bladder may occasionally allow the eventual development of very satisfactory function. Although closure is carried to and includes the vesical neck, the decision to attempt vesical neck correction should be postponed. Continuation of incontinence at an early age is not a problem, and, although the small bladder will ultimately be sacrificed, its temporary retention will provide a protective temporary conduit as well as providing material for the development of a subsequent prostatic fossa. Very occasionally, a carefully selected case may be considered for retention of the bladder and for attempted repair of the anteriorly separated sphincteric structure. This is an ideal goal that is not often attained, but it is not obviated by this plan of treatment.

Very satisfactory abdominal wall reconstruction may be accomplished without the necessity of osteotomy, nor has osteotomy been considered necessary for the correction of the frequently described gait abnormality. Experience and observation have repeatedly demonstrated that the locomotion disability associated with exstrophy is insignificant and not disabling, and it is quite doubtful that significant improvement or change could be accomplished by osteotomy. Osteotomy has not been considered necessary for plastic penile reconstruction nor for the occasional reconstruction of the bladder neck; both can be effectively accomplished by rearrangement of the existing abdominal wall structure.

Urinary diversion may be required in most instances of epispadias with exstrophy. Ureterosigmoidal diversion has been used to good effect as a temporary or a permanent form of diversion and urine transport. This form of diversion may be performed concurrently with abdominal wall rearrangement. The ileal conduit provides a very effective means of urinary diversion. However, previous rearrangement of the abdominal wall is a distinct aid to the subsequent positioning and functioning of the ileostomy. For these several reasons, the postponement of partial cystectomy and diversion for a year or even much longer is recommended.

Plastic correction of epispadias is time-consuming, and it requires separate consideration if an adequate functional and cosmetic result is to be attained. Postponement to an elected time provides the additional advantages of an increased size of the organ and cleanliness of operative field. Plastic reconstruction for epispadias can, in fact, be performed at any age.

The less frequently encountered forms of epispadias require the formation of a distal urethra only, and these may be readily corrected by procedures described by Cantwell [1], Young [5], and others. However, in all instances, existing chordee correction is definitely assisted by extensive rearrangement of the penile integument, including the preputial apron. The short dorsal surface of complete penile epispadias limits the tissue available for possible urethral formation from this area. The principle of formation of a urethral tube flap on the dorsum of the penis, with subsequent rotaton between the separated corpora cavernosa, may present possible limitations to the correction of chordee and interfere with adequate erection. The ideal corrective procedure should provide ample tissue for development of a urethral tube from the penopubic orifice to the tip of the glans after chordee correction.

Surgical Technique

Two silk sutures are placed through the glans for traction, thus emphasizing the restricting effects of ventral chordee. A circumferential incision is made about the vesical neck or the residue of the bladder that is planned for formation of a prostatic fossa. Parallel incisions are made on the dorsum of the penis from the circumscribed orifice or prostatic fossa to the glans. The incisions are carried about the glans, allowing a cuff of several millimeters in width to be attached to the glans (Fig. 17-1). The preputial apron, which is characteristic of all cases of epispadias, is preserved and left attached to the ventral integument. The penis is completely denuded, preserving all possible blood supply. The broad band of fibrous tissue between the corpora cavernosa, including the wedge of fibrous intercavernosal tissue, is resected down to the ventral fascia. The excision must be carefully performed in order to eliminate all possible areas of constriction from the level of the corona to the infundibulum (Fig. 17-2). The penis thereafter becomes signifi-

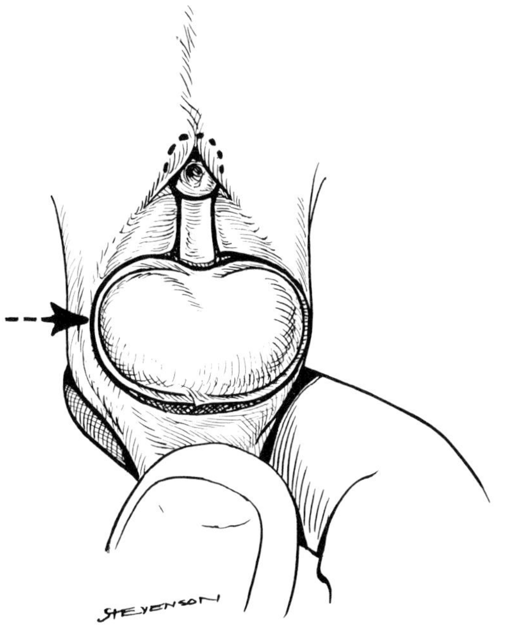

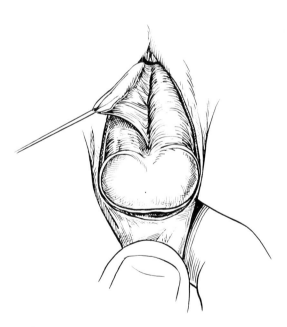

FIG. 17-1. Circumferential incision about the vesical neck or prostatic fossa, parallel ventral incisions, and paraglandular incision. The preputial apron is demonstrated.

FIG. 17-2. Excision of ventral and intercavernosal restricting tissue. Denudation assists chordee correction and elongation of the penis.

cantly more pliable and the length is appreciably increased. Chordee correction may be further aided by dissection about the base of the penis and partially incising the suspensory fascia. The dorsal vessels are usually separated and must be preserved; the attachment of the corpora to the separated pubes must be left undisturbed.

The epithelial layers of the preputial apron are carefully separated by sharp and blunt dissection, preserving all possible blood supply. This maneuver creates a single layer of epithelium that is appreciably more extensible than is apparent. The epithelial pouch thus produced is developed into a single flap by lateral incisions which open the pouch to produce the greatest possible length (Fig. 17-3).

A short transverse incision is made through the ventral fascia into the intercavernosal sulcus immediately proximal to the corona. The fascial opening is enlarged sufficiently to allow the development of the subsequent unrestricted passage of the urethral tube (Figs. 17-3 and 17-4).

The preputial flap is formed into a tube, the epithelial surface is turned inward, and the edges, beginning at the end of the flap, are approximated using interrupted sutures of 4-0 or 5-0 atraumatic catgut. As the urethral tube is developed, it is drawn through the ventral incision beneath the glans and

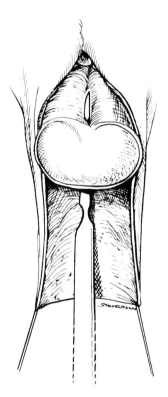

FIG. 17-3. Development of the preputial apron into a single-layered epithelial flap. Ventral fascial incision is carried to the intercavernosal sulcus.

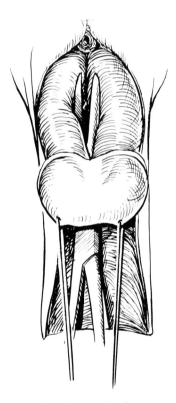

FIG. 17-4. Maximum chordee correction and elongation. Development of the subglandar tunnel and the relationship to the preputial hood.

diagonally upward between the corpora (Fig. 17-5). The urethral tube thus created from the preputial flap is usually of sufficient length to extend from a hypospadial position to the anteriorly positioned vesical neck or the preserved prostatic fossa. This tube may be developed about a section of rubber tubing of adequate length and diameter. Occasionally, if the vesical neck is intact, a catheter of adequate size may be used for drainage; this is particularly applicable to older patients. When bladder diversion is indicated, it must be via the suprapubic route. A nephrostomy tube, such as the Cummings type, that serves the combined purpose of suprapubic drainage and as a mold for urethral development has been used effectively.

A variation of the procedure may be considered which utilizes a portion of the dorsally derived epithelium that is formed into a proximal tube combined with the preputial-flap urethra as described. Although this provides additional urethral length, the requirement of midpenile anastomosis and the rather deficient blood supply of the dorsally derived epithelium should be kept in mind. Generally, the use of the preputial flap has been found sufficient.

The newly formed urethra is approximated to the infundibulum using interrupted sutures reinforced by a second suture layer. The widely separated corpora cavernosa are drawn together over the diagonally placed urethra using interrupted sutures. This reconstitutes the fascial plane and encloses the newly formed urethra in its entirety from the hypospadial position of the orifice to the anteriorly located vesical neck or prostatic fossa (Fig. 17-6).

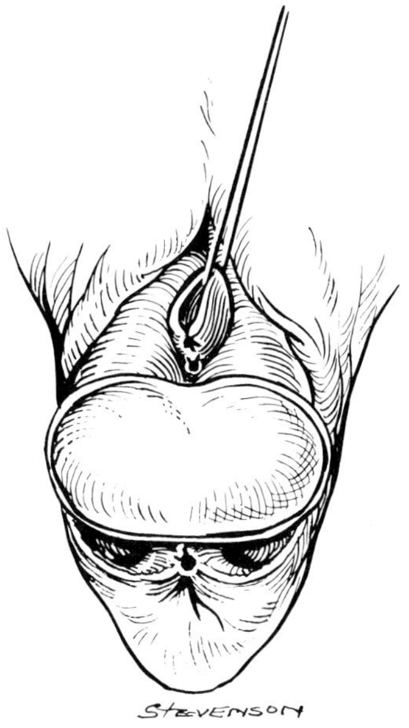

STEVENSON

FIG. 17-5. Development of the urethra from the preputial flap. The flap is trimmed to appropriate size. The urethra is drawn between the corpora.

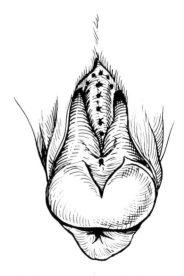

FIG. 17-6. Anastomosis of the urethral tube to the prostatic fossa or vesical neck. The diagonal course of the urethra from the hypospadial position to the vesical neck is illustrated, as is the approximation of the corpora cavernosa. The spadic glans deformity is corrected.

A triangle of epithelium is excised from the broad anterior surface of the glans. The penis is reinvested using interrupted sutures about the coronal cuff and in the midline anteriorly from the dorsal surface of the glans to the base of the penis. Short relaxing incisions may be required for adequate reinvestment without tension. The penis is extended by attaching the glans stay sutures to either thigh, using an elastic band and adhesive (Fig. 17-7).

Results and Complications

The hypospadial position of the newly created urethral orifice is a distinct advantage. The voiding position is quite satisfactory, and there is a lessened tendency to restriction and curvature when erect. The subsequent transfer of the meatus to the tip of the glans is feasible, but this requires additional surgery of dubious value.

The most probable complication is fistula formation over the point of anastomosis. Constriction may occur at the vesical neck area in instances of sphincteric reconstruction. There are distinct advantages gained by a deliberately postponed and separate operation for the correction of epispadias, particu-

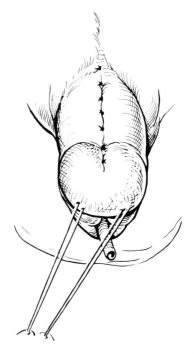

FIG. 17-7. Epithelial reinvestment of the penis. Glans sutures attached to the thigh assist chordee correction.

larly when vesical neck surgery or diversion is required; fewer complications and a better functional and cosmetic result may be anticipated.

References

1. Cantwell, F. V. Operative treatment of epispadias by transplantation of the urethra. *Am. J. Surg.* 22:689, 1895.
2. Hinman, F., Jr. A method of lengthening the penis in exstrophy of the bladder. *J. Urol.* 79:237, 1958.
3. Marshall, V. F., and Meucke, E. C. Variations in exstrophy of bladder. *J. Urol.* 88:766, 1962.
4. Mays, H. B. Epispadias with incontinence: A method of treatment. *J. Urol.* 60:749, 1948.
5. Young, H. H. A new operation for epispadias. *J. Urol.* 2:237, 1918.

Hypospadias

18

Introduction

CHARLES E. HORTON
CHARLES J. DEVINE, JR.

Hypospadias is a congenital defect in which there is incomplete development of the urethra. It occurs about three or four times in 1,000 live male births. It is manifested by an abnormal urethral opening that occurs either proximal to its normal location on the ventral surface of the penis or in the perineum. The skin on the ventral penile surface is thin and covers a broad band of fibrous tissue. The tissue extends in a fan-shaped area from the abnormal meatus to the glans. This band shortens the ventral aspect of the penis, causing a curvature or *chordee*.

Various classifications of hypospadias have been described. Elaborate classifications are not essential and we prefer the following: glandar, distal penile, proximal penile, penoscrotal junction, and perineal hypospadias.

The structures that form the bulk of the substance of the penis are the three erectile bodies consisting of the paired *corpora cavernosa penis* and the *corpus spongiosum penis*, which lies ventrally in the groove between the two corpora cavernosa. They are surrounded by a fascial covering, the *tunica albuginea*, trabeculae of which form the blood spaces within the corpora. Central arteries are located within the corpora cavernosa and bring blood into these structures. The urethra traverses the penis in the corpus spongiosum, emerging at the distal end in the conical enlargement of the corpus called the *glans penis*. The structures covering the erectile bodies from the outside are, first, the skin, which covers the penis and at its distal end is folded on itself to cover the glans with the prepuce. Below the skin is the *dartos fascia*, which is a loose layer of connective tissue. Superficial lymphatics and the superficial dorsal veins are located in the fascia. Beneath the dartos fascia is *Buck's fascia*, which extends distally to the free margin of the prepuce. Buck's fascia surrounds the corpora cavernosa. It splits to contain the corpus spongiosum separately. The paired dorsal arteries and nerves, as well as the deep dorsal vein and lymphatics, are beneath this layer in the groove between the corpora cavernosa.

The *venae profundae penis* are on the ventral side in the groove lying between the corpora cavernosa and the corpus spongiosum. Encircling veins and lymphatics run from the dorsal group to the venae profundae along the entire length of the shaft. The hypospadial penis differs from the normal penis in that the urethra and corpus spongiosum are absent. The fibrous band that causes chordee replaces Buck's fascia and the dartos fascia. The skin on the ventral surface is thin. The prepuce is deficient ventrally and forms a dorsal hood over the glans.

Pictorial History of Hypospadias Repair Techniques

CHARLES E. HORTON
CHARLES J. DEVINE, JR.
NAMIK BARAN

These illustrations were carefully constructed on the basis of our interpretation of the original techniques of pioneer surgeons. Many of the original illustrations appeared to be incomplete or misleading, and individual interpretations have been attempted in such cases.

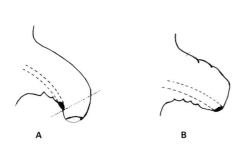

FIG. 18-1. The first hypospadias surgery (Heliodorus and Antyllus; A.D. 100–200) consisted of amputation distal to the existing meatus.

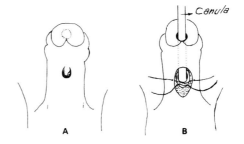

FIG. 18-2. Dieffenbach (1838) [12] pierced the glans to the normal urethra and allowed a canula to remain in position until the channel became lined with epithelium. This operation was not successful.

237

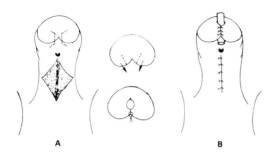

FIG. 18-3.   Mettauer in 1842 [19] suggested that the "organ be liberated by multiple subcutaneous incisions." Bouisson (1861) [6] was the first to suggest a transverse incision at the "point of greatest curvature," and, after straightening the organ, to close the defect by skin grafts or flaps.

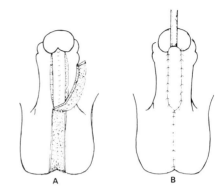

FIG. 18-4.   Bouisson [6] in 1861 was apparently the first to report the use of scrotal tissue to reconstruct the urethra. The diagrams do not adequately explain the resurfacing of the ventrum of the penis.

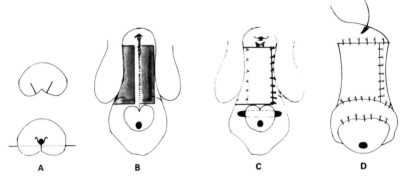

FIG. 18-5.   Thiersch (1869) [26] first described the use of local tissue flaps to repair epispadias. B.   This technique was later used in hypospadias. He was the first to suggest that perineal urinary diversion be done to temporarily direct urine away from the side of urethral reconstruction.   C   and D.   Thiersch did the first button-hole flap in the prepuce to allow resurfacing of the penis with the prepuce.

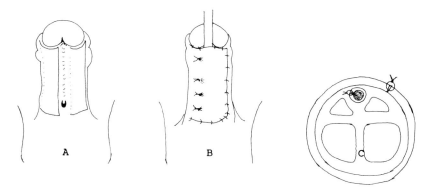

FIG. 18-6. Thiersch [26] suggested the use of broad flaps with their bases on opposite sides of the penis and emphasized the need to overlap the flap edges. The cross section of the penis is as Thiersch originally illustrated the operation. The smaller paired bodies near the urethra were not identified.

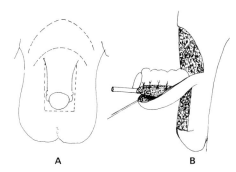

FIG. 18-7. Moutet (1870) [20] reconstructed the urethra from the scrotum and covered the raw penile undersurface with a bipedicled abdominal flap.

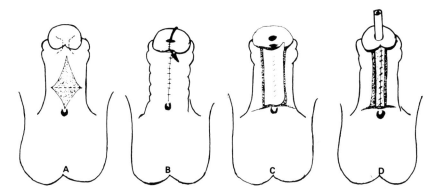

FIG. 18-8. Duplay (1874) [13] used Bouisson's technique of release of chordee. He later formed a central flap which was tubed, and then covered with lateral penile flaps. Duplay stated that it did not matter if the central tube was incompletely formed, and he believed that epithelialization would occur to form a channel if the incomplete tube was buried under the lateral flaps.

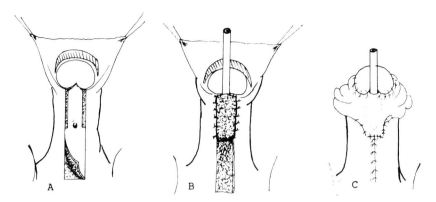

FIG. 18-9. Wood (1875) [27] described a flap based distally on the urethra to be turned over to form the floor of the urethral channel. He combined this with a Thiersch-type button-hole flap to cover the raw surface.

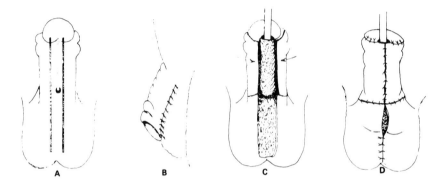

FIG. 18-10. Rosenberger (1891) [25], Landerer (1891) [16], and Bidder (1892) [4] used scrotal tissue for urethroplasty, and for the first time described burying the penis in the scrotum to obtain skin coverage.

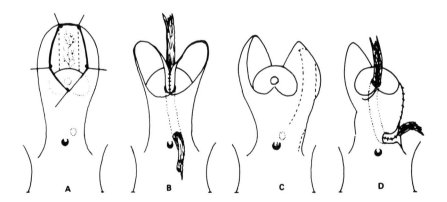

FIG. 18-11. Hook (1896) [15] first described a vascularized preputial flap for urethroplasty (A and B). He further suggested the use of a lateral oblique flap from the side of the penis (C and D) for urethral reconstruction.

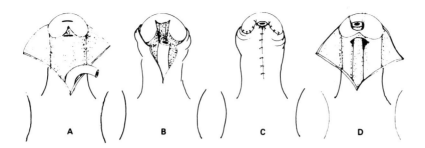

FIG. 18-12. Beck [2] and Hacker (1897) undermined and advanced the urethra into the glans.

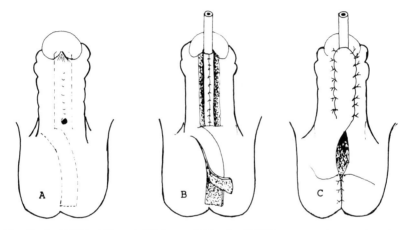

FIG. 18-13. Beck (1897) [2] and White and Martin (1917) suggested a urethroplasty similar to that of Duplay, but used an adjacent rotation flap from the scrotum for resurfacing.

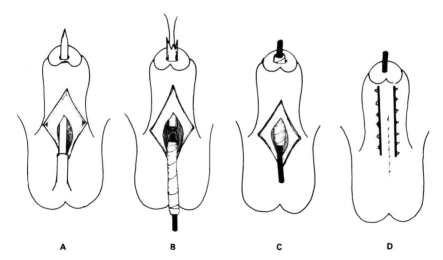

FIG. 18-14. Nové-Josserand [21, 22] was the first surgeon to report (1897; 1914) attempts to repair hypospadias with a free graft (split-thickness).

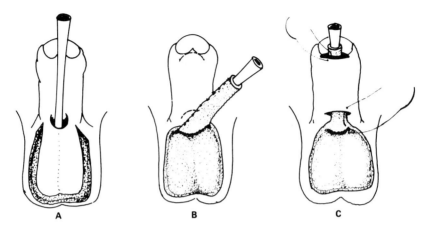

FIG. 18-15.   Rochet (1899) [24] used a large, distally based scrotal flap for urethroplasty. This flap was buried in a tunnel on the ventral surface of the penis.

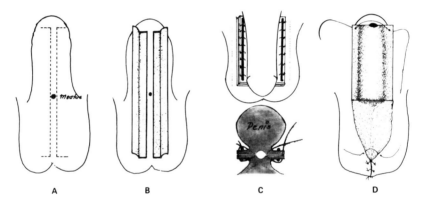

FIG. 18-16.   Bucknall (1907) [8] described an operation similar to that of Rosenberger [25] in that the urethra was partially constructed of scrotal skin and the penis was buried in the scrotum to obtain later skin coverage.

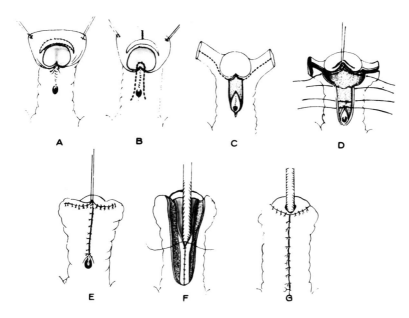

FIG. 18-17. Edmunds (1913) [14] was the first surgeon to transfer the skin of the prepuce to the ventral surface of the penis at the time of the release of chordee. Using this abundant skin, he was able to complete a Duplay-type urethroplasty at a later stage.

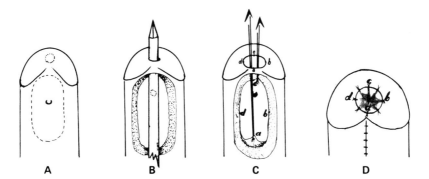

FIG. 18-18. Bevan (1917) [3] carried a flap based on the urethral meatus through a glandar channel to repair distal hypospadias.

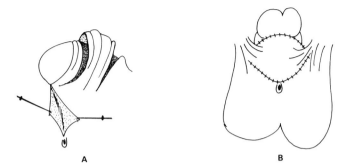

FIG. 18-19. Beck (1917) [2] used a bipedicled preputial flap to resurface the raw ventral penile area that remains after the release of chordee.

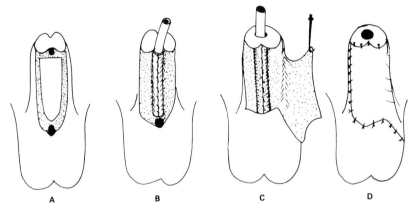

FIG. 18-20. At a second stage, Beck (1917) [2] formed the urethra from the abundant ventral skin, and covered the area with one large lateral penoscrotal flap.

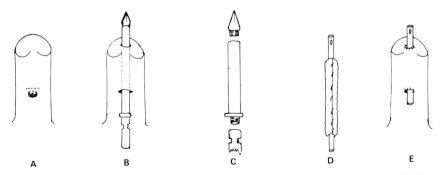

FIG. 18-21. McIndoe (1937) [18] used a special trochar to introduce a split graft for urethroplasty.

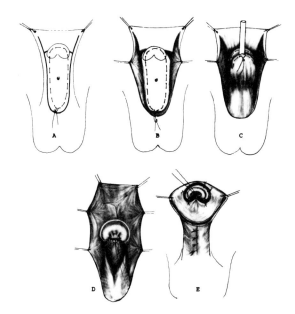

FIG. 18-22. Ombrédanne (1932) [23] used a large sacculated penile flap for urethroplasty and resurfaced the area with a button-hole preputial skin flap.

FIG. 18-23. Blair and Brown (1933) [5] built the urethra from ventral penile skin and resurfaced the area by using a laterally based scrotal flap that was "set in" in two operations.

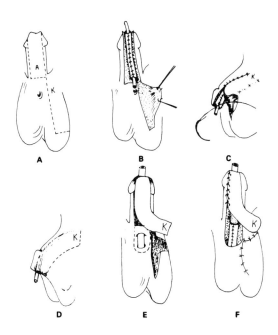

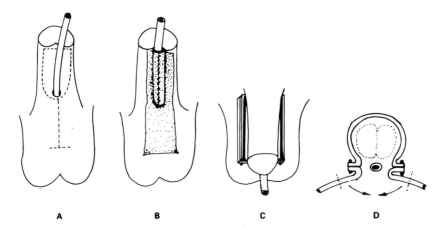

FIG. 18-24. Cecil (1952) [10] and Cabot (1935) [9] used a modification of the Rosenberger-Bucknall operation following reconstruction of the urethra from ventral penile skin.

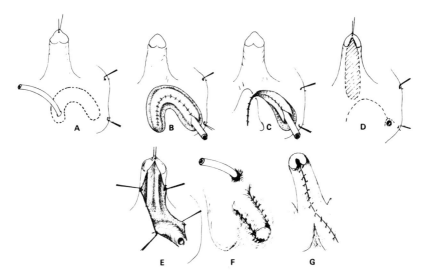

FIG. 18-25. Lowsley and Begg (1938) [17] constructed a urethral tube from scrotal skin and sutured the raw ventral penile surface to the scrotum.

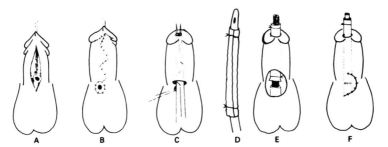

FIG. 18-26. Young and Benjamin (1948) [28] used a two-stage repair utilizing a split-thickness skin graft from the anterior medial aspect of the upper arm for urethroplasty.

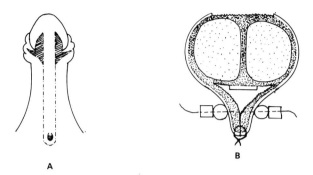

FIG. 18-27. Denis Browne (1950) [7] used a buried strip of skin that tubed itself to form a channel.

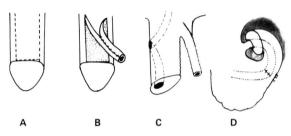

FIG. 18-28. Davis (1950) [11] utilized a tube of skin from the dorsum of the penis for urethral reconstruction. The penis was bent dorsally to bring the tip of the glans to the base of the pedicle of the tubed flap.

References

1. Anger, M. Th. L'hypospadias: A récemment presénté à la société de chirurgie (*seance du 21 janvier 1874*). Reported by M. F. Guyon in *Bull. Soc. Nat. Chir.* 1:188, 1815.
2. Beck, C. Hypospadias and its treatment. *Surg. Gynecol. Obstet.* 5:511, 1917.
3. Bevan, A. D. A new operation for hypospadias. *J.A.M.A.* 68:1032, 1917.
4. Bidder, A.: Eine Operation der Hypospadie mit Lappendildung aus dem Scrotum. *Dtsch. Med. Wochenschr.* 10:208, 1892.
5. Blair, V., and Brown, J. B. The correction of scrotal hypospadias and of epispadias. *Surg. Gynecol. Obstet.* 57:646, 1933.
6. Bouisson, M. F. De l'hypospadias et de son traitement chirurgical. *Trib. Chir.* 2:484, 1861.
7. Browne, D. A comparison of the Duplay and Denis Browne techniques for hypospadias operation. *Surgery* 34:787, 1953.
8. Bucknall, R. T. H. A new operation for penile hypospadias. *Lancet* 2:887, 1907.
9. Cabot, H. An improved operation for hypospadias. *Proc. Mayo Clin.* 10:796, 1935.
10. Cecil, A. B. Modern treatment of hypospadias. *J. Urol.* 67:1006, 1952.
11. Davis, D. The surgical treatment of hypospadias, especially scrotal and perineal. *Plast. Reconstr. Surg.* 5:373, 1950.
12. Dieffenbach, J. F. The simple canalization

method. In *Dictionnaire encyclopédique de médicine,* 1838. Biblioteque Nat. Paris, France.

13. Duplay, S. De l'hypospadias périnéo-scrotal et de son traitement chirurgical. *Arch. Gen. Med.* 1:513, 657, 1874.

14. Edmunds, A. An operation for hypospadias. *Lancet* 1:447, 1913.

15. Hook, W. V. A new operation for hypospadias. *Ann. Surg.* 23:378, 1896.

16. Landerer. *Dtsch. Z. Chir.* 32, 1891.

17. Lowsley, O. S., and Begg, C. L. A three-stage operation for the repair of hypospadias: Report of cases. *J.A.M.A.* 110:487, 1938.

18. McIndoe, A. An operation for the cure of adult hypospadias. *Br. Med. J.* 1:385, 1937.

19. Mettauer, J. P. Practical observations on those malformations of the male urethra and penis, termed hypospadias and epispadias, with an anomalous case. *Am. J. Med. Sci.* 4:43, 1842.

20. Moutet De l'uréthroplastie dans l'hypospadias scrotal. *Montpellier Med.* May, 1870.

21. Nové-Josserand, G. Traitement de l'hypo-spadias; nouvelle méthod. *Lyon Méd.* 85:198, 1897.

22. Nové-Josserand, G. Résultats éloignés de l'uréthroplastie par la tunnelisation et la greffe dermo-épidermique dans les formes graves de l'hypospadias et de l'épispadias. *J. Urol. Med. Chir.* 5:393, 1914.

23. Ombrédanne, L. *Précis clinique et opération de chirurgie infantile.* Paris: Masson, 1932. P. 851.

24. Rochet, W. Nouveau procédé pour refaire le canal pénien dans l'hypospadias. *Gaz. Hebd. Med. Chir.* 46:673, 1899.

25. Rosenberger. *Dtsch. Med. Wochenschr.* P. 1250, 1891.

26. Thiersch, C. Ueber die Entstehungsweise und operative Behandlung der Epispadie. *Arch. Heilkunde* 10:20, 1869.

27. Wood, J. Quoted by C. H. Mayo. *J.A.M.A.* 36:1157, 1901.

28. Young, F., and Benjamin, J. A. Repair of hypospadias with free inlay skin graft. *Surg. Gynecol. Obstet.* 86:439, 1948.

Current Concepts
of Treatment

J. BARCAT

I have personally operated on about 600 cases of hypospadias. As a recent moderator of a symposium on this subject arranged by the French Society of Children's Surgery [1], I was able to benefit from the experience of many of my French and foreign colleagues, who have observed almost 4,000 hypospadiacs.

Although the different anatomicoclinical types of hypospadias are listed by other contributors to this chapter, I prefer the classification defined below. I maintain that the type of hypospadias cannot always be defined by the original site of the meatus. The position of the meatus is affected by lesions associated with the shaft of the penis and the glans; a torsion may twist it laterally, or chordee may bring it close to the tip of the glans. Similarly, a stricture of the meatus that will require an upward meatostomy may make it necessary to consider it to be more posterior than it seemed at first. Consequently, I classify hypospadias not according to the original site of the meatus but rather according to the new location of that site after the correction of the associated malformations.

Classification of Hypospadias

1. *Anterior hypospadias* (70 percent of cases)
   a. Balanic (meatus situated on the inferior surface of the glans).
   b. Balanopenile (meatus situated in the balanopenile furrow).
   c. Anterior penile (meatus situated in the distal third of the shaft).

2. *Middle hypospadias* (7 percent of cases)
   a. Middle penile (meatus situated in the middle third of the shaft).

3. *Posterior hypospadias* (20 percent of cases)
   a. Posterior penile (meatus situated in the posterior third of the shaft).
   b. Penoscrotal (meatus situated at the base of the shaft in front of the scrotum).
   c. Scrotal (meatus situated on the scrotum or between the genital swellings).
   d. Perineal (meatus situated behind the scrotum or behind the genital swellings).

These posterior forms are often associated with a bifid scrotum and suprapenile insertion of the genital swellings. Cryptorchidism may be present. In addition, there may be hypoplasia of the penis, which occurs in about 10 percent of the posterior hypospadias cases.

4. There are also a few atypical forms: hypospadias with complete prepuce, penile chordee without hypospadias, and double urethra with a single hypospadial meatus.

General Treatment Principles

There is no *one* good method for all hypospadias treatment. The technique must be adapted for each individual case. Therefore, one ought to have at his disposal a rather large range of procedures in order to be prepared for all possible eventualities.

The psychological status of hypospadic children should not be ignored. Sometimes it is perfectly normal, but quite often there may be retardation in their intellectual development. Moreover, this kind of shortcoming easily engenders an inferiority complex which may even appear before school age but which particularly may develop at puberty. For this reason, I endeavor to operate on children when they are very young.

One must try to counterbalance prudence, which calls for the safest technique, with the desire to simplify treatment, that is, to try to avoid multiple-stage operations and thereby reduce the psychological trauma to a minimum. One-stage operations are preferable whenever they show a reasonable chance for success. We do not hesitate, however, to use multiple-stage methods should they appear to be necessary.

Finally, one should never undertake urethroplasty without having first rebuilt the normal architecture of the external genital organs. Specifically, this should never be done without having corrected stenosis of the meatus, chordee, torsion, webbing, or cryp-

torchidism. Reestablishing the normal morphology must be the objective of the preliminary operations before urethroplasty.

Preliminary Operations

STENOSIS OF THE MEATUS

In my observations, 46 percent of anterior, 41 percent of middle, and 15 percent of posterior hypospadias cases exhibit this deformity. I never use simple meatotomy, since cicatrization often causes relapse; I prefer meatostomies with mucocutaneous sutures (Fig. 18-29).

PROXIMAL (OR DOWNWARD) MEATOSTOMY

The posterior edge of the meatus is incised in the direction of the axis of the shaft. Then the mucosa edge and the skin edge on each side are sutured to each other. This causes the meatus to retract the full length of the incision (2 to 3 mm, generally). Whenever the urethral floor is thin, the meatostomy should be prolonged over the full length of this avascular stretch, which will probably be unsuitable for any kind of plastic surgical work. This can bring about a retraction of 2 to 3 cm.

DISTAL (OR UPWARD) MEATOSTOMY

This procedure can only be used in balanic hypospadias associated with a narrow

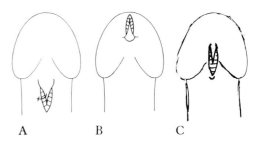

FIG. 18-29. A. Proximal meatostomy. B. Distal meatostomy. C. Special meatostomy (Culp) on a supernumerary meatus. (From *Rev. Pédiatrie,* Nov.–Dec., 1965.)

meatus. It consists of incising the protuberance formed by the glans in front of the meatus. The two edges of the incisions must be sutured. Occasionally, this allows the urinary stream to become normal without need for urethroplasty.

SPECIAL MEATOSTOMY

This is required only for supernumerary meatus. The septum that closes off a blind-ending canaliculus is simply incised so that all recesses are eliminated in the urethral floor.

CURVATURES (PRIMARY)

These have been found in 15 percent of anterior, 46 percent of middle, and 70 percent of posterior hypospadias cases.

For a long time, I used the Ombrédanne technique to lengthen the penis in such cases; this technique consists in making a transverse incision below the meatus and resecting all the fibrous tissue up to the albuginea of the corpora cavernosa as well as the longitudinal fibrous link that represents the remains of the supraurethral groove. Once straightening is obtained, the transverse incision becomes a longitudinal wound that is sutured in the direction of the main axis of the shaft. Occasionally, however, the longitudinal suture becomes hypertrophic and contracts.

I now prefer the following technique (Fig. 18-30): An arciform incision with posterior concavity is made below the meatus, keeping 2 to 3 mm of skin around the latter to avoid its being caught up in the scar. Freeing of the corpora cavernosa and removal of the fibrous tissue is accomplished as in the Ombrédanne procedure. A Z-plasty is then completed for ventral closure. A suture of No. 2 nylon is placed through the glans, which is fastened to the skin of the abdomen to make sure the penis remains extended for about 10 days.

I do not employ lengthening techniques

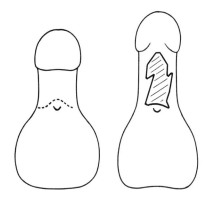

FIG. 18-30. Technique for lengthening the penis. (From *Rev. Pédiatrie,* Nov.–Dec., 1965.)

which make use of the prepuce to fill the cutaneous wound, since I feel that the prepuce should be thought of as a tissue reservoir that can be useful during urethroplasty and it ought not to be sacrificed until after the latter has been successful.

No matter what technique is used, although the lengthening operation eliminates the curvature, it increases the length of the inferior surface of the shaft, puts the glans farther away from the meatus, and does not touch the urethra.

There are cases in which the lengthening can only be accomplished by dividing the urethra that is situated in front of the chordee to be resected (chordee without hypospadias). This also occurs in residual curvatures following urethroplasty either because the curvature has relapsed or because the surgeon has reconstructed the urethra without having first corrected the curvature. In either case, if the urethral canal is of good quality, I am reluctant to section it; rather than correct the curvature by lengthening the inferior surface of the shaft, I prefer to shorten its superior surface. We call this *dorsal straightening* (Fig. 18-31). A longitudinal median incision is made on the dorsal surface above the dorsal vein (which is preserved). Dissecting under-

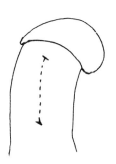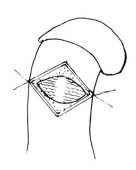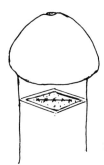

FIG. 18-31. Technique for dorsal straightening of the penis.

neath the vein, the albuginea of the corpora cavernosa is excised, following an ellipse with its major axis transverse and its size proportional to the amount of straightening desired. After resection of the ellipse, the two edges of the gap are sutured with nonabsorbable thread, thus obtaining the straightening of the shaft. The original cutaneous incision is closed and the excess skin resected. To avoid hemorrhage during the operation, I place a tourniquet at the base of the shaft. A pressure dressing, which is removed on the fourth day, is used.

The indications for dorsal straightening are not common: in 3 years I have performed the operation six times. Nesbit has used this technique in certain minor forms of hypospadias with chordee [7].

TORSIONS

Of our cases, 12 percent had torsion. Whenever this is slight, it does not warrant correction. If it is greater than 20 or 25 degrees, I perform a detorsion. If the torsion is less than 40 degrees, I do a simple overlapping autoplasty (Fig. 18-32): Two flaps are cut into an N, one with its superior base centered on the meatus, the other with a penoscrotal inferior base. After the flaps are dissected, their overlapping makes detorsion possible.

If the torsion is greater than 40 degrees, I use detorsion circumcision at the base of the shaft (Fig. 18-33). In spite of early fears, I have never observed difficulties in vascularization. Cutaneous sutures are made in hypercorrection.

CONCEALED PENIS (ANTERIOR SCROTUM)

This exists only in posterior hypospadias (18 percent) and is almost always associated with chordee.

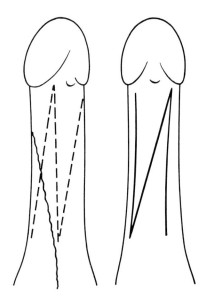

FIG. 18-32. Technique for detorsion by overlapping autoplasty. (From *Rev. Pédiatrie,* Nov.–Dec., 1965.)

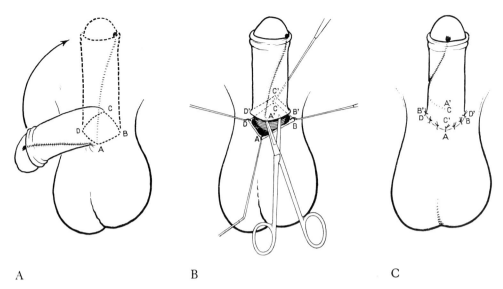

A	B	C

FIG. 18-33. Technique of detorsion circumcision (Caucci). A. Balanic hypospadias with 90 degrees torsion to the left. The circumcision is indicated by the dotted lines at the base (A, B, C, D). B. Incision of the skin and dartos fascia until the fascia penis superficialis is uncovered. On the line A, B, C, D, small orientation incisions may be made on the skin or silk stitches may be placed. A full décollement is executed at the root of the shaft. C. Completed hypercorrection (180 degrees). The circumcision is sutured to the base in separate stitches with silk thread. (From *Ann. Chir. Infant.* 10:287, 1969.)

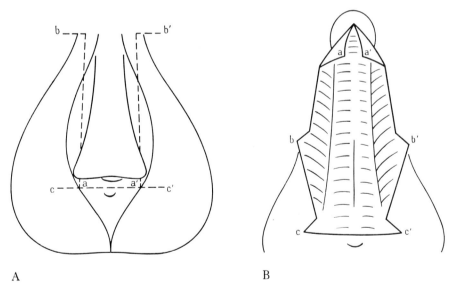

A	B

FIG. 18-34. Liberation of a congenitally concealed or adherent penis. A. Incision lines. B. View of the flaps after the penis has been raised. Points *b b'* correspond to the penoscrotal groove and are sutured to each other, as are points *a a'*. If the scrotum is bifid, suture *c c'* makes it possible to join the separated pouches. Otherwise, line *c c'* is sutured to the inferior part of lines *b c and b' c'*. (From *Rev. Pédiatrie*, Nov.–Dec., 1965.)

The correction must raise the shaft, bring the genital swellings down below it, and join them together (Fig. 18-34). It involves three incisions: A transverse premeatic incision that divides the internal rim of the genital swellings and the skin of the perineum that connects them (line cc' in Fig. 18-34). Two incisions perpendicular to the first delimit the shaft laterally. This is then raised by sectioning all fibrous tissue until the corpora cavernosa are free. The incision is closed longitudinally to reconstruct the sheath of the penis and to bring the genital swellings together.

WEBBED PENIS

This is very rare (2 percent of our cases).

Urethroplasty Techniques for Anterior Hypospadias

BALANIC HYPOSPADIAS

I do not think that these cases should be operated on if the canal is of sufficient caliber and the urinary stream is only slightly deviated.

If the meatus is small, I do a distal meatostomy which, by enlarging the top of the orifice, brings it closer to the summit of the glans and corrects the direction of the stream. Occasionally, one is forced to do an upward meatostomy that causes the orifice to recede and changes it into a balanopenile one.

BALANOPENILE AND ANTERIOR PENILE HYPOSPADIAS

I prefer always to use a perineal urethrostomy. The catheter is left in place for 10 days. I use a tourniquet at the root of the penis to prevent bleeding. This is removed after a pressure dressing has been applied. The bandage is removed on the fourth day.

I prefer two surgical techniques, both derived from the procedures described by Mathieu in 1932 [6]. One technique utilizes a penile flap with a superior perimeatal hinge that is raised and sutured to the internal lip of two paramedian balanic incisions. The cover is assured by direct suture of the external edges of the incisions of the glans and skin (Fig. 18-35).

This simple procedure has the disadvantage of seldom producing an apical meatus, for very often the last stitches of the suture give way so the urethra opens up on the inferior surface of the glans. Furthermore, it often confronts the surgeon with a difficult dilemma: either the flaps of the urethroplasty are large and the widely separated cover edges are difficult to bring together, running the risk of separation; or, in order to get a good cover, the flaps are cut narrowly, thus producing the risk of having a canal with insufficient caliber. I therefore prefer an alternate technique in anterior cases: the necessary cover for the urethra is obtained from the thickness of the glans. The urethral canal is constructed by two pedicle flaps—penile and balanic—and is buried in a trench-like cavity cut in the glans. The urethra is covered by the sides of the cavity (Fig. 18-36). I called this technique the balanic groove technique.

The penile flap is identical with the one described in the Mathieu procedure [6]. It must be slightly longer than the distance separating the meatus from the summit of the glans so its free edge can be turned back into a collar on the inferior edge of the new meatus.

Two paramedian incisions onto the glans outline this flap as in the Mathieu procedure, but the glans mucosa flap is detached from the glans so the flap below can be turned down around the meatus. Sutures are tied with the knots inside the urethra, and the ends of each

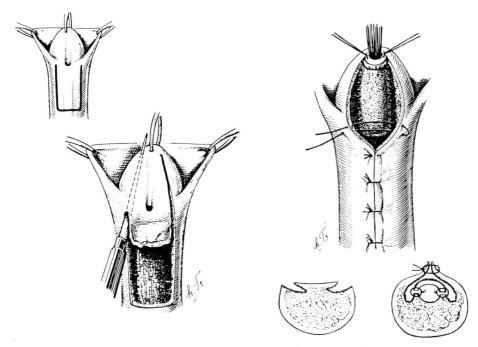

FIG. 18-35. Mathieu technique. (From *Rev. Pédiatrie,* Nov.–Dec., 1969.)

suture are allowed to protrude through the meatus.

In order for the area of the meatus to be buried deeply, the glandar incision and groove must go behind the meatus and the terminal part of the urethra. The superior surface of the latter is, therefore, separated from the supraurethral gutter for 10 to 15 mm in order to make the original urethra and the new canal both moveable (see Fig. 18-36C). A long vertical trench is created on the bottom, on which the urethra can be rested. It is enclosed there by suturing the sides of the groove (that is, from top to bottom), the glans, the balanopenile furrow, and the sheath. It is wise during this phase to calibrate the canal with a sound or catheter of the appropriate size.

An apical meatus is thus obtained, as well as a urethra that is transbalanic and that can be made as full as desired, since there is no lack of cover.

Two dangers are to be avoided: (1) The trench should be carried sufficiently low behind the original meatus, otherwise it will not provide sufficient tissue for cover and may produce fistulas; (2) A penile flap that is cut too short to be turned down at its extremity will produce a circular suture line where it meets the meatus and incurs the risk of causing a secondary stenosis.

RESULTS

Of 267 case reports collected for the above-mentioned symposium, the balanic groove technique showed primary success in 80 percent of the patients. The results were excellent in 192 cases, with a perfectly apical meatus, a urethra of good caliber, and a glans that appeared normal (Fig. 18-37); the results in 21 cases were moderately good, with a somewhat retracted meatus and a tendency to stricture (this was corrected by dilatation).

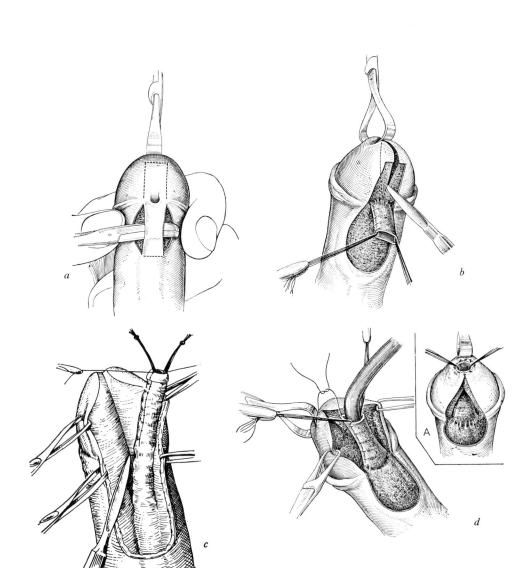

FIG. 18-36.   Balanic groove technique. (From *Ann. Chir. Infant.* 10:311, 1969.)

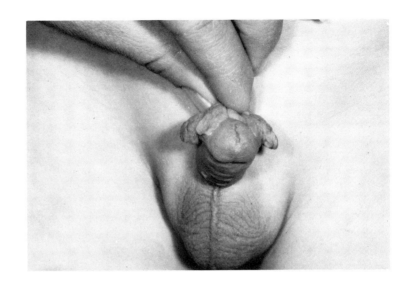

FIG. 18-37. Result of the balanic groove technique. The prepuce still has to be resected.

Of the 20 percent that were failures, the patients were most frequently troubled by fistulas. This problem has become more rare since we have been making regular use of the perineal diversion of urine.

FÈVRE TECHNIQUE FOR ANTERIOR HYPOSPADIAS

Instead of covering the new canal by burying it in the thickness of the glans, our teacher, Marcel Fèvre, thought of covering it by folding an extra-long penile flap back on itself (Fig. 18-38).

STAGE I: PENILE FLAP INCISION (SEE FIG. 18-38A AND B)

This flap must be at least twice as long as the canal to be constructed. Therefore, it must be cut with particular care to preserve vascularization despite its length.

The sides of the flap are outlined on both sides of the median line on the skin. The shaft is then held between the thumb and index finger of the left hand, stretching the skin in a circular manner. Layer by layer, the skin and subcutaneous tissue are incised until

the corpora cavernosa are completely free. The full thickness of all vascular tissue is left attached to the flap. When the two incisions are completed, a grooved sound is placed in the urethra to serve as a guide. The point of a blunt scissors is slipped through next to the urethra below the flap to free the remaining tissue. The inferior extremity of the flap is then sectioned and brought back along its superior perimeatic path.

In order to preserve the vascular supply to the maximum degree, one must be careful not to continue the dissection of this pathway too high.

STAGE II: (SEE FIG. 18-38C)

Two paramedian incisions on the glans delimit the balanic flap that remains adherent to the glans, as in the standard Mathieu procedure. The penile flap is sutured to the internal lips of these balanic incisions.

STAGE III: COVERAGE (SEE FIG. 18-38D)

In the balanic region and down below the original meatus, cover is obtained by folding back the penile flap, which is first sutured to the external lips of the balanic incisions.

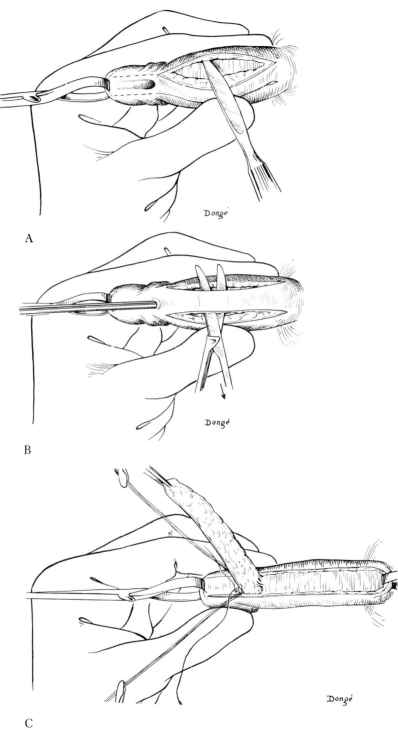

A

B

C

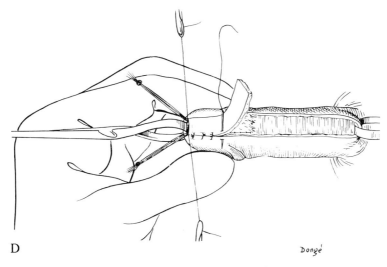

D

Dongé

FIG. 18-38. Fèvre technique utilizing a large Mathieu-type flap. A and B. First stage. Incision and dissection of the large flap. C. Second stage. The flap is sutured to the internal edges of the incisions of the glans. D. Third stage. The flap is folded back to cover the canal. (From *J. Chir.* 81:562, 1961.)

Lower down, it is sutured to the penile skin edges, and still farther down, the latter are connected directly to each other.

It is often helpful to make a relaxing incision behind the shaft to relieve tension in the last part of the suture.

RESULTS

This procedure seems to offer a great deal of security: in 55 cases, 46 were primary successes (84 percent). Fistulas were rare (5 percent). Failures were due only to mistakes in the dissection of the flap: if it does not contain sufficient tissue, it will be poorly vascularized and will run the risk of becoming gangrenous.

The results are esthetically acceptable but not as good as those of the balanic groove technique (Fig. 18-39). The indications for these two procedures are very similar. They apply exclusively to anterior hypospadias (balanopenile and anterior penile hypospadias).

I prefer to use the balanic groove procedure (1) if the inferior surface of the glans is

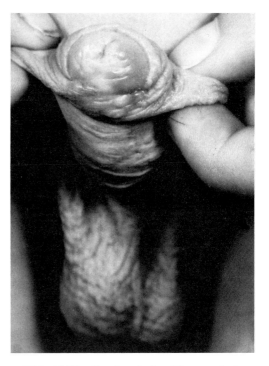

FIG. 18-39. Result of the Fèvre technique (large Mathieu-type flap technique) for balanopenile hypospadias (after meatostomy).

convex and if there is no deep fossa navicularis, or (2) if the shaft has already been subject to a lengthening procedure for correction of chordee or a detorsion. Here, the scarred skin cannot provide a long flap with adequate blood supply.

The large Mathieu-type flap is usually indicated if the inferior surface of the glans has already been excavated and especially if it already presents a deep fossa navicularis.

Urethroplasty for Middle and Posterior Hypospadias

Whenever there is enough scrotal tissue behind the meatus, I regularly use the procedure which in France is called *Leveuf première manière* (Leveuf I). This well-known two-stage procedure very closely resembles the technique described by Bucknall in 1907. The first stage is shown in Figures 18-40 and 18-41. The second stage (penoscrotal libera-

tion stage) can be performed 3 months later. We always perform a perineal urethrostomy in conjunction with the first stage.

Of the middle hypospadias cases, only 62 percent were primary surgical successes. On the other hand, when posterior penile or penoscrotal forms were involved, a 77 percent cure rate was obtained.

This technique has been criticized because of the risk of hair developing in the canal after puberty. The possibility of this danger appears to be rather remote provided that the scrotal flap is not too wide and is carefully limited to the vicinity of the median raphe where there are few hair follicles.

Sometimes I also use the *Leveuf deuxième manière* (Leveuf II), which was inspired by Cecil's technique. With this method, there is less chance of hair developing, since the canal is taken from the skin of the sheath. For this, however, the shaft and the glans must be quite well developed, and it seems to be difficult to perform before the onset of puberty.

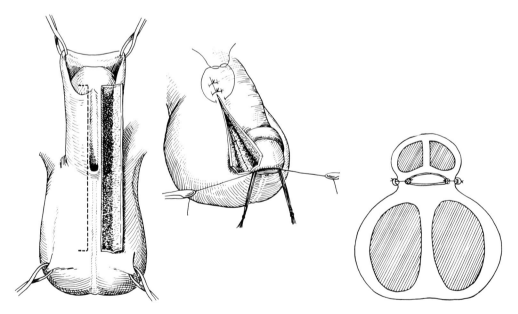

FIG. 18-40. "Leveuf I" procedure for urethroplasty. A. Outline of autograft flaps. B. Surface-joining stage. C. Completed operation (cross-sectional view). (From *Rev. Pédiatrie,* Nov.–Dec., 1965.)

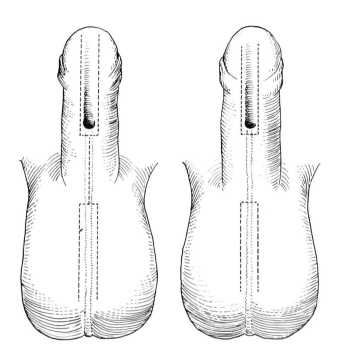

FIG. 18-41. "Leveuf I" procedure for urethroplasty. Variation of the outline of autograft flaps for a case of midpenile meatus. (From *Rev. Pédiatrie*, Nov.–Dec., 1965.)

If the scrotal tissue is in short supply because of original aplasia (or as a result of the failure of preceding surgery), the Leveuf technique cannot be used. For us, the procedure of choice is then the Denis Browne operation; however, this operation has provided primary success in only 53.5 percent of our cases.

SCROTAL OR PERINEAL HYPOSPADIAS

Often this is accompanied by an aplasia of the scrotum, which makes it impossible to consider any other repair but one of the Duplay or Denis Browne type, at least for the later stage that will bring the canal close to the root of the penis. Even if the scrotum is well developed, the meatus may be located too posteriorly to use the Leveuf procedure.

For such difficult cases we now use what is called the *cross-flap technique,* which was described by Boularan and Cahuzac at the above-mentioned symposium in 1967 (Fig. 18-42). This technique makes it possible to bring the urethra to the base of the penis and

thus obtain a penoscrotal meatus. Three months later, the urethroplasty is completed by a Leveuf-type operation.

Cahuzac [2] applied the principle of separation of suture lines, which has been recommended by Thiersch and which Cecil had proposed as a modification of the Duplay operation. Cahuzac cuts two rectangular flaps from the scrotum: on one side, a deep flap with an internal base to pivot on this base to form the anterior wall of the canal; on the opposite side, a superficial flap with an external base to be slipped over to cover the preceding one. The suture lines are thus clearly defined, since each flap is sutured to the opposite.

In Figure 18-42, parts 1 and 2 show the outline of the deep flap (incised on the left scrotal area) and the superficial crossing flap (incised on the right scrotal area). Between the two, there remains a cutaneous strip whose left edge corresponds to the base of the deep flap. The two flaps are of the same length, but the posterior extremity of the deep flap is cut back so it will fit over the urethral orifice without forming a cul-de-sac.

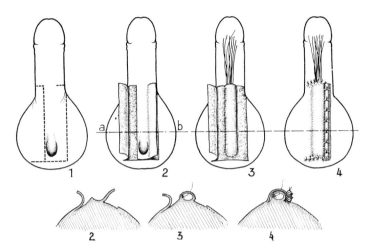

FIG. 18-42. First stage in the correction of scrotal hypospadias by the Boularan-Cahuzac cross-flap technique. Cross sections (a-b) are shown below.

In part 3 of Figure 18-42, the deep flap is seen folded back and sutured to the right side of the median cutaneous strip. Finally (part 4), the superficial flap, which is dissected broadly and is very elastic, is slipped over to cover the canal.

Out of eight cases operated on by this technique, Cahuzac had only one separation and one fistula that healed spontaneously. I have used this procedure four times, three of which were successful; I believe that the Boularan-Cahuzac procedure is a valuable contribution.

Perineal urethrostomy is helpful in this procedure, but it is not indispensable. Posterior hypospadias cases are usually coincidental with a poorly developed, short, narrow perineum. Cendron [3] pointed out that these are the only cases in which repeated urethrostomies cause trouble (eight fistulas occurring in 18 cases). Therefore, it is very important to be able to avoid perineal diversion in this first stage so it may be used in later stages.

Optimum Age at Operation

Preliminary operations present no problem as to age. In the case of stenosis of the meatus, the meatostomy should be performed as early as possible, sometimes at birth if the stenosis is tight. I operate for chordee, detorsion, and concealed penis in patients as young as the age of one. For urethroplasties, the question of optimum age is much more debatable, and some of our European colleagues tend to delay surgery until puberty.

There are two contrary factors in determining the optimum age: the psychological factor and the security factor. Psychologically, the malformation can be a source of problems as early as school age and even earlier. At adolescence in particular, the patient may develop serious complexes from which he is not always successful in freeing himself when he becomes an adult. Even if he has been operated on, a purely psychological impotence can result. The psychological aspect, therefore, points out the importance of operating early so treatment will be completed before school age and, in any event, before puberty.

On the other hand, the security factor would provide grounds for delaying surgery, since the operation would appear to be more successful on a well-developed organ with ample tissue.

Personally, I do not think that the young

age of my patients has been responsible for any poor results, and I attach such importance to the psychological factor that I am a very strong advocate of early operations. I

perform urethroplasties on patients as young as the age of five and sometimes even earlier if the shaft is sufficiently developed.

References

1. Barcat, J. Symposium sur l'hypospadias. 16th meeting of the French Society of Children's Surgery. *Ann. Chir. Infant.* 10:287, 1969.
2. Cahuzac, M., Claverie, J. P., and Cahuzac, J. P. Notre expérience de la cure de l'hypospadias. Techniques chirurgicales à propos de 195 cas. *Mem. Acad. Chir.* 98:143, 1972.
3. Cendron, J. Traitement des hypospadias par la technique modifiée de Leveuf. *Ann. Chir. Infant.* 2:84, 1961.
4. Leveuf, J., and Godard, H. La greffe temporaire de la verge sur le scrotum dans la cure de l'hypospadias. *J. Chir.* 48:328, 1936.
5. Leveuf, J. Le traitement de l'hypospadias. *J. Chir.* 62:96, 1946.
6. Mathieu, P. Traitement en un temps de l'hypospadias balanique et juxta-balanique. *J. Chir.* 39:481, 1932.
7. Nesbit, R. M. The surgical correction of minor hypospadias with chordee. *Pediatrics* 42:471, 1968.

One-Stage Repair—I

THOMAS RAY BROADBENT
ROBERT M. WOOLF

The management of the patient with hypospadias requires correct sex determination and assignment. The parents are advised against having the boy circumcised at birth, since the preputial skin is essential to any repair and, especially, to a one-stage repair of hypospadias. Surgical correction is postponed until the patient is 5 to 5½ years of age to allow for the growth of a frequently small penile organ. However, correction should be provided before the patient begins school in order to avoid undue emotional stress. A boy must be able to stand and void like his male classmates if he is to avoid curiosity and embarrassment [1].

One-stage correction is preferred because it offers the patient minimal scarring, minimal hospitalization and costs, and comparable functional and esthetic results to multiple-stage procedures. In any repair of hypospadias, one must:

1. Correct the state of chordee so that the penis is normal during erection as well as when flaccid;

2. Construct an adequate sized urethra free of hair, obstructing bands, and stricture;

3. Produce a urethra capable of growth and distention, free of fistula, and with a meatal orifice near or at the tip of the glans penis [2].

Hypospadias of the midshaft and penoscrotal and perineal varieties can be successfully corrected in one stage with a buried, vascularized, skin-strip technique. This repair is not recommended for coronal and balanic varieties [3].

Surgical Technique

Preoperative preparation, medication, general anesthesia, and surgical positioning, cleansing, and draping are as preferred by the surgeon.

Diversion of the urinary stream is produced by a perineal urethrostomy that is performed by cutting down on a meatal sound in the urethra, grasping and everting the urethral mucosa, and slipping a No. 12 Foley catheter into the bladder.

Bleeding is controlled (the position of the hypospadial opening permitting) with a soft rubber drain placed as a tourniquet at the base of the penile shaft. Blood is squeezed from the penis, the rubber drain is drawn snugly but not harshly about the penis, and the drain is held tight with a clamp.

Dye (brilliant green) is used to outline the incisions. A skin strip is marked that extends around the hypospadial meatus and extends distally along the ventral aspect of the penis. The strip deviates slightly to the right (or to the left) and runs onto the dorsum of the distal penile skin (prepuce) to just beyond the dorsal midline (Fig. 18-43). The skin strip is wide enough to encompass a No. 12 French catheter loosely, that is, about one-third the circumference of the penis. Caution is taken to ensure this width of tissue at the

hypospadial meatus and at the corona, which are the two most likely sites for fistula formation if the closure is unduly tight.

The incision along the distal edge of the strip on the dorsum of the penis is extended along the edge of the prepuce and around the penis to contact with itself ventrally near the midline. The preputial skin, except for the skin strip, can then be mobilized as required for shifting and rotation to the ventral surface. This tissue will be used to cover the new urethra (tubed skin strip).

The fibrous tissue that causes the chordee is excised. Correction of chordee and straightening of the penis always allows the hypospadial opening to retract toward the scrotum. It is essential that the previously outlined skin strip be long enough to accommodate for this apparent lengthening of the

FIG. 18-43. A. Outline of skin strip to be utilized in urethral reconstruction. B. Strip extends proximal to hypospadial opening and should be kept wide at this level and at the corona. C. The skin strip to be tubed for urethral reconstruction extends to, or beyond, the dorsal midline. (From T. R. Broadbent and R. M. Woolf, *Br. J. Plast. Surg.* 18:406, 1965.)

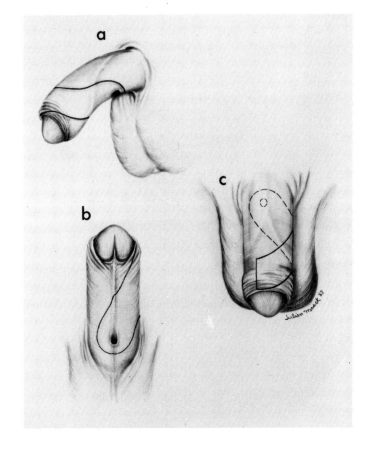

penis and thus the extension of the strip to or slightly beyond the dorsal midline is necessary.

If the glans penis is large enough, it is tunneled or even cored out to receive the new urethra. If, as is usually the case, it is too small, it is split along the ventral midline to its tip so the new urethra may lie in the substance of the glans.

The skin strip is not undermined but is left attached to its "mesentery" of loose areolar tissue and vessels. The skin strip is tubed with a continuous 5-0 catgut suture, and a reinforcing layer of nonabsorbable 6-0 Dacron sutures further buttresses this tubing (Fig. 18-44). The distal portion of the tubed skin strip is pulled gently from its dorsal position, avoiding all but the slightest distal mobilization, and is threaded into or laid into the glans penis. The meatal orifice is fixed at the tip of the penis with interrupted 5-0 or 6-0

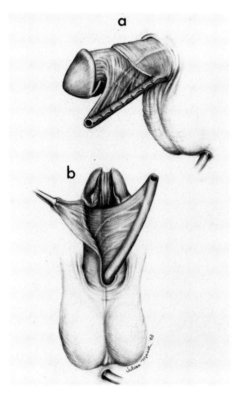

FIG. 18-44. A. Skin strip has been tubed. The "mesentery" and vessels in the areolar tissue remain attached to the strip. B. Remaining preputial skin, grasped with a forceps, has been freed and shifted ventrally for covering the new urethra. The skin strip has been tubed to form the new urethra. The glans is either cored or, as shown here, split and cored to receive the urethra that will be laid into it. (From T. R. Broadbent and R. M. Woolf, *Br. J. Plast. Surg.* 18:406, 1965.)

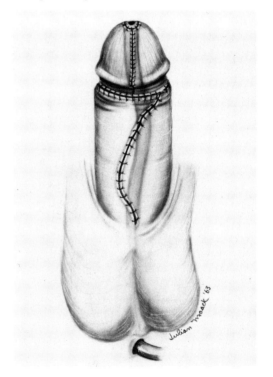

FIG. 18-45. The skin strip has been tubed, laid into its new bed, and brought to the tip of the glans. The glans is closed over if there is sufficient tissue, but if not, the loose preputial skin, which was shifted to the ventral surface of the penis and covers the new urethra, may be extended up onto the glans. Perineal urethrostomy is used for diversion of the urinary stream. (From T. R. Broadbent and R. M. Woolf, *Br. J. Plast. Surg.* 18:406, 1965.)

catgut sutures. The rubber drain tourniquet is removed, and hemostasis is meticulously accomplished with electrocoagulation. Only then may the closure be safely completed; seemingly unavoidable edema in these tissues can be frightening, but a hematoma is disastrous to normal healing. The remaining previously mobilized preputial skin is rotated to the ventral surface and used to cover the new urethra, extending when necessary onto the glans penis. Closure is effected with subcutaneous 6-0 Dacron sutures. The skin may be closed with a subcuticular nylon pull-out suture or a continuous or interrupted suture of 6-0 catgut (see Figs. 18-43 to 18-45).

The penis, including the glans, is bandaged with fine mesh petroleum gauze and Tensoplast tape, which is applied with modest tension and arranged so that the penis remains in an erect position, thereby enhancing venous drainage. Postoperatively, the patient remains in bed for 10 to 12 days. Bladder irrigation is not used; only over-the-bed sterile drainage is employed. At the end of 10 days, the dressings are removed. Two days later, the perineal catheter is removed, and voiding is allowed through the new urethra and the perineum. The perineal urethrostomy opening closes spontaneously in 3 to 4 days.

References

1. Broadbent, T. R., and Woolf, R. M. Hypospadias: One-stage repair. *Br. J. Plast. Surg.* 18:406, 1965.
2. Broadbent, T. R., and Woolf, R. M. Hypospadias—one-stage repair—two-stage repair. *Rocky Mountain Med. J.* 68:35, 1971.
3. Broadbent, T. R., Woolf, R. M., and Toksu, E. Hypospadias: One-stage repair. *Plast. Reconstr. Surg.* 27:154, 1961.

One-Stage Repair—II

JOHN D. DESPREZ
LESTER PERSKY

The almost simultaneous, independent publication of three methods of one-stage repair of hypospadias in 1961 by Broadbent, Woolf, and Toksu [1], Horton and Devine [3, 4] and DesPrez, Persky, and Kiehn [2] suggested a practical and advantageous approach to a problem that had previously been solved by multiple operations. Whereas techniques may vary, the results over the past 10 years have substantiated this initial unanimity of enthusiasm for the correction of hypospadias by one operation.

The repair of hypospadias involves the elimination of fibrous chordee to straighten the penile shaft and glans, retropositioning the meatus, and construction of an intact distal meatus. The correction of grade I, or coronal hypospadias, is indicated only when there is considerable "cobra head" angulation of the glans during erection or when the angulation is sufficient to cause downward spraying during urination. Mild distal hypospadias with little angulation is best left alone.

The repair is generally initiated at 3 years of age or when the penis is sufficiently large to accommodate at least a No. 10 Foley catheter within the newly constructed urethra. Repair should be completed by the time the child enters school.

Surgical Technique

A full-thickness skin strip is outlined proximally from the urethral meatus along the ventral shaft of the penis and outward onto the inner surface of the prepuce. The length of this skin strip is not determined initially but is deferred until after the fibrous tissues causing the chordee have been excised. The width of the strip should be at least 1.5 cm or more in order to be tubed comfortably around a No. 10 or No. 12 Foley catheter.

This skin strip is completely elevated from the shaft. The incision is carried completely around the meatus, leaving a small cuff of skin, together with the strip, attached to the meatal margin. The urethra is freed posteriorly, using extreme care, from its fibrous attachment, and the meatus is allowed to recess to its normal position (Fig. 18-46).

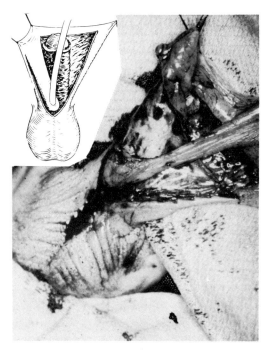

FIG. 18-46. The skin strip has been developed and the chordee is corrected.

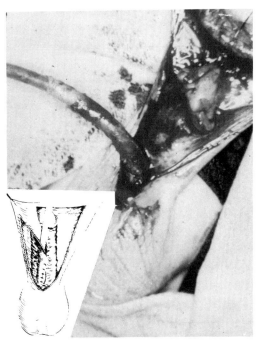

FIG. 18-47. The skin strip has been tubed around the catheter.

Thus, access to the chordee-causing tissue is achieved. Resection of this fibrous tissue, which is particularly heavy in the median raphe between the corpora cavernosa but which may extend well laterally, is carefully and completely achieved. If the glans is angulated, the fibrous frenulum is removed, thus opening the glans by forming a trough. Penetration of the underlying tunica albuginea covering the corpora should be carefully avoided to prevent significant bleeding.

The skin strip and proximal cuff are tubed around an indwelling Foley catheter by careful invagination with 4-0 chromic catgut sutures (Fig. 18-47). The desired length of this skin tube may now be determined, and the tube is cut free distally from the prepuce. The skin tube is rotated so that the suture line abuts deeply against the corpora and is

snubbed down in the desired position. The distal end is brought to the glans or fixed to the tip within the trough opening (Fig. 18-48).

The new distal urethra is then covered by a wrap-around flap or a dorsal hood flap (Fig. 18-49). If the new urethra is long, the remaining skin covering the entire shaft of the penis and unfolded prepuce is mobilized and brought diagonally around the circumference of the penis in order to cover the new urethra with intact skin and to avoid superimposed suture lines. In the more distal deformity, the new urethra is short and is covered by the dorsal hood flap brought down by passing the glans through a slit to cover the volar area with a bipedicle U-shaped flap, sutured well laterally and ventrally away from the urethra.

The skin is closed with 4-0 chromic catgut,

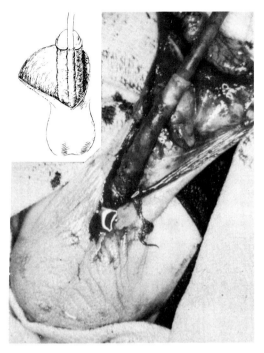

FIG. 18-48. The skin urethra is positioned against the corpora and proper length is determined.

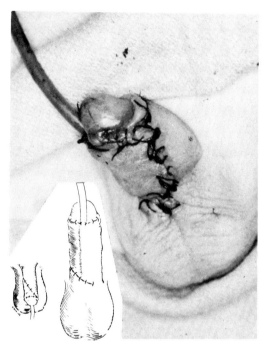

FIG. 18-49. The remaining penile skin is mobilized and wrapped around to cover the urethra.

and a secure tie-on stent dressing of moist cotton reinforced with Elastoplast is applied. This dressing is not removed for 7 to 10 days; the indwelling catheter remains for 12 to 14 days. Gantrisin (sulfisoxazole) is given for 3 weeks. The child is immobilized for a week of bed rest to safeguard the catheter and dressing.

Results

The results of some 65 cases during 10 years of experience have been gratifying but not entirely devoid of difficulty. Two-thirds of the cases healed primarily and resulted in correction by the one-stage procedure. In the remaining one-third, a small urethral fistula developed that necessitated a secondary minor surgical procedure, thus completing the repair in two stages. One total failure occurred due to hematoma about the skin tube which resulted in scar formation and tortuosity and necessitated excision and multiple-stage repair. Fistulas were most common in grade I, or distal hypospadias cases, and least common in grade III, or scrotal perineal hypospadias cases. Although the constructed urethral tube was much longer in the latter cases, closure was more secure since the tube was buried deeply beneath layers of soft tissue.

Meatal stricture was not uncommon following attempts to bring the new urethra to the tip of the glans. Some strictures required meatotomy or Z-plasty, whereas others responded to dilatation, a procedure that re-

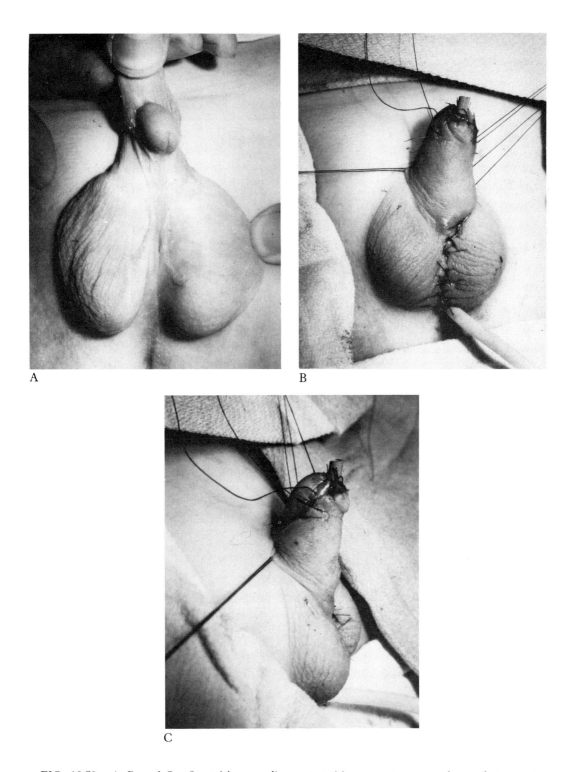

A

B

C

FIG. 18-50. A, B, and C. Scrotal hypospadias corrected by a one-stage procedure utilizing perineal urethrostomy and a distal rubber stent.

quires general anesthesia in this age group. On occasion, if the tube were brought only to the corona and not anchored to the base of the glans, the meatus was observed to slide somewhat proximally with the growth of the penis, necessitating later revision or even additional lengthening of the urethra to correct spraying. Urethral obstruction, stricture, stone formation, or cystitis has not been observed during the follow-up period.

Patients that have been previously circumcised require the addition of a skin graft to complete the coverage of the penis. In these patients, there is usually insufficient skin to construct a urethra and cover it adequately. Stretching is readily achieved but is almost certain to result in fistula formation.

A diverting perineal urethrostomy and rubber tube urethral stent have been employed in several cases instead of an indwelling catheter. The incidence of fistula formation is essentially the same. However, on occasion, the temporary, but not always complete, diversion of urine by urethrostomy from the operative area may have merit (Fig. 18-50).

The same technique has been applied to five cases of chordee without hypospadias, or the so-called congenitally short urethra, and to two cases of hypospadias without chordee. The latter rare situation is managed similarly, and the procedure is facilitated by being able to build a urethra without the necessity of removing the fibrous bands. If the urethra is "short," mobilization of the entire penile urethra and removal of the underlying fibrous tissue permits lengthening and corrects the bent shaft without cutting and splicing the urethra. The urethra is replaced essentially as a free graft and is covered by a wrap-around or dorsal hood flap of intact skin. This avoids sectioning of the urethra, suture splicing, and staged procedures.

The principle of one-stage repair of hypospadias has been tested and found to be satisfactory. Careful surgical technique, complete release of all fibrous bands, meticulous hemostasis, adequate skin mobilization for tubing, careful invagination of the tube suture line with buttressing against the corpora, coverage of the new urethra with a well-mobilized skin flap, avoidance of superimposed suture lines, well-placed supportive dressing, and attentive postoperative care should give excellent results.

References

1. Broadbent, R. T., Woolf, R. M., and Toksu, E. Hypospadias—one-stage repair. *Plast. Reconstr. Surg.* 27:154, 1961.
2. DesPrez, J. D., Persky, L., and Kiehn, C. L. One-stage repair of hypospadias by island flap technique. *Plast. Reconstr. Surg.* 28:405, 1961.
3. Devine, C. J., Jr., and Horton, C. E. A one-stage hypospadias repair. *J. Urol.* 85:166, 1961.
4. Horton, C. E., and Devine, C. J., Jr. Film: A one-stage hypospadias repair. Eaton Laboratories, 1957.

One-Stage Repair — III

CHARLES E. HORTON
CHARLES J. DEVINE, JR.

To begin the surgical repair, a black silk suture is placed through the glans penis doral to the tip. Tension on this suture and dorsal pressure on the penis aids in dissection and reduces bleeding. The desired incisions are marked on the skin. The injection of 1 to 2 ml of lidocaine with adrenalin 1:100,000 into the operative area also aids in hemostasis. A perineal urethrostomy or suprapubic cystostomy is usually done for urinary diversion.

An incision is made around the urethral meatus and is extended down the urethral groove to the corona; it is then carried around the penis. The fibrous tissue and abnormal skin distal to the urethral meatus are excised. The lateral flaps of normal skin are undermined and retracted. It is imperative that skin edges be handled with hooks instead of forceps; nowhere in the body is the tissue more susceptible to trauma from rough handling than in this area. The execution and technique of handling tissue are as important as the planning of this operation. Buck's fascia is incised near the corona lateral to the point where fibrous bands can be palpated. It is removed by dissecting toward the urethra and the midline. It has been found that dissection in this direction aids in preventing damage to the corpus cavernosum. If the corpus cavernosum is inadvertently entered, the defect is repaired with 6-0 chromic catgut sutures. Absolute hemostasis is essential. Coagulation of discrete bleeding points rather than ligation of large masses of tissue promotes primary healing.

Buck's fascia and the dartos fascia in the area of the defect must be excised, and the corpora cavernosa are meticulously cleaned. The importance of complete removal of all tissue contributing to the abnormal curvature cannot be overemphasized. Beneath Buck's fascia, there are numerous small vessels called the venae profundae. Bleeding from these vessels should not be mistaken for bleeding from the corpus cavernosum, thus discouraging adequate removal of the fascia and the fibrous tissue. The tunica albuginea of the corpora cavernosa should be clean and glistening at the conclusion of the procedure.

With the penis under tension and dorsiflexed, palpation of the shaft may reveal other bands of fibrous tissue that should be excised.

There must be no restricting tissue left when urethroplasty is combined with the release of the chordee. Recurrence of chordee with the urethra completely reconstructed would present a situation that is difficult to correct. The proximal attachment of the abnormal fascia surrounds the existing meatus. The urethral meatus must be separated from the corpora cavernosa, and the abnormal fibrous tissue surrounding the urethra must be removed. However, excessively extensive dissection around the urethra may open the normal corpus spongiosum and thus cause excess bleeding. The urethral meatus will retract beneath the intact skin when the fibrous tissue causing the chordee has been adequately removed. After the coronal incision is continued around the penis about 2 mm proximal to the glans, the prepuce is unfolded into a single layer and the skin of the penis is elevated from the shaft for a distance of 2 to 3 cm. The desired length and width of prepuce for the urethral graft is excised. The length of the graft is determined by measuring from the existing urethra to the tip of the penis; the graft width is determined by the size of the normal urethra. If a size 12 French catheter fits the urethra, the graft must be 12 mm wide. The skin graft is sutured loosely over a stent catheter, with the raw surface outward. A running suture of 6-0 chromic catgut is used to form a free, full-thickness graft tube. The graft is kept moistened with saline.

Preputial skin is ideal for the free skin graft tube to replace the urethra. In circumcised cases, full-thickness skin grafts from the inner, hairless portion of the upper arm or groin can be used, but preputial skin is thinner, pliable, and more desirable. The width of the prepuce has not failed to furnish a graft of sufficient length in our cases. We would not hesitate to piece two sections of skin together if necessary to produce an adequate length of graft. A large, elliptical proximal anastomosis is formed by beveling the urethra and skin graft tube. The stent catheter is then inserted 3 to 4 cm into the distal urethra. The graft is positioned with its seam deep against the groove between the corpora cavernosa. A triangular midline glandar flap is incised, elevated, and thinned. This is easily done by dissection between the glans and corpora cavernosa where a good cleavage plane will be found. The lateral wings of glandar tissue are mobilized by undermining. The triangular flap can be interposed into the distal suture line, preventing circular contracture. It is sewn to the tunica albuginea of the corpora cavernosa and to the elliptical opening of the distal skin graft tube with 6-0 chromic catgut. The lateral glandar wings are then elevated and brought together over the distal urethra. This changes the flat, spatulate shape of the glans to a more normal conical configuration.

The urethral meatus is located exactly at the tip of the glans. The skin defect ventrally must then be covered, using local tissue in the form of a flap. An incision may be made in the remaining prepuce and a hood flap—described first by Ombrédanne and popularized by Nesbit—is constructed. This flap is brought to the ventral surface of the penis by inserting the glans through the incision in the prepuce. This flap will cover the entire ventral surface of the penis; however, if more proximal coverage is desired, a small scrotal flap can be elevated and used in conjunction. Frequently, instead of an Ombrédanne-type hood, the prepuce will be divided in the midline and brought to the ventral surface of the penis in the form of two lateral flaps. To prevent displacement of the tube graft, the black silk retraction suture is placed through the stent catheter (Figs. 18-51–18-63)

For perineal and scrotal hypospadias with bifid scrotum, the repair differs in that the chordee can be resected via ventral excision, and, anterior to the meatus, a usable strip of

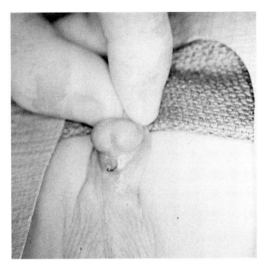

FIG. 18-51. Preoperative penile hypospadias.

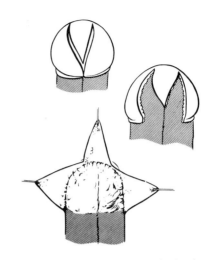

FIG. 18-53. Incisions are made in the glans to produce lateral wings and a midline triangular flap.

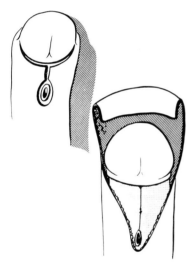

FIG. 18-52. Incision on the shaft is continued around the prepuce.

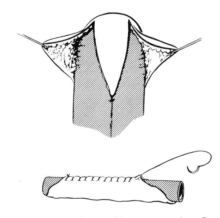

FIG. 18-54. The midline triangular flap is thinned and resutured to the corpora.

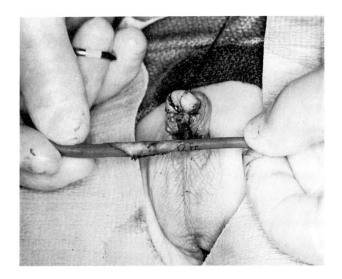

FIG. 18-55. Skin graft tube taken from the prepuce.

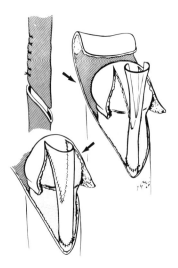

FIG. 18-56. Elliptical anastomoses are made proximally to the normal urethra and distally to the midline flap.

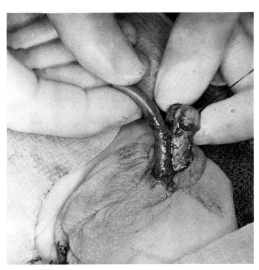

FIG. 18-57. Anastomosis of the skin graft tube.

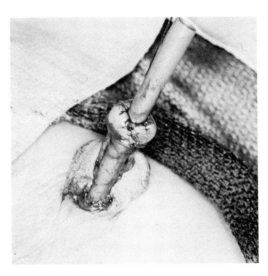

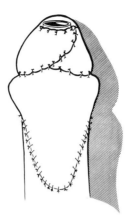

FIG. 18-58. Ventral surface deficit. Glandar wings have been approximated ventral to the urethral meatus.

FIG. 18-59. Ombrédanne-type coverage is obtained via an incision in the prepuce.

FIG. 18-60. Prepuce has been opened.

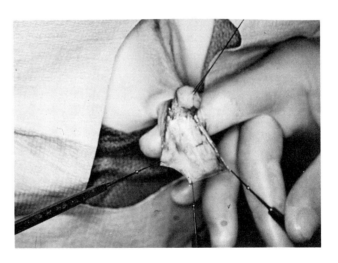

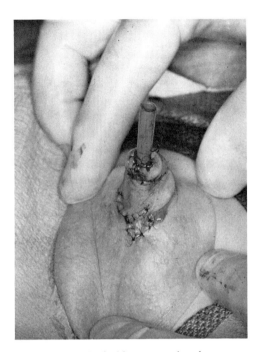

FIG. 18-61. Ombrédanne-type hood coverage of the ventral surface. Note the meatus at the tip of the glans.

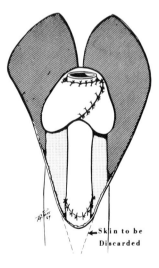

FIG. 18-62. An alternative coverage is obtained by splitting the prepuce.

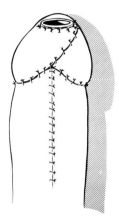

FIG. 18-63. Skin closure following the method shown in Figure 18-62.

hairless mucosa-like skin is present for a distance of 2 to 4 cm before it is involved with the chordee (Fig. 18-64). Therefore, if chordee release underneath and distal to this area is accomplished, the penis is straightened adequately. We then tube this skin to elongate the proximal urethra to the base of the penile shaft (Fig. 18-65). A full-thickness skin graft is anastomosed to this tube and completes the urethral repair distally (Figs. 18-66 and 18-67). Coverage is accomplished by excising all excess scrotal skin left in the scrotal cleft and by closing the scrotum in the midline in layers to form a normal appearing organ (Fig. 18-68). An Ombrédanne hood can be used for ventral coverage, or Byars' preputial flaps may be preferred.

Because we have been encouraged by the reports of Mustardé, we have been utilizing a Bevan-type flap based distally on the urethra for distal penile hypospadias. This flap is folded anteriorly to meet the large median glandar flap in minor degrees of hypospadias (Figs. 18-69 to 18-74). This makes it unnecessary to use a free graft, and there is a complete urethra to the glans tip. Coverage is either by

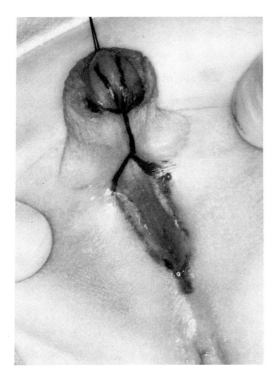

FIG. 18-64. These incisions are used for scrotal and perineal hypospadias cases.

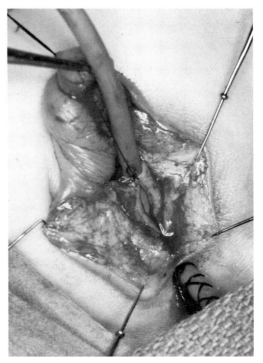

FIG. 18-65. A proximal skin flap is tubed to bring the urethra to the base of the penis.

an Ombrédanne flap or by a Byars' preputial shift. A Foley catheter is inserted through the reconstructed urethra to the bladder for drainage. No perineal diversion is necessary. The catheter is removed on the fourth or fifth postoperative day.

Following the surgery, the repair is covered with fine mesh nitrofurazone-impregnated gauze, and an occlusive Elastoplast dressing is applied (see Fig. 18-74). Care is taken to see that this does not compromise the blood supply. The outer dressing is removed on the third day, and the patient is placed in a tub of sterile water three times a day thereafter to soak away the final layers of gauze covering the wound. The stent catheter is removed on the seventh postoperative day. No sounding or calibration is done unless symptoms indicative of stricture or fistula formation occur.

The meatus is kept lubricated with antibiotic ointment three times daily to prevent dry crusts from plugging the outlet. After removal of the stent, the tip of an ophthalmic tube is inserted into the urethral meatus for gentle dilatation three or four times a day. Approximately 75 percent of all primary cases operated are cured in one operation by these techniques (Figs. 18-75 and 18-76).

The V-shaped glandar flap is a useful technique to use in conjunction with either a Duplay or Denis Browne urethroplasty. By advancing the triangular flap into the central strip of skin to be used for the urethral reconstruction, the meatus can be placed at the tip of the penis. Lateral coverage is obtained by using the glandar wings and the lateral skin of the shaft of the penis (Figs. 18-77 to 18-81).

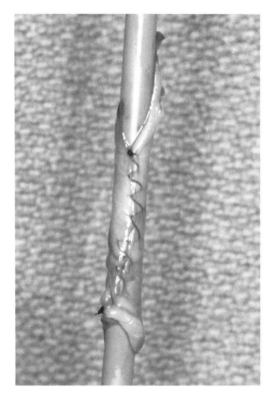

FIG. 18-66. Full-thickness skin graft tube.

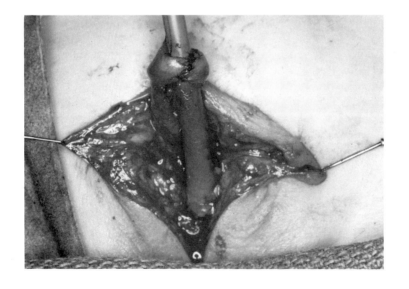

FIG. 18-67. Urethral reconstruction is accomplished by anastomosis of the skin graft tube to the glans and the proximally reconstructed urethra.

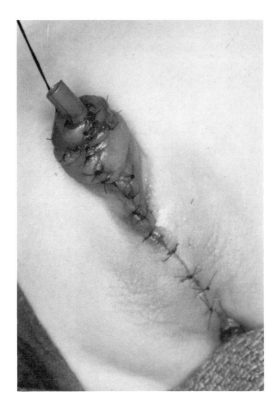

FIG. 18-68. Closure of the scrotum for proximal coverage and the use of Byars-type preputial flaps for penile coverage.

FIG. 18-69. Preoperative distal hypospadias.

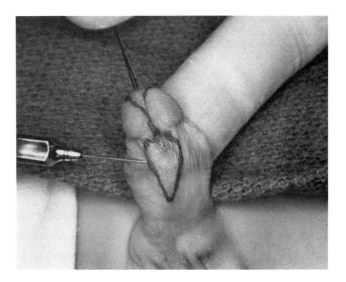

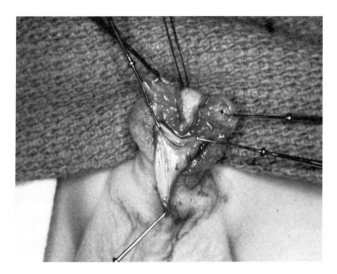

FIG. 18-70. A flap is elevated.

FIG. 18-71. A Bevan-type flap is based on the urethral meatus.

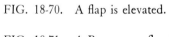

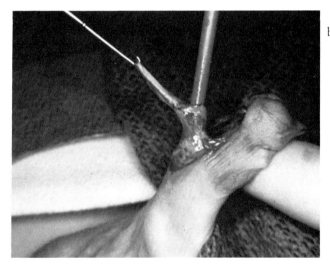

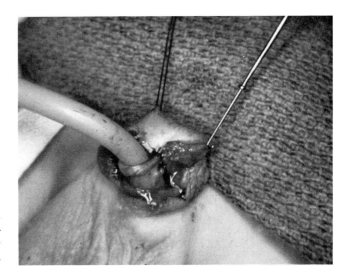

FIG. 18-72. The flap is sutured to the midline glandar flap to construct the urethra skin closure by transfer of prepuce to ventral surface.

FIG. 18-73. The prepuce is split and brought to the ventral surface.

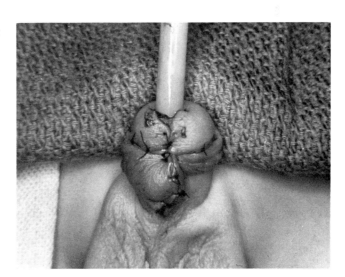

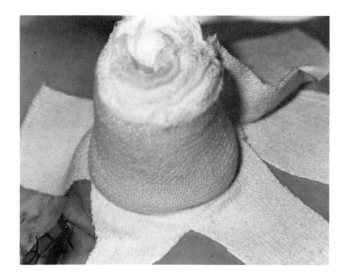

FIG. 18-74. Bandage of Elasto-plast.

FIG. 18-75. Typical chordee and distal hypospadias in an adult male.

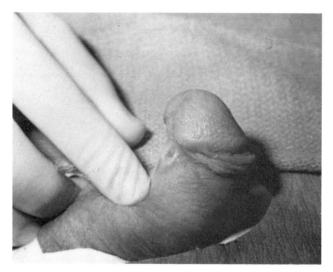

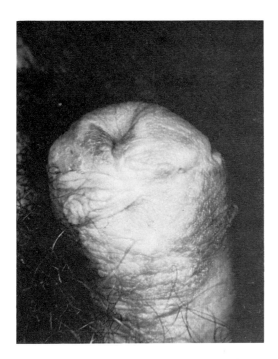

FIG. 18-76. Postoperative view of case shown in Figure 18-75. Meatus is at the tip of the glans.

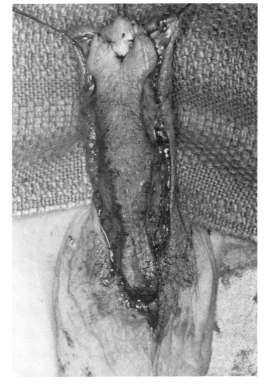

FIG. 18-77. V-shaped glandar flaps are anastomosed to the central strip of skin to produce a meatus at the tip. The central strip of skin can be left to tube itself (method of Denis Browne), or it can be tubed with sutures (method of Duplay). See Figs. 18-79 and 18-80.

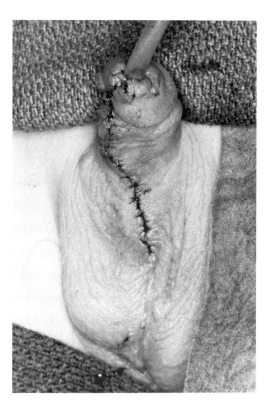

FIG. 18-78.   Closure is accomplished with the meatus at the tip.

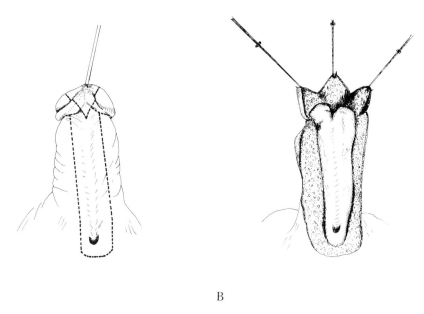

A   B

FIG. 18-79.   Midline glandar flap technique will produce a meatus in the tip of the glans in Duplay, Byars, or Denis Browne-type operations.   A.   Central strip of skin is outlined on the ventral surface of the penis.   B.   A midline glandar flap is elevated. The midline incision is at the tip of the ventral strip of skin. The lateral glandar wings are retracted.

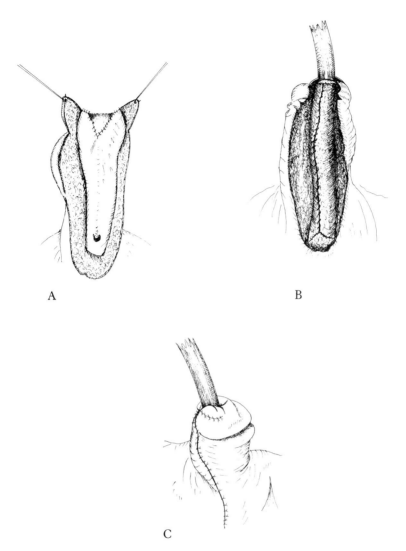

A

B

C

FIG. 18-80. A. A midline glandar flap is sutured to the midline incision in the ventral skin strip. B. Completion of the tube for the urethra. The lateral glandar wings are to be brought medially for reshaping of the glans and coverage of the distal urethra. C. Completed repair. The meatus is at the tip of the glans.

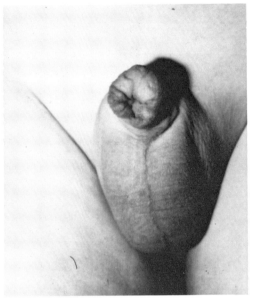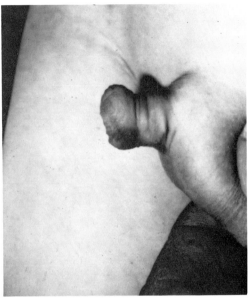

FIG. 18-81. Catastrophies may occur even in careful hypospadias repairs. This patient, who was operated on elsewhere, had the glans slough away after surgery.

References

1. Backus, L. H., and DeFelice, C. A. Hypospadias—then and now. *Plast. Reconstr. Surg.* 25:146, 1960.
2. Bevan, A. D. A new operation for hypospadias. *J.A.M.A.* 68:1032, 1917.
3. Bucknall, R. T. H. A new operation for penile hypospadias. *Lancet* 2:887, 1907.
4. Byars, L. T. Surgical repair of hypospadias. *Surg. Clin. North Am.* 30:1371, 1950.
5. Cecil, A. B. Surgery of hypospadias and epispadias in the male. *J. Urol.* 27:507, 1932.
6. Cloutier, A. M. A method for hypospadias repair. *Plast. Reconstr. Surg.* 30:368, 1962.
7. Culp, O. S. Experiences with 200 hypospadias: Evolution of a therapeutic plan. *Surg. Clin. North Am.* 39:1007, 1959.
8. Devine, C. J., and Horton, C. E. One-stage hypospadias repair. *J. Urol.* 85:166, 1961.
9. Edmunds, A. An operation for hypospadias. *Lancet* 1:447, 1913.
10. Fogh-Andersen, P. Hypospadias: Thirty-four completed cases operated on according to Denis Browne. *Acta Chir. Scand.* 105:414, 1953.
11. Horton, C. E., and Devine, C. J., Jr. Film: A one-stage hypospadias repair. Eaton Laboratories, 1959.
12. Horton, C. E., and Devine, C. J., Jr. A One-Stage Hypospadias Repair. In Broadbent, T. R. (Ed.), *Transactions of the Third International Congress of Plastic Surgery.* Amsterdam: Excerpta Medica, 1963.
13. Horton, C. E., and Devine, C. J., Jr. Hypospadias. In *Modern Trends in Plastic Surgery,* Vol. 2, Section IV. London: Butterworth, 1966.
14. Humby, G. A one-stage operation for hypospadias. *Br. J. Surg.* 29:113, 1941.
15. McCormack, R. M. Simultaneous chordee repair and urethral reconstruction for hypospadias. *Plast. Reconstr. Surg.* 13:257, 1954.
16. Mustardé, J. C. One-stage correction of dis-

tal hypospadias: and other people's fistulae. *Br. J. Plast. Surg.* 18:413, 1965.

17. Nesbit, R. M. Plastic procedure for correction of hypospadias. *J. Urol.* 45:699, 1941.

18. Nové-Josserand, G. Nouvelle technique pour la restauration en une séance des hypospadias étendus par la tunnelisation avec greffe dermo-epidermique. *J. Urol.* 8:449, 1919.

19. Russell, R. H. Operation for severe hypo-

spadias. *Br. Med. J.* 2:1432, 1900.

20. Smith, D. R. Surgical treatment of hypospadias. *J. Urol.* 73:329, 1955.

21. Wehrbein, H. L. Hypospadias. *J. Urol.* 50:335, 1943.

22. Young, F., and Benjamin, J. A. Preschool age repair of hypospadias with free inlay skin graft. *Surgery* 26:384, 1949.

One-Stage Repair — IV

JOHN C. MUSTARDÉ

It may be questioned whether it is justifiable to subject a child to an operation when that child suffers from one of the minor but very common forms of hypospadias that involves only the terminal one-fifth of the penis and the coronal area. Much will depend on the likelihood of complete success of such an operation, the risks involved to the child, and the possibility of offering a one-stage procedure of reasonable simplicity. The technique to be described [4] has been in continuous use for 6 years.

The operation is performed, if possible, when the patient is 1 year old. Babies appear to suffer less physical discomfort at this age, and they are less affected psychologically than later on. Before the age of one, the penis may be very small and more difficult to work with. The operation is designed to correct any chordee that may be present, and it should eliminate the hooded prepuce as well as producing a new urethra that opens on the tip of the glans.

Surgical Technique

Preliminary posterior urethrostomy may be carried out, or an indwelling nonrubber cath-eter may be inserted during the operation. The penis is held by a suture passed through the glans dorsal to the proposed urethral opening, and a rectangular flap is outlined that is 15 mm wide and as long as will be required to reconstruct the urethra once the chordee has been completely corrected (Fig. 18-82). The flap should be based 1 or 2 mm distal to the existing urethral opening, and it is incised around down to the layer of loose connective tissue. Undermining is carried out except for a distal strip that represents about one-fourth to one-third of the end adjacent to the urethra, which must not be punctured during this dissection (a metal probe can be inserted to show the location of the urethra). It is important to ensure that the two distal corners of the attaching strip are quite free and untethered without actually being under-mined (Figs. 18-83 and 18-84).

The distal incision is now carried around the corona. Access is thereby provided for the careful dissection and removal of all the con-nective tissue on the ventral surface that causes the chordee. This having been done, the urethral opening will now be 1 cm or more from the glandar skin, but if the dis-tance should be less, some glandar skin should be excised to effect this.

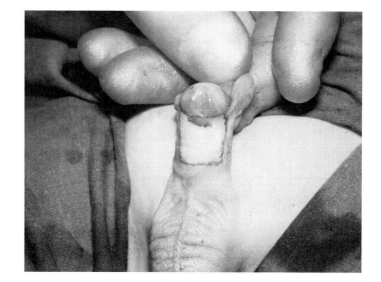

FIG. 18-82. Outline of the flap on the ventral surface of the penis. (Figures 18-82 to 18-90 are from J. C. Mustardé [Ed.], *Plastic Surgery in Infancy and Childhood,* Edinburgh and London: Churchill/Livingstone, 1971.)

Fig. 18-83 Incision along the distal edge of the flap allows the chordee to be corrected, and the urethral opening slides proximally.

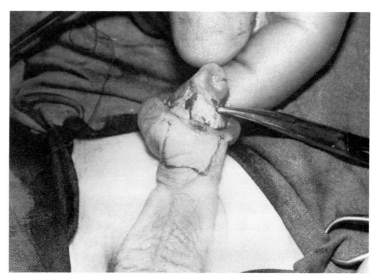

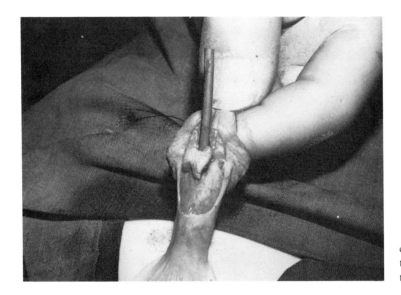

FIG. 18-84. The flap is completely incised around; the distal quarter is left attached as a vascular base.

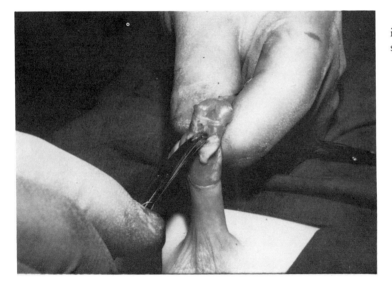

FIG. 18-85. Tunneling is performed through the shaft and glans.

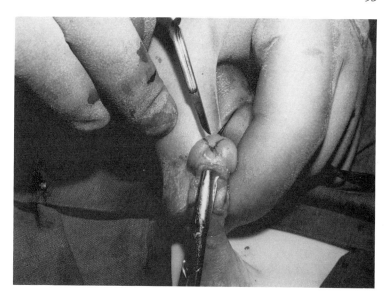

FIG. 18-86. Opening is made in the tunnel by a Horton-Devine-type V-shaped incision.

An incision 6 to 7 mm in width is made in the tissue immediately distal to the urethral opening (Fig. 18-85). Using blunt-ended scissors, a tunnel is created up into the glans, where a wide V-shaped opening is made as in the procedure of Horton and Devine [2] (Fig. 18-86). If a posterior urethrostomy has been used, a 10 cm length of catheter is passed via the urethral opening as far into the urethra as possible; if no urethrostomy has been carried out, a nonrubber self-retaining catheter is passed into the bladder. The flap is tubed over the catheter, except for the terminal 1 cm, using 6-0 catgut. The two free corners are sutured temporarily to the length of catheter (or tied to it if an indwelling catheter is used) (Fig. 18-87), and the tubed flap on its length of catheter is passed via the tunnel onto the surface of the glans (Fig. 18-88). The two free corners are sutured to the upper incision of the V, and the tongue of the latter is sutured to the last stitch used for tubing the flap (the suture should be left long

for this purpose). Using 6-0 catgut, the rest of the flap is sutured with great care to the V opening to minimize formation of scar tissue and later contraction. One or two 6-0 catgut sutures may be inserted in the loose superficial connective tissue to ensure that the skin tube is completely buried in the tunnel at the proximal end.

Attention is now turned to covering the raw area of the ventral surface. This is done by opening out the prepuce, button-holing it, and bringing it forward after the manner of Ombrédanne (Fig. 18-89); the sutures are 6-0 or 5-0 catgut (Fig. 18-90). The very thin skin from the inner aspect of the prepuce can usually be discarded.

Light pressure is applied to the penis—I use a two-way stretch, open-weave material (Lastonet) wrapped twice loosely around the penis—to prevent excessive edema of the preputial skin. The catheter, the length of tubing in the urethra (if one has been used), and the dressings are removed in a warm

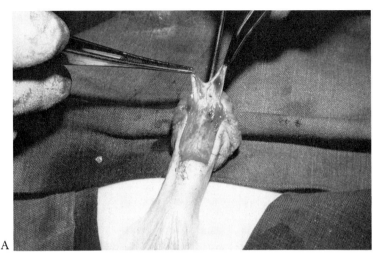

A

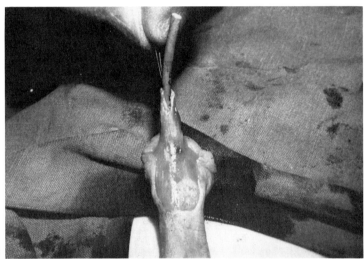

B

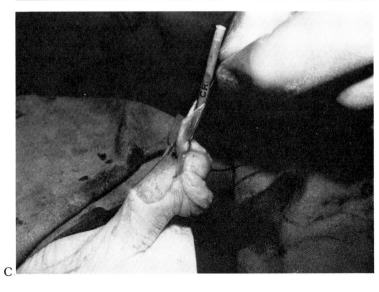

C

FIG. 18-87. A, B, and C. A flap is raised and partially tubed around a length of catheter that is passed into urethra.

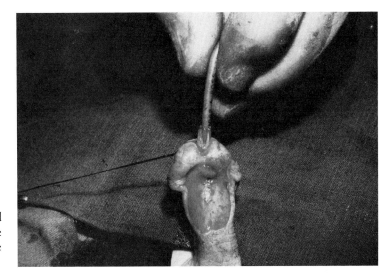

FIG. 18-88. The tubed flap is brought through the tunnel and out onto the surface of the glans.

FIG. 18-89. Ombrédanne-type of flap, using preputial skin.

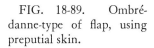

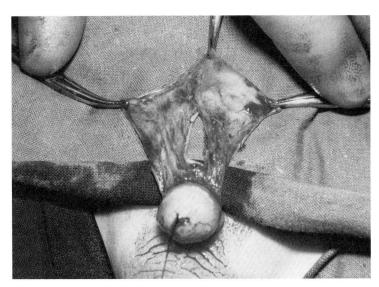

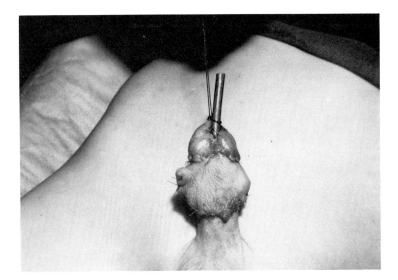

FIG. 18-90. The flap is brought over onto the ventral surface of the penis and is sutured in place.

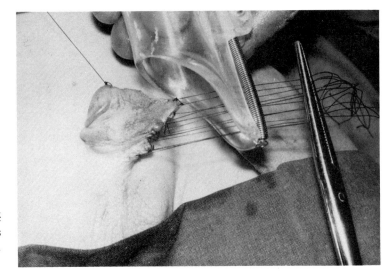

FIG. 18-91. Mustardé clamp for holding sutures in hypospadias or fistula repair.

bath 9 days after surgery. If a perineal urethrostomy has been used, the child is kept in the hospital until the opening is closed.

During the past 2 years, I have combined the long, proximally based Broadbent flap [1] and its vascular "mesentery" with my own tunneling technique in the distal one-third of the shaft and the glans for those patients with more severe degrees of hypospadias. In about a third of the patients, a fistula has occurred at the proximal end of the reconstructed urethra, requiring a secondary operation for its closure [3] (Fig. 18-91).

References

1. Broadbent, J. R., Woolf, R. M., Toksu, E. Hypospadias—one stage repair. *Plast. Reconstr. Surg.* 27:154, 1961.
2. Horton, C. E., and Devine, C. J., Jr. Hypospadias and epispadias. *Clin. Symp.* 24:3, 1972.
3. Mustardé, J. C. One stage correction of distal hypospadias: and other people's fistulae. *Br. J. Plast. Surg.* 18:413, 1965.
4. Mustardé, J. C. Hypospadias in the Distal Third of the Penis. In *Transactions of the Fifth International Congress of Plastic and Reconstructive Surgery.* Melbourne: Butterworth, 1971. P. 356.

One-Stage Repair — V

ESAT TOKSU

In the treatment of hypospadias, many procedures have been used in obtaining the ultimate goal; namely, acceptable esthetic appearance, functional integrity, and simplicity of the surgical technique. This one-stage procedure was developed with the same purposes in mind and can be described as an island tubed-flap procedure. The island tubed flap is located on the ventral surface of the prepuce and is used to replace the missing anterior urethra. The transfer of the island tubed flap is provided through a button-hole on the dorsal skin, as in the Nesbit procedure [8]. The procedure is illustrated in Figures 18-92 to 18-98.

The procedure provides an anatomical location for the meatus and a transfer of flexible tissue with good blood supply that is a histological match for the missing urethral segment. This procedure has been utilized only for distal hypospadias in the last 8 years. Twenty-four such operations have been performed. Nineteen of these cases healed primarily. Four patients had complications with fistula formation; these were easily closed secondarily. One patient developed severe cellulitis and lost the flap.

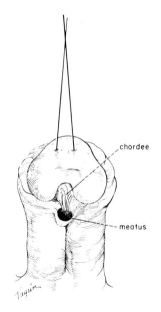

FIG. 18-92. A traction suture is placed through the glans penis. (From E. Toksu, *Plast. Reconstr. Surg.* 45:365, 1970. Copyright © 1970, The Williams & Wilkins Co., Baltimore.)

298

FIG. 18-93. A. Traction sutures are placed at the lateral distal margins of the prepuce, and an incision line is outlined on the ventral surface of the prepuce for the formation of a tube flap. B. The formation of the tube flap is carried out with minimal undermining of the skin edges, which is easily accomplished because of the looseness of the areolar tissue in this location. (This minimal undermining is an important step in this procedure for the preservation of the vascularity of the flap.) A 2 mm Silastic rod is placed in the tube flap. The fibrous tissue causing the chordee is removed, and a V-shaped incision is made in the glans penis as first described by Horton and Devine [6]. (From E. Toksu, *Plast. Reconstr. Surg.* 45:365, 1970. Copyright © 1970, The Williams & Wilkins Co., Baltimore.)

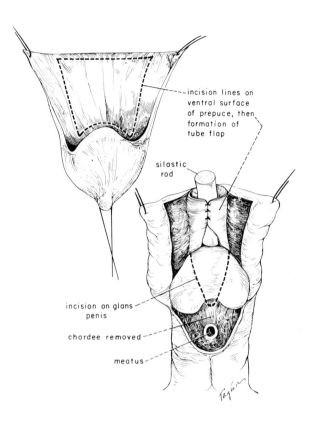

FIG. 18-94. The central V-shaped flap retracts upward on release of the chordee, and the lateral flaps are slightly undermined at the level of the fascia penis. (From E. Toksu, *Plast. Reconst. Surg.* 45:365, 1970. Copyright © 1970, The Williams & Wilkins Co., Baltimore.)

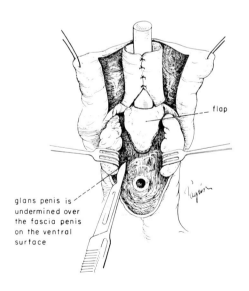

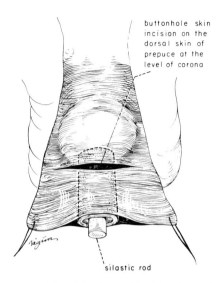

FIG. 18-95.   A horizontal incision is made on the dorsal skin of the prepuce at the level of the proximal end of the tube flap and the future site of the corona. All the vessels, including the superficial dorsal vein, that are located in the areolar tissue are retracted laterally. The dartos fascia is incised and the button-hole is made. (From E. Toksu, *Plast. Reconstr. Surg.* 45:365, 1970. Copyright © 1970, The Williams & Wilkins Co., Baltimore.)

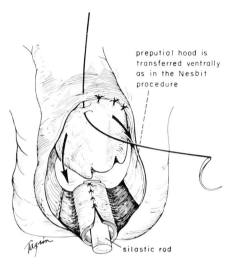

FIG. 18-96.   The preputial hood containing the tube flap is transferred ventrally through the button-hole, as in the Nesbit procedure [8]. (From E. Toksu, *Plast. Reconstr. Surg.* 45:365, 1970. Copyright © 1970, The Williams & Wilkins Co., Baltimore.)

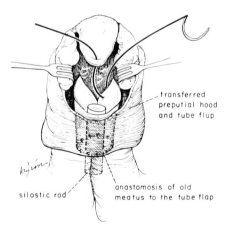

FIG. 18-97.   The proximal and distal ends of the tube are sutured to the old meatus as well as to the tip of the penis to match the triangular flap as part of the dorsal floor. (From E. Toksu, *Plast. Reconstr. Surg.* 45:365, 1970. Copyright © 1970, The Williams & Wilkins Co., Baltimore.)

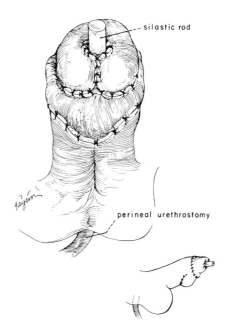

FIG. 18-98. The lateral flaps that are developed from the glans penis are then sutured together over the tube flap to make the new meatus. The skin incisions are closed, and the excess "dog ears" are removed. The Silastic rod is then passed through the anastomosis to provide splinting as well as drainage of mucosal secretions and blood. It also provides an exit for possible leakage of urine into the operative area from around the routine urethrostomy catheter. (From E. Toksu, *Plast. Reconstr. Surg.* 45:365, 1970. Copyright © 1970, The Williams & Wilkins Co., Baltimore.)

References

1. Backus, L. H., and DeFelice, C. A. Hypospadias then and now. *Plast. Reconstr. Surg.* 25:146, 1960.
2. Broadbent, T. R., Woolf, R. M., and Toksu, E. A. Hypospadias—one-stage repair. *Plast. Reconstr. Surg.* 27:154, 1961.
3. Davis, D. M. Surgical treatment of hypospadias. *J. Urol.* 65:595, 1951.
4. DesPrez, J. D., Persky, L., and Kiehn, C. L. One-stage hypospadias repair by island flap technique. *Plast. Reconstr. Surg.* 28:405, 1961.
5. Horton, C. E., and Devine, C. J., Jr. Film: A one-stage hypospadias repair. Eaton Laboratories, 1959.
6. Horton, C. E., and Devine, C. J., Jr. Hypospadias. In T. Gibson (Ed.), *Modern Trends in Plastic Surgery.* London: Butterworth, 1967.
7. Mustardé, J. C. One stage correction of distal hypospadias: and other people's fistulae. *Br. J. Plast. Surg.* 18:413, 1965.
8. Nesbit, R. Plastic procedure for correction of hypospadias. *J. Urol.* 45:699, 1941.

Method of Cronin
and Guthrie

THOMAS D. CRONIN
THOMAS H. GUTHRIE

Hypospadias, a congenital deformity in the anatomical bailiwick of the urologist, requires strict adherence to the principles of plastic surgery for its correction. Having recognized this thirty years ago, the authors —a plastic surgeon (Dr. Cronin) and a urologist (Dr. Guthrie)—decided to work together as a surgical team in the correction of hypospadias in order to provide the greatest benefit to the patient.

It is our preference to see the patient when newborn, at which time the future plan of treatment can be explained to the parents. At the time of the initial examination, whether in the hospital or office, the patency of the displaced meatus is determined, and if needed, meatotomy is performed. The patency of the urethra is determined to rule out obstructive uropathy. In the severe perineal form of hypospadias in which the sex of the infant is in doubt, studies must be carried out to determine the proper sex assignment.

In the two-stage procedure, correction of chordee is usually performed at $1\frac{1}{2}$ to 2 years of age. The second stage follows, as a rule, at between 3 and 4 years of age. It is desirable, whenever possible, to have the patient out of diapers before the second stage procedure, and, hopefully, the repair can be completed prior to kindergarten or school age. In any event, at least 4 to 6 months should intervene between stages to permit full revascularization and softening of the tissues.

Early repair has the advantage of preventing the patient from feeling abnormal or different from other little boys. Erections in this age group are not as great a complicating factor in postsurgical recovery as in older boys. Also, when there is ventral chordee, it is difficult—and sometimes impossible—to correct this in the teenage group, because the entire shaft of the penis is involved in the curvature.

The urologist participates in the treatment program in the following ways:

1. To correct meatal stenosis and to rule out other lower tract obstruction.
2. To order and to interpret excretory urograms.

3. To perform urethrography and endoscopy to rule out the presence of urogenital sinus or utricle (müllerian duct) cyst.
4. To order and interpret buccal smear studies for sex chromatin, and, if indicated,
5. To order chromosomal study and hormonal assays, such as those for 17-ketosteroids.
6. To perform gonadal biopsy or pelvic exploration as indicated.
7. To perform perineal urethrostomy either at the time of a second stage procedure or during a one-stage procedure.
8. To supervise catheter care, fluid intake, urinary output, and so on.
9. To observe urinary flow by flow rate studies performed in the postoperative period, and, whenever possible, after the patient has gone through his adolescent development.

The plastic surgeon is charged with:

1. Performing the surgical correction of the hypospadias in one, two, or more stages, as needed.
2. Postoperative care, including maintenance of dressings and attention to complications such as hemorrhage and flap necrosis.
3. Responsibility for follow-up care (such as dilatations, if needed) and the repair of fistulas or strictures.

Surgical Technique

Because of the thinness and delicacy of the penile tissues, a nontraumatic technique is imperative. The use of small skin hooks for traction, Adson or similar tissue forceps for handling the tissues, and small eye scissors for dissection is recommended. Heavy chromic catgut sutures cannot be absorbed by the thin tissues involved and almost certainly will be extruded, with resulting fistula formation. Minimal amounts of 4-0 or 5-0 plain catgut are used as buried sutures. Continu-

ous, pull-out sutures of 4-0 monofilament material may be even better. An understanding of the methods of formation and shifting of the skin flaps is essential, especially in the more severe degrees of hypospadias and in patients who have been unsuccessfully operated on previously.

Most of our repairs have been based on the technique described by Blair, Brown, and Hamm [2] and later modified by Byars [4]. Variations have been employed that seemed best in individual cases, such as changes in the transfer of flaps, leaving the strip of skin untubed at the second stage (Browne [3]), the use of free full-thickness skin grafts (McCormack [6]), and a one-stage technique (Bevan [1]).

CORRECTION OF CHORDEE

A traction suture of 4-0 catgut is inserted through the glans and tagged with a mosquito forceps. The subcutaneous tissues are infiltrated sparingly with 1 to 2 ml of 0.25 percent Xylocaine (lidocaine) with 1:400,000 adrenalin (to 1 ml of 1 percent Xylocaine with 1:100,000 adrenalin, add 3 ml of normal saline solution). The blood vessels in this area appear to be particularly susceptible to the action of adrenalin. A delay of about 10 minutes in incising the skin permits the adrenalin to take effect.

The proposed line of incision is marked with methylene blue (Fig. 18-99). Skin hooks are used to retract the skin flaps laterally, and attention is given to the removal of all fibrous bands from the ventral surface of the penis, exposing the corpora cavernosa in the area from the glans to the meatus and as far laterally as necessary. As a rule, it is necessary to continue the dissection proximally. As the shaft is freed up and straightened, the meatus and urethra assume a more posterior position with respect to the glans. This dissection may be carried out with a knife, a

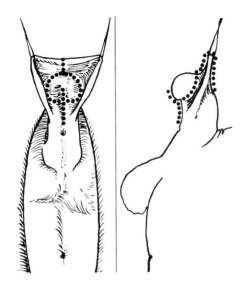

FIG. 18-99. The incision extends from the meatus distally through the groove in the glans to the tip. Another incision is made through the inner layer of the prepuce about 3 to 4 mm from the glans. The dorsal slit is not made until after the prepuce has been unfolded. See Figure 18-101. (From T. D. Cronin, T. Guthrie, and D. Herr, Experiences in the surgical correction of hypospadias. *Amer. J. Surg.* 110:818, 1965.)

small curved iris scissors, or a combination of both.

Attention is next directed to the incision in the glandar groove (Fig. 18-100). Tiny skin hooks are inserted in the mucosal margins in the depth of the groove, and the mucosa is delicately dissected laterally using a No. 15 blade. Sometimes a traction suture is more efficient than the skin hook. When the dissection of the mucosal lining of the groove has been completed, an amazingly large raw surface will have been created in the glans (see Figs. 18-99 and 18-100).

Bleeding is minimal because of the adrenalin treatment. When vessels are seen and cut, however, it is well to clamp them with a mosquito hemostat and either ligate them

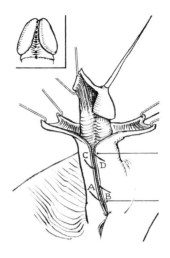

FIG. 18-100. Mucosa of the glans is dissected laterally. Inset shows incision in the glandar groove.

with 5-0 plain catgut or use electrocoagulation.

Preputial flaps should be developed by unfolding the double-layered prepuce (Fig. 18-101). Two tiny hooks are inserted in the edge of the skin on the dorsum produced by the circumcision and are lifted upward. The prepuce can be transilluminated by directing the surgical light at the prepuce from the head of the table while the surgeon dissects carefully with small eye scissors. The blood vessels can be seen and avoided as the prepuce is unfolded. Many delicate connective tissue bands must be cut before the unfolding is completed. This single preputial flap is divided in two by a dorsal slit. The flaps are swung around to the ventral surface to cover the raw area previously created in the glans and shaft (Fig. 18-102). Sutures of 4-0 plain catgut are inserted through the preputial and glandar flaps and are left long enough to tie over a bolster to ensure that the preputial flaps are firmly spread out in the glandar defect. Before the bolster is applied, however, the two preputial flaps are sutured down the

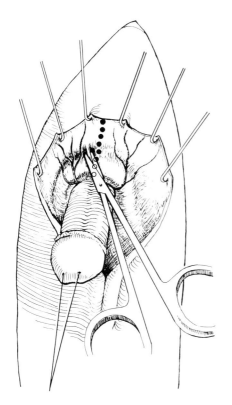

FIG. 18-101. Prepuce being unfolded. Vessels, as seen by transillumination, can be avoided in the dissection and in making the dorsal slit.

midline with a continuous mattress suture of 4-0 plain catgut. A meatotomy is performed to change the meatal opening from a round one, which is subject to contracture and stenosis, to an elongated, oblique opening that is resistant to stenosis as healing occurs. After tying the bolster in place, a Foley catheter of about size F-14 or F-16 is inserted. While an assistant holds the penis perpendicular to the pubic area by the traction suture, a circular gauze dressing is applied.

Catheter drainage is continued for about one week, at which time healing is usually complete.

SECOND-STAGE OPERATION

Since the chordee is usually corrected at about 1½ to 2 years of age and since there is no urgency in completing the second stage, this operation is usually not performed until the following year. However, a minimum of 4 to 6 months would be indicated, in any event, to permit the tissues to soften and relax.

We believe the newly constructed urethra should be put at complete rest during the healing period, and, therefore, the urine should be diverted by an indwelling Foley catheter. This is not passed via the new urethra because of the frequency of urethral infection when a catheter is left in place for a week or more. We have used perineal urethrostomy (Fig. 18-103) exclusively, since there is less chance of urinary flow through the newly constructed anterior urethra as a consequence of bladder spasm with involuntary voiding than would occur with suprapubic diversion.

Again, the subcutaneous tissues are sparingly infiltrated with 0.25 percent Xylocaine with 1:400,000 adrenalin, and a traction suture is inserted through the glans. In the child under 5 or 6 years of age, a size F-16 urethra should be planned. A piece of catgut is cut of sufficient length to wrap *exactly* once around an F-16 sound. This piece of suture, held in the middle with a mosquito forceps, is used to measure the distance (16 mm) between the parallel lines and hence the width of the flap (Fig. 18-104).

The edges of the flap are very slightly undermined, and the flap is tubed using a continuous suture of 5-0 plain catgut or a continuous pull-out suture of 4-0 monofilament (Fig. 18-105). Sometimes a small wedge or two of skin needs excision as the area of the meatus is sutured. Skin hooks are inserted along the lateral skin edges, and, with scis-

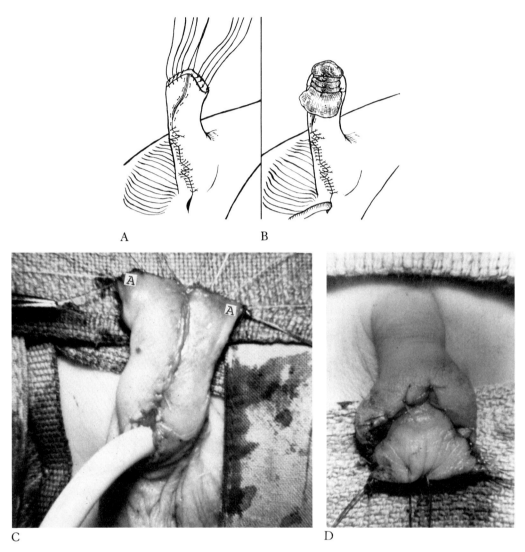

FIG. 18-102. A. The preputial flaps have been used to cover the raw area on the glans and penile shaft. Note that sutures have been left long to tie over the bolster. B. The bolster is essential to ensure complete spreading and adherence of the flaps over the raw surface of the glans. C. The Foley catheter has been inserted and is ready for the bolster. The preputial flaps (*A*) cover the raw area of the spread out glans and of the penile shaft. D. Dorsal view of the glans. (A, B, and C from T. D. Cronin, T. Guthrie, and D. Herr, Experiences in the surgical correction of hypospadias. *Amer. J. Surg.* 110:818, 1965.)

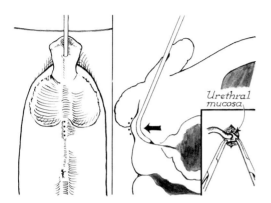

Urethral mucosa

FIG. 18-103. Perineal urethrostomy. While an assistant presses firmly with the curve of a sound against the perineum, the urologist stretches the perineal skin firmly over the sound with his thumb on one side and his fingers on the other side, thereby efficiently preventing bleeding as he makes a half-inch incision down to the sound with his right hand. Then, still maintaining pressure unrelentingly with the left hand, the cut edge of the urethral mucosa is grasped firmly with a mosquito forceps on each side—not until this moment can the thumb-finger pressure be released. A Foley catheter, about size F-16, is then inserted. The hemostats are removed, and a deep bite with a 4-0 catgut suture is taken for hemostasis and wound closure. (From T. D. Cronin, T. Guthrie, and D. Herr, Experiences in the surgical correction of hypospadias. *Amer. J. Surg.* 110:818, 1965.)

sors, a plane superficial to Buck's fascia is opened up by spreading and occasionally cutting with the scissors. The flaps thus formed should be so sutured as to separate the two suture lines as much as possible (see Fig. 18-105). Most often, vertical distance has been utilized, as shown in Figure 18-105, by the use of a cotton roll that has been moistened in mineral oil to keep it from getting hard from dried blood. Extreme care should be taken to avoid tying the mattress sutures of 4-0 plain catgut too tightly, since this could result in pressure necrosis of the skin flaps.

We have also approximated these skin flaps with two or three continuous 4-0 monafilament pull-out sutures; one or two sutures are inserted in a serpentine manner in the subcutaneous tissues, each end being brought out through the skin and left long. The last suture is placed immediately beneath the skin. At the distal end, some interrupted sutures may be indicated. Sometimes the preputial skin flaps may be better utilized by rotating one across the midline to cover the new urethra (see Figs. 18-105B and C); the other flap is trimmed where necessary. In this situation, interrupted vertical mattress sutures of catgut are needed.

The penis is bandaged as in the first stage. The dressing is inspected and changed, if necessary, on about the fifth day. The perineal catheter is usually removed on about the eighth to tenth day, and hot sitz baths two to three times daily are suggested for a week or more to help resolve the swelling. Occasional dilatation with a sound may be indicated during the first several weeks. Rarely, a small meatotomy has been indicated and is usually performed as an office procedure.

At times the Denis Browne [3] procedure of leaving an untubed, flat strip of skin beneath the covering skin flaps has been used. This has been done most often when there has been a shortage of skin, since Johanson [5] has shown that the circumference of the resulting urethra may be increased as much as one-third. Sometimes the distal skin for the urethra is tubed, leaving that near the base of the penis untubed, since the later is the area where the circumferential skin of the penis is tightest. The dorsal relaxation incision advocated by Browne has been used only when there was definite circumferential tightness of the skin. Although healing without scar contracture doubtlessly occurs in most cases, we have seen one such contracture and would advise a skin graft if the dorsal wound is unusually large.

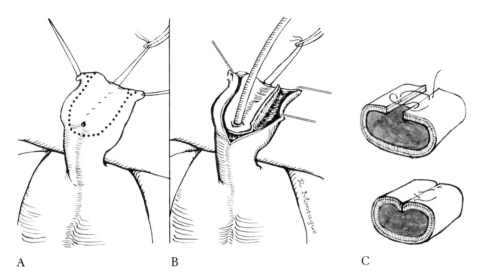

A   B   C

FIG. 18-104. A. A flap 16 mm in width (20 to 24 mm for teenagers) is outlined and is shown ready to be tubed and sutured. B. The skin flap has been tubed from the meatus to the tip. C. A continuous, inverting suture is used to form the urethra. (A and B from T. D. Cronin, T. Guthrie, and D. Herr, Experiences in the surgical correction of hypospadias. *Amer. J. Surg.* 110:818, 1965.)

ONE-STAGE REPAIR

When the meatus is at or near the coronal groove with mild or no chordee, the repair may be completed in one stage. The usual procedure, after removal of any contracting fibrous tissue, has consisted of the elevation of a flap on the ventral surface of the penis, as demonstrated in Figure 18-106. This is a very satisfactory method since the suture line is buried against the shaft of the penis and thus there is very little chance of fistula formation. This "flip-flop-flap," because of its thinness and narrow pedicle, probably acts as a free full-thickness skin graft to a considerable extent. Realization of this has suggested the frank use of a free full-thickness graft of the prepuce (Fig. 18-107A). A piece of prepuce of adequate width and length is trimmed from the prepuce and sutured, raw surface outward, around an F-16 catheter. The meatus is incised longitudinally, and the end of the tubed skin graft is cut obliquely to minimize the possibility of stricture at the anastomosis. This free graft must be covered by a healthy flap from which much of its blood supply must come. Hemostasis is particularly important with a free graft, since a hematoma could easily prevent the graft from contact with its source of blood supply and result in its partial or complete loss.

Complications

FISTULA

Fistula formation has not been a frequent problem, but it is most likely to occur in the penoscrotal, scrotal, or perineal types of hypospadias in which there is a deficiency of skin available for repair. Repair has usually been

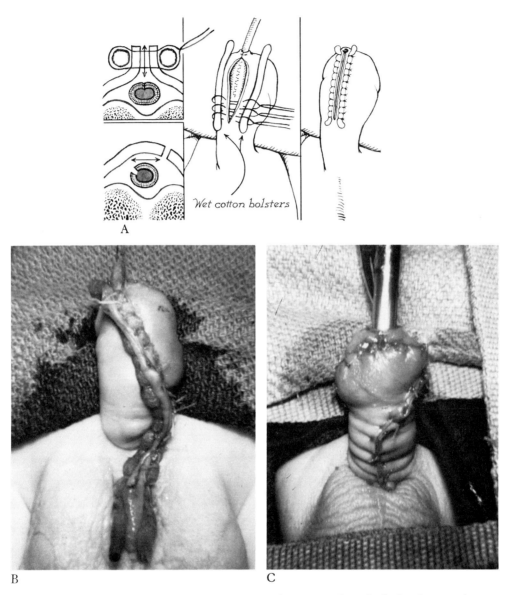

FIG. 18-105. A. Inner and outer suture lines can be separated vertically by the use of mattress sutures over cotton bolsters, as was used most frequently in this series, or horizontal separation may be used, as shown in lower left inset, which is achieved by making the urethral skin flap to one side of the midline. B. Vertical separation of suture lines. C. Use of a rotational flap produces a horizontal separation of the suture lines. (From T. D. Cronin, T. Guthrie, and D. Herr, Experiences in the surgical correction of hypospadias. *Amer. J. Surg.* 110:818, 1965.)

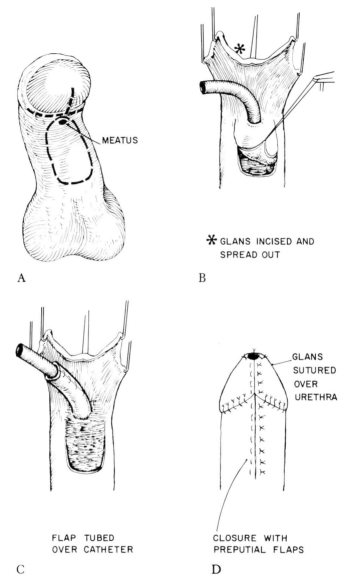

A

B

**✳ GLANS INCISED AND
SPREAD OUT**

FLAP TUBED
OVER CATHETER

CLOSURE WITH
PREPUTIAL FLAPS

C   D

FIG. 18-106.   Lines of incision to open up glans, correct chordee, and form the flap for the urethra.   B.   The glans has been dissected open, as shown in Fig. 18-100.   C.   The flap has been tubed
around a catheter, which will be removed when a perineal urethrostomy has been done.   D.   The
penile defect is closed with preputial flaps that are formed as shown in Figure 18-101. The glans can
usually be closed over the new urethra, but there is an abundance of preputial skin available if needed.

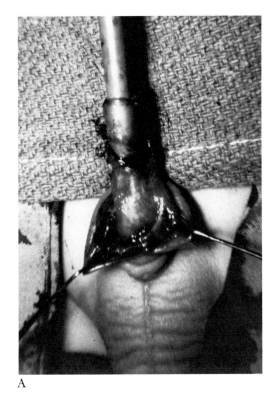

A

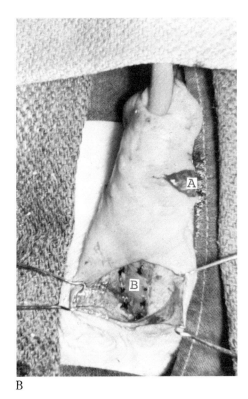

B

FIG. 18-107. A. A free full-thickness skin graft forms the distal urethra. It is sutured around a Silastic tube as a stent, which is left in place for about 5 days and then removed. B. A free full thickness skin graft (marked with dots of methylene blue) to relieve a stricture. Note the donor site on the side of the penis. (From T. D. Cronin, T. Guthrie, and D. Herr, Experiences in the surgical correction of hypospadias. *Amer. J. Surg.* 110:818, 1965.)

delayed until the tissues have returned to a normal degree of softness, and it has then been carried out by a circular incision and inversion of the skin edges with 5-0 plain catgut. The second layer is accomplished either with cotton rolls and mattress sutures of catgut, or, in some instances, by rotation of a flap large enough to cover the first line of closure to a generous degree, the flap being sutured with vertical mattress sutures.

HEMATOMA

There is usually some postoperative oozing of blood about which nothing need be done.

However, if bleeding is profuse after surgery, the patient should be taken back to the operating room, the wound opened, and all clots removed. Bleeding points are clamped and tied or coagulated. Unrecognized hematomas may result in loss of skin grafts or flaps.

Infection has presented no problem in our series.

STRICTURE

Slight tightness of the meatus has been treated by dilatation, and meatotomy has been employed for more definite strictures.

The extent of urethral strictures has been

determined by sounding and urethrography. If repeated dilatation has failed, the stricture is relieved surgically. A curved incision long enough to expose the area of tightness is made well to one side of the midline on the ventral surface of the penis, and the flap thus formed is dissected laterally, exposing the urethra. The largest sound that the normal portion of the patient's urethra will admit is gently inserted into the area of stricture. The urethra is incised with a knife as the sound is passed. The incision is extended a few millimeters on each side of the narrow portion of urethra to ensure complete release. An elliptic pattern of the urethral defect is made from a piece of paper or rubber dam.

Using this pattern, a full-thickness skin graft is taken, preferably from the penis itself (see Fig. 18-107B). If there is insufficient skin on the penis, an area of thin hairless skin, such as from the back of the ear or the inner side of the arm, is chosen. The graft is then carefully sutured in place with continuous 5-0 plain catgut sutures, and the covering skin flap is sutured. A short piece of Silastic tubing of proper size, coated with an antibiotic ointment, is left in the urethra for about 5 days, by which time the graft should have become well fixed in place and the catheter can be removed. Urinary diversion by means of a perineal urethrostomy is advisable for about 10 days.

In certain more extensive or recurrent strictures, we have used the Johanson procedure [5] of laying open the stricture area and suturing the urethral edges to the external skin edges; two to three months later, a urethra is constructed in the usual manner.

Results

From 1940 until the present (1972), we have operated on 190 patients with hypospa-

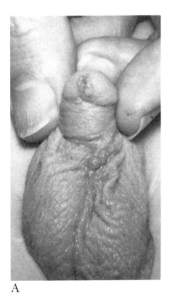 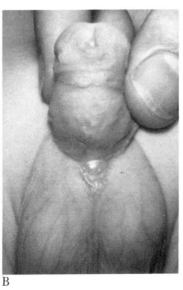 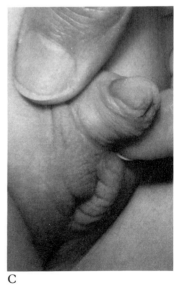

A   B   C

FIG. 18-108. Results of two-stage operation: A. penile, B. penoscrotal, and C. scrotal types of hypospadias. (From T. D. Cronin, T. Guthrie, and D. Herr, Experiences in the surgical correction of hypospadias. *Amer. J. Surg.* 110:818, 1965.)

TABLE 18-1. Operations and Complications (Jan. 1, 1965–Dec. 31, 1969)

	Number	Percent
Patients	56	—
One-stage operations	25	45%
Two-stage operations	31	55%
Total operations	99	—
Total complications	16	16%[a]
Patients with complications	14	25%[b]
Patients without complications	42	75%

[a] Percentage of 99 operations.
[b] Percentage of 56 patients.

dias and have performed 304 staged procedures. Some of the recent cases requiring more than one stage have not yet been completed. There were 52 (17 percent) complications requiring surgical correction (Fig. 18-108). Of the above, 138 patients had 207 staged procedures without any complications.

The complications can be broken down as follows: fistula alone, 26; fistula as the result of postoperative hemorrhage, slough, stricture, or wound separation, 11; stenosis, 6; slough of flaps after the first stage procedure, requiring an additional procedure before the second stage could be done, 5.

A one-stage repair was performed on 72 patients, with 12 complications or about 17 percent. The majority of these patients had minimal to moderate chordee, or the urethral meatus ended in the distal penile, coronal, or glandar area, or both.

Three of the 26 patients with penoscrotal hypospadias were also diagnosed as pseudohermaphroditic.

Statistics regarding hypospadias repair on patients 12 years of age or older were also compiled. Thirteen patients in this category had 19 procedures with 9 complications (47 percent). The majority of repairs in older patients were performed early in the series.

Subdividing the overall series into more recent statistics, 122 patients had 195 procedures from 1960 to 1969. There were 29 complications (15 percent): fistula occurred in 14 patients, stenosis in 6, and flap necrosis in 5.

Beginning in 1961, local anesthesia with adrenalin has been used as an adjunct to minimize bleeding during dissection. Since then, 171 operations have been performed, with 26 complications (15 percent). These complications consisted of fistula in 11 cases,

TABLE 18-2. Types of Cases and Complications (1965–1969)

	Cases	Procedures	Complications
Scrotal and penoscrotal	5	10	0
Penile	37	72	14 (19%)
Near corona or glans	14	17	2 (12%)
Breakdown of Complications:			
Fistula	5		
alone	3		
secondary	2		
Stenosis	3		
Flap necrosis	4		
Postoperative bleeding	1		
Short meatus	1		
Separative wound	1		
Excess skin at meatus	1		
Total	16		
Number of stage one patients with complications	6		
Number of stage two patients with complications	8		

stenosis in 5, slough in 5, and wound separation in 2.

From these data, one can deduce that 26 procedures in the recent series have been carried out without the use of local anesthesia, with only three complications (12 percent). These less favorable results for local anesthesia may be due to the fact that early in its use, the local anesthetic was not diluted. In the past 5 years, however, we have used diluted local anesthesia, and there has been a complication rate of 16 percent.

In the last 5 years, the majority of patients have been in the younger age group. All but 10 of 56 patients were 6 years old or less. Only one patient was over 12 years of age; he was 16 and the result was good even though a fistula formed that closed spontaneously.

Of these 56 patients, 25 were 3 years old or less at the time of the first or only operation. It is probably significant to note that of these 25 patients, only two (8 percent) had a sufficiently serious complication to warrant an additional operation. One of these patients

developed flap necrosis requiring a skin graft, and the other developed postoperative bleeding requiring a return to the operating room. Conversely, 30 patients between the ages of 4 and 10 had a total of 12 complications (40 percent) that required an additional procedure. These data seem to indicate the advisability of operating on these children as early as possible. The explanation for the 32 percent difference may be because children in the older age group have a greater tendency to erection, especially around ages 5 and 6.

Associated congenital anomalies were noted only in the penoscrotal or scrotal hypospadias group. Of these 26 patients (of the total series of 190 patients), six had other anomalies. Three were found to be hermaphrodites, two patients had congenital heart disease, and one had an inguinal hernia. One of the patients with congenital heart disease also had malrotation of the gut, congenital flexion contractures of the fingers with syndactylism, and a unilateral kidney (Tables 18-1 to 3).

TABLE 18-3. Comparison of Early and Later Results (1940–1964 and 1965–1969)

	Cases	Procedures	Complications			
Scrotal and penoscrotal	21 (5)[a]	46 (10)[a]	11 (0)[a]	24%	(0%)[a]	
Penile	44 (37)	67 (72)	12 (14)	18%	(19%)	
Near corona or glans	69 (14)	92 (17)	13 (2)	14%	(12%)	

[a] Numbers in parentheses: 1965–1969 group.

References

1. Bevan, A. D. Hypospadias. *J.A.M.A.* 68: 1032, 1917.
2. Blair, V. P., Brown, J. B., and Hamm, W. G. The correction of scrotal hypospadias and of epispadias. *Surg. Gynec. Obstet.* 57:646, 1933.
3. Browne, D. An operation for hypospadias. *Proc. R. Soc. Med.* 42:466, 1949.
4. Byars, L. T. Functional restoration of hypospadias deformities. *Surg. Gynec. Obstet.* 92:149, 1951.
5. Johanson, B. Reconstruction of the male urethra in strictures. *Acta. Chir. Scand.* Suppl. 176, 1953.
6. McCormack, R. M. Simultaneous chordee repair and urethral reconstruction for hypospadias; experimental and clinical studies. *Plast. Reconstr. Surg.* 13:257, 1954.

Hypospadias with and without Chordee

ORMOND S. CULP

Hypospadias with Chordee

When the customary hooded prepuce is still present, the simple method of correcting chordee, shown in Figure 18-109, is employed. If the original meatus is of adequate caliber, it should be preserved to avoid postoperative meatal stenosis. If the patient has been circumcised, some form of Z-plasty is utilized to obtain sufficient ventral skin. Too frequently, straightening operations have been too conservative. Thorough dissection is imperative. Fine Mersilene sutures (4-0) in the skin minimize scarring along the closure.

The type of dressing after this type of operation is important (Fig. 18-110). A layer of Telfa (to expedite removal), held in place by conforming gauze and covered with Elastoplast, prevents edema and controls oozing. If the Elastoplast is applied too tightly, healing of the skin edges may be impaired. Secondary closure was necessary in 5 percent of the early cases.

The catheter is left indwelling for only a day or so unless the original meatus has been revised or compromised; then, it remains in situ until the dressing and the skin sutures are removed on or about the tenth postoperative day. Earlier removal of the dressing results in undesirable edema.

This type of straightening has been used successfully on patients from 1 to 45 years of age. The ideal age for operation seems to be around the age of 18 months. Persistent chordee required repetition of the operation 6 to 12 months later in 4 percent of the cases managed in this fashion. Most of these failures were in individuals beyond puberty who were plagued by uncontrollable postoperative erections. Six of these patients had ventral clefts or contractures of the corpora cavernosa that required partial excision of the undersurface of the corpora before straightening could be accomplished. Only skin and the pressure dressing were used to cover the exposed vascular channels in these cases, but subsequent erections were normal.

After all chordee had been corrected, the

315

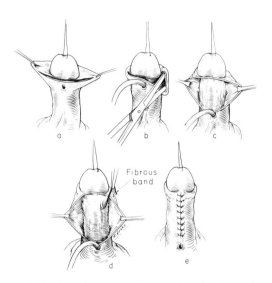

FIG. 18-109. Correction of chordee. A. Transverse incision distal to meatus is extended into the hooded prepuce. B. The prepuce is freed with blunt scissors. C. The urethra is freed from the corpora with an indwelling catheter as a guide. D. All constricting tissue is excised after freeing the penile skin laterally. The meatus gravitates to the most convenient position. E. The penile skin is closed longitudinally with interrupted sutures. (From O. S. Culp, Surgical correction of hypospadias. *Trans. Am. Assoc. Genitourin. Surg.* 49:57, 1957. Copyright © 1957, The Williams & Wilkins Co., Baltimore.)

urethral meatus was at or distal to the penoscrotal juncture in almost three-fourths of the patients. Under no circumstances should additional urethra be constructed until the penis is truly straight, the displaced meatus is of adequate caliber, and at least 6 months have elapsed since the last operation. The ideal age of urethroplasty seems to be about 5 years, but of late more patients have been operated on during the 12 months preceding this age without difficulty or regrets. The degree of genital growth has been a potent motivating factor.

When the meatus is at or just distal to the penoscrotal juncture, the modification of the Cecil operation that is shown in Figure 18-111 is employed. The size of the indwelling catheter is dictated by the amount of tissue available at the contemplated site of the new meatus and not by the caliber of the remainder of the new urethra. Usually a 10-F or 12-F catheter is used for 1 week in children, and a 16-F or 18-F is employed in teenagers. Chromic catgut (4-0) is used throughout the operation. It is important to wrap the deep scrotal tissue snugly over the new urethra and attach it high on the corpora (Fig. 111C′) in order to avoid potential periurethral pockets and to ensure having a long tract if a fistula develops. Reinforcing sutures around the new meatus help prevent meatal retraction.

The penis and new urethra are freed from the scrotum after an interval of at least 2 months (Fig. 18-112). A longer period of attachment is advisable if there were earlier unsuccessful operations. The catheter or sound is used only during the dissection. It is prudent to provide ample strips of scrotal skin on each side. These can be trimmed or sacrificed entirely if redundant, but lateral freeing of the skin is not advisable if the first stage was followed by a temporary fistula. The old tract may not be obliterated at this time. Meticulous hemostasis in the scrotum is essential. Since this may be deceptive, a dependent scrotal drain is employed for 2 or 3 days. This has prevented hematomas, which occurred in 6 percent of early cases. Mersilene skin sutures are removed after 1 week.

If the meatus is on the penile shaft and well removed from the penoscrotal juncture (30 percent of all cases), only the distal portion of the penis is attached to the scrotum (Fig. 18-113). It is also imperative to bury at least 1 cm of normal urethra to avoid a possible fistula in the unattached recess at the

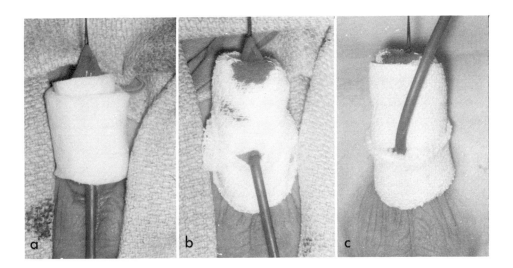

FIG. 18-110. Dressing after correction of chordee. A. Layer of Telfa. B. Conforming gauze. C. Covering of Elastoplast. (From O. S. Culp, Struggles and triumphs with hypospadias and associated anomalies: Review of 400 cases. *J. Urol.* 96:339, 1966. Copyright © 1966, The Williams & Wilkins Co., Baltimore.)

base. The free penoscrotal angle greatly simplifies the second-stage operation.

The two-stage Cecil-type operations have been preferred because they have eliminated persistent postoperative fistulas. If leakage occurs after removal of the catheter, the long tract heals spontaneously. The second stage also affords an opportunity to correct inadequacies that may follow the first stage. Many of these otherwise might be ignored or discredited.

These techniques should be confined to penile and penoscrotal degrees of hypospadias. It is impractical to bury a new pendulous urethra in apposition to a new scrotal urethra. Even if the integrity of both components is maintained, freeing is notably difficult.

The Denis Browne principle has been employed when the meatus is scrotal or perineal (Fig. 18-114). Urine is diverted by perineal urethrostomy. An attempt is made to advance the meatus onto the glans by suturing the lateral skin flaps to denuded areas on the glans with 4-0 chromic catgut. Similar sutures are used in the skin edges.

By replacing the conventional double-stop sutures with mattress ones of Mersilene (4-0) placed around strips of 8-F rubber tubing, the incidence of persistent fistula was reduced from 30 percent to 15 percent. The through-and-through drain near the penoscrotal juncture provides a better safety valve than do the simple stab wounds of the original technique. This drain is removed on the third day, and the Mersilene sutures are taken out routinely on the seventh postoperative day. Experience has shown that leaving them in place longer can create fistulas.

The perineal catheter is removed 10 to 12 days after operation. If a pendulous defect has developed, prolonged diversion of urine alone will not close it. The scrotal segment always heals. Fistulas in the pendulous portion can be managed in a variety of ways.

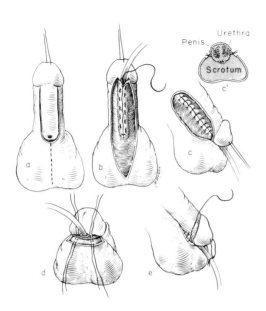

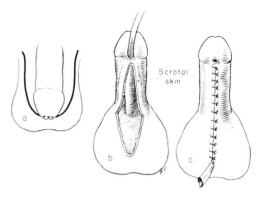

FIG. 18-111. First stage of Cecil-type urethroplasty (modification I). A. Location of incisions. B. New urethra is constructed over an indwelling catheter with a continuous suture of 4-0 chromic catgut. C. The new urethra is buried in the scrotum with interrupted fine catgut sutures. C'. Sutures are attached high on the lateral aspect of the corpora, and scrotal tissue is wrapped snugly against the new urethra. D. Interrupted sutures reinforce the approximation of the glans and new meatus to the scrotum. E. The skin is closed with subcuticular sutures of fine catgut. The original silk traction suture in the glans helps anchor the indwelling catheter. (From O. S. Culp, Surgical correction of hypospadias. *Trans. Am. Assoc. Genitourin. Surg.* 49:57, 1957. Copyright © 1957, The Williams & Wilkins Co., Baltimore.)

FIG. 18-112. Second stage of Cecil-type urethroplasty. A. Incisions in the scrotum are joined at the new meatus. B. Using a catheter or sound for orientation, the urethra is freed from the scrotum. C. The skin closed with Mersilene sutures, and a rubber drain is left in the dependent portion of the scrotum. (From O. S. Culp, Surgical correction of hypospadias. *Trans. Am. Assoc. Genitourin. Surg.* 49:57, 1957. Copyright © 1957, The Williams & Wilkins Co., Baltimore.)

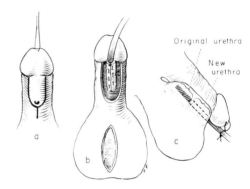

FIG. 18-113. Modification II of Cecil-type urethroplasty. A new urethra is constructed from the penile meatus (A) over a catheter (B), and a corresponding incision is made in the scrotum. C. Some normal as well as reconstructed urethra is buried in the scrotum in the usual manner. The penoscrotal region is left free. (From O. S. Culp, Surgical correction of hypospadias. *Trans. Am. Assoc. Genitourin. Surg.* 49:57, 1957. Copyright © 1957, The Williams & Wilkins Co., Baltimore.)

Hypospadias without Chordee

Hypospadias without chordee is usually extremely mild and seldom requires treatment. Some patients need only meatotomy. These have meatal stenosis, coronal hypospadias, and no chordee. Each has a distal opening or indentation which, on probing, com-

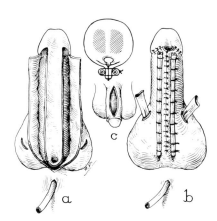

FIG. 18-114. Modified Denis Browne method. A. Urine is diverted by a perineal urethrostomy, and a central strip of skin is isolated. B. Fine Mersilene mattress sutures are tied over 8-F rubber tubing and are used instead of conventional double-stop sutures. A through-and-through drain is inserted at the penoscrotal juncture. C. Customary dorsal slit. (From O. S. Culp, Experiences with 200 hypospadiacs: Evolution of a therapeutic plan. *Surg. Clin. North Am.* 39:1007, 1959. By permission of W. B. Saunders Company.)

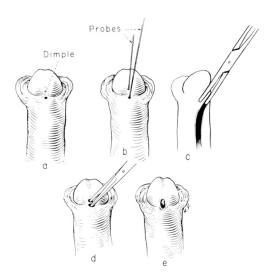

FIG. 18-115. A. Mild hypospadias with meatal stenosis but no chordee. B. The dimple on the glans communicates with a separate short channel parallel to the normal urethra. C. The intervening septum is crushed with a mosquito clamp and (D) divided with scissors, thereby enlarging the meatus (E) without sacrificing any urethra. (From O. S. Culp, Surgical correction of hypospadias. *Trans. Am. Assoc. Genitourin. Surg.* 49:57, 1957. Copyright © 1957, The Williams & Wilkins Co., Baltimore.)

municates with a separate, vestigial, terminal urethra parallel to the one through which the urine passes (Fig. 18-115). By crushing and dividing the intervening septum, the caliber of the meatus can be increased without sacrificing any of the normal urethra.

These stenoses do not tend to recur and rarely require subsequent dilatations. Since there is no chordee and the meatus is in a satisfactory functional position, the only further treatment necessary in most of these cases is circumcision.

The exceptional individual without chordee but born with a significant degree of penile hypospadias is managed by the method shown in Figure 18-113.

Deliberate termination of the urethra on the base of the glans poses no functional limitations. The urinary stream can be directed normally. Furthermore, several patients in this series are now proud fathers. Extending the urethra to the tip of the glans is fraught with hazards that more than offset any added cosmetic effect.

Results

A dependable, foolproof operation for correction of hypospadias and associated anomalies remains elusive. The incidence of complications depends upon the degree of critical appraisal of results. Too frequently, surgeons have ignored postoperative shortcomings more easily than the victims have been able to tolerate them.

In this series, 20 percent of the 500 individuals had minor annoyances that were corrected without additional operations. Most of these were urinary fistulas that healed spontaneously or mild meatal strictures that were eliminated by a few dilatations.

Major complications necessitated additional surgical procedures in 22 percent of all cases. The new urethral meatus slipped posteriorly after 10 percent of the Cecil-type operations and after 17 percent of the Denis Browne procedures. Any time the patient is unable to direct his urinary stream satisfactorily and sprays urine instead, revision of the new meatus is mandatory. This can be accomplished during the second stage of the Cecil plan. Urine usually is diverted by perineal urethrostomy. Additional terminal urethra is constructed by the Thiersch-Duplay method, and the skin is closed in the modified Browne manner. The same type of advancement has been effective after deficient Browne-type operations. Most of the gaping postoperative meatuses following a Browne-type operation,

however, have required reconstructions similar to modification II of the Cecil-type operation (see Fig. 18-113). During many of the second-stage Cecil-type procedures, the urethra has been advanced as much as 1 cm successfully without diversion of the urine.

Although fistulas became extinct after properly executed Cecil-type operations, and more meticulous suturing around the new urethral meatus promptly reduced the incidence of meatal retraction, meatal strictures became the counterpart which occurred in 15 percent of the patients. The meatus did not constrict after Browne-type operations; it tended to gape instead. Enlarging a meatus proved to be much simpler than reducing the caliber of one that sprayed.

Although it is the inalienable right of every boy to be a "pointer" instead of a "sitter" by the time he starts to school, only 32 percent of the patients were seen early enough to complete their treatment during the preschool period. Indeed, only 70 percent were cured before 12 years of age. There is urgent need for widespread missionary work on behalf of hypospadiacs.

References

1. Culp, O. S. Early correction of congenital chordee and hypospadias. *J. Urol.* 65:264, 1951.
2. Culp, O. S. Experiences with 200 hypospadiacs: Evolution of a therapeutic plan. *Surg. Clin. North Am.* 39:1007, 1959.
3. Culp, O. S., and McRoberts, J. W. Hypospadias. In Alken, C. E., Dix, V. W., Goodwin, W. E., Weyrauch, H. M., and Wildbolz, E. W. (Eds.), *Handbook of Urology.* Berlin: Springer-Verlag, 1968, pp. 307–342.

Belt Technique

FOSTER FUQUA

A technique for hypospadias repair has been employed in 54 cases with gratifying results. Prior to 1956, I used either a modification of the two-stage Thiersch-Duplay technique or the Denis Browne procedure for hypospadias repair, and I encountered the expected incidence of fistula and stricture formation. In 1956 I became aware of a technique employed by Dr. Elmer Belt [1] which differed from previously described methods and which seemed to combine simplicity of performance with predictable acceptable cosmetic and functional results. This technique had been employed by Dr. Belt for some years with good results, and it is suitable for the repair of most hypospadiac cases. In my experience, the Denis Browne [2, 3] procedure is now reserved for those cases with insufficient skin due either to loss from previous operation or to injudicious circumcision, or for the more severe scrotal or perineal types of hypospadias.

The Belt method basically consists of transposition of the entire foreskin to the ventrum of the penis by an exaggerated button-hole technique at the time the chordee is corrected as the initial procedure. After a lapse of at least one year, a portion of the transposed foreskin is used to fashion a tube of appropriate length and diameter to reach the end of the penis. This new urethra is then drawn through a tunnel on the ventrum of the penis so it is completely covered by intact subcutaneous tissue and the remainder of the foreskin. For this technique to be applicable, it is necessary either for the existing external urethral meatus to be on the shaft of the penis after the initial straightening procedure or for it to have been advanced to the peno-scrotal junction if perineal hypospadias was present originally. It is also important that the second stage be planned specifically at the time of the first-stage procedure.

In carrying out the first stage, the foreskin is rearranged, allowing this preputial skin to lie on the ventral surface of the penis where it later becomes available for extension of the urethra. There are two layers of the preputial skin: a soft mucosal layer that formerly lay against the glans penis and a second layer of true skin. These two layers are approximately equal in length and, in most cases, afford the exact amount needed for adequate construction of the new urethra. Experience shows

321

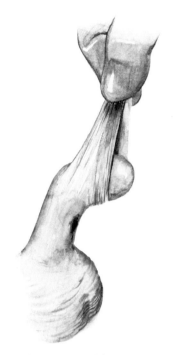

FIG. 18-116. A case of hypospadias, showing the two layers of preputial skin.

that the normal uncircumcised foreskin of a hypospadiac patient is always long enough to permit the fashioning of a flap equal to the full length of the penis, if need be, as far back as the penoscrotal junction (Fig. 18-116).

Surgical Technique

A circumferential incision is then made in the usual manner just proximal to the corona, reserving a small amount of mucous membrane adjacent to the glans (Fig. 18-117). Further dissection of this non-hair-bearing skin is done as illustrated. This exposure affords an excellent opportunity to correct the chordee. In the preparation of the two layers of the prepuce, it is important not to jeopardize the blood supply to the mucosa-like layer or the skin layer as separation of these two is carried out.

Following this dissection, a button-hole is then made on the dorsum a little farther back toward the base of the penis than ordinarily done. This ensures adequate tissue on the ventral surface of the penis for the second-stage repair (Fig. 18-118).

The penis is then transferred through this button-hole (Fig. 18-119), and approximation of the skin and mucous membrane is carried out with interrupted 4-0 catgut sutures. The closure of the transplanted dorsal hood on the ventral surface (Fig. 18-120) is performed in order to gain adequate skin for the second-stage procedure. A small Foley catheter is left indwelling, and a modified pressure dressing is utilized for 4 or 5 days postoperatively.

After a minimum time lapse of 1 year, the second-stage repair is done (Fig. 18-121). Figure 18-122 demonstrates the use of a strip of the former preputial skin (with its mucosa-like surface) to form the distal urethra. When the first incision for this step is made, it should extend down the entire length of the mucosa-like undersurface of the transplanted skin flap up to the edge where the skin meets the mucosa. In this illustration, it may appear that too little tissue is present, resulting in foreshortening of the new distal urethra, but in fact there is usually an abundant amount of tissue available for making this new tube any length required. Bringing the incision close to the original external meatus at this point permits the urethra to be turned in more easily and lessens the chance of fistula formation and sacculation. Once the outline of the new urethral tube has been formed, the distal portion is freed and the epithelial strip is then fashioned into the new distal urethra using fine, interrupted 4-0 catgut sutures to approximate one raw edge to the other.

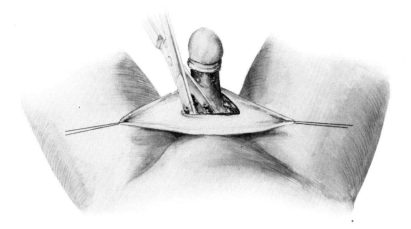

FIG. 18-117. Circumferential incision adjacent to corona and dissection of skin, allowing correction of chordee.

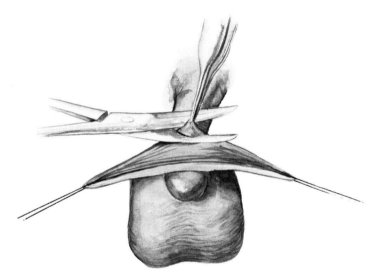

FIG. 18-118. A button-hole is made on the dorsum farther back toward the base of the penis than is ordinarily done to ensure adequate tissue on the ventral surface for the second-stage repair.

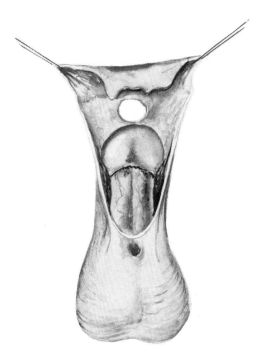

FIG. 18-119. Chordee has been excised, and the two layers of preputial skin are separated.

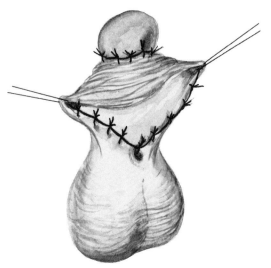

FIG. 18-120. The penis is transferred through the button-hole, and the skin and mucous membrane are approximated with 4-0 or 5-0 chromic catgut sutures.

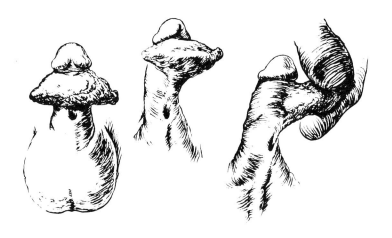

FIG. 18-121. Belt's original drawings show an abundance of transplanted skin available on the ventral surface for utilization in the second-stage procedure.

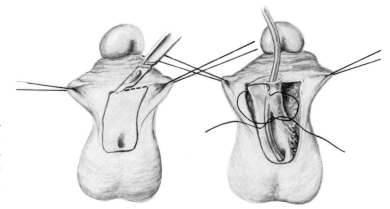

FIG. 18-122. The ure-
thral tube is formed with
the above incision and sutured with 4-0 or 5-0
chromic catgut over a catheter of appropriate size.

Preparation of the tunnel through which the new distal urethral tube is to pass to the glans penis is then performed (Fig. 18-123). The tunnel is made to extend the channel adjacent to the corpora cavernosa out to the glans. Attempts to channel the glans proper usually result in stricture formation, and it is preferable to incise the existing rudimentary meatus or ventral sulcus and to utilize this site for the patient's external urethral orifice. The final step consists of drawing the newly formed distal urethral tube through the tunnel to its permanent exit on the glans penis (Fig. 18-124).

The suture line of the new tube is completely covered by the tunnel composed of

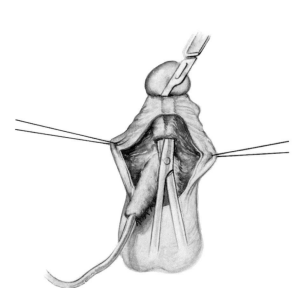

FIG. 18-123. Preparation of new urethral meatus and tunnel through which the new urethral tube is to pass out to the glans penis.

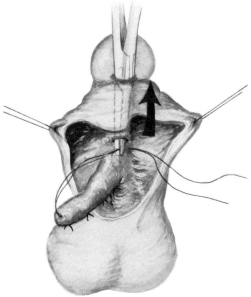

FIG. 18-124. The urethral tube is pulled through the tunnel to its exit on the glans.

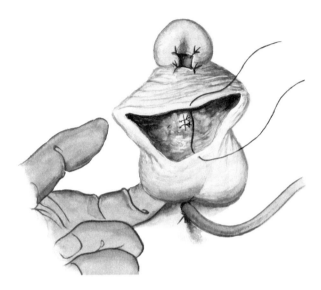

FIG. 18-125.   The new meatus is secured with quadrant sutures, and skin closure is accomplished with 4-0 or 5-0 chromic catgut.

intact fascia and subcutaneous tissue, thus effectively minimizing the chance of urinary leakage with resultant fistula formation. Any excess or redundant skin should be excised, and the ventral flap should be sutured in an appropriate manner with interrupted sutures (Fig. 18-125). Urinary diversion is done at the outset of the procedure, either by perineal urethrostomy or by suprapubic cystostomy; in either event, it is maintained for a minimum period of 2 weeks [5]. I personally prefer the use of perineal urethrostomy.

Results

In 54 cases throughout the period from 1956 to 1970, the only complication encountered was one small fistula. This operation is relatively simple to perform, is less likely to result in fistula formation than other procedures used, and has not been accompanied by the complications of stricture or meatal stenosis. It has proved to be a most gratifying technique in my hands, resulting in excellent functional and cosmetic results.

References

1. Belt, E.   Personal communication, November 1956.
2. Browne, D.   An operation for hypospadias. *Lancet* 1:141, 1936.
3. Browne, D.   An operation for hypospadias. *Proc. R. Soc. Med.* 42:466, 1949.
4. Creevy, C. D.   The correction of hypospadias, a review. *Urol. Survey* 8:2. 1958.
5. Glenn, J. F., and Boyce, W. H.   *Urologic Surgery.* New York: Harper & Row, 1969. P. 512.

Utilization of the
Prepuce for Repair

HOWARD B. MAYS

The treatment of hypospadias that utilizes preputial tissue for reinvestment of the straightened penis and the development of a complete tubular urethra produces a very satisfactory functional and cosmetic result [3, 5, 10]. The plethora of rearranged preputial tissue is adequate for correction of all degrees of penile hypospadias and most cases of penoscrotal deformities. When combined with one of several effective principles, the procedure may be adapted to the correction of the rarer instances of scrotal and perineal deformities.

Several favorable factors suggest the utilization of the prepuce. The most important property is that the tissue exists without necessary purpose and is available as an ideal material to be utilized in the correction of hypospadias. The tissue is hairless, is quite elastic, and possesses an ample blood supply. A very extensible flap may be developed and yet the vascularity may, with care, be almost completely preserved. A urethral tube thus created tends to grow in diameter and length

in proportion to the penile enlargement. Keloid formation seldom if ever occurs, and there is a gratifying minimum of scar tissue after surgery. A rapid assumption of relatively normal appearance may be expected.

The principle that the hypospadiac patient, regardless of degree of deformity, should not be circumcised until the possible need of this tissue is excluded is generally and widely accepted. Seldom, if ever, is there justification for early elective circumcision of any case of hypospadias, with the questionable exception of the very simple juxtaglandar type, and only then when the penis has been clearly demonstrated to be free of chordee. Adequate evaluation of a newborn infant with an apparently minor degree of chordee and hypospadias presents a difficult decision; therefore, circumcision is to be postponed until a final decision is reached regarding the possible usefulness of the preputial tissue. Usually the degree of chordee may be effectively determined by the end of the first year.

The decision to perform either a single or a

multiple-stage procedure is usually based upon the primary estimate of the eventual location of the urethral orifice after chordee correction, with the understanding that there will be an appreciable retraction of the urethra following extensive penile denudation and straightening. The most desirable age for correction of chordee and integument rearrangement is usually about 1 to 2 years of age, although a patient presenting much later may be treated with the expectation of a very satisfactory result. When a multiple-stage procedure is selected, the second operation may be performed after an interval of 6 months; the most effective results, however, may be expected following an interval of a year or even much longer, depending upon the size of the genitalia. There appears to be no demonstrable advantage to earlier surgery.

Lesser degrees of deformity, such as those in which the orifice is located in the distal third of the penis and there is only a moderate degree of chordee, should be spared surgery for several years because of the distinct advantage presented by a larger organ and the additional benefit of more effective transurethral urinary drainage. The use of a catheter of adequate caliber for direct urethral drainage and as a mold for urethral development is an undeniable advantage, particularly when dealing with the lesser deformities requiring correction.

Two-Stage Operation

FIRST STAGE

The first-stage operation involves far more than chordee correction. Extensive denudation of the penis will allow more effective excision of restricting fascia and connective tissue. Rearrangement of the penile integument, including the preputial tissue, is used to cover completely the exposed straightened penis. Both the simultaneous formation of a glandar urethra and the preservation of ample tissue for the subsequent employment of any of a variety of second-stage methods are feasible and practical. If desired, a grooved glans may readily be substituted, or, at a later date, a glandar tunnel may be converted to a sulcus extending beyond a juxta-glandar urethra.

The existing urethral orifice is calibrated and, if necessary, dilated sufficiently to accommodate an indwelling catheter of appropriate size. The penis is extended using stay sutures placed on either side of the tip of the glans. A circumferential incision is made about the corona, providing a cuff several millimeters in length; particular attention is given to the preservation of the cuff on the undersurface (Fig. 18-126A). Parallel incisions are made on either side of the midline and are extended from the glans-encircling incision nearly to the existing urethral orifice. The epithelium immediately adjacent to the urethral meatus should be preserved, thus lessening the possibility of subsequent stricture in this area. All restricting tissue of the rudimentary corpus spongiosum or thickened Buck's fascia is removed; this may require dissection of some portion of the intercavernosal septum. Short transverse incisions in the tunica albuginea may assist elongation, but exceptional care is required to preserve the corpora cavernosa intact and undisturbed. The attainment of a maximum degree of unrestricted extension may require still further correction; therefore, nearly complete denudation of the penis is accomplished by blunt and sharp dissection while carefully preserving the vascular supply. Thus, one large hood-like flap is developed that is attached chiefly about the base of the penis. The hood-like double-layered prepuce is placed under tension and separated into a single layer of epithelium and subcutaneous tissue by blunt and sharp dissection. Again,

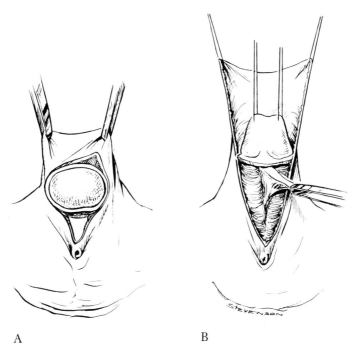

A   B

FIG. 18-126. A. Circumferential and ventral incision for correction of chordee. B. Denudation of the shaft and development of the preputial flap.

careful attention to the preservation of all possible blood supply is mandatory (Fig. 18-126B).

The distance from the base of the penis to the coronal cuff is determined, and the amount of skin required to cover the dorsum of the penis without tension is estimated. It should be kept in mind that the tissue is quite elastic and that the ultimate purpose of this step is to provide integument for the ventral surface of the penis. Adequate tissue will be available to cover the ventrum to the retracted urethra in instances other than the occasional case of significant scrotal or perineal hypospadias. With the flap extended, a transverse stab incision is made at this predetermined point. The length of the transverse incision is approximately the same as the diameter of the glans. The length of the inci-

sion should be conservative and may be increased later as required. A flap is then formed by two lateral incisions extending from the ends of the transverse incision distally and, in length, a little more than is deemed necessary to provide for the formation of the glandar urethra (Fig. 18-127A). The base of this trapdoor-like flap is thus in a distal position. The length should be determined by estimating the amount of tissue that is sufficient to form into the glandar urethra, allowing enough for extension several millimeters beyond the tip of the glans. The width of the flap must be sufficient to form a tubular urethra. The preputial flap is then drawn over the glans (Fig. 18-127B).

A tunnel is formed in the glans by piercing from a position deep in the intercavernosal groove; one must be careful to preserve the

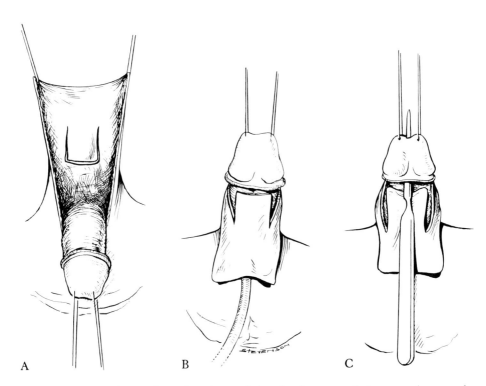

FIG. 18-127. A. A flap is formed to be used for development of the transglans urethra. B. The preputial flap is drawn over the glans. C. Development of the glans tunnel.

previously formed cuff of skin of the frenulum area. Penetration of the glans may be accomplished by use either of a pointed instrument, such as a small myringotomy knife, or of a small circular punch of appropriate diameter, such as a sharp-edged dermatology punch. The canal may be enlarged by stretching it sufficiently with a hemostat to allow passage of a sound of adequate size (Fig. 18-127C). Excision of a small circle of epithelium about the sound at the new external meatus in the tip of the glans is important for the prevention of stenosis.

The distal urethra is formed by approximating the edges of the flap, meticulously using interrupted sutures of 5-0 atraumatic catgut. These sutures should not penetrate the epithelial surface. A short section of rubber or plastic tubing, varying in size in accordance with the patient's age and genital size, is selected to serve as a form for the urethra. The pedunculated tube is drawn through the glans canal to a position slightly beyond the tip and the protruding urethra is sutured to the margins of the glans neostomy (Fig. 18-128A).

The remainder of the flap is used to cover the ventral surface of the penis, and, in most instances of penile and penoscrotal deformities, it should be of sufficient length to reach the retracted urethral orifice. The epithelial margins are sutured with 3-0 or 4-0 absorb-

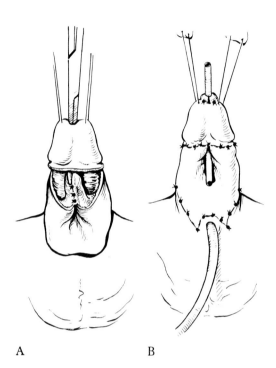

A   B

FIG. 18-128. A. Development of the glans urethra. B. Penile integument rearrangement. The first stage is now completed.

able material. Lesser degrees of deformity require far less tissue than may be available. Excision of excess skin should be roughly in accordance with need but without particular attention to appearance, taking care not to sacrifice any tissue that might subsequently be utilized. It is noteworthy that this large flap, which completely surrounds the distal portion of the penis and forms a majority of the ventral covering, eventually acquires an appearance and texture quite indistinguishable from the normal tissue, and displays scarcely noticeable scarring.

The penis is overextended by suturing the two stay sutures previously placed in the glans to the abdominal wall. A bolster of gauze may be used to accentuate chordee correction. Usually a light gauze dressing will suffice, although an elastic occlusion dressing may be desirable (Fig. 18-128B).

Dissection throughout the procedure is performed with care; therefore, bleeding is not generally a significant feature. Occasionally a rubber band tourniquet may be helpful. Ice may be used intermittently, but the continuous use of cold applications for a prolonged period is unwise. Small children are restrained for several days. The urethral catheter and the small tube used as a form for the glandar urethra are removed between the third and fifth postoperative day. Unnecessary postoperative dressing should be avoided; however, if elastic occlusion dressing has been used, it should be replaced after the first day with a light dry dressing.

SECOND STAGE

The second-stage operation should be performed after an appropriate interval of at least 6 months or preferably much longer. During this period, reestablishment of adequate blood supply will have occurred, and the transposed tissue will have become soft and pliable. Should the penis be small, the second-stage procedure should be postponed to allow sufficient growth of the genitalia. Chordee having been corrected, there is no advantage to be gained by an early second-stage operation. Calibration of the newly formed urethra during this period should demonstrate satisfactory patency and aid in the decision of whether to carry the completed urethra to the tip of the glans or to provide a temporary or permanent distal urethra in the juxtaglandar position.

Diversion of the urine is generally essential. Although most surgeons apparently prefer perineal diversion, experience has suggested possible advantages of the combination of cystostomy and urethral drainage either using a small nephrostomy-type catheter, such as the McIver type, or, preferably, using the Cummings nephrostomy tube. Either will provide ample suprapubic drainage, and the distal portion of the tube may serve as a form about which the penile urethra may be loosely constructed. This recommended procedure is quite simple and serves the same purpose as a combined suprapubic and perineal drainage. A small sound of appropriate size, preferably with a perforated tip, is inserted into the partially distended bladder and depressed, presenting the tip suprapubically. A short cut-down incision is made, carefully securing the edges of the bladder to ensure that inversion of the bladder does not occur. The tip of the catheter is sutured to the sound and drawn into proper position in the bladder, thus providing a cystostomy and urethral-tube combination. The urethral portion of the combined tube is usually tied after having been drawn through the previously formed glans tunnel. Formation of the penile urethra by slight variation of the methods described by Duplay [4] and Thiersch is recommended, but the modifications suggested by Denis Browne [2] or a number of other procedures may also be effectively employed. Significantly, however, by employing the procedure as described, there is nearly always more than ample tissue from which to develop a completely formed tube.

Parallel incisions are placed sufficiently wide apart to develop a tension-free tube. These incisions are joined proximally and distally by carefully developed U-shaped incisions about the proximal and distal orifices (Fig. 18-129A). Dissection under the medial and lateral aspects of the incisions need be only minimal. Closure of the urethral tube is

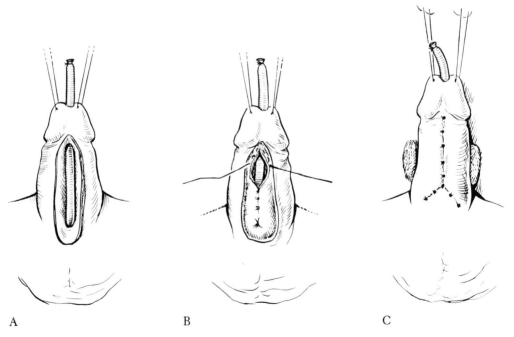

A   B   C

FIG. 18-129. Second stage. A. Formation of the penile urethra. The Thiersch-Duplay modification is shown. B and C. Closure and overextension by abdominal wall sutures.

accomplished by closely spaced interrupted atraumatic 4-0 or 5-0 sutures that should not penetrate the epithelial surface. Closure of the distal ends of the penile urethra is accomplished by semi-purse-string sutures (Fig. 18-129B). Reinforcing fascial sutures are recommended. All demonstrated constriction and tension must be relaxed by free dissection of the penile integument. Occasionally, lateral incisions near the base of the penis and, rarely, a longitudinal dorsal incision may be indicated in anticipation of possible postoperative edema. Skin margins are reapproximated with interrupted absorbable suture material. The use of an inverted Y closure at the penile scrotal area, using scrotal tissue freely, may greatly lessen the possibility of tension (Fig. 18-129C).

Stay sutures in the glans are used to extend

the penis, securing it to the abdominal wall rather loosely. A light gauze dressing or an elastic pressure dressing is used. Restraint for all younger patients for at least 24 hours or longer is recommended. Urinary drainage is maintained for 5 days or longer.

Single-Stage Operation

Many of the lesser degrees of penile hypospadias and selected cases of juxtaglandar deformity with notable chordee may be effectively corrected in a single stage.

The previously described glans-encircling incision is made, and all constricting tissue causing acute angulation is carefully removed, particularly on the ventral surface (see Fig. 18-126A). A flap is developed,

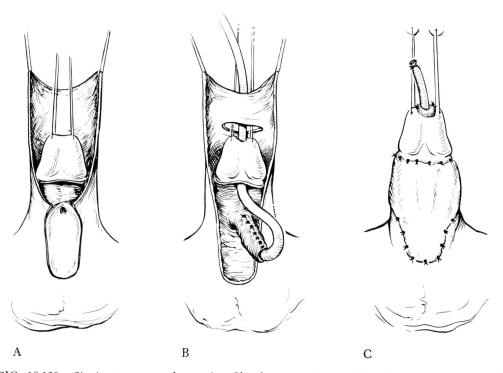

A   B   C

FIG. 18-130. Single stage procedure. A. Chordee correction and development of a preputial flap. B. Development of the transglans urethra. C. Penile reinvestment.

which is similar to that described by Bevan [1], around the retracted meatus. This is done with extended parallel incisions that are sufficient in width and length to create an adequate epithelial-lined tube several millimeters longer than the measured distance from the retracted orifice to the tip of the glans (Fig. 18-130A). A transglans tunnel is developed as previously described (Fig. 18-130B). Closure of the urethral tube is accomplished about the indwelling catheter by meticulously placed interrupted 4-0 or 5-0 absorbable sutures. The newly formed tube is drawn through the glans several millimeters beyond the tip and is sutured to the glans. The glans tunnel must be properly developed and of adequate size to eliminate pressure.

The integument deficiency created by the chordee correction and penile lengthening is covered by a dorsally derived flap (Fig. 18-130C).

Correction of Chordee without Hypospadias

Chordee associated with a normally placed orifice is rarely encountered. Should the urethral length appear to be insufficient to allow proper straightening, the dorsally derived preputial flap procedure is readily adaptable to the correction of this unusual anomaly. The basic penile incisions are made as previously described (see Fig. 18-126A). If, during elimination of all constricting tissue, the urethra is found to be insufficient in length, it is severed and the ends are allowed to retract as complete extension and chordee correction is performed (Fig. 18-131A). The denuded penis is covered with the dorsally derived flap after the glans is drawn through the transverse incision. Careful approximation of the skin flap to the two urethral orifices created by severence ensures a smooth continuity of

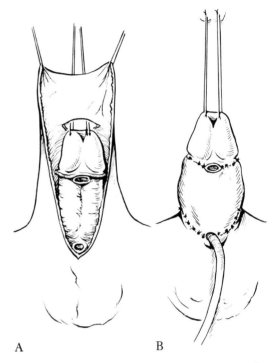

FIG. 18-131. Correction of chordee with normally placed urethral meatus. A. Chordee correction and severence of the urethra. B. Penile reinvestment.

the urethra that is later to be developed. Drainage is recommended for a few days through the retracted urethral orifice (Fig. 18-131B). Essentially, this procedure creates a situation closely akin to the desired result of the first stage of the two-stage procedure previously described. Following an appropriate interval, the second stage is undertaken as previously described (see Fig. 18-129).

Rarely, one may encounter significant chordee in which the urethra is long enough that curvature may be corrected unrestricted by urethral length and leaving the urethra intact. All constricting tissue is released, and the required degree of denudation of the penis is performed to overcorrect the deformity. The preputially derived flap is readily adaptable as a pliable covering to assist in the reinvestment of the shaft. An exceptionally satisfactory functional and cosmetic result may be anticipated.

Complications

The possibility of some form or degree of complication should be anticipated in every case of hypospadias repair, and in some measure this prediction is nearly always realized. It is obviously necessary to understand that an entirely uncomplicated primary result is a desired but infrequently attained goal, regardless of the procedure employed. It is good practice to discuss with the parents the possible complications that might well require additional surgical effort beyond the basic one or two stages proposed.

Hemotoma as a complication of surgery should rarely occur and is best prevented by attention to hemostasis. Fulguration, if used, should be light and minimal. Postoperative use of an elastic pressure dressing for a brief period is useful. Any use of cold applications should be intermittent and discontinued after a few hours.

Postoperative extravasation as the result of forceful voiding despite adequate urinary diversion may occasionally occur, with the possibility of some loss of flap tissue. Fortunately, the preputially derived skin has very good regenerative ability, and there is little tendency to scar tissue formation.

The most common complication of urethroplasty is fistula formation, and this may be expected fairly frequently. Undeniably, the probability of this is increased by efforts to create a normal positioning of the urethral orifice. The probability of fistula formation may be reduced by anticipating a less than optimal result, i.e., by accepting or converting to a juxtaglandar orifice or a glans groove. A fistula developing in this area in the presence of a satisfactorily formed transglandar urethra may be later corrected to a very satisfactory result. Fistula formation understandably appears most often at the juncture of the old and new urethra, and it may occur anywhere along the course of the newly created tube. However, the nature of the preputially derived integument lends itself readily to closure.

Postoperative stricture may occur at the juncture of the new and old urethra or at the new external meatus. Stenosis at the terminal urethra may occur as a result of a restricting glans tunnel or a terminal urethra that is too small. Periodic gentle dilatation may be required; however, once a satisfactory urethral caliber has been established, recurrent late stricture has been only infrequently encountered. The preputially derived urethra possesses the remarkable ability to grow in proportion to penile growth. Patients seen again many years after hypospadias correction have been found to be without constriction and with a normal urethral caliber.

Urethral diverticulation may occur and is likely to appear more often following single-stage procedures. It is less likely to occur, however, if the completely formed tube of the urethra is reinforced by fascial covering. Persistent diverticulation usually results in dribbling and may encourage infection and possible calculus formation. Plication of fascial reinforcement and, occasionally, excision of redundant tissue may be required. This complication is fortunately rarely encountered following the described procedures.

cavernosa is pierced, bleeding will result that is difficult to stop and postoperative swelling will be maximal.

Narrowing of the meatal opening must be checked for before the urethra is sutured to the surrounding skin, and a generous meatotomy should be performed whenever necessary; it is most important to ensure a wide meatal opening at this stage of the operation.

The best skin with which to resurface the raw area exposed by removal of the fibrous band is the nonhirsute distensible skin of the prepuce and the penis. To mobilize this, incisions are made along the line of the coronal sulcus on each side, thus creating two flaps that can be advanced to the midline ventrally and sewn to each other. Once again, meticulous attention must be paid to hemostasis on the raw surfaces so created on the penis and on the undersides of the flaps (Fig. 18-132).

In most cases, it is not necessary to carry the subcoronal incisions around the penis so they meet on the dorsum. Occasionally, however, in very severe cases in which the penis is so deformed that the glans is virtually tethered into the perineum, so much skin may be needed on the ventral surface that there is no alternative. If it is decided that this is necessary, the inner skin surface of the prepuce should be incised vertically from its midpoint dorsally to its free border, and the two preputial surfaces are separated to create winged flaps to advance onto the ventral surface (Fig. 18-133).

The operation is completed by a dorsal slit, which takes care of the unavoidable postoperative swelling and ensures that this does not hinder proper healing of the suture line. It causes no increase in surgical difficulty when the urethra is reconstructed. A catheter is inserted through the meatus and maintained for a week to keep the suture line dry. Opinion is divided as to whether the penis should be dressed and strapped to the ab-

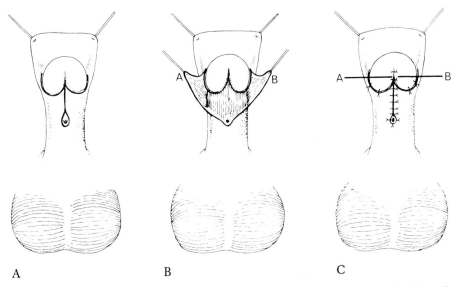

A   B   C

FIG. 18-132. Correction of flexion deformity—Mild case. A. Incisions. B. The flaps are reflected. C. The flaps are inset.

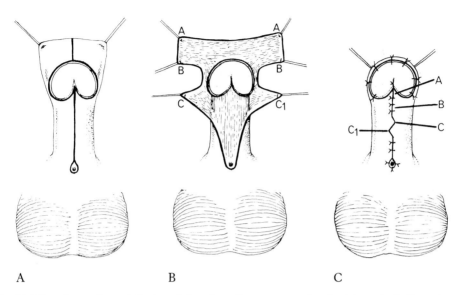

FIG. 18-133. Correction of flexion deformity—Severe case A. Incisions, including the vertical incision of the inner layer of the prepuce. B. The flaps are reflected. C. The flaps are inset.

dominal wall or whether it should be left entirely free. It probably makes little difference in the end result and, having tried both methods, it is the author's preference to leave it free because (1) constricting bandages are potentially dangerous to the circulation in the flaps if tension develops, (2) leaving the suture line uncovered minimizes the chances of infection developing, and (3) the child is more comfortable.

Many attempts have been made by surgeons to combine the operation for removal of the flexion band with the operation to restore the urethral channel, but so far none has been completely successful in terms of the results. Either the correction of chordee has been incomplete, or the complications of urethral restoration have been increased; more often both have occurred. It is the author's firm belief that the two objectives are best realized by separate operations and that they should be separated by an interval of at least 6 months.

Restoration of Urethral Tube

The multiplicity of methods advocated is convincing proof of the difficulties and complications of this operation. It is common knowledge that in minor cases many methods have an equal chance of success. Preputial transference based on the Ombrédanne operation [7], which has been most recently modified by the excellent technique of Elliott Blake [1], gives satisfactory results, but in cases involving the penile shaft, the peno-scrotal junction, and the perineum, these techniques do not provide sufficient material for success. After having tried skin inlays, as described by Nové-Josserand [6] and more recently by McIndoe [5], and flaps of the type described by Edmunds [3], the author has relied entirely upon the Denis Browne [2] operation for the last 15 years.

This procedure consists of suturing local skin flaps over a buried strip of skin extending from the meatus to the glans. It relies

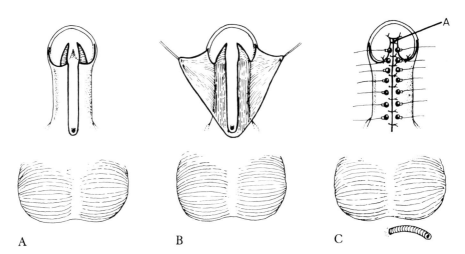

FIG. 18-134. Restoration of the urethral tube (Denis Browne technique). A. Incisions, including the excision of triangular areas on the glans. B. The flaps are raised. C. The flaps are inset using beads and metal stops. *A* indicates the junction point of the two flaps held with a silk stitch. A perineal catheter is in place.

upon the growth of epithelium from the edges of the buried strip onto the undersurface of the covering flaps to complete the urethral tunnel (Fig. 18-134). Its merits are that it is a simple operation to perform and that it is no more difficult for a severe case than for a minor one. It has been criticized on account of its leading to fistula formation; it is certainly not free of this complication, but it is no more vulnerable in this respect, if properly performed, than other procedures, and perhaps less so than some. The essential prerequisite to success is satisfactory urinary diversion by means of a self-retaining catheter through a perineal urethrostomy for 2 weeks. Almost all fistulas are due to the failure of complete urinary diversion during this postoperative period.

The urethrostomy is best made by passing the end of the catheter down the urethra on a small hemostat (after placing the bulb in the bladder) and cutting down onto the tip of

the hemostat in the perineum (Fig. 18-135). Successful drainage is accomplished by passing the hemostat far enough back into the perineum before cutting down onto it to ensure that the emerging catheter is not looped or curved but emerges in a straight line from the bladder.

The only other likely cause of fistula formation is failure to take heed of Denis Browne's insistence [2] that the suture line must be sewn sufficiently loosely to allow for the inevitable postoperative swelling. To minimize the chances of stitches becoming tight and cutting out, Denis Browne advocated the use of beads held by short cylindrical lengths of metal pinched onto fine nylon sutures. The rounded surfaces of these beads certainly do help by presenting a smooth surface to the skin. The operation can be equally successful with ordinary sutures, providing these are tied loosely. If the beads are used, the stitches should transfix the skin

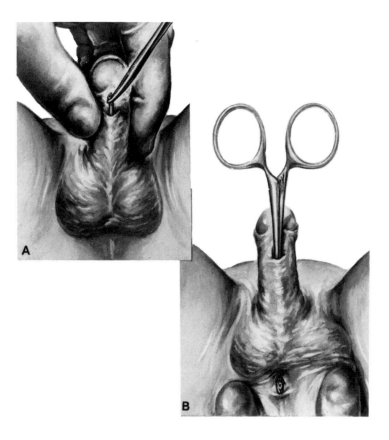

FIG. 18-135. Perineal urethrostomy. A. The catheter is grasped with a hemostat. B. The catheter is passed down the urethra with the hemostat to present in the perineum. (Courtesy of *Modern Trends in Plastic Surgery,* edited by Thomas Gibson, Butterworth, 1966.)

flaps at least 3 mm from their edges so the beads do not overlap them.

The theoretical prognostication that reliance upon the growth of the epithelium to complete the tunnel would result in a narrow, strictured urethra is not born out in practice. Perhaps this is because of the regular stretching of the tube by the passage of urine. The only place where stricture may occur is at the tip of the glans; this results from leaving a too narrow strip of skin in the glandar furrow by cutting the apices of the triangular excisions too close to each other. These triangular excisions are made to pro-

vide raw surfaces to which the covering flaps can become attached along the ventral surface of the glans, and they are essential to the operation; great care, however, must be taken not to approximate their tips too closely. If this mistake is made and a meatal stricture results, a meatotomy is the only solution. Dilatation does not give lasting relief.

The operation should always be completed by a dorsal slit, and the wound should be left open to scab over. It heals in about 10 days. The sutures are removed between the eighth and tenth days, depending on the amount of swelling, and the catheter after 2 weeks. The perineal wound takes 48 hours to heal and leaves no stricture, provided the incision is made along the line of the urethra. No drains should be inserted beneath the skin flaps; they are unnecessary if hemostasis is meticulous; they rarely drain a significant amount of blood; they do nothing to mitigate against postoperative edema; and the stab wounds that they require may reduce the blood supply to the flaps.

One final word of warning in the management of these difficult cases is appropriate: it is wise to determine the sex of every child cytologically before any operation is undertaken. Mistakes involving female pseudohermaphrodites of the adrenogenital type are not as uncommon as might be supposed, nor is it too difficult to be mistaken in a male pseudohermaphrodite when the penis is very small and tethered into the perineum.

References

1. Blake, H. E. In Robb, C., and Smith, R. (Eds.), *Operative Surgery Service*. London: Butterworth, 1965. Part XV, p. 53.
2. Browne, D. Hypospadias. *Postgrad. Med. J.* 25:367, 1949.
3. Edmunds, A. An operation for hypospadias. *Lancet* 1:447, 1913.
4. Matthews, D. N. A tribute to the services of Sir Archibald McIndoe to plastic surgery. *Ann. R. Coll. Surg. Engl.* 41:403, 1967.
5. McIndoe, A. H. An operation for the cure of adult hypospadias. *Br. Med. J.* 1:385, 1937.
6. Nové-Josserand, G. Traitement de l'hypospadias: Nouvelle méthode. *Lyon Méd.* 85:198, 1897.
7. Ombrédanne, L. *Précis clinique et operatoire de chirurgie infantile* (3rd ed.). Paris: Masson et Cie, 1932.

"Large Fistula" Modification

JAIME PLANAS

The Denis Browne operation [1, 2] for the repair of hypospadias, in which a narrow strip of skin is buried along the shaft of the penis, was a great advance in the treatment of those conditions in which sufficient penile skin is not available and no useful substitute for it can be found. The large percentage of fistula formation in our cases and in the experience of others, as well as the impossibility of obtaining a properly located distal meatus at the tip of the glans (even with Browne's modification of resecting two mucosal triangles on the ventral surface of the glans) led us to develop a new procedure based on Browne's principle. Our procedure is designed to overcome the danger of the pressure of the beads over the skin flaps and to provide a terminal meatus at the summit of the glans.

The operation is performed in two stages with a minimum interval of 6 months between them. In the first stage, the chordee is corrected and the intraglandar portion of the urethra is created. In this way, a straight penis is obtained with the glans tunnelized (Fig. 18-136). The deformity may be compared in this stage to a normal penis with a large fistula [3].

Closure of this large fistula is made at the second stage by leaving a strip of skin along the two openings, which is covered with the lateral flaps. Apposition of the lateral flaps is obtained by means of two superimposed running sutures in the subcutaneous tissue; these are withdrawn after 10 days. In this way, no pressure over the skin surface is exerted by beads, thus avoiding necrotic points and fistula formation. A perineal urethrostomy is performed previous to the second stage in order to obtain a dry field for 7 to 10 days.

First-Stage Operation

Using the Blair-Byars technique, the hood of the prepuce is grasped with two forceps at its mucocutaneous junction and is split with scissors to within 1 to 2 mm of the coronal sulcus (Fig. 18-137A). An incision is made in the mucous membrane on each side, a few millimeters from the coronal sulcus (Fig. 18-137B). By undermining the mucous mem-

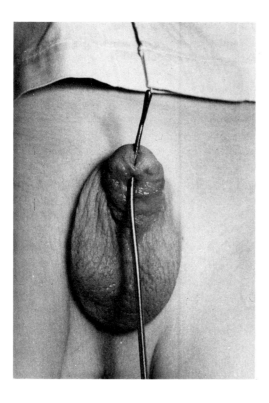

FIG. 18-136. Glans is tunnelized after the first stage of the operation.

brane, two ample wings of prepuce are thus created (Fig. 18-137C). Resection of the tissue causing the chordee elongates the penis (Fig. 18-137D). The glans is then split vertically in half (Fig. 18-137E). The cut should be deep, and if made in the midline, an almost dry field will be found (in the embryo, the glans closes through this plane). The wings of prepuce are carefully inspected, and any distal part of them whose color indicates defective circulation is discarded. One of the wings is applied directly to the raw surface of the split glans and secured by a stitch to the deepest part of it. With the aid of a catheter, a short preputial tube is made by folding the flap around it, raw surface outward, and securing it with a few stitches (Fig. 18-137F).

The stitches are placed with the knots in the lumen of the tube and tied firmly to assist their spontaneous elimination. The cutaneous tube is buried into the glans by suturing the two sides of the glans with two or three stitches (Fig. 18-137G).

The piece of catheter is left in place for a few weeks after the operation to maintain the shape and patency of the tube. The raw surface of the shaft of the penis is covered with the other preputial wing. An indwelling catheter is also maintained for several days following surgery. The penis is wrapped with wet gauze to absorb postoperative oozing.

Second-Stage Operation

After 6 months, the urethroplasty is performed. This procedure consists only of the closure of the large fistula. This is done by an incision down each side that meets at both ends (Fig. 18-138A). This type of closure eliminates the possibility of distal breakdown, which may occur in the Denis Browne operation [1]. The two parallel incisions on the ventral surface of the penis are 4 mm apart, leaving a central strip of skin as in Denis Browne's procedure. Two lateral flaps are undermined. Undermining should be deep and close to the corpora cavernosa so the lateral flaps are as thick as possible. The cutaneous strip is buried by approximation of subcutaneous tissue using two superimposed running sutures. The first suture enters the skin at the base of the penis or through the scrotum, into the wound, and leaves the penis through one side of the glans (Fig. 18-138B; see Fig. 18-139). A small piece of tube is threaded on the suture to protect the glans (Fig. 18-138C). A second running suture is placed to enter the opposite side of the glans (Fig. 18-138D) and to leave through the base of the penis or the scrotum (Fig. 18-138E).

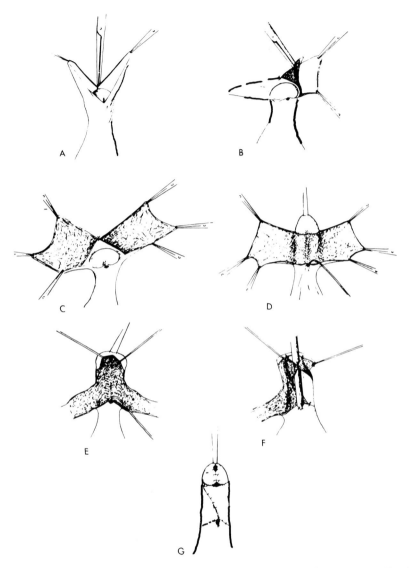

FIG. 18-137. First-stage operation. A. Splitting the hood of the prepuce. B. Incising the mucous membrane of the prepuce to prepare the wings. C. Preputial wings are created. D. The penis is elongated. E. The glans is split vertically in half. F. Forming a cutaneous tube with one of the preputial wings. G. The cutaneous tube is buried in the glans after suturing the two sides of the glans.

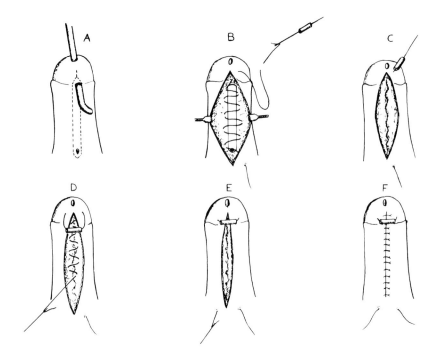

FIG. 18-138. Second-stage operation. A. Parallel incisions, 4 mm apart, meet at both ends of the "large fistula." B. Approximation of subcutaneous tissue with the first running suture. C. After tightening the first running suture, the cutaneous strip is covered. A small piece of tube is threaded on the suture to protect the glans. D. Insertion of the second running suture, which (E) leaves through the base of the penis or the scrotum. F. Skin borders are closed with fine silk sutures.

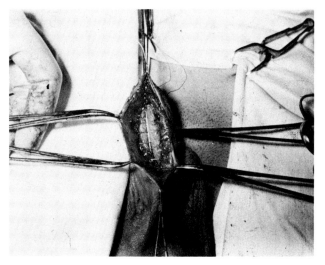

FIG. 18-139. Insertion of the first running suture (second stage of the operation) to close the "large fistula."

Skin borders are closed with fine silk sutures (Fig. 18-138F). The penis is again wrapped with wet gauze. Supramid 2-0 is used for the running sutures.

Perineal urethrostomy, using Denis Browne's technique, is performed before starting the second stage. The running sutures are removed approximately 10 days after the operation. The loop protected by the piece of tube is cut, and the sutures are tractioned from the base of the penis [4].

References

1. Browne, D. An operation for hypospadias. *Proc. R. Soc. Med.* 42:466, 1949.
2. Browne, D. Hypospadias. *Postgrad. Med. J.* 25:376, 1949.
3. Planas, J. L'hypospadias. *Acta Urol. Belg.* 30:357, 1962.
4. Planas, J. Hypospadias. In *Transactions of the Fifth International Congress of Plastic and Reconstructive Surgery*. Melbourne, Australia: Butterworth, 1971. P. 263.

Byars' Technique

PETER RANDALL

The contributions of Dr. Louis T. Byars to the field of hypospadias repair can be divided into two categories: first, a surgical viewpoint that is particularly applicable to this type of work, and second, a plan of treatment that is outstanding for its simplicity and directness. His results, though modestly expressed in his writings, were excellent [1–4].

Byars taught that there are many ways in which this deformity can be corrected. Some are simple and straightforward, some are more complex, and some are unbelievably complicated. All of them can be made to work, particularly in the hands of a surgeon who is skilled and who is anxious to demonstrate that a particular plan is a good one. In general, however, the more simple and direct approaches will have a higher rate of success than the more complicated ones. The overall results will therefore be better in a greater number of patients if the technique is not too intricate.

He also pointed out that this type of surgery involves the handling of small structures, including some of the thinnest skin and most delicate tissues a surgeon has to work with. As a result, it must be treated with great care. Small instruments and fine suture material are needed. Some surgeons are adept at working with these tissues, others simply are not. They are accustomed to bigger structures, heavier sutures, and rougher techniques; they will thus have difficulty in the field of hypospadias repair regardless of what plan of reconstruction they follow.

Surgical Technique

Byars preferred to initiate the first step in reconstruction when the patient was about 3 years of age. He excised the chordee (Fig. 18-140) and rotated two preputial flaps to the ventral side of the penis. The night before surgery and the morning of surgery, the genitalia are thoroughly cleaned with a surgical soap, and care is taken that the area is well rinsed off after the soap is applied. In the operating room, the surgical preparation is a very weak tincture of iodine cleaned off with alcohol. A 4-0 silk stitch is placed through the glans for traction and stabilization. The tissues causing chordee are completely excised, including any overlying atrophic skin.

348

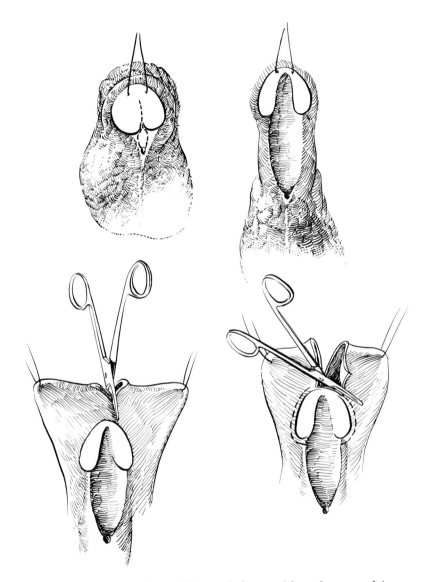

FIG. 18-140. The chordee is excised widely, including excision of any overlying atrophic skin. The incision is carried up into the glans in the midline to allow the skin urethra to be reconstructed well into this area. The preputial skin is incised as in a "dorsal slit," and then is incised around the glans to leave a cuff adjacent to the corona.

The natural urethral opening will then assume a more proximal position. The distance to be bridged by a reconstructed skin tube will necessarily appear to be greater than before the chordee correction.

He noted that chordee was not really a "bow-string" contracture, because if one were to cut the string of a bow at any point, the bow would straighten out just as much as it would if the entire string were removed. In hypospadial chordee—as in Dupuytren's contracture—the contracted tissue is attached to the adjacent structures for its entire length. If one simply incises the fibrous tissue, some residual contraction will remain, and in fact further contraction will occur as the incision heals. Correction of this type of deformity requires complete excision of the contracted tissue. Care should be taken not to incise into the corpora.

The distal end of the proximal urethra is placed in a position where closure can be achieved without tension on the urethra. If a stenosis of the distal end of the urethra is noted, it is widely incised longitudinally. Frequently, however, an apparent stenosis is made of very elastic tissue that will admit a large sized catheter and will not have to be incised.

Next, a ventral incision is made in the glans that allows the two halves of the glans to fall apart. One of the skin flaps can be placed well up into this structure so the reconstructed urethra may extend all the way to the end of the penis. This incision is in a natural plane and does not enter the spongy tissue. The skin flaps are constructed by making a dorsal longitudinal incision in the preputial skin. The base of this incision is sutured with a single stitch. A second preputial incision is then made around the penis about 2 to 3 mm proximal to the glans. This T-shaped incision leaves two rectangular flaps, one on either side of the vertical part of the T (corresponding to the dorsal incision), and each flap is folded on itself. Considerable

tissue is obtained by unfolding these flaps. The circulation in these flaps is occasionally impaired distally; questionable areas should be excised (Fig. 18-141).

The flaps are rotated to the ventral side of the penis, and either they are interdigitated so that the corner of one extends to the tip of the incision in the glans and the other covers the proximal denuded area, or they are approximated end-to-end in the midline. With a minimal midshaft to distal hypospadias, only one flap need be used and the other can be left in place. In a case of severe penoscrotal or perineal hypospadias, these flaps should still supply sufficient tissue to allow a redundancy of skin on the ventral side. No dorsal relaxing incision is needed. By interdigitating the two flaps diagonally, their junction forms a zig-zag incision on the ventral side that will prevent the possibility of a subsequent contracture. For suture material, 5-0 chromic catgut is preferred, but fine silk can be used if the surgeon does not mind the toil of removing the sutures. The ends of the sutures are left long on the ventral side of the glans to allow the placement of a tied-on dressing in the glans, thus keeping the skin flaps well up into the incision in this area [2].

A catheter is placed in the bladder and secured with a skin suture. The dressing includes fine mesh Xeroform gauze on the suture line and several layers of cotton gauze in the area of the incisions. These are not carried farther around the shaft, thus allowing skin-to-adhesive contact. Wrap-around strips of elastic adhesive are placed snugly around the entire shaft of the penis, leaving a tiny amount of glans exposed. The proximal turns are looser and include the catheter. The degree of snugness is about as tight as would be comfortable on one's finger. By leaving a small amount of the glans exposed, it is possible to check the circulation by simply touching the tissue to determine if sensation is present. It is not usually possible to detect any color changes in this tissue, but should

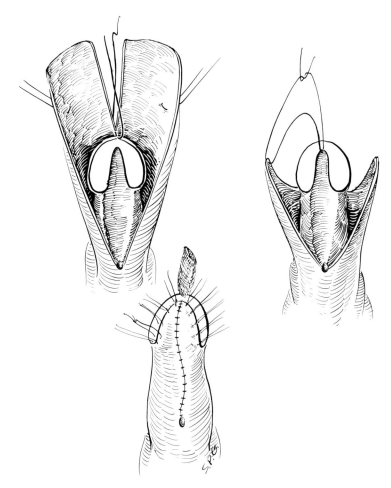

FIG. 18-141. Two large flaps of skin are developed from the prepuce. Skin with dubious circulation is judiciously trimmed. The flaps are repositioned on the ventral side of the penis. In the region of the glans, the sutures are left long so they can be tied over a bolus of gauze.

the sensation be lost, the dressing is removed.

The catheter is never occluded but is allowed to drain into several cotton "abdominal pads" that are secured to the leg by tape and cotton ribbon ties. These pads are changed as necessary. In children the catheter is not connected to straight drainage: if long rubber tubes are used, they are easily kinked, and if kinked, bladder spasm and straining can force urine around the catheter into the area of the repair. Catheters can also be dis-

lodged inadvertently in children when attached to drainage tubes. The catheter is irrigated three times a day with 30 ml of sterile saline, and it is left in place for 6 days, at which time the dressing is removed and tub baths are started twice a day. Patients are kept on an antibiotic such as Gantrisin (sulfisoxazole) while the catheter is in place.

The next stage can be done anytime after 2 months, but an interval of 1 year is preferred. It consists of making a skin-lined ure-

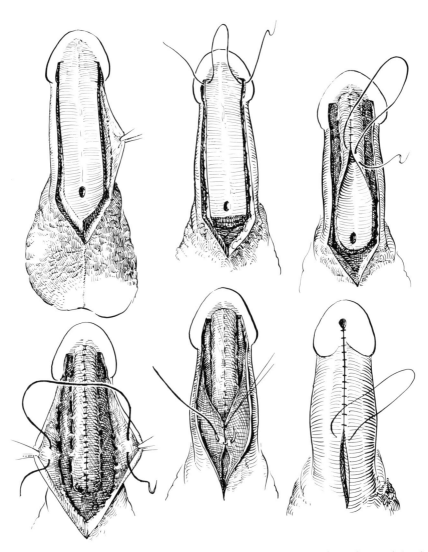

FIG. 18-142.   A skin strip with a width of three times the diameter of a catheter of the desired urethral size is outlined and tubed with a running fine chromic catgut inverting stitch. The skin is closed in depth over the newly constructed skin urethra. Urine is diverted through a perineal urethrostomy.

thra, covering this reconstructed tube with adjacent skin, and connecting it to the proximal urethra. In more severe cases, Byars initially would separate these steps into two procedures, the last step consisting of connecting the reconstructed tube to the proximal urethra, but in later years he usually combined them in one operation, thereby completing the reconstruction in two stages.

For this stage, a perineal urethrostomy is done. The catheter again is secured with a stitch. The dressing, the use of the catheter, and the time of the suture removal are the same as described above. At no time does a catheter transgress the newly constructed urethra, so reaction to foreign structures is minimized.

The urethral skin tube is constructed by making two parallel incisions in the midventral skin from the proximal urethra to the glans. The width of this strip of skin is of critical importance and should be three times the diameter of the intended urethra or roughly three times the width of a No. 10 catheter for a child. The incisions are marked with methylene blue, incised to subcutaneous tissue, and simply tubed with a continuous inverting stitch of 5-0 chromic catgut. The edges do not have to be undermined. The closure is started at the glans to ensure a good position of the distal end.

The incisions for the skin tube are extended around the distal end of the proximal urethra (Fig. 18-142). Closure is achieved with continuous 5-0 chromic catgut sutures. Careful tailoring is needed in the region of

the urethral meatus to prevent redundancy of tissue or a possible stricture at this location. The knot on this suture is placed proximal to the skin tube-urethral junction to minimize the possibility of a fistula at this point.

The skin lateral to this ventral strip must be closed in depth over the newly created skin tube. Accordingly, this skin must be undermined and mobilized. Closure is achieved either with several layers of tiny subcutaneous 6-0 silk stitches and 5-0 chromic catgut mattress sutures on the skin, or with 5-0 chromic throughout [3].

The connection of the skin tube and the distal end of the proximal urethra can be carried out as a third stage. If so, the steps in technique, including the perineal urethrostomy, are still the same. The perineal catheter is left in about 7 days, and when withdrawn, the resulting fistula is left open and allowed to close spontaneously.

Results

Byars' approach to the repair of hypospadias is simple, sound, and straightforward. It requires about 14 days of hospitalization. It may take one or even two steps more than other techniques, but it is a very reliable method. Byars reported only one fistula in 69 consecutive cases in which there had been no previous surgery [4]. To my knowledge, this is the lowest incidence of fistula formation in a significant series of cases with any technique thus far reported.

References

1. Blair, V. P., and Byars, L. T. Hypospadias and epispadias. *J. Urol.* 40:814, 1938.
2. Byars, L. T. Functional restoration of hypospadias deformities. *Surg. Gynecol. Obstet.* 92:149, 1951.
3. Byars, L. T. A technique for consistently satisfactory repair of hypospadias. *Surg. Gynecol. Obstet.* 100:184, 1955.
4. Byars, L. T. Hypospadias and Epispadias. In Converse, J. M. (Ed.), *Reconstructive Plastic Surgery.* Philadelphia: Saunders, 1964. Pp. 2021–2036.

Method of Ricketson

GREER RICKETSON

The surgical procedures for the correction of hypospadias vary with the extent of the deformity and with the technique of the operating surgeon. The procedures that I use are not completely original, since I have combined various maneuvers previously described by other authors, though with a personal touch here and there, particularly in the second stage of reconstruction. The criteria for good reconstruction of a hypospadial penis are (1) it must be corrected so that it will carry out its dual function as normally as possible and (2) the appearance must be as near to normal as possible in order to alleviate the anxiety of the patient.

In order to meet the first criterion, the patient must be enabled to urinate properly, to have proper erections, and at the same time, to ejaculate effectively in the normal place for the purposes of reproduction. The penis must be straightened by correcting the ventral chordee. The urethra must be constructed of material that will continue to grow at the same rate as the penis. It must be material that is free of foreign matter, such as hair, that will cause fistulas, infection, or possible stone formation, and, in order to prevent the possibility of strictures and diminution of urethral size, it should be a material that will not contract.

The consideration of appearance is probably as important to the growing boy as is the first. The urinary stream should emerge from the normal site so the child can stand and void like other boys. The penis should be free of excessive scars or rosettes of skin. It should produce a stream of urine with a normal spiral, rather than the fan-shaped spray that is produced by an irregular and abnormal sized urethra. Excessive scars around the scrotum and abdominal areas should be eliminated if possible.

In order to correct the chordee and straighten the penis, the ventral fibrous band must be completely excised. The band consists of thin, friable skin extending from the base of the glans back to the urethral opening. Beneath the skin, dense fibrous tissue is found which is the remnant of the urethra, including Buck's fascia and the maldeveloped corpus spongiosum. Excision of this mass of tissue should be done by sharp dissection, completely removing it back from and slightly proximal to the urethral opening.

354

The dense band is not completely removed until the urethral opening has been released from its position and allowed to contract to a more proximal position. An adequate dissection will leave the corpora cavernosa completely bare.

Following the straightening procedure, it is necessary to obtain satisfactory coverage of the ventral surface by the transfer of tissue in some manner. The best material for coverage is the skin of the dorsum of the penis, since it meets all the requirements of texture and color. In addition to transferring sufficient skin to the area for coverage, I find it advisable to consider the second stage—the reconstruction of the urethra—at this time. It is my belief that the mucosal section of the prepuce is as near to being ideal skin for the reconstruction of the urethra as can be obtained. Therefore, both the dorsal skin and preputial mucosa are transferred to the ventral surface at this stage in order to have sufficient tissue for coverage as well as sufficient tissue for later reconstruction of the urethra.

As stated previously, there is an abundance of skin on the dorsal surface. I prefer to transfer this tissue to the ventral surface as a bipedicled visor flap in order to prevent a central longitudinal scar on the ventral surface. This type of shift of tissue allows the muscosal portion of the prepuce to be sutured to the urethral opening and to be used later for the reconstructed urethra, and it leaves the skin portion to be used for coverage of the reconstructed urethra and the ventral defect during the second-stage operation. This provides tissue that is soft, that will stretch, that does not contain hair, and that will not contract when used as a pedicle flap.

This principle of first-stage reconstruction and correction of chordee has been previously described by Beck [1], Nesbit [8], and perhaps others. No attempt is made to reconstruct any portion of the urethra at this time.

It is my belief that the visor flap of skin acts not only as a coverage for the ventral surface, but also to a certain extent as a sling to help hold the distal portion of the penis in a more nearly straight position during the healing process. I do not find it necessary to attach a suture to the glans and abdomen in order to hold the penis straight.

A catheter is placed in the urethra and a pressure dressing applied to the penis distal to this. The catheter is left in place for about 48 hours, after which the patient is allowed to void as he did prior to the operation. The dressing is usually removed in about 5 to 6 days. There is always some swelling after the removal of the dressing, but this swelling subsides in time.

The second stage of reconstruction is the construction of the urethra, which may be carried out any time after 3 or 4 months following the first stage, or it may be delayed for as many years as desired. The second-stage operation can be performed as soon as the skin has healed satisfactorily, all edema has subsided, the blood supply has reached normal, and the skin on the ventral surface is normal in appearance, pliable, and soft.

The second-stage repair may be considered to be a combination of the Thiersch-Duplay procedure and my own contribution based on the study of other methods. The proximal portion of the reconstructed urethra is of the Thiersch-Duplay type in that the parallel incision extending approximately to the urethral opening produces a flap of tissue that is sufficiently wide to be approximated as a tubed pedicle. These parallel incisions are extended to approximately the midportion of the shaft of the penis rather than extending out to the glans. The incisions are then carried in a lateral oblique manner, creating two lateral flaps that are approximately one-half the size of the desired urethra. The flaps are based at the midline on the ventral surface and remain attached to the skin that is to be used for the reconstructed urethra. This in essence creates a Y-shaped portion of the skin on the ventral and lateral surfaces. Most of the skin is made up of the mucosal prepuce that has been previously shifted from the dorsal side. The arms of the Y are elevated, starting from the distal point and extending back to the ventral surface of the penis. These flaps are then sutured together, creating a free end of the reconstructed tube.

A tunnel is then made beneath the remaining portion of the distal ventral skin of the penis, through the glans, and with an exit at the normal urethral opening. The free end of the reconstructed urethra is then passed through this tunnel and sutured to the glans at the urethral opening, thereby producing a completely closed urethral tube from the bladder to the tip of the penis. Recently, I have elected to use the glandar flap as described by Horton and Devine [5] in order to break up the circular suture line at the distal urethral opening, thereby adding an extra safety valve against possible stricture at this point. The remaining portion of the skin on the ventral surface distal to this construction, which had previously been transferred from the dorsal side, is elevated and pulled down over the reconstructed urethra and the defect created by the surgery. This, which I have described as a "window shade" type of procedure, eliminates the necessity of two overlying suture lines on the ventral surface.

The catheter that was placed in the urethra and used as a stent for reconstruction of the distal urethra is now removed. A one size smaller catheter is inserted in order to alleviate pressure and, at the same time, to maintain normal contour of the healing reconstructed urethra. A pressure dressing is applied and left in place for approximately a week. The patient is then allowed to void normally. I do not find it necessary to make any attachment of the penis to the abdomen or to use any special device like a splint.

First-Stage Operation

A 4-0 Dermalon suture is placed through the dorsal surface of the glans in order to control movement of the penis and for dorsal extension during the course of the operation. Parallel incisions are made on the ventral surface, just to each side of the ventral fibrous band, that extend from about 0.5 cm proximal to the glans to a position about 0.5 cm proximal to the urethral opening (Fig. 18-143). A U-shaped incision incorporating the ends of these parallel incisions is made just distal to the urethral opening. Starting at the base of the glans, the entire fibrous band is excised, as previously described. Special attention is paid to the fibrous band just at the base of the glans. Once this is removed, the glans is allowed to straighten considerably, and, as the fibrous band is gradually dissected out, the penis will attain normal extension and straightening. Bleeding is controlled as much as possible by clamps and ligature (using 5-0 plain catgut), or by the use of cautery.

The dorsal foreskin is drawn proximally, after which an incision is made that completely encircles the penis about 0.5 cm proximal to the glans. The foreskin is then drawn distally, and an estimate is made of how much skin should be left on the dorsal side for normal coverage without undue tension. A horizontal or slightly U-shaped buttonhole incision is made through the skin and superficial fascia. The button-hole is made large enough so it will completely encircle the base of the penis without tightness. By blunt dissection, a small channel is made from the button-hole incision to the base of the glans. No attempt is made to elevate all the skin of the penis completely, as is described in some cases.

The glans of the penis is threaded through the button-hole, thereby transferring the excess dorsal skin and dorsal mucosal prepuce

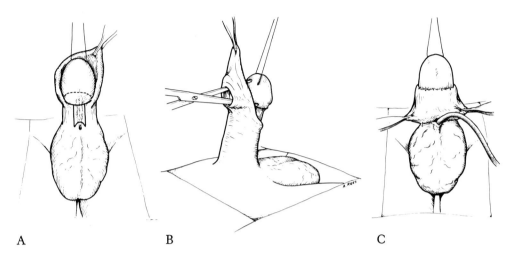

A   B   C

FIG. 18-143. First-stage operation. A. Excision of chordee and incision around the base of the glans. B. Button-hole in the dorsal foreskin. C. The prepuce and skin are sutured over the ventral defect.

to the ventral surface. The skin edges of the button-hole are then sutured around the base of the glans to the 0.5 cm of remaining mucosa with 5-0 chromic catgut. Careful attention is paid to include the superficial fascia in the suture as well as the skin, which will help control bleeding as well as prevent undue stretching of the skin. I believe that a limited amount of dissection on the dorsal side between the button-hole and the glans ensures a more adequate blood supply to the visor flap that is transferred to the ventral surface. When the visor flap is shifted, the tight ventral skin is allowed to retract laterally, eliminating the necessity of dart-type incisions or relaxation.

The central portion of this visor flap is then attached to the distal side of the urethral opening with interrupted sutures of 5-0 chromic catgut; this is the mucosal portion of the prepuce. Using a similar type of suture material, the closure is then extended laterally on each side, and the visor flap is approximated to the raw skin edges. A mattress-type suture is frequently used in order to approximate the skin edges more accurately. A pressure dressing is then applied to the penis. If one suspects that hemostasis has not been controlled adequately, it is perhaps wise to place small drains beneath the flap for drainage.

Second-Stage Operation

A 4-0 Dermalon suture is again placed in the dorsal side of the glans for control. A catheter is placed in the urethra. With the penis held in dorsal extension, the excess skin on the ventral side is pulled distally and spread out as much as possible (Fig. 18-144). It may be held with sutures, if desired, or by forceps. Parallel incisions are made from the midportion of the penis proximally and are then joined together around the urethral opening on the proximal side. At the distal point, these incisions are carried laterally and obliquely far enough to gain tissue of adequate length to reach the end of the glans without stretching. An incision is then made

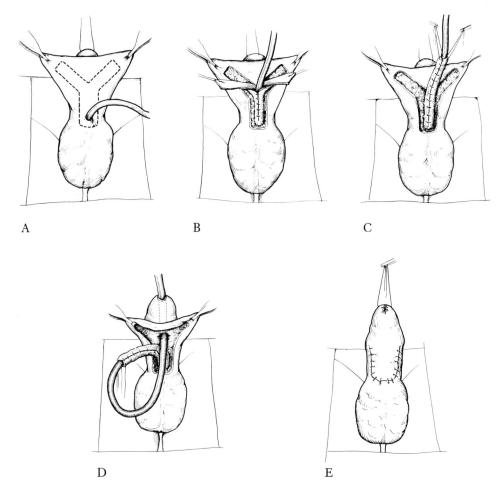

FIG. 18-144. Second-stage operation. A. Outline of incisions for the Y flap. B. Partial tubing of the pedicle flap around a catheter. C. Completion of the tubed flap. D. Insertion of the catheter and reconstructed urethra through the channel under the distal skin and through the glans. E. Suture of the urethra at the glandar opening and coverage of the ventral defect with the "window shade" flap.

parallel to these Y-shaped incisions, producing flaps that are approximately one-half the width of the desired urethral size. These flaps are cut across at the most distal portion and are elevated by blunt dissection from the underlying bed, which is based in the midline on the ventral surface. The parallel skin edges of the central flap are brought together to incorporate the catheter and are sutured into position with 6-0 chromic catgut. These sutures may be either interrupted or continuous, as desired. The sutures are actually placed in the subcutaneous tissue rather than in the skin itself. The Y-shaped flaps are likewise incorporated around the catheter with sutures on the dorsal and ventral sides of the catheter. I find it advisable to leave the long end of the sutures attached to the most distal portion of this tube in order to facilitate its transferal beneath the skin flap to the end of the glans.

By blunt dissection with sharp-pointed scissors, a channel is made under the remaining portion of the skin on the ventral surface distal to the reconstructed urethra, to the base of the glans, and out through the glans to the tip at the normal urethral opening site. A glandar flap is elevated, which is based on the dorsal side at the new urethral opening. I find it advisable to use a small scalpel to incise dorsally through the glandar portion of this dissected tunnel. An effort must be made to make the canal slightly to the dorsal side in order to prevent the possibility of tearing of the glandar mucosa at its tip. A hemostat is then placed through the glans to pick up the catheter and the ends of the remaining sutures; these are drawn through the canal along with the reconstructed urethra. The distal end of the reconstructed urethra is sutured to the mucosal edge of the glans and to the glandar flap with interrupted sutures of 5-0 chromic catgut.

The remaining skin distal to the reconstructed urethra, which was transferred to the ventral surface at the previous stage, is now drawn down like a window shade over the urethra and ventral defect. It is sutured along the skin margins with 5-0 chromic catgut. I find it advantageous to place a few subcutaneous stitches in order to facilitate better approximation. Sometimes it is necessary to perform a little blunt dissection of the skin flap before it can be drawn proximally to a sufficient length for coverage. When the Thiersch-Duplay parallel incisions are made, the skin margins retract laterally and dorsally and leave room for the skin flap, which is shaped similar to a V once the Y arms for the urethra have been elevated. Should insufficient skin be present for adequate coverage of the ventral defect, the proximal portion of the reconstruction of the urethra can be covered

by Z-shifting of the skin flaps of the penis, and the remaining portion can be covered by the excess distal skin.

The previously placed catheter is then removed, and a catheter one size smaller is then inserted through the reconstructed urethra into the bladder for drainage. This catheter is tied by the 4-0 Dermalon suture that had been placed in the end of the glans to maintain stability and position of the catheter. A pressure dressing is then applied to the entire penis.

Comments

I believe that a satisfactory method for the repair of penile and scrotal hypospadias has been developed by using the most successful techniques of other surgeons in conjunction with my own ideas. I believe that in this method, the best skin available is used for the reconstruction, and that the Beck-Nesbit [1, 8] type of visor flap produces less scarring on the ventral surface at the first stage than does the Edmunds [4] method of transferring the dorsal skin laterally. My method permits total reconstruction of the urethra at the second stage rather than requiring the connection of the reconstructed urethra at different stages. It is my belief that the urethra constructed of tubed pedicles allows for more normal growth and less possibility of contracture than do the free skin grafts described by Nové-Josserand [9], McIndoe [7], and McCormack [6], Horton [5], and others. My type of repair also creates a reconstructed urethra of uniform size throughout. I believe that this allows for a more normal flow of urine than does the Ombrédanne [10] technique, whereby a sac-type urethra is formed at the distal portion. My operation produces a glandar urethra similar to that described by Davis [3] but without the back-bending maneuver that is necessary with his technique. The method I have described eliminates the necessity for scrotal skin, as used by Bucknall [2], and thereby avoids the possibility of hair-bearing skin being used in the reconstructed urethra.

It is my belief that the first stage should be carried out when the patient is approximately 1 year of age; however, it can be satisfactorily performed at any age thereafter. The early operation allows for normal growth of the penis without the hindrance of chordee. In most cases, the second-stage operation has been carried out when the patient is approximately 4 to 5 years of age. I believe it is particularly important to finish the reconstruction before these children reach school age [10]. The psychological problems that confront them when they find it necessary to void in the public school toilets, frequently in front of other children, are insurmountable [5].

References

1. Beck, C. Hypospadias and its treatment. *Surg. Gynecol. Obstet.* 24:511, 1917.
2. Bucknall, R. T. A new operation for penile hypospadias. *Lancet* 2:887, 1907.
3. Davis, D. M. The surgical treatment of hypospadias, especially scrotal and perineal. *Plast. Reconstr. Surg.* 5:373, 1950.
4. Edmunds, A. Pseudo-hermaphroditism and hypospadias. *Lancet* 1:323, 1926.
5. Horton, C. E., and Devine, C. J., Jr. Hypospadias and epispadias. *Clin. Symp.* 24:3, 1972.
6. McCormack, R. M. Simultaneous chordee repair and urethral reconstruction for hypospadias. *Plast. Reconstr. Surg.* 13:257, 1954.
7. McIndoe, A. H. The treatment of hypospadias. *Am. J. Surg.* 38:176, 1937.
8. Nesbit, R. M. Plastic procedure for correction of hypospadias. *J. Urol.* 45:699, 1941.
9. Nové-Josserand. G. Traitement de l'hypospadias; nouvelle méthode. *Lyon Méd.* 85:198, 1897; Apropos du traitement de l'hypospadias. *Bull. Soc. Chir. Lyon* 7:325, 1904.
10. Ombrédanne, L. Hypospadias pénien chez l'enfant. *Bull. Soc. Chir. Paris* 37:1076, 1911.
11. Ricketson, G. A method of repair for hypospadias. *Am. J. Surg.* 95:279, 1958.
12. Russell, R. H. Operation for hypospadias. *Ann. Surg.* 46:244, 1907; Operation for severe hypospadias. *Br. Med. J.* 2:1432, 1900.

Blair-Wehrbein-Duplay Technique

DONALD R. SMITH

In the 1930s, perusal of the literature describing the most popular methods of hypospadias repair was, for the most part, discouraging. Flaps were developed that were far too long for their bases; hair-bearing skin was often utilized in the formation of the new urethra; the methods described for correction of chordee often failed to afford a straight organ. In contrast, however, was the article written by Blair et al. in 1938 [2]. Their method of straightening the penis seemed sound: a complete urethral tube was formed of non-hair-bearing penile and preputial skin and the integument used for urethroplasty was replaced by a flap of scrotal skin. I treated 18 patients in this manner, with very satisfactory results [10].

In order to reduce the procedure from three to two stages, I then applied the technique suggested by Wehrbein [11] wherein a scrotal tubed pedicle is formed in conjunction with the first-stage operation. This in no way violated the tenets espoused by Blair, and it has worked well for me in the repair of this defect in 140 patients.

Observations made at the operating table during the reduction of chordee in 190 patients have led me to disagree with the generally accepted cause for the deformity [8]. The strip of skin just distal to the hypospadial orifice is devoid of subcutaneous tissue and is therefore plastered to the shaft. Wide separation of this skin from the corpora cavernosa requires sharp dissection. Once this has been accomplished, a significant degree of chordee has been reduced. When this adherent ventral skin has been freed back to the meatus, a normal, very vascular corpus spongiosum can be seen coursing from beneath the subcutaneous urethra to the glans. The curvature is further corrected by displacing the distal portion of the urethra proximally (see Fig. 18-147), below. It is possible, with a pair of small dissecting scissors, to develop a cleavage plane between the corpus spongiosum and the urethra down to the point where the urethra finally enters the body of the corpus spongiosum. This dissection reveals that the subcutaneous urethra is firmly attached to the sulcus between the three corpora cavernosa by two thin pillars of fibrous tissue. When these are divided, thus freeing the urethra from the corpora, the remainder of the chordee has been reduced. It is unusual to find any residual fibrous bands that require resection.

Surgical Technique

Figures 18-145 to 18-149 depict the first-stage procedure. First, a probe should be passed down the urethra. Often the most distal urethral wall and overlying skin are tissue-paper thin. This requires meatotomy down to the point of normal tissue. If this is not done, the surgeon, in making the flap for the new urethra at the second stage, is sure to cut into the urethra just proximal to the hypospadial orifice. Should meatotomy be done, the parents must be instructed to dilate this orifice once a day for a month to prevent stenosis.

Recently, I suggested that the preputial flaps, swung onto the ventrum, should be closed in a Z fashion [9]. I have since learned that this was an error, because later, when forming the U-shaped flap for the formation of the urethra, one finds the knife coursing through an area of scar on either side. At these points, it is difficult to invert the skin when forming the new urethra. A midline closure does not produce the threat of contracture and reformation of chordee; penile skin is most kind.

I prefer to correct the chordee when the patient is 18 months of age, and to perform the urethroplasty when he is 4 years of age. This leaves time for any revisions that might prove necessary, yet the deformity is still corrected before the boy enters school.

At the second operation, the new urethra is formed (Figs. 18-150 and 18-151). It is essential that the central flap be wide enough so

that it can be closed loosely over the indwelling catheter. Minimal undermining of the edges of this flap is necessary so the tube can be formed without tension. At points where it proves difficult to invert the edges, the squamous cell epithelium can be leveled off with small scissors. The edges of the urethral flap distally should converge toward each other so that a relatively small meatus will be formed (see Fig. 18-150). This allows an increased ability to direct the stream during urination.

Since formation of the new urethra has left the ventrum denuded, the skin of the scrotal tube is used in replacement. The end of the tube that is attached to the dependent portion of the scrotum is divided, and the tube is opened on its anterior surface. It is then swung up to cover the raw area of the penis.

When beginning my explorations in the field of hypospadias repair, I utilized perineal urethrostomy as a diversionary procedure. It proved not to be a simple operation. It was necessary to close the defect secondarily in two cases, and, in two other cases, stricture developed at the site. After I started using the small indwelling urethral catheter, I observed no increase in the incidence of complications. Recently, as an alternative to the urethral catheter, I have placed two Intracaths as cystostomy tubes. No decreased incidence of fistula formation was noted.

At the conclusion of the operation, a pressure dressing is used. The penis is covered with petroleum gauze, and fluffed gauze is placed over the penis. A spica of 6-inch stockinette is applied and is reinforced with adhesive tape. The dressing and the catheter are removed on the seventh day. I have never used prophylactic antimicrobial medication because of the presence of the indwelling catheter. The urine of these patients becomes spontaneously sterile within a few weeks.

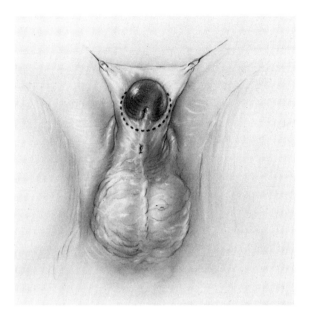

FIG. 18-145. First-stage operation. A skin incision is outlined that encircles the penis just proximal to the corona. (From D. R. Smith, *Trans. Amer. Assoc. Genitour. Surg.* 58:15, 1966. Copyright © 1966, The Williams & Wilkins Co., Baltimore.)

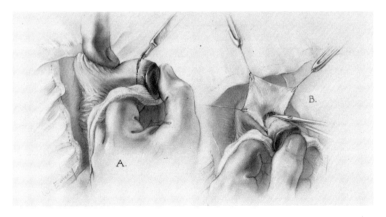

FIG. 18-146. A. The penis is sharply ventriflexed over the index finger, and countertraction is applied. An incision is made 5 mm from the coronal edge. Ventrally, the incision should course distally into the area of the frenum, but it must not encroach on the urethral orifice since the suture line on the edge of the orifice will, with later closure of the skin, lead to stenosis. B. With countertraction on the proximal skin edge by the use of double hooks, the skin on the dorsal and lateral surfaces is dissected off the shaft for a distance of about 3 cm. This is done by spreading the subcutaneous tissues with small scissors and snipping the resulting bands. The preputial skin fold is opened in a similar manner. (From D. R. Smith, *Trans. Amer. Assoc. Genitour Surg.* 58:15, 1966. Copyright © 1966, The Williams & Wilkins Co., Baltimore.)

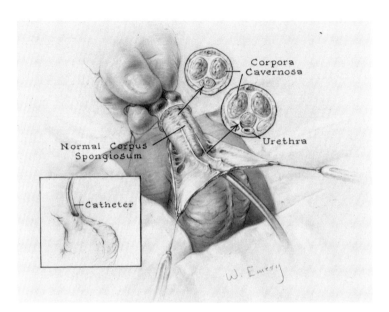

FIG. 18-147. A 12F Robinson catheter is passed to the bladder. The skin between the hypospadial orifice and the frenular area, which strongly adheres to the corpus spongiosum, must be freed by sharp dissection. This maneuver corrects the chordee to a great extent. A cleavage plane can be found with the points of a small scissors between the urethra and the corpus spongiosum. This is developed by spreading the scissors down to the point where the urethra plunges into the corpus spongiosum. The skin lateral to the corpus spongiosum can be easily freed. The two pillars of fibrous tissue that attach the urethra to the crevices between the three corpora are divided, thus displacing the orifice more proximally. Remnants of those pillars may require resection. The catheter protects the urethra from injury during the dissection. Bleeders are electrocoagulated with a needle-tipped electrode or tied with 4-0 plain catgut. (The cross sections show anatomy: the corpus spongiosum is normally placed; the urethra is subcutaneous and lies on the corpus spongiosum. (From D. R. Smith, *Trans. Amer. Ass. Genitour. Surg.* 58:15, 1966. Copyright © 1966, The Williams & Wilkins Co., Baltimore.)

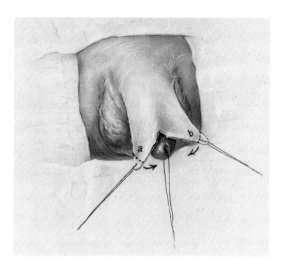

FIG. 18-148. Two stay sutures are placed in the center of the dorsal foreskin. A dorsal 3 cm slit is made, and the resulting flaps are swung to the ventrum. If more skin is required, the dorsal slit is deepened. The tips of the flaps are later resected. (From D. R. Smith, *Trans. Am. Assoc. Genitourin. Surg.* 58:15, 1966. Copyright © 1966, The Williams & Wilkins Co., Baltimore.)

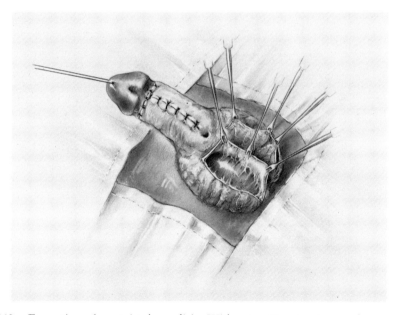

FIG. 18-149. Formation of scrotal tube pedicle. Without putting tension on the scrotal skin, two parallel incisions are outlined by stabbing the skin with a No. 25 needle dipped in methylene blue. The superior ends of the incisions should be level with the penoscrotal junction. The length of the incisions is equal to the distance between the urethral orifice and the frenum. The width of the flap is about 2.5 cm for a 2-year-old boy. A narrow tube is useless. The skin of the flap is freed by sharp and blunt dissection. The catheter must be in place to protect the urethra when the scrotal septum is incised; bleeders here require 4-0 plain catgut ties.

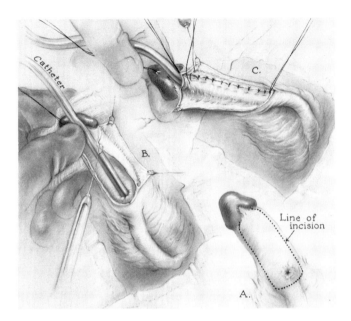

FIG. 18-150.   Second-stage operation.   A.   The line of incision is outlined by stabbing the skin with a No. 25 needle dipped in methylene blue. The flap should be 2 to 2.5 cm wide to form a tube size of 14F to 16F, allowing for inverting sutures. The edges of the epithelium can be beveled with fine scissors to facilitate inversion of the skin edges. A 12F Robinson catheter is placed in the bladder.   B and C.   The urethra is formed with interrupted Lembert sutures or a running inverting suture of 4-0 (urethral) chromic catgut. (From D. R. Smith, *Trans. Am. Assoc. Genitour. Surg.* 58:15, 1966. Copyright © 1966, The Williams & Wilkins Co., Baltimore.)

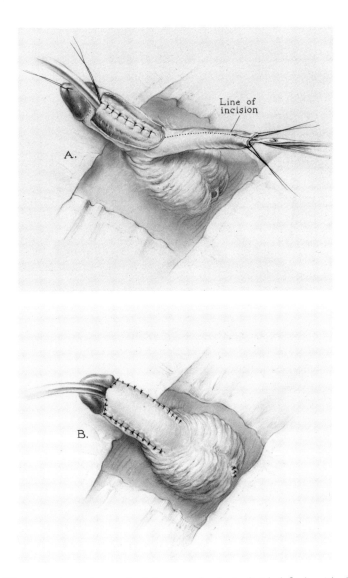

FIG. 18-151.   The most dependent end of the scrotal tube is divided flush with the scrotum. Two stay sutures are placed at the edge of the upper surface. Sharp pointed scissors are used to develop the cleavage plane down the core of the tube, which is then opened.   B.   The scrotal flap covers the ventral defect. Closure is done in two layers with interrupted 4-0 plain catgut. A pressure dressing is applied; the dressing and catheter are removed 7 days later. The parents must dilate the meatus with an oral thermometer daily for 1 month. (From D. R. Smith, *Trans. Am. Assoc. Genitourin. Surg.* 58:15, 1966. Copyright © 1966, The Williams & Wilkins Co., Baltimore.)

Complications

Some incidence of complications seems inevitable. These include fistula formation, retraction of the urethral orifice, gaping meatus, and stricture, both deep and meatal. Table 18-4 analyzes the complications I have observed in the 120 preschool boys who have been subjected to the described technique. These patients required a third (usually minor) operation.

If a fistula forms, it is usually at the site of the junction of the new urethra with the original urethra. Small fistulas are apt to close spontaneously. If they do not, it is best to wait at least 3 months before closure is attempted. I repair a fistula by making an elliptical incision about it; the island of squamous epithelium surrounding the fistula is excised with small scissors, and the urethral opening is closed with interrupted Lembert sutures of 4-0 (ureteral) chromic catgut. The covering skin is approximated with vertical

TABLE 18-4. Analysis of Complications in 120 Blair-Wehrbein Operations

Operation	Complications	
	No.	%
First stage		
Meatal stenosis requiring meatotomy	3	2.5
Incomplete correction of chordee	1	0.8
Second stage		
Fistula	14	11.7
Retraction of meatus	8	6.6
Gaping orifice	6	5.0
Stenosis of meatus	1	0.8
Deep stricture	2	1.6
Totals	35	29.0

mattress sutures of the same material. In my experience, this technique rarely fails. Should two fistulas be very close together, it is best to divide the bridge between them and close them as one fistula.

If the meatus ends up being proximal to the point desired and if there is some redundancy of skin about the distal part of the penis, the usual U-shaped incision can be made in a manner similar to that described for the original urethroplasty. Their distal ends should converge upon one another to ensure the formation of a relatively narrow meatus. The skin lateral to the defect is then undermined and closed over the new urethra with vertical mattress sutures. If redundant skin is absent distally, the urethra can be advanced by utilizing the principles of the Denis Browne operation [4].

If the urethral meatus gapes, leading to a poorly directed stream, an incision is made through the skin of the meatal ring. The urethra is freed from the overlying skin for a distance of 1 cm. On one side, a wedge of urethral wall is excised, and the resulting edges are sutured with 4-0 (ureteral) chromic material. On the other side, a wedge of skin is excised, and its edges are closed. I do not employ an indwelling catheter when I repair these complications.

Meatal stenosis responds well to meatotomy. Meatal dilatations carried out by the parents, using an oral thermometer, keep the meatus open. Of the two deep strictures I observed, one was relieved by a single urethral dilatation; the other was cured by internal urethrotomy.

The Blair-Wehrbein-Duplay operation lends itself well to penile or penoscrotal hypospadias repair. When the orifice is proximal to the penoscrotal junction, there is not enough scrotum from which to form a scrotal tube. Furthermore, the wide central flap that is necessary for the formation of a complete urethra is not obtainable, since such a urethra would incorporate hair-bearing scrotal integument. Only the Denis Browne technique is applicable in this instance.

In the situation where the meatus is located on the corona and where there is no chordee of the shaft but significant ventral tipping of the glans, the procedure described by Allen and Spence [1] affords an excellent cosmetic result.

The indications and complications of the operation I espouse apply equally to the excellent Cecil operation, which is particularly advocated by Culp [5]. If the Cecil operation has any disadvantage, it is that all patients are subjected to three operations, whereas with the Wehrbein technique, only 30 percent of my patients required a third operation. The one-stage procedures [3, 6, 7] have the advantage of requiring a second stage in only 30 percent of cases. Should these operations prove to afford a result equal to the more commonly used two- and three-stage techniques, their future is assured.

References

1. Allen, T. D., and Spence, H. M. The surgical treatment of coronal hypospadias and related problems. *J. Urol.* 100:504, 1968.
2. Blair, V. P., and Byars, L. T. Hypospadias and epispadias. *J. Urol.* 40:814, 1938.
3. Broadbent, T. R., Woolf, R. M., and Toksu, E. Hypospadias—one-stage repair. *Plast. Reconstr. Surg.* 27:154, 1961.
4. Browne, D. An operation for hypospadias. *Proc. R. Soc. Med.* 42:466, 1948.
5. Culp, O. S. Struggles and triumphs with hypospadias and associated anomalies: Review of 400 cases. *J. Urol.* 96:339, 1966.
6. Horton, C. E., Devine, C. J., Jr., Crawford, H. H., and Adamson, J. E. Hypospadias. In Gibson, T. (Ed.), *Modern Trends in Plastic Surgery.* London: Butterworth, 1966. Pp. 268–284.
7. Persky, L., Kiehn, C. L., and DesPrez, J. D. A one-stage hypospadias repair. *J. Urol.* 88:259, 1962.
8. Smith, D. R. Hypospadias: Its anatomic and therapeutic considerations. *J. Int. Coll. Surg.* 24:64, 1955.
9. Smith, D. R. Repair of hypospadias in the preschool child: A report of 150 cases. *Trans. Am. Assoc. Genitourin. Surg.* 58:15, 1966.
10. Smith, D. R., and Blackfield, H. M. A modification of the Blair procedure for the repair of hypospadias. *J. Urol.* 59:404, 1948.
11. Wehrbein, H. L. Hypospadias. *J. Urol.* 50:335, 1943.

Preoperative and Postoperative Evaluation

LARS AVELLÁN
BENGT JOHANSON

In comparison with the abundance of publications on the operative procedures that are recommended for the treatment of hypospadias, the scientific works dealing with preoperative and postoperative problems are rather scarce. We have studied these problems and developed certain principles that have given satisfactory results in our clinical practice.

General Problems

In order to carry out rational treatment of hypospadias according to a fixed treatment schedule, the first problem, namely an early diagnosis, must be solved.

The ideal solution is to make the diagnosis at the maternity clinic immediately after delivery. In countries such as Sweden where a central registration of congenital malformations has been established, a pediatrician associated with the maternity clinic is responsible [4]. The preliminary information afforded the mother by the pediatrician at the maternity clinic is of great importance. Apart from the fact that the best consolation to a mother who has given birth to a malformed child is information about the malformation, its treatment, and the possible results, it is essential that she also be told to which clinic the baby should be remitted for treatment. The first visit to this clinic should, in our opinion, be at the age of 1 to 2 years, at which time the degree of hypospadias, meatal stenosis, and chordee can be determined. At this consultation, the surgeon informs the mother in detail about the malformation and also about the schedule practiced at the clinic.

In the extensive literature on hypospadias, the opinions vary considerably as to the ideal time for the initial surgical treatment.

The objectives in the correction of hypospadias are to enable the boy to urinate in a normal manner during early childhood and to enable a normal development of the penis so that it may become a sexually functional organ in adulthood. The following

370

TABLE 18-5. Treatment Schedule

Test	Age	Operation
Uroflometry	3 (Stage I)	Meatotomy
Urography		Resection of valves
Cystourethrography		Straightening or urethral construction
	4 (Stage II)	Urethral construction
Uroflometry	5	
Uroflometry	12	
Cystourethrography	17	

schedule (Table 18-5) has been developed in order to realize these objectives.

The fact that the time of the initial surgery has been fixed at the age of 3 years is the result of the following investigations and clinical experiences.

The only absolute indication for an operation at this age is an obstacle to urination. In our primary series such an obstacle was present in 41 percent of the cases, which was caused by meatal stenosis in 33 percent, by urethral valves in 5 percent, and by meatal stenosis and urethral valves in 3 percent. At this age, no acquired change of the urinary tract was found in connection with the above-mentioned obstacles; however, it has been noted that this has taken place when the diagnosis was made later. Thus, it is essential to make certain whether there is any functioning obstacle.

Since clinical estimation of the urinary stream and the caliber of the meatus is difficult and unreliable, an objective measurement of the flow of urine is necessary. Timed micturition [3] has provided satisfactory measurements in older children and adults, but it is not adequate for the age group in question. We therefore use uroflometry. For measurement of flow, a modified Brotherus' uroflometer (Fig. 18-152) has been employed,

the accuracy of which depends on the fact that the kinetic energy is almost entirely eliminated [1]. The maximal flow is measured in minimum differences of 5 ml per second, and the course of miction is registered in the form of a curve (Fig. 18-153). The lowest normal value in children was found to be 15 ml per second in a control series. Since the maximal flow depends on the fullness of the bladder, the volume of miction should reach an amount, varying between 100 ml and 200 ml, that is determined for each age group. For measurement of the flow in small children, a specially designed chair has been employed. The measurements can be made without any discomfort to the child, and the physician need not be present (see Fig. 18-152). The lowest acceptable flow value in preoperative uroflometry has been set at 15 ml per second. When at least two measurements have revealed an impairment of the maximal flow, there is an obstruction preventing urination.

In order to localize the obstacle in the urethra, cystourethrography should be performed. As mentioned above, the most common obstacle is meatal stenosis. In the cases in which a congenital urethral valve causes the obstruction, there is a prestenotic dilatation of the urethra. If there is indication of an acquired obstacle to flow, trabeculae in the bladder are diagnosed. The investigations carried out at our clinic show that if an obstacle still remains after the age of 3 years, formation of trabeculae is found in a number of cases. This, no doubt, is caused by the fact that the boys at this age have developed urinary continence.

Since other congenital malformations associated with hypospadias may occur in the upper urinary tract, all cases of hypospadias should be subjected to urography, in addition to preoperative cystourethrography, in order to obtain a complete survey.

From the preoperative estimation of func-

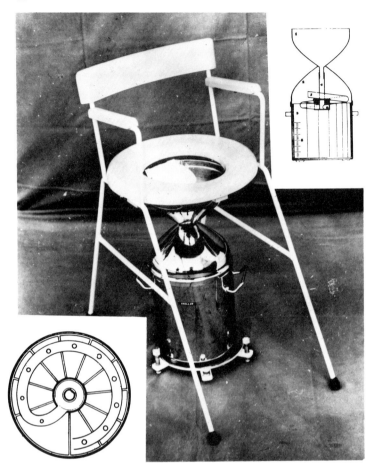

FIG. 18-152. Components of the uroflometer with chair-pot. *Upper right:* Sagittal section of segmented collector with scale in each compartment. *Lower left:* Transverse section of spiral distributing tube with outlets into compartments.

tion and the status of the urinary tract, the following indications for operation can be established. If the flow value is lower than 15 ml per second and the cystourethrographic examination reveals no urethral valves or a urethral valve without prestenotic urethral dilatation, meatotomy is indicated. On the other hand, if there is a urethral valve with prestenotic dilatation, transurethral resection of the valve has to be performed, combined with meatotomy if indicated. In order for the boy to be able to urinate in a normal way in early childhood, curvature and torsion, when present, have to be corrected at the same time as the obstacle that is impairing urination is removed.

In our primary series, curvature was found in 66 percent and torsion in 16 percent of the cases. The diagnosis of curvature may involve difficulties. The case history given by the parents is important though not always reliable, since an abundant dorsal preputial excess of skin and a hooded prepuce can sometimes simulate curvature. It has been found that observation of the penis in the morning, when the child awakens and normally a physiological erection occurs, can provide an idea of the amount of curvature.

Different degrees of torsion in the penile shaft are not an unusual observation. Severe torsion, especially in childhood, may cause difficulties in urination since the child easily

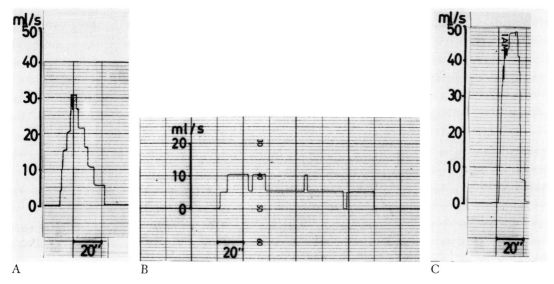

FIG. 18-153. Examples of miction curves. A. Miction curve for a normal 3-year-old boy with maximal flow of 30 ml per sec. B. Preoperative flow registration in a 3-year-old boy with hypospadias and meatal stenosis. Maximal flow is 10 ml per sec. C. Postoperative flow registration in the same patient as in B after meatotomy, straightening, and urethral construction. Maximal flow is now 50 ml per sec.

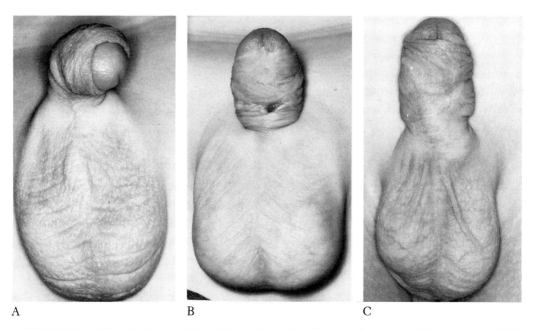

FIG. 18-154. Glandar hypospadias with torsion. A. Preoperative state with curvature and 45° torsion (3 years of age). B. Same case after straightening and correction of torsion. C. Same case after urethral construction at 4 years of age.

sprinkles his clothes with urine. Torsion has mostly been found in the distal forms of hypospadias and can also occur in those cases in which curvature is absent.

Correction of curvature has to be carried out in all cases where it is observed, even in those cases in which only a glandar curvature is present. An ignored and untreated glandar curvature can cause sexual difficulties in adulthood. Torsion must also be corrected in all cases in which it is observed (Fig. 18-154).

Although of less importance than those referred to above, other factors that favor the initial surgery being performed not later than at 3 years of age are postoperative erection, the effect of pain, and psychic aspects. Experience in surgical treatment of hypospadias has shown that healing is disturbed by erection. A physiological erection in the morning as a result of a full bladder can occur at all ages, from infanthood up to and including senility, whereas the purely sexual erection occurs at the prefertile and fertile ages. Before the age of 3 years, an erection does not disturb the postoperative healing. No effective erection preventive has so far been introduced.

All surgeons who have performed operations on the penis have probably discovered that the patients in early childhood are remarkably less affected by pain compared to children 7 or 8 years of age and older.

The child's keen power of observation, especially with respect to differences and deviation from the normal genital organs, is well known. At school a visible and functional anomaly will rapidly arouse the interest of school-mates, and the hypospadiac will be subjected to ridicule.

The postoperative controls can be classified in two groups: (1) those carried out in immediate connection with the operation and (2) those carried out at a later date. Regarding the first group, it should be noted that uroflometrics have to be performed both before and after Stage II (see Table 18-5). The minimum demand at that point is a flow of 20 ml per second. The controls in the latter group are considered necessary and are carried out at the ages of 5, 12, and 17 years, using uroflometrics and cystourethrography (Fig. 18-155).

If preoperative cystourethrography reveals the presence of urethral valves without prestenotic urethral dilatation, it is essential that in the tests at the ages of 12 and 17, special attention be given the valves. An obstacle to flow at these periods of life may arise as a result of the unchanged diameter of the valve in the normally increasing caliber of the urethra. At the age of 17, seminal analysis has been carried out routinely. In our series, this has revealed only normal findings.

Special Problems

Each particular method of treatment often involves special problems. At our clinic, hypospadias has been treated since 1957 according to the following principles.

MEATOTOMY

When meatal stenosis is present, the urethra is cut in a proximal direction for approximately 1 cm or until a normal lumen is reached. Even if a nearly adequate meatus is found, meatotomy is still carried out in order to avoid the occurrence of stricture between the original and the constructed urethra. Experience has shown that formation of such a stricture is caused in most cases by the surgeon not having incised enough in the meatotomy. Furthermore, urethral construction in Stage II yields a better result when the meatus is localized more proximally and not closely behind the coronal sulcus.

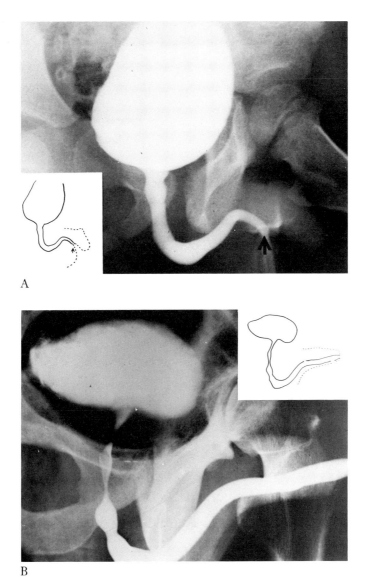

FIG. 18-155. Cystourethrography in hypospadias. A. Preoperative state at 3 years of age. The adequate meatus in the penoscrotal angle is indicated by the arrow. B. Same case at 17 years of age after straightening and urethral construction; adequate meatus is localized at the tip of the glans.

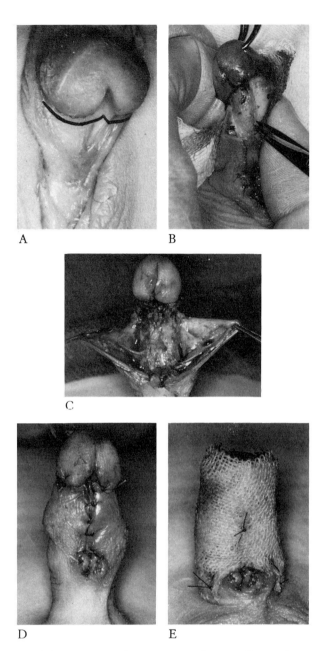

FIG. 18-156. The straightening procedure in penile hypospadias with curvature. A. The incision, including half of the circumference of the penile body on the ventral side, is indicated. B. After meatotomy, a towel clip is placed in the glans in order to put the penile body under outmost tension by bending the penis in a direction opposite to the curvature. This will allow the fibrospongioid plate to come into view. The fibrospongioid plate is divided with multiple, short cuts. C. A complete release of the penis shaft is obtained, and bilateral penile skin flaps are raised. D. The bilateral flaps are brought together. E. The penis is wrapped in a ribbon gauze bandage, which is sutured through the skin to the penile fascia.

RESECTION OF THE URETHRAL VALVES

If cystourethrography shows the presence of a urethral valve with prestenotic dilatation of the urethra, transurethral resection of the valve is performed by diathermic cutting.

STRAIGHTENING

This has been done by making an incision just proximal to the coronal sulcus, including half of the ventral circumference (Fig. 18-156). The fibrospongioid plate, which causes the curvature and which lies on the underside of the penis, is broken with small, multiple cuts, and, without excision of the so-called chordee, the tunnica albuginea is carefully left intact. When complete release is obtained, the defect on the underside is covered with bilateral inner-layer preputial flaps. The torsion of the penile shaft is caused by a thin fibrous layer running from the base distally and far laterally along the whole ventral aspect. The torsion is totally released by careful excision of this fibrous tissue; working under magnification facilitates the procedure.

URETHRAL CONSTRUCTION

In a few cases in which the meatus is adequate and curvature is absent, the only surgical procedure performed at Stage I is construction of the urethra according to the Denis Browne method [2]. In principle, Stage II is carried out one year after Stage I. When the meatus is found to fulfill the above-mentioned requirements and the scar on the underside of the penis is soft and satisfactorily healed, urethral construction according to the Denis Browne method is performed in all cases.

If the glandar groove is of normal depth (Fig. 18-157), an adequate, vertically positioned meatus in the glans will be obtained. If the glandar groove is shallow or merely noticeable (Fig. 18-158), a retardation of the flaps occurs that results in a transversally positioned meatus either in the coronal sulcus or directly proximal to this. As the method of treatment has been standardized, this result has been accepted and glandar groove reconstruction has been avoided, the importance and results of which have been disputable. In a normal penis, an intact frenulum will act as a shutter on the meatus on erection. Hypospadiacs lack the frenulum and thus also the ability to close the meatus tightly. The vertically positioned meatus at the tip of the glans allows closure of the meatus as the cavernous tissue of the glans is expanded on erection. However, with the transversally positioned meatus in the coronal sulcus, this ability is lacking. Every hypospadiac must be made aware of the risk of contamination from coitus. At the routine control when the patient is 17 years old, he is informed of this fact as well as about the importance of proper hygiene and the necessity of urinating postcoitally.

Results

The best evaluation of the principles elucidated above may be to review the results of our clinical series. The data comprises 204 primary cases with hypospadias that were treated and followed-up during the period from 1957 to 1966. The distribution according to grade of hypospadias is shown in Figure 18-159. Curvature was noted in 134 cases (65.6 percent) and torsion in 34 cases (16 percent). In 23 instances, the meatus was considered adequate and there was no need for surgery. Congenital urethral valves were found in 23 cases (11 percent); prestenotic dilatation was found in 10, and these were treated with transurethral diathermic cutting of the valves.

The large majority of the hypospadias pa-

normal urethra and to the distal glandar triangular flap. We have found that it is easy to produce this tunnel by dissecting with sharp-pointed scissors, then dilating it with clamps and sounds. Tissue must be excised from the deep portions of the glans so that stricturing will not occur later. It is easier to attach the skin graft tube to the glandar V-shaped flap and then pass the proximal end through the tube to make the anastomosis between the urethra and the skin graft tube.

The proximal anastomosis can be covered with a scrotal rotation flap (Fig. 20-1B). This procedure will correct most hypospadias cripples in a one-stage operation (Figs. 20-1 and 2).

If the skin is considerably scarred and deficient, modifications of the Cecil or Denis Browne operations can be done. All scar tissue should be excised from the normal meatus distally on the ventral side of the penis. A full-thickness untubed graft of hair-

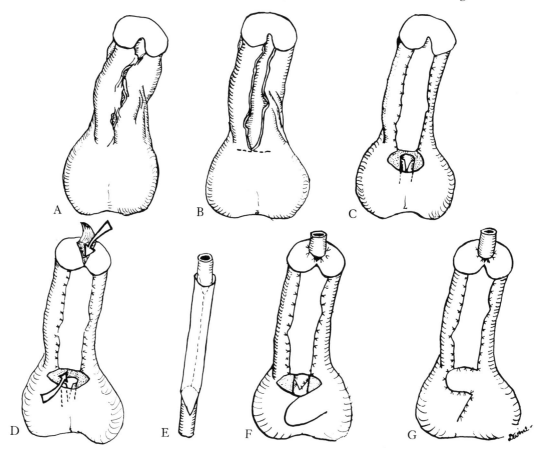

FIG. 20-1. A. Old scarred urethra. B. Incision down the midline. C. The urethra is opened and sutured laterally. The proximal urethra is exposed. D. A glandar flap is elevated, and a tunnel is made beneath the old urethra. E. The skin graft tube. F. Elliptical anastomosis of the tube proximally and distally. G. A rotation flap from the scrotum covers the anastomosis. (From C. E. Horton and C. J. Devine, Jr., *Plast. Reconstr. Surg.* 45:425, 1970. Copyright © 1970, The Williams & Wilkins Co., Baltimore.)

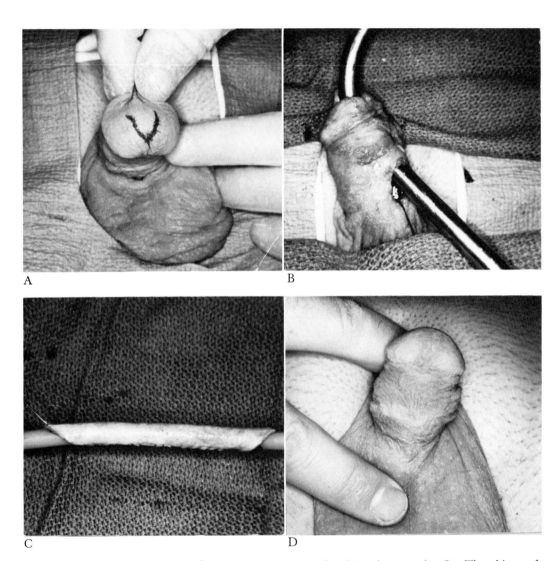

FIG. 20-2. A. The glandar flap. B. A sound is placed in the tunnel. C. The skin graft tube. D. Postoperative appearance. The urethral meatus is at the tip of the penis. (From C. E. Horton and C. J. Devine, Jr., *Plast. Reconstr. Surg.* 45:425, 1970. Copyright © 1970. The Williams & Wilkins Co., Baltimore.)

less skin can be sutured from the meatus to the tip of the penis, or a tubed skin graft can be constructed for urethral reconstruction. Coverage of the ventral raw surface and the urethra should be secured by opening the scrotum and burying the penis in the scrotum. Once initial healing has occurred, another stage to separate the penis and scrotum is necessary (Fig. 20-2).

In general, once complications have oc-curred in hypospadias repairs, the surgeon has a tendency to attempt small operations, hoping to convert failure into success with a minimum of effort. This generally makes matters worse. In most crippled cases, exten-sive resection of scarring, major shifts of tissues, and meticulous reconstruction will usually be found necessary to transform a difficult problem into a therapeutic success.

References

1. Backus, L. H., and DeFelice, C. A. Hypo-spadias—then and now. *Plast. Reconstr. Surg.* 25:146, 1960.
2. Culp, O. S., and McRoberts, J. W. Hypo-spadias. In Alken, H. von C. E., et al. (Eds.), *Handbook of Urology.* New York: Springer-Verlag, 1968.
3. Devine, C. J., Jr., and Horton, C. E. Hypo-spadias. In Goldwyn, R. M. (Ed.), *The Un-favorable Result in Plastic Surgery: Avoid-ance and Treatment.* Boston: Little, Brown, 1972.
4. Horton, C. E., and Devine, C. J., Jr. A one-stage repair for hypospadias cripples. *Plast. Reconstr. Surg.* 45:425, 1970.

The Retrusive Hypospadial Meatus

CHARLES E. HORTON
CHARLES J. DEVINE, JR.

21

IN THE PAST, most hypospadias repairs have not brought the meatus to the end of the glans. Many surgeons attempted reconstruction of the urethra to the tip, only to encounter distal urethral strictures and proximal "blow-out" fistulas [2, 3]. These failures have included techniques in which both free grafts and local tubes have been used for urethra substitutes. We believe there are two reasons for such complications. The first difficulty occurs in attempting to create a circular or even stellate-shaped glandar meatus. Here, by creating a circular anastomosis, a well-known principle of surgery is violated. A circular suture line will contract and a diminished opening will occur. The epithelium of the glans seems to contract more than other body surface areas. The second difficulty occurs because usually no attempt is made to core out the solid glans to accommodate the soft, easily compressible urethra. Therefore, the distal urethra is compressed postoperatively by the firm glans and heals in a restricted environment [6].

Because elongating the urethra to the tip of the glans resulted in many complications, authors have frequently advocated leaving the meatus at the corona and have preferred not to bring the urethra to the end of the penis. Occasionally after the hypospadias repair is completed, the subglandar urethral meatus may appear to regress proximally, perhaps from minor suture disruptions at the distal end of the urethral graft or tube or from additional growth of the penile shaft. This frequently changes a nearly acceptable result to an unacceptable condition. Retrusion of the urethra has received little attention because of the difficulties encountered in distal urethral construction and because many believe the subglandar meatus to be acceptable. Impregnation is possible in this circumstance, and little concern is given to the psychological problems that admittedly must be present when the penis is obviously deformed.

In 1966 we first described the use of triangular flaps to produce an elliptical anastomosis of the distal urethra to the glans [4]. This has resulted in a technique that can be adapted to any type of hypospadias repair and that has significantly reduced the problems of bringing the urethra to the tip of the penis. The distal elliptical anastomosis that is possible with this technique prevents circular contracture of the suture line. The triangular flaps originally described were formed from the side of the groove in the glans and were sutured in the center. We have since modified our technique and now form one large central triangular flap with the wide base ending at the exact tip of the glans where the meatus is desired [5]. When this triangular flap is elevated, a core of glandar tissue can be removed to accommodate the urethral tube, and all elements of abnormal fibrous tissue

causing chordee at the shaft-glans angle can be excised.

An additional advantage of this technique is that the spatulate glans, which is uniformly flattened in hypospadias, can be reshaped by elevating and transposing the lateral portions of the glans located on each side of the triangular flap. When the lateral glandar wings are undermined, they will usually be adequate to interdigitate and cover the ven-

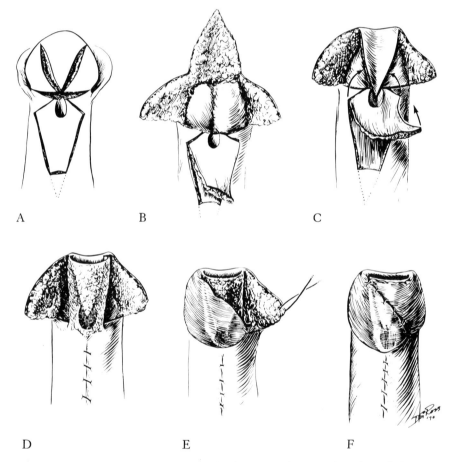

FIG. 21-1. A. Glandar flaps are outlined. The flap from the ventral surface of the penis is based distally on the urethral orifice. B. The glandar flaps are elevated, and the elevation of the penile flap is begun. C. The dorsal incision in the meatus allows the insertion of the midline glandar flap to enlarge the meatus and provide a roof for the distal urethra. D. The penile flap is sutured to the midline glandar flap to form a urethra that ends at the tip of the glans. E. The lateral glandar wings are used to close the ventral defect and to reshape the glans. F. Closure is accomplished.

tral surface of the newly constructed urethra. This contours the glans into the desired conical shape and covers the distal urethra at the penile tip.

To correct the retracted meatus problem or the minor distal hypospadias case, an operation has been devised using the principle of the original Bevan flap [1] in conjunction with our original triangular and lateral glandar flap operation (Fig. 21-1).

A 4-0 black silk traction suture is first placed in the dorsum of the glans above the site where the meatus is to be constructed. A distally based flap is marked on the ventrum of the penis; this is based on the existing meatus. The flap is designed with a sharp, distally retrograde end, which is later to be trimmed as desired. This flap is elevated, and care is taken to preserve adequate tissue at the meatal flap base to carry an adequate blood supply into the flap. A triangular glandar flap is then elevated, a central core of glans is removed, and the lateral wings are mobilized.

The urethral meatus is then incised on its dorsal surface to produce an ellipse at the end. If the meatus was previously constricted, this meatotomy allows an adequate opening without impairing the nourishment of the base of the skin flap for urethral reconstruction. If chordee is present, all abnormal tissue can be removed at this time. Hemostasis with cautery should be obtained. The tip of the glandar V-shaped flap is then sutured into the dorsal meatal groove to reconstruct the dorsum of the urethra. The penile diamond-shaped flap is turned to provide ventral urethral skin. The wider edges of the base of the penile-shaft flap fit into the narrow tip of the V-shaped flap to allow adequate urethral caliber in the reconstruction. As the triangular flap becomes wider near the tip of the glans, the penile skin flap becomes more narrow, thus allowing a channel of consistent size to be constructed by uniting the two

flaps. The pointed end of the penile flap is appropriately trimmed and discarded. All sutures are tied with the knots in the lumen of the urethra. The V flap edges should be anchored to the underlying tissue along the depth of the lateral suture lines. When the urethra has been completed, the lateral wings of the glans are interpolated and united ventral to the meatus to reshape the glans. The distal ventral end of the urethra is sutured to the glandar wings, repositioning the meatus at the exact tip of the glans.

The remaining prepuce is then incised around the coronal sulcus, leaving a 2 mm edge of mucosa on the glans. The prepuce is unfolded and a dorsal incision is made to divide the prepuce into two equal parts. This incision is continued to the point where the dorsal penile skin appears to be of desired length (as in circumcision). The preputial skin is then brought to the ventral surface of the penis to resurface the uncovered urethra. Most frequently, the two flaps are sutured together in the midline, and the excess length of each of the preputial flaps is discarded. Occasionally, only one of the preputial flaps will be used to resurface the ventral raw area, and the other flap will not be utlized.

A Foley catheter is left indwelling for 3 to 4 days. A pressure Elastoplast dressing is applied for 2 days. Thereafter, the patient is placed in a sterile saline tub bath three times a day while in the hospital. The usual period of hospitalization required is 5 days. The patient is given instructions to soak and lubricate the suture line while recuperating at home.

When the catheter is removed, Neosporin from an ophthalmic tipped tube is used to lubricate and soften the meatal crusts. The tube tip is used to keep the meatus open and prevent the formation of dry crusts that would plug the urethra.

Postoperatively, the urinary stream has been found to be adequate and no dilatation of the repair has been required. It has always been possible to place the urethral opening at the tip of the glans with this technique, thus providing a more normal appearing and functional organ. No serious complications have been encountered, although one hematoma and one small area of devitalized ventral penile skin flap have been seen. In spite of this, all cases have healed spontaneously, and no further surgery has been necessary.

This technique has been performed on eight postoperative cases that had been operated on elsewhere and required uethral elongation, as well as in many primary hypospadias repairs. It should be considered when lengthening of the distal urethra is desirable, and it is useful in selected cases only (Fig. 21-2).

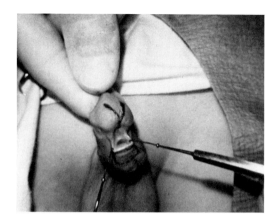

FIG. 21-2. Typical case of postoperative retrusion of the urethral meatus. This result is not desirable, and a secondary operation should be done. A glandar flap for bringing the urethra to the tip is marked out.

References

1. Bevan, A. D. Hypospadias. *J.A.M.A.* 68:1032, 1917.
2. Culp, O. S., and McRoberts, J. W. Hypospadias. In Alken, H. von C. E., et al. (Eds), *Handbook of Urology.* New York: Springer-Verlag, 1968.
3. Devine, C. J., Jr., and Horton, C. E. Hypospadias. In Goldwyn, R. M. (Ed.), *The Unfavorable Result in Plastic Surgery: Avoidance and Treatment.* Boston: Little, Brown, 1972.
4. Horton, C. E., and Devine, C. J., Jr. Hypospadias. In T. Gibson (Ed.), *Modern Trends in Plastic Surgery.* London: Butterworth, 1966. Pp. 268–284.
5. Horton, C. E. Hypospadias. In Mustardé, J. C. (Ed.), *Plastic Surgery in Infancy and Childhood.* Philadelphia: Saunders, 1971.
6. van der Meulen, J. C. H. M. *Hypospadias.* Springfield, Ill.: Thomas, 1964.

Urethral Fistulas

CHARLES E. HORTON
CHARLES J. DEVINE, JR.

22

URETHRAL FISTULAS can be caused by infection, tumor, trauma, or, most commonly, by poor healing following urethroplasty. The treatment of fistulas caused by tumor formation becomes secondary to the treatment of the tumor itself and will not be discussed here.

Urethral fistulas following hypospadias repair are not uncommon, usually occurring in 15 to 45 percent of cases. It is desirable to design and execute urethral surgery so that primary and complete healing occurs. From a practical point of view, it will probably be impossible to achieve that goal.

Initial Care

When inflammation, trauma, or urinary extravasation first occur, the paraurethral tissues quickly become edematous and friable. Limited subcutaneous tissue is present beneath the thin penile skin. There is little use to attempt to close a newly formed fistula by secondary suturing, and, in fact, further inflammation will inevitably result in a larger fistulous opening. Therefore, we recommend that if fistula formation occurs following surgical repair of trauma to the urethra,

inflammation, or urethroplasty, then (1) a Foley catheter be inserted into the bladder for drainage, (2) appropriate antibiotics be given if infection is present, and (3) the patient be followed conservatively until the induration of the tissues disappears and softening occurs.

The catheter should remain indwelling for 10 to 14 days, and, if it is more expedient, the patient can be sent home and followed by visits to the office during this time.

If the catheter is left in the urethra and bladder for 2 weeks, epithelial healing will occur to cover raw surfaces, and extending the time of catheter retention will not aid in the healing of the fistula. Once epithelialization of the raw edges of the fistula occurs, spontaneous closure cannot be expected. The fistulous openings, however, are circular, and it is well known that fistulas will diminish in size from their initial circumference since all scar tissue shortens and contracts as it matures. Occasionally, the openings will become so small that they can be seen only on close inspection and will leak only under high pressure during micturition. Once a fistula has formed and adequate initial treatment (an indwelling catheter for 2 weeks and antibiotics, if necessary) has been given, it is recommended that no surgical repair be considered for 3 to 6 months. We feel it is necessary for this much time to elapse in order to allow the damaged tissue to return to normal and to allow resolution of all adjacent scar tissue as far as possible.

Repair of the Mature Fistula (Simple)

Before attempting any repair of a fistula, the urethra should be carefully calibrated to determine that no distal stenosis is present. If such is the case, this must be corrected simultaneously with the fistula repair for obvious reasons. We prefer the use of a median glandar flap that is advanced into the urethra for meatal stenosis, and the use of full-thickness preputial skin grafts for deeper urethral strictures. When an adequate urethral channel is assured, surgical repair of the fistula can be attempted.

In cases of very small fistulas, it is occasionally possible to induce spontaneous closure by applying a small flake of silver nitrate or inserting a probe painted with trichloroacetic acid within the fistulous opening. This destroys the circular epithelium and produces an eschar in the tract. Frequently, epithelialization of the tract openings will occur and

the fistula will close. This can be used only on minute fistulas and is not always successful. Since it is an office procedure, however, little is lost if the attempt fails. This technique can be used in the late postoperative period when a fistula is first suspected if an indwelling catheter is in place.

In the usual case of small fistulas, no diminution in the size of the urethra at the site of the fistula will occur if a direct closure of the fistulous edges is performed (Figs. 22-1 to 22-4). If, however, the fistula is over 2 mm in size, a closure of the edges without producing more urethral surface will cause a narrowing of the urethra at that site (Fig. 22-5). To prevent this, a turnover flap based on the fistula edge should be designed to reconstruct

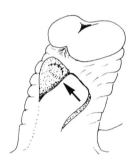

FIG. 22-2.   Closure of the fistula.

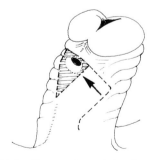

FIG. 22-1.   Preparation of the flap for fistula closure.

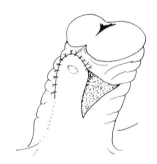

FIG. 22-3.   Transfer of the flap.

the urethral wall. This flap is dissected to the scar edge, preserving the blood supply in this area to nourish the flap. The opposite fistulous edges are then pared, and the uroepithelium is separated from the surface epithelium over a wide distance. The continuity of the urethral epithelium must be restored, and all edges are brought into the urethra (Figs. 22-6 and 22-7). We have found that this is best done by using magnification and by suturing the urethral edges with 6-0 chromic catgut, burying the knots inside the urethra. To make certain that all epithelium

is inverted, it has been suggested that the suture ends be brought out the urethra externally through the meatus.

Once urethral continuity has been reestablished, the outer skin defect must be covered. Direct imposition of the skin suture line over the urethral suture line should be avoided.

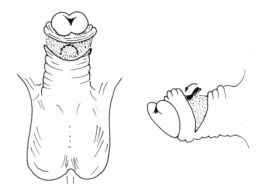

FIG. 22-6. Closure of the fistula with the local turnover flap.

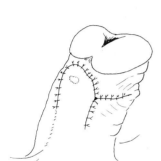

FIG. 22-4. Flap closure.

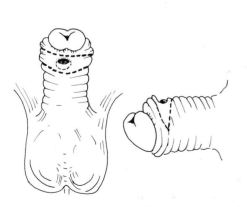

FIG. 22-5. A larger fistula requiring local turnover flap to reconstruct the urethral lumen.

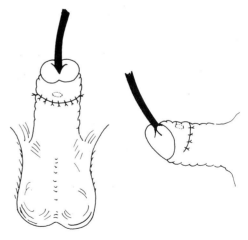

FIG. 22-7. Skin closure. The suture lines are not adjacent.

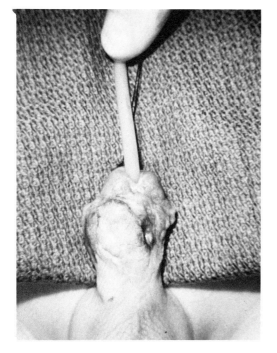

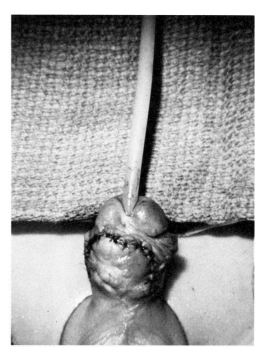

A   B

FIG. 22-8.   A.   Fistula occurring after operation for hypospadias.   B.   Flap closure of the fistula.

Certain authors advocate tenting the skin over the fistula repair and closing with several subcutaneous layers to produce a considerable distance between the skin suture line and the urethral suture line ("closing in depth"). This repair has the disadvantage of producing a bulky tag on the penile surface. Since there is usually an abundance of skin available on the penis, we prefer the use of a wide rotation flap that is taken adjacent to the point of fistula repair. This requires the sacrifice of skin surrounding the fistula for a distance of 1 to 1.5 cm in each direction in order for the large flap to extend well to each side of the fistula repair. This produces a flat, normal penile skin surface, and in our experience, it has given better results than multiple

layers of sutures over the urethral repair (Fig. 22-8). The use of a dermal graft to reinforce the area may be desirable (Fig. 22-9). Occasionally an island of epithelium on a dermal flap can be helpful in fistual repairs [6] (Fig. 22-10).

Repair of the Multiple Fistulas

Occasionally, the hypospadias cripple who has had multiple stages of unsuccessful repairs is encountered [5]. When several fistulas are present and the adjacent skin is scarred, it is futile to attempt repair with local tissues [4].

It is not uncommon for a surgeon to oper-

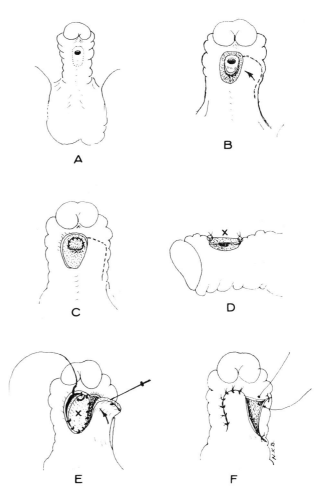

FIG. 22-9. A. Outline of incisions for fistula closure. B. Turnover flap based on fistula edge. C. The turnover flap is sutured to the uroepithelium. D. A free dermal graft (with the epidermis removed) is used to interpose and reinforce at the fistula area (*x*). (Horton and Devine technique.) E. The free dermal graft is sutured to subcutaneous tissue (*x*). F. Skin closure is accomplished with a rotation flap.

ate to close fistulas on one, two, or even more occasions. Although the surgical technique appears simple, a word of caution is necessary to advise the patient that this "small procedure" is indeed difficult, and a successful repair, while anticipated and desired, is occasionally elusive.

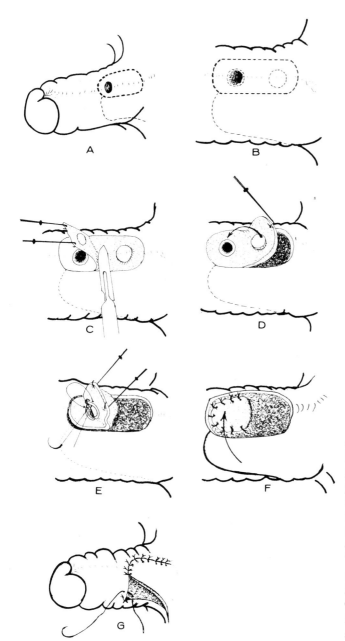

FIG. 22-10. A. Outline of incisions for fistula closure (Hecker and Mathes). B. Same incisions in greater detail, showing central plug prepared. C. Epithelium is removed from all areas except the central "plug" that is to be used to resurface the urethra. D. Elevation of the dermal flap carrying the "epidermal plug." E. The epidermal plug is sutured to the uroepithelium. F. The dermal flap is then sutured to subcutaneous tissues. G. Skin closure can be accomplished in many ways, e.g., with flaps or by simple straight-line approximation.

References

1. Cecil, A. B. Repair of hypospadias and urethral fistula. *J. Urol.* 56:237, 1946
2. Culp, O. S. Experiences with 200 hypospadiacs. *Surg. Clin. North Am.* 39:1007, 1959.
3. Devine, C. J., Jr., and Horton, C. E. Hypospadias. In Goldwyn, R. M. (Ed.), *The Unfavorable Result in Plastic Surgery: Avoidance and Treatment.* Boston: Little, Brown, 1972.
4. Horton, C. E., and Devine, C. J., Jr. A one-stage repair for hypospadias cripples. *Plast. Reconstr. Surg.* 45:425, 1970.
5. Horton, C. E., and Devine, C. J., Jr. Hypospadias. In Mustardé, J. C. (Ed.), *Plastic Surgery in Infancy and Childhood.* Philadelphia: Saunders, 1971.
6. Mellin, P. *Urologic Surgery in Infancy and Childhood.* Stuttgart: Georg Thieme, 1970.

Urethral Diverticula

CHARLES J. DEVINE, JR.
CHARLES E. HORTON

23

WHEN dribbling occurs after micturition, a diverticulum should be suspected. Examination during urination may reveal a dilated urethral pouch; urethrograms are diagnostically conclusive. Prior to surgery, a cystoscopic examination and careful evaluation of the urethra are mandatory. Often there may be blind passages and urethral folds that are unsuspected, or hair growth and concretions may produce unexpected problems. When the cystoscope is in the urethra, the meatus can be manually closed, and the urethra dilatated with fluid (Fig. 23-1). The cystoscope light will illuminate the dilatated urethra and pouch to allow accurate demarcation of the disorder prior to actual surgery [1].

The distal urethra should be carefully inspected to make certain no distal stenosis or stricture is present. Distal problems must be corrected simultaneously with or prior to the repair of the diverticulum [2].

When the extent of the diverticulum has been determined, a longitudinal incision adjacent but lateral to the area should be made and the urethra opened. An appropriate sized Foley catheter is then placed through the urethra, and all pouches and abnormalities are excised. The existing urethral epithelium can be contoured to the desired channel size and sutured with 5-0 chromic catgut with the knots tied inside the lumen. The penile skin closure should be made lateral to the urethral closure to prevent superimposition of suture lines and possible fistula formation (Fig. 23-2.

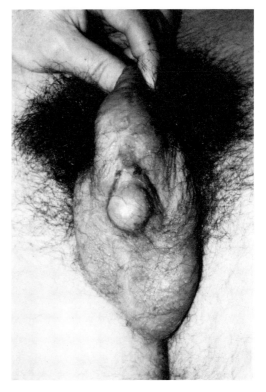

FIG. 23-1. Diverticulum of urethra.

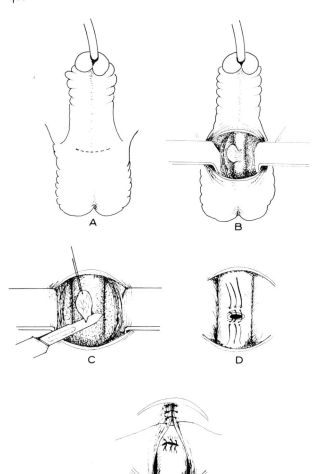

FIG. 23-2. A. Outline of incisions. B. Exposure. A bulb syringe can be inserted in the urethra to fill the urethra with fluid to distend the diverticulum. C. Excision. D. Inversion of the uroepithelium. E. Closure of the subcutaneous tissue prior to the placement of skin sutures.

We prefer to keep the catheter indwelling for one week postoperatively and to give the patient bacteriostatic medication to prevent urinary infection. An occlusive dressing is recommended for 3 days after surgery [3].

References

1. Culp, O. S., and McRoberts, J. W. Hypospadias. In Alken, H. von C. E. (Eds.), *Handbook of Urology*. New York: Springer-Verlag, 1968.
2. Devine, C. J., Jr., and Horton, C. E. Hypospadias. In Goldwyn, R. M. (Ed.), *The Unfavorable Result in Plastic Surgery: Avoidance and Treatment*. Boston: Little, Brown, 1972.
3. Horton, C. E., and Devine, C. J., Jr. A one-stage repair for hypospadias cripples. *Plast. Reconstr. Surg.* 45:425, 1970.

Congenital Absence of the Vagina

JOHN T. HUESTON
IAN A. McDONALD

24

ALTHOUGH the fundamental problems of congenital absence of the vagina are anatomical, its significance is both physiological and psychological. Its physiological importance is that from puberty the patient does not menstruate and suffers sexual incapacity. It is psychologically significant for the teenager, who feels that she is abnormal and cannot fulfill the need to identify herself as a complete female, and later for the bride, who becomes frustrated because normal coitus is impossible. A combined approach by a gynecologist and a plastic surgeon is essential, since the assessment and treatment of the condition are aimed at the whole patient and not at the solitary facet of the absent organ.

Etiology

The causes of developmental absence of the vagina may be considered in the chronological order of their possible action:

1. Genetic
2. Hormonal
3. Failure of end-organ response
4. Iatrogenic (pharmaceutical)
5. Psychological (transexualism)

GENETIC

Disjunction of the sex chromosomes at fertilization may produce an aberration of sexual differentiation. The XO combination that produces gonadal agenesis is associated with a person who remains sexually immature, e.g., as in Turner's syndrome (Fig. 24-1). Another aberration, the XXY trisomy (Klinefelter's syndrome), usually results in the infant being reared as a male. The XXX trisomy ("super female") is associated with the development of a normal vagina.

The partial aberrations or mosaics may pose a problem because the external genitalia alone may be deficient, and, since most of these individuals are reared as females, a vagina may need to be constructed for them in later life. Such abnormalities, however, are rare. Azoury and Jones [1], in reviewing the cases of congenital absence of the vagina at Johns Hopkins Hospital, showed that all their cases had a normal chromosomal pattern.

HORMONAL

At the fifth week of intrauterine life, the primitive gonad differentiates into either a

407

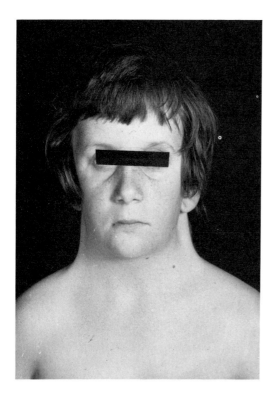

FIG. 24-1. A case of Turner's syndrome showing the characteristic webbing of the neck.

testis or ovary. The differentiated gonad of the embryo produces chemical substances, or evocators, that stimulate or inhibit development of the appropriate genital duct system depending upon the genetic sex of the individual. The testis produces a wolffian stimulator and a müllerian inhibitor.

The wolffian stimulator may be absent, and the individual, though a genetic male, takes on the characteristics and phenotype of a female. The female internal genitalia are often deficient in such an individual.

Case 1. An individual of rather coarse but definitely female phenotype (Fig. 24-2) presented at the age of 23 because of amenorrhea and the inability to achieve coitus. She was found to have only a small dimple where the vagina should be but otherwise had normal female external genitalia. Chromosomal studies revealed a karyotype 44/XY (Fig. 24-3), confirming that she was a genetic male. The serum testosterone was also at the male level. At a laparotomy, gonads were found adjacent to the internal inguinal rings. Frozen section revealed that these were normal testes. They were excised. A vaginal cavity was manufactured at the same time as the laparotomy by the McIndoe technique [3].

Subsequently this patient was given oral estrogens. She softened and became entirely feminine.

Occasionally, neither type of internal genital tract develops. We have seen patients in whom normal ovulating ovaries were present, but they had failed to stimulate a fully developed müllerian system. These patients had no vagina, uterus, or fallopian tubes, and the round ligaments ended at the pelvic brim. The ovaries, though normally developed, had failed to descend into the pelvis and were found on the posterior abdominal wall in front of the psoas major muscles.

Another hormonal abnormality that can produce deficient sexual development in the female child is the adrenogenital syndrome. In this condition, a high concentration of androgenic corticosteroid, which arises from the fetal adrenals and is secreted in utero in a normally developing female, inhibits normal müllerian development. The labia become hypertrophied and often fuse in the midline to produce a pseudoscrotum. The vagina, though present, is only a rudimentary organ, remaining small and very narrow, and the müllerian system above is perfectly formed but undeveloped. The clitoris hypertrophies, but hypospadias usually persists (Fig. 24-4). The child has the physical appearance of a hairy male (Figs. 24-5 and 24-6), and if reared thus, an operation to create a vaginal cavity may not be desirable, especially in an older person. Such an individual can be

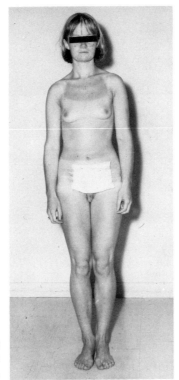
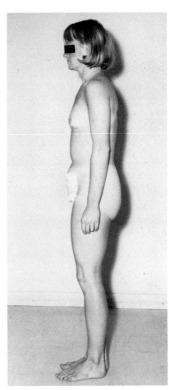

FIG. 24-2. Female phenotype with absence of vagina and a male karyotype (see Fig. 24-3).

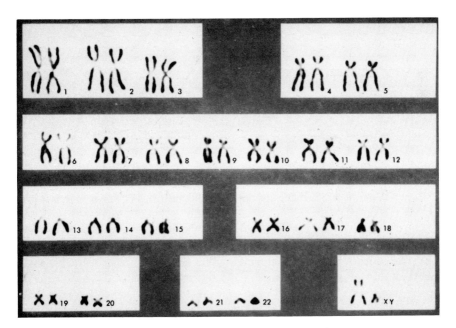

FIG. 24-3. Karyotype 44/XY confirms that despite the female phenotype, the patient in Figure 24-2 is a genetic male.

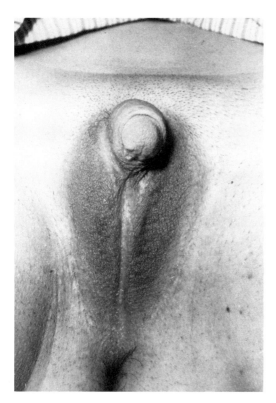 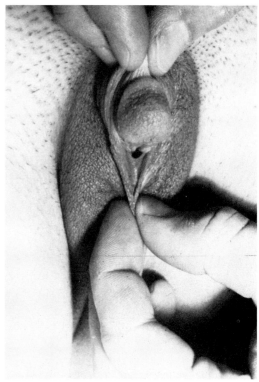

FIG. 24-4.   A case of adrenogenital syndrome showing hypertrophied labia and clitoris, a rudimentary vagina, and virtual hypospadias.

helped by treating the hypospadias, removing the ovaries, and replacing the hormones with testosterone and cortisone.

Most patients with an adrenogenital syndrome should be rendered female. Cortisone will be required, followed occasionally by estrogen therapy to stimulate müllerian development, and the surgical construction of a vaginal cavity is undertaken. Vant and Horner [14] described an adrenogenital patient who subsequently became pregnant and had a normal baby by cesarean section.

Occasionally, the gonad fails to differentiate completely into one side or the other and remains as an ovotestis. Such an organ may be bipartite in its secretions, producing the hormones of both sexes. In early development, the androgenic hormones take precedence, and the individual tends to develop predominately along male lines but with bisexual stigmata such as hypospadias, fused labia, or labial gonads. It is easier to rear such an individual as a female, since plastic reconstruction of the female external genitalia certainly is simpler than reconstruction of those of the male. Parents are advised after birth that the sex of rearing should be female. This will require division of the labia and removal of the genital tubercle at an early age, preferably before the age of 3 years. The creation of a vaginal cavity is postponed until maturity is reached and the child has decided to identify totally as a woman. Many authorities advocate the removal of the ovotestis in infancy to

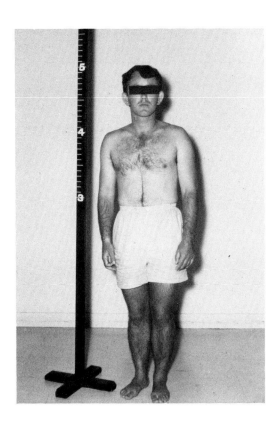

FIG. 24-5. Same case as shown in Figure 24-4. The physical appearance of a hairy male rules against the construction of a vagina.

overcome the bipartite nature of its secretion and to avoid the possibility of a dysgerminoma, a highly malignant tumor that is said to occur with great frequency in the ovotestis. The appropriate sexual hormones, in most cases estrogen and progesterone, are prescribed orally at puberty, and this treatment is continued throughout the remainder of the sexually active life of the individual.

FAILURE OF END-ORGAN RESPONSE

Sometimes the gonads are normally developed but the end organ, the wolffian ducts or the müllerian ducts, fails to respond to their secretions.

In the case of testicular feminization, the normal hormones are produced but the external genitalia remain undeveloped. The child has the external appearances of a female and is usually reared as a girl. When maturity occurs, the breasts develop as does a rudimentary external genital system of the female type. The vagina is usually present only in the lower portion from the urogenital sinus. Chromosomal examination of these individuals shows that they possess a normal autosomal configuration but have a male-type XY sex chromosome pattern. Hormonal investigations will reveal that testosterone is produced by testes that remain undescended in the abdomen. These individuals frequently become very beautiful women and many are to be found in night clubs and on the theatrical stages of the world (Fig. 24-7).

A laparotomy and biopsy of the gonads reveals a normal though rather atrophic testis with spermatogenesis halted at the primary spermatid stage; spermatozoa usually are not identified. Most authorities recommend that the testes be removed at laparotomy and that extrinsic estrogen be given orally after puberty to ensure breast development. A vaginal cavity is constructed at the time of sexual maturity.

In the opposite variety—with ovarian development—the end organs may fail to be stimulated by an as yet unknown and undemonstrated müllerian evocator of a normal ovary. In this circumstance, the müllerian ducts remain absent and the vagina fails to form except at the caudal end. The ovary develops normally and possesses a normal morphological appearance; ovulation apparently occurs and a corpus luteum is to be found (Fig. 24-8). This appears to be a relatively common form of developmental absence of the vagina.

Another common form occurs when the vagina fails to recanalize after fusion of the lower ends of the müllerian ducts. In such a

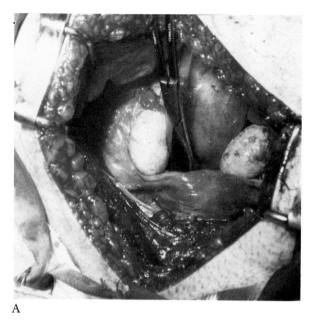

A

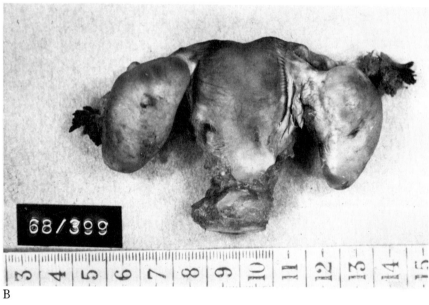

B

FIG. 24-6. A. On operation, female internal genitalia were found in the patient shown in Figures 24-4 and 24-5. B. Operation specimen showing overaies and a small uterus.

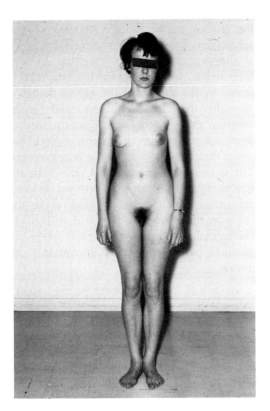

FIG. 24-7. Female phenotype with male XY chromosome pattern, intraabdominal testicular development, and no müllerian elements present.

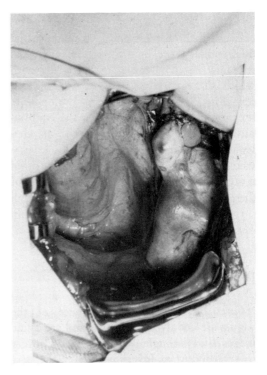

FIG. 24-8. Case showing ovarian development but the absence of müllerian duct elements. A corpus luteum can be seen at the upper pole of the large ovary on the right side of the illustration. Uterus and tubes are absent.

case, the uterus, fallopian tubes, and ovaries develop along normal lines, but the vagina is represented only as a solid block of tissue lying beneath the cervix. It is possible that pregnancy can occur after surgical construction of a vagina, and such cases have been recorded [7].

IATROGENIC (PHARMACEUTICAL)

If a woman has been prescribed a contraceptive pill containing androgenic hormonal preparations and unwittingly becomes pregnant due perhaps to omitting only a single day's dose, she may continue to take these androgens during the time of differentiation of the gonads in the fetus or for the next few weeks while the müllerian or wolffian systems are developing. This may interfere with the linear sexual development of a female embryo and produce bisexualism; it will have no effect on a male embryo. The female fetus thus afflicted, though of female phenotype, will have an enlarged phallus, fused labia, and an absent vagina. Reared as a female, the infant will require clitoridectomy and division of the labia before the age of 3 years. Later, a vaginal cavity is constructed. These individuals usually possess normal female fertility.

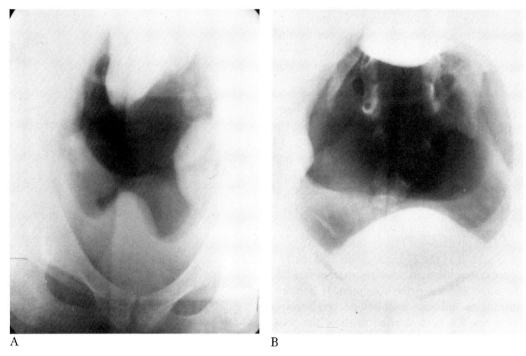

A   B

FIG. 24-10. A. Gynecogram of the pelvis that is shown at operation in Figure 24-8. A large ovarian mass can be seen on the right side of the illustration. The bladder is behind the symphysis, but there is no uterus or tubes. B. Gynecogram showing the bladder anteriorly, the rectum posteriorly, and the complete absence of internal female genitalia.

ful instrument in the investigation of vaginal absence.

LAPAROTOMY

Laparotomy, "the final court of appeal," should be performed in almost every case of developmental absence of the vagina when surgical correction is contemplated. This operation should be combined with the construction of a vaginal cavity; not only can the abdominal surgeon assess the deviations in sexual development but he can also assist the perineal surgeon in the proper placement of the mold and graft without too much pressure on pelvic viscera and peritoneum.

In the uncommon but most important case of an absent vagina with a normal uterus, tubes, and ovaries, synchronous combined surgery can obviously enhance the patient's chances of successful conception.

Treatment

The first decision to make in the treatment of developmental absence of the vagina is whether to operate.

Surgical construction of a vagina is not necessary in those female individuals who prefer to appear or respond as a male or if they have no sexual drive whatsoever. Rarely, in a case of testicular feminization syndrome, repeated pressure on the urogenital sinus dimple from a male partner's phallus may produce a serviceable cavity and no surgery may be required.

The second decision regards when to operate. The appropriate time is dictated by the presence or absence of the clinical symptoms of cryptomenorrhea, the psychological need to identify as a female, or when a marriage is contemplated.

Some individuals, for psychological reasons, need to have a vagina constructed even without the prospects of matrimony.

Case 2. A highly trained and intelligent tutor obstetrical nurse presented at the age of 25 years. She stated that she wished to have a vagina constructed, knowing well that she did not possess this organ, and that she felt introspective and depressed because she knew she was not the same as other women. Although she had no prospect of matrimony, she was profoundly frustrated each day in the delivery room during her work with normal women during their confinement.

A vaginal cavity was constructed and thereafter she kept it continuously dilated for many years using a glass mold. She was now able to identify and behave like a woman, her depression was resolved, and, although she has never married, she states that she has benefited considerably from the operation.

The third decision is how to operate. Three different methods of treatment have been described:

1. Baldwin's classic operation (1904) [3], which uses an isolated loop of bowel (either lower ileum or sigmoid colon) was the first modern method of surgical creation of a vagina. The operation requires bowel resection and anastomosis. It is, however, associated with a definite morbidity and even mortality due to the extent of the surgical procedure. Patients are also frequently embarrassed by a profuse mucus discharge from the secretory epithelium of the gut. Pratt and Smith [12] are enthusiastic modern protagonists of the method, but their operations have mostly followed excision of the vagina for cancer.

2. The Frank principle [7] utilizes a firm acrylic mold that is pressed against the urogenital dimple by a means of a harness; thus, the sinus gradually deepens and inverts. This method often fails, but it has been modified by Wharton [15], who surgically opened a plane of cleavage at the vaginal site and inserted molds of increasing size into the cleft. Local urogenital epithelium grows in to cover the granulating deficiency. When the same result can be achieved in a single surgical grafting procedure, there seems to be little reason in modern practice for retaining this outdated technique [4].

3. The McIndoe method of inlay grafting secures primary healing with a skin graft of the surgically created vaginal cavity. The present technique of the authors is based on that developed at the Royal Chelsea Hospital for Women in London by the combined surgical endeavors of Sir Archibald McIndoe as plastic surgeon and Sir Charles Read as gynecologist [9-10.]*

Surgical Technique

The operation for vaginal construction is conducted under the same anesthetization as the laparotomy for gonadal biopsy. The advantages of such a combined approach are several: the plastic surgeon gains first-hand knowledge of the internal genitalia; there is bipolar control of the pelvic dissection for the new vaginal cavity, allowing modification of mold size; precision of placement of the graft to an existent uterus is possible; and, of course, the patient is grateful to have only one anesthetization for both abdominal and perineal procedures. The cooperation of two different surgical specialists operating together on the same problem will enhance the

* The present authors wish to acknowledge with gratitude and great respect the personal tuition that each has received in his specialty from these great teachers.

mutual understanding of the condition and promote a stable continuity in the management of these patients, which is so important in obtaining the best long-term result [4].

PREOPERATIVE PREPARATION

The perineum is shaved; however, the thighs are not in order to allow selection of hairless skin for the inlay graft.

Three soft molds are prepared either from soft foam rubber or from plastic quarter-inch sheets that are cut and rolled so that they can be inserted inside a plastic condom (Fig. 24-11). Another reinforcing condom is applied over this, and both are tied to retain the sponge. Although maximum volume is attempted, the length and breadth of such molds vary from about 12 by 3 cm to 8 by 4 cm.

Before entering the hospital, the patient purchases a firm and snug-fitting panty-girdle for postoperative support of the vulva in retaining the mold.

POSITION

The lithotomy position allows access to the three areas required: the suprapubic area for laparotomy and gonadal biopsy, the vulva for vaginal construction, and the inner aspect of the left thigh from which the split skin-thickness graft is usually taken.

INCISIONS

For laparotomy, a horizontal incision is made just within the pubic hair-bearing skin and parallel to its upper border; this allows access to the lower abdomen without leaving a disfiguring abdominal scar.

For vaginal construction, an inverted V shaped incision is favored (Fig. 24-12). This doubles the length of the junctional scar with

the graft and thus lessens the risk of stenosis that may follow a single vertical incision.

The inverted V is preferred over a cruciform incision because when the V-shaped flap is laid into the posterior wall of the new vaginal orifice, it provides an intact path of entry that is well adapted to the subsequent mild trauma occurring to this posterior vaginal lip during mold changes and, most importantly, during coitus. A transverse scar margin at this posterior margin may, if tight, cause discomfort.

DISSECTION OF THE CAVITY

A metal catheter is placed in the urethra to ensure its identification during dissection (Fig. 24-13), and the left index finger is placed in the patient's rectum to define the posterior visceral limit of dissection. A cavity is then made in the loose pelvic areolar tissue by a combination of scissor and digital dissection.

The opening of the peritoneal cavity for gonadal biopsy allows direct inspection of the upper limit of dissection to the subperitoneal plane. When the dissecting fingers force up the peritoneum from the pouch of Douglas, the longest mold is inserted that can be retained without producing blanching of the peritoneum.

It is important to limit the extent of lateral dissection to that required for only the 3 or 4 cm diameter mold. Excessive lateral dissection will create recesses that are not needed for the vagina and are not likely to be filled by the mold, as well as incur the risk of hematoma and graft failure.

Hemostasis is occasionally difficult, but, after 5 minutes packing, inspection of the cavity using a Sims's speculum will facilitate diathermic coagulation of the remaining bleeding.

The volume of the cavity is the most im-

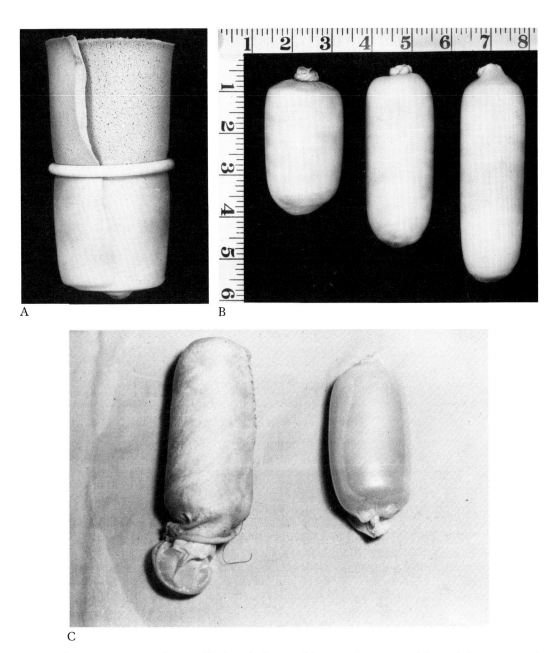

FIG. 24-11. A. A condom is filled with foam rubber or plastic. B. Three different sizes of soft molds made by sponge rubber tied inside condoms. C. On the left is shown a thick split-thickness skin graft sutured around the larger and longer of these molds.

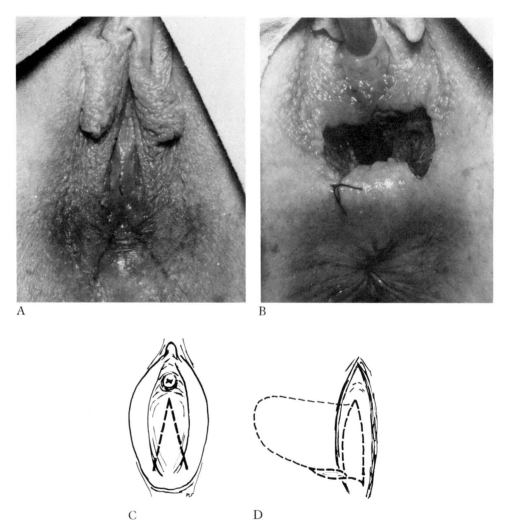

FIG. 24-12.   A and B.   An inverted V-shaped incision is outlined with the apex near the external orifice.   C and D.   The incision is dropped back into the posterior wall of the new vaginal cavity.

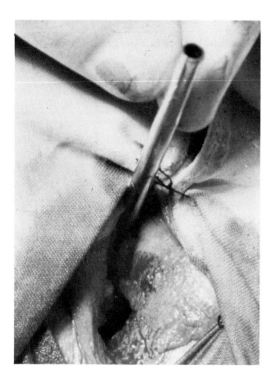

FIG. 24-13. A metal catheter, placed temporarily in the urethra, assists in its identification during dissection.

portant aspect. If a long (12 by 3 cm) mold cannot be fully inserted, a shorter (8 or 10 cm) but broader (4 cm) mold is used. This ensures the introduction of the maximum area of skin graft. For practical coitus, the vaginal function will finally be determined by the surface area of its lining.

The metal catheter is then changed to a 5 ml Foley indwelling catheter, and the dissected cavity is packed during application of the graft onto the mold.

THE GRAFT

McIndoe [8] in 1949 advocated the use of thin grafts since they took more readily and there was less inclusion of dermal epithelial elements. However, these are no longer used; it was the very thinness of these grafts that allowed the subsequent rapid contraction of the inlay-grafted cavities.

Thicker grafts are now favored because the degree of contraction of a free graft is inversely proportional to the amount of dermis carried on the graft. The donor site is selected to minimize the number of hair follicles and sebaceous glands. Usually, the inner aspect of the thigh is suitable as well as convenient. If the thigh is hairy, the buttock may be preferred. The very last choice would be the abdomen, but we have not yet been forced to mutilate this esthetically important area in seeking a suitable donor site.

The easier take of the thinner grafts over thick grafts should not be totally ignored in selecting a donor site. It is relevant that the inner aspect of the thigh, having the thinnest skin available between the navel and the knee, is preferred, since a greater proportion of dermis is provided for a three-quarter thickness, and hence thin, graft from this area than from any other local donor site. Usually, therefore, most of the dermis is included in our three-quarter thickness split-thickness skin graft from the inner aspect of the thigh. A very thin split-thickness skin graft from the adjacent thigh is used over the primary donor site to expedite its healing and thus minimize local scar disfigurement.

The graft is not glued to the mold but is draped over it lengthwise and sutured with several continuous silk sutures, leaving the knots on the inner aspect of the "graft condom."

The simpler technique of Polycratis [11] depends on the integrity of this seam stitching, and although this packing technique allows the graft to be applied to all the cavity walls, these may not be regular in interior contour. The value of introducing such a simple packing technique has been to demonstrate that the previously favored rigid mold is not essential, and hence its drawbacks—the risk of urethrovaginal and rectovaginal fistulas, the danger of vault hematoma, and the patient's discomfort—need no longer be encountered in this operation.

The soft mold used in our technique is adjustable to pelvic movements and avoids the shearing effect produced by such movements when a rigid mold is in place. The risk of hematoma is least if the dissection has not been extended laterally beyond the mold requirements. The application of the fascial aspects of the pelvic viscera to the graft-covered mold has been adequate to prevent hematoma and has permitted complete take of the graft in all patients since the time this technique was adopted.

Retention of the Graft

The graft-covered mold will protrude past the vestibular incision, and marginal healing will occur by overlap. Extrusion of the mold must be prevented, and McIndoe's suggested use of a labial suture to construct a perineal bridge is the most reliable method of retention.

The free margins of the labia minora are incised and sutured together with layered interrupted fine catgut and silk sutures across the introitus and behind the emerging catheter. A firm dressing is held in place by a T-binder, and the knees are gently bandaged together before the patient is returned to her bed.

Postoperative Management

The patient lies flat for 3 or 4 days with the knees gently bandaged and the catheter draining continuously to a bedside bag. The bowels are confined.

After 3 days, it can be presumed that the graft has taken, but care is necessary to avoid anything that may cause movement of the soft mold and thus dislodgement or shearing of the graft. The patient may sit up but not leave the bed. Neomycin bladder washouts are performed every 6 hours, and the pad and T-binder are changed at least daily. Nitrofurantoin (50 mg) and a combination of oral penicillin and tetracycline are given prophylactically. Sufficient laxatives are used to allow defecation without forceful bearing down; the patient is warned against such efforts.

The first dressing is applied 2 weeks postoperatively. With the patient under general anesthesia and in the lithotomy position, the labia are divided, the mold is gently extracted, and the grafted cavity is inspected with a Sims's speculum. Silk sutures and redundant necrotic tags of graft are removed, and a general toilet of the grafted cavity is completed. After changing the Foley catheter, a fresh mold is inserted. A pad is retained by a T-binder until later the same day when the patient changes her preordained snuggly fitting panty-girdle.

For one week after the first dressing, the patient is kept in bed and instructed on the technique of mold changing. The catheter is removed. She changes the mold temporarily, if necessary, to micturate during this early postoperative phase. By the fourth week, the patient is usually sufficiently proficient and confident in her personal welfare to leave the hospital.

Prolonged retention of the mold for 4 to 6 months was necessary when thin grafts were used. Now, this unpleasant period can be avoided by the use of thick grafts that can be dressed after 2 weeks. It is necessary that the patient be warned that contraction of the cavity, sufficient to render it unserviceable, will occur rapidly unless a full-size mold is worn continuously for at least 6 months and, after that, nightly for the rest of her sexual life. Daily or twice daily, the patient can remove the mold temporarily for a vaginal douche if necessary.

Coitus can safely be performed 6 weeks postoperatively if the junctional scar in the introitus is soft, the graft sound, and her partner considerate. However, it is suggested that the operation be carried out 3 to 6 months prior to the patient's incurring any marital obligations in order to allow regional postoperative resolution and the maximum restoration of female confidence. Only if Bartholin's glands are not present or not functioning will any lubrication be necessary, but none of our patients has required this.

Complications and Results

Structural changes have been reported in the skin grafts lining the new vaginal canal; in particular, glycogen staining of the stratified squamous epithelium has occurred. This histological change, indicating some local estrogen effect, may be associated with even more extensive changes that allow sufficient distention in the skin-grafted canal for vaginal delivery of babies. Moore [9] reported a patient who has thus delivered three babies *per via naturalis* after this operation.

The review by Simmons [12] of 101 patients treated by our mentors, McIndoe and Read, has confirmed that inlay skin grafting is a safe, sure method of constructing a vaginal cavity.

References

1. Azoury, R. A., and Jones, H. W., Jr. Cytogenetic findings in patients with congenital absence of the vagina. *Am. J. Obstet. Gynecol.* 94:178, 1966.
2. Baldwin, A. F. *Ann. Surg.* 40:398, 1904.
3. Booney, V., and McIndoe, A. H. Unique constructive operation. *J. Obstet. Brit. Emp.* 51:24, 1944.
4. Castañares, S. Plastic construction of artificial vagina. *Plast. Reconstr. Surg.* 32:368, 1963.
5. Counsellor, V. S. Diverticulitis; symptoms, complications and management, particularly in females. *Am. J. Obstet. Gynecol.* 33:256, 1948.
6. Frank, R. T. Formation of artificial vagina without operation. *Am. J. Obstet. Gynecol.* 35:1053, 1938.
7. McIndoe, A. H. The treatment of congenital absence and obliterative conditions of the vagina. *Br. J. Plast. Surg.* 2:254, 1949.
8. McIndoe, A. H., and Banister, J. B. Operation for cure of congenital absence of vagina. *J. Obstet. Brit. Emp.* 45:490, 1938.
9. Moore, F. T., and Simonis, A. A. Per via naturalis following reconstruction of the vagina. *Br. J. Plast. Surg.* 22:378, 1969.
10. Polycratis, G. S. A Safer Technique for Vaginal Construction. In *Transactions of the First International Congress of Plastic Surgeons*. Baltimore: Williams & Wilkins, 1957.
11. Pratt, J. H., and Smith, G. R. Vaginal reconstruction with a sigmoid loop. *Am. J. Obstet. Gynecol.* 96:31, 1966.
12. Simmons, C. A. Vaginoplasties at Chelsea Hospital for Women, 1938–1958. *Proc. R. Soc. Med.* 52:953, 1959.
13. Turunen, A. Ovarian stroma in a patient with congenital absence of the vagina. *Ann. Chir. Gynaecol. Fenn.* 46:359, 1957.
14. Vant, J., and Horner, H. Adrenogenital syndrome: Absence of the vagina with pregnancy and successful delivery. *Am. J. Obstet. Gynecol.* 85:355, 1963.
15. Wharton, L. R. Simple method of constructing a vagina: Report of 4 cases. *Ann. Surg.* 107:842, 1938.

Secondary Procedures for Vaginal Reconstructive Failures

CHARLES E. HORTON
JEROME E. ADAMSON
RICHARD A. MLADICK
JAMES CARRAWAY

25

MANY COMPLICATIONS can occur after reconstruction of the vagina. Skin grafts occasionally will not grow, and the resulting vaginal cavity may be smaller than desirable due to secondary scar contracture. The patient may, in spite of adequate presurgical counseling, remove the vaginal mold too soon, or if the mold is firm and ill-fitting, pressure ulceration of the urethra may occur, forcing early removal of the vaginal stent with resulting graft contracture. If for any reason an inadequate vagina is encountered after previous surgery, a secondary procedure is indicated, provided the patient is cooperative and desires help (Fig. 25-1A).

Although the well-vascularized intestinal pouch may be considered for use in secondary cases, we prefer to reenlarge the vaginal cavity by sharp and blunt dissection through incisions in the shallow existing vagina. The use of adrenalin (1:100,000) injected into the tissues facilitates dissection and lessens bleeding. Because of the previous surgical scarring, at least 6 and preferably 12 months should elapse before secondary reconstruction is attempted. A split-thickness skin graft from the medial thigh or buttocks is again procured and fitted over an appropriate mold (Fig. 25-1B).

Either a sponge covered with a condom, a hollow acrylic mold with an appropriate urethral groove and eyelet, packing, or an inflatable balloon mold can be used to retain the graft in the cavity (Fig. 25-1C). The balloon-type stent has much to offer in that the release of the fluid inside the balloon causes the stent to collapse, and it can be withdrawn from the vagina for cleaning with neither the pain nor need for anesthesia. When the vagina and stent have been cleaned, the balloon can be reinserted and inflated with saline to produce pressure against the vaginal cavity. Silastic molds retain odors and are expensive; however, heavy rubber balloons are usable if the former are unobtainable.

The retainer should be worn for 6 weeks

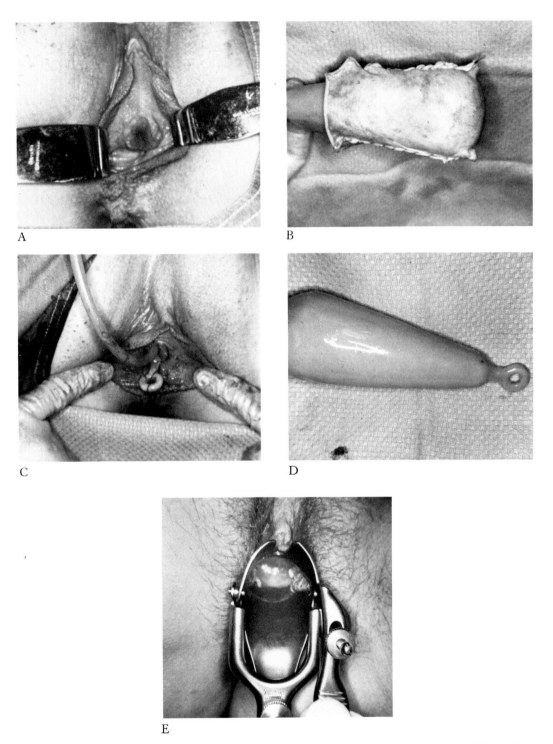

FIG. 25-1. A. Secondary stenosis of vaginal reconstruction (for congenital absence of the vagina) due to early removal of the stent by the patient. B. Skin graft is sutured over a hollow acrylic stent. C. Skin graft and stent in place. D. The stent is used as a retainer. E. Postoperative result. The adult speculum is inserted to its full length.

with removal only for cleaning (Fig. 25-1D). Thereafter, the stent can be removed for coitus or for 1 hour each morning and evening until 3 months have elapsed. We then advise the patient to wear the retainer for 12 hours every day until married and frequent intercourse occurs, or if necessary, i.e., if tightening of the new vagina commences, to wear it more frequently. Not until 6 months after surgery is it safe to be without the tampon for any period of time (Fig. 25-1E).

Patients who have had one failure at reconstruction and who sincerely desire help are much more likely to cooperate and be aware of the necessity of wearing the stent for prolonged periods. No unusual technical difficulties are anticipated in the scar dissection of the previously operated field, although occasionally a long shallow tube of contracted skin can be identified in the operative area. We believe that all of the old skin graft should be excised and a new graft inserted, rather than attempting to join the new graft to the older, stenotic skin canal.

References

1. Abbe, R. New method of creating a vagina in case of congenital absence. *Med. Rec.* 54:836, 1898.
2. Blocker, T. G., Jr., Lewis, S. R., and Snyder, C. Plastic construction of artificial vagina: Further experiences. *Plast. Reconstr. Surg.* 11:177, 1953.
3. Braley, S. A. Do-it-yourself vaginal molds of silicone rubber. *Plast. Reconstr. Surg.* 47:192, 1971.
4. Castañares, S. Plastic construction of artificial vagina. *Plast. Reconstr. Surg.* 32:368, 1963.
5. Conway, H., and Stark, R. B. Construction and reconstruction of the vagina. *Surg. Gynecol. Obstet.* 88:37, 1949.
6. Howell, J. A. Congenital Absence of the Vagina. In Grabb, W. C., and Smith, J. W. (Eds.), *Plastic Surgery: A Concise Guide to Clinical Practice.* (2nd ed.) Boston: Little, Brown, 1973.
7. McIndoe, A. The treatment of congenital absence of obliterative conditions of the vagina. *Br. J. Plast. Surg.* 2:254, 1949–1950.
8. Owens, N. Suggested Pyrex form for support of skin grafts in construction of artificial vagina. *Plast. Reconstr. Surg.* 1:350, 1946.
9. Stark, R. B. Congenital Absence of the Vagina and Other Abnormalities of the External Female Genitalia. In Converse, J. M. (Ed.), *Reconstructive Plastic Surgery.* Philadelphia: Saunders, 1964. P. 2076.
10. Wilde, J. Reconstruction of vagina following Wertheim operation. *J. Plast. Reconstr. Surg.* 22:322, 1958.

Techniques for Circumcision and Urinary Diversion

JOSEPH G. FIVEASH, JR.

26

VARYING DEGREES of redundant foreskin are seen in the normal newborn male. The presence of a foreskin is not an indication for circumcision, although smegma and urinary alkaline encrustations may collect under a partially retractable prepuce and cause severe local irritation [1]. Evidence is widespread that carcinoma of the penis develops almost exclusively in the uncircumcised male. Circumcision must be done in childhood, however, if successful prophylaxis against this often invasive squamous cancer is to be achieved. Early allegations that continued presence of the foreskin results in an increased incidence of masturbation, nightmares, and malnutrition are without foundation [2].

When the distal opening in the prepuce is so contracted that the visceral surface of the foreskin cannot be retracted back over the glans penis, the condition is known as *phimosis*. Rare reports from the early urological literature implied uremic death has resulted from this unusually severe form of distal urethral obstruction. More likely, complications occurred that were due to continued and recurrent local irritation of the glans, leading to ulcerative balanoposthitis or to urethral meatal stenosis. A dorsal slit of the prepuce provides temporary relief by improving cleanliness of the area; permanent cure, however, is effected by circumcision.

Local application of antibiotic ointment to the glandar ulcers hastens healing, but a urethral meatal stenosis may persist. Mild meatal stenosis may be treated by gentle dilatation of the meatus alone. If it is more severe, a ventral meatotomy can be performed under local anesthesia as soon as the inflamed tissues have reverted to normal.

Circumcision is definitely contraindicated in the male with any degree of hypospadias. The hairless skin of the prepuce is ideally suited for reconstruction of the urethra, and this potential donor site should not be diminished in size needlessly until the final surgical procedure has been completed. Cases of chordee without hypospadias should not be circumcised until after the penis has been surgically straightened, since occasionally the straightening procedure results in injury or avascular necrosis to the urethra, with resultant urethral slough or urethrocutaneous fistula formation. Circumcision in Jewish infants born with hypospadias should be delayed until the urethral reconstruction has been completed.

Surgical Technique

The prepuce consists in part of a parietal surface that is a continuation of the squamous epithelium covering the penile

429

shaft. Distal to the glans penis, it is folded on its longitudinal axis to form a velvety visceral surface that inserts circumferentially around the penile shaft just proximal to the corona. Both the parietal and visceral skin surfaces are completely free of hair follicles.

Adhesions between the proximal surface of the corona and the visceral surface of the prepuce must be thoroughly broken by retracting the foreskin over the shaft of the penis. Sufficient stretching of the visceral prepuce should be produced to allow the deep purple proximal corona to be completely visible. Cream-colored particles of smegma or small calcifications should be removed [3].

After the foreskin has been retracted proximally over the glans penis to free any adhesions, it is drawn distally back past the tip of the glans and grasped securely in the 3 o'clock and 9 o'clock positions with Allis clamps or hemostats. A vertical incision is made from the tip of the foreskin along its dorsal surface to a point just proximal to the corona. Incisions through both the parietal and visceral prepuce are carried circumferentially and obliquely around either side of the penile shaft, paralleling the corona and joining at the frenulum. Brisk bleeding may be encountered, and this may be controlled by carefully placed ligatures of small plain catgut. After hemostasis is complete, the skin of the penile shaft is sutured to the resected

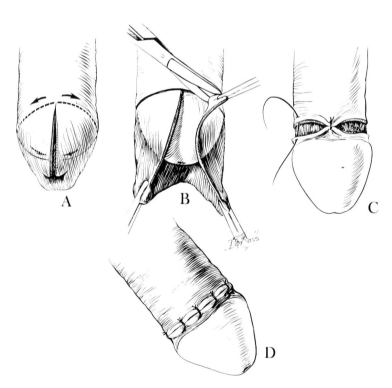

FIG. 26-1.   Method 1.   A.   A dorsal slit is made up to the corona.   B.   Circumferential incisions are made around the penile shaft.   C.   The skin of the penile shaft is sutured to the resected margin of the visceral prepuce.   D.   Closure.

margin of the visceral prepuce using four-quadrant sutures of 3-0 chromic catgut on an atraumatic needle (Fig. 26-1). Multiple sutures of 3-0 plain catgut, tied so as not to indent the skin, are used to complete closure of the incision. A circumferential strip of gauze covered with antibiotic ointment is applied to the incision line and held in place by loose gauze wrapped around the penis. An ice pack is applied for 12 hours to reduce pain and swelling. The patient is discharged on the day following surgery, and daily tub sitz baths are started.

Rarely, elderly patients may have difficulty voiding the night of circumcision. This is often relieved by hot sitz baths; urethral catheterization should be avoided unless absolutely necessary.

An alternative method of circumcision is shown in Figure 26-2.

Urinary Diversion

Diversion of the urethral stream is easily accomplished in the female by means of a standard Foley balloon catheter attached to a closed urinary drainage bag. The catheter employed should be the smallest size that is consistent with adequate and complete drainage of urine from the bladder.

It is impossible to irrigate a catheter repeatedly without introducing bacteria into the bladder. Consequently, routine irrigation of indwelling catheters is contraindicated. By maintaining an oral or intravenous intake of approximately 3 liters daily, a urinary output of 1.5 liters can be produced by the average adult. This quantity of urine will often prevent particulate matter from plugging the catheter and will tend to "wash off" concretions that form in the lumen of the catheter. Acidification of the urine by the oral administration of ascorbic acid (vitamin C) will also help to keep a catheter lumen free of

obstruction. If there is a preexisting bladder infection by a urea-splitting organism, alkaline concretions may form rapidly and occlude the catheter within 3 or 4 days. In this unique situation, irrigations twice daily with 1 ounce of Suby Solution G* will help maintain a patent catheter.

Diversion of the urethral stream in the male is complicated by the anatomy of the lower urinary tract. The anterior portion of the male urethra is divided into a relatively narrow portion—the pendulous urethra—which is distal to the suspensory ligament of the penis and whose stratified columnar epithelium is perforated by the secretory glands of Littre. In the normal state, these glands produce a minute but constant source of lubrication within the pendulous urethra that drains through the urethral meatus. When the lumen of the urethra is partially obstructed by an indwelling catheter, the secretions of the glands of Littre cannot easily escape and may pool around the catheter, forming an ideal culture medium for bacterial growth. A purulent urethritis with local and systemic toxic manifestations may result. Generous application of antibiotic ointment to the urethral meatus three or four times daily will reduce the incidence of bacterial infection within the urethra. Daily cleansing of the catheter and glans with soap and aqueous benzalkonium will also decrease the bacterial population.

The bulbous urethra in the male is that portion located between the urogenital diaphragm (external sphincter) and the suspensory ligament. It is cavernous in shape, averages between 12 and 18 mm in diameter, and lacks the glands of Littre found in the pendulous urethra. Consequently, this portion of the urethra tolerates an indwelling drainage catheter without the hazard of purulent urethritis.

* Cutter Laboratories, Inc., Berkeley, Calif.

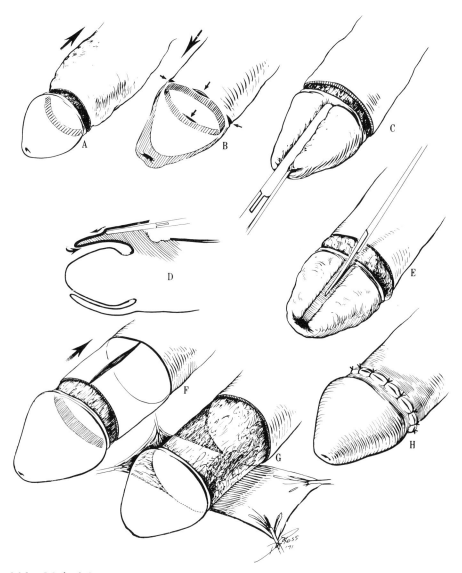

FIG. 26-2. Method 2. A. A circumferential incision is made in the visceral prepuce. B. The foreskin is drawn distally over the glans; four-quadrant nicks have been made in the penile skin over the corona. C. The circumferential incision in the penile skin is completed; a straight clamp is closed on the dorsal foreskin. D. The crushed foreskin is elevated from the underlying tissue. E. A longitudinal strip of crushed foreskin is incised on the parietal and visceral surfaces. F. The foreskin is retracted; the three incisions are shown. G. The foreskin is separated by sharp dissection from the underlying tissue. H. The skin of the penile shaft is sutured to the resected margin of the visceral prepuce.

Insertion of a catheter into the bladder via the bulbous urethra is known as a *perineal urethrostomy*. The technique of perineal urethrostomy varies slightly with the type of drainage catheter utilized. The procedure is done under general or regional anesthesia immediately preceding the operation that resulted in the need for urinary diversion.

TECHNIQUES OF PERINEAL URETHROSTOMY

FOLEY BALLOON CATHETER

The patient is placed in the lithotomy position, and the perineum is prepared and sterilely draped. A Robinson (red rubber) catheter or Van Buren sound is gently inserted into the bladder through the urethra. While an assistant steadies the perineum, a vertical incision approximately 2 to 3 cm long is made over the bulbous urethra in the median raphe between the base of the scrotum and the anus. The procedure becomes quite simple when the incision is very carefully deepened so that each layer of fascia is meticulously retracted to ultimately expose an adequate length of urethra containing the catheter or sound. A vertical incision is made in the urethra, and traction sutures of 4-0 atraumatic silk or catgut are placed through the full thickness of the urethra on either side of the urethrostomy. Handling the urethral edges with forceps is to be avoided at all times. When precise control of the urethral edges has been obtained, the catheter or sound is removed from the urethra; the definitive Foley catheter, properly lubricated, is gently inserted into the urethrostomy in the bulbous urethra and advanced in retrograde fashion into the bladder. After the balloon has been inflated, the perineal wound should be closed with appropriate suture material. When the catheter is no longer needed, it is removed. The perineal stoma will close quickly provided there is no distal obstruc-tion, and suturing of the wound is unnecessary.

ROBINSON (RED RUBBER) CATHETER

By the use of this catheter, the irritating effect of the Foley balloon on the trigone of the bladder is avoided, and the incidence of bladder spasms is theoretically reduced. With the patient in the lithotomy position, a catheter of proper size is gently introduced into the bladder on a lubricated catheter guide so only 2 to 3 cm of the catheter are within the bladder. While an assistant holds the catheter immobile at the meatus, the guide is withdrawn until its tip is in the bulbous urethra. The guide is then turned 180 degrees so that its tip bulges visibly against the perineal skin. A small midline incision is made down to the catheter, which is firmly grasped with a clamp. The guide is removed and that portion of the catheter distal to the urethrostomy is carefully pulled back through the pendulous urethra in retrograde fashion until the catheter hangs free from the perineal urethrostomy. It is essential to hold the proximal part of the catheter immobile while the distal portion is being withdrawn back through the pendulous urethra. The catheter must be anchored securely to the adjacent skin with strong silk sutures to prevent its inadvertent removal.

Complications of the procedure are infrequent but may include urethrocutaneous fistulas, wound infection, or urethral stricture at the operative site.

If urinary diversion is to be maintained for many months, a suprapubic cystostomy is the most satisfactory method.

Urethral Meatotomy

If the urethral meatus is normally located in the glans penis but is of inadequate caliber, it should be surgically enlarged. A local anesthetic agent containing Xylocaine is infiltrated into the ventral tip of the glans. The glandar tissue between the urethral meatus and the ventral aspect of the glans is crushed with a straight clamp. The crushed tissue is subsequently incised in the midline with a scalpel or fine scissors. Usually there is no bleeding, and sutures are not required. Daily dilata-

tions of the meatus with the blunt tip of a tube of ophthalmic antibiotic ointment are useful until healing is complete.

If there is stenosis of a hypospadial meatus, a ventral meatotomy should never be done, since this serves only to increase the extent of the hypospadias.

References

1. Calnan, J., and Copenhagen, H. Circumcision for the newborn. *Br. J. Surg.* 53:427, 1966.
2. Preston, E. N. Whither the foreskin? A condition of routine neonatal circumcision. *J.A.M.A.* 213:1853, 1970.
3. Shulman, J., Ben-Hur, N., and Neuman, Z. Surgical complications of circumcision. *Am. J. Dis. Child.* 107:149, 1964.

Obesity of the Genital Area

CHARLES E. HORTON
JEROME E. ADAMSON
RICHARD A. MLADICK
NAMIK K. BARAN

27

THE MOST COMMON result of excessive weight gain is the pendulous abdomen. When massive increase in size is noted, the abdomen may drop to cover the pubic area, and the genitalia (male or female) may appear to recede deep within excess folds of pubic, inguinal, and abdominal fat and skin. Intertrigo and maceration causing itching, malodor, and various other symptoms may result. In addition, the excessively fat individual may have some difficulty in performing sexually because of the bulky tissues surrounding the genital areas. Even after the obese person has lost weight, the skin usually will not have sufficient elasticity to retract with the weight loss, and it will remain hanging in front of the genitalia [1].

A simple operation consisting of amputation of the excess abdominal tissues can be offered to these individuals. In cases of less severity, an incision from iliac crest to iliac crest, keeping above the pubic hair line in the midline, will allow undermining of the lower abdomen, appropriate excision, and primary closure (Fig. 27-1). Usually, the umbilicus is lowered, but does not have to be violated. In women who desire cosmetic tightening of a stretched but not excessively obese abdominal wall, a vertical midline excision can be made at the umbilicus, and a triangle of abdominal skin is removed to tighten the wall laterally as well as vertically (Fig. 27-2A). A midline abdominal scar is not as objectionable to females as is loose and baggy abdominal tissue, since a scar is connotative of necessary surgery and not the aging process [2].

When the abdominal pendulosity is large, the umbilicus is situated lower than normal and must be either excised or elevated. Excision is not desirable. To elevate the umbilicus, an incision is made around the umbilical opening and the stalk is dissected down to the abdominal fascia. The umbilical stalk has longitudinal blood vessels within its wall that supply adequate vascularity. The abdominal skin is then undermined to the desired height (keeping on the fascia in a relatively avascular plane) and is pulled down to the iliac-pubic-iliac incisional line, where excess skin is then amputated. The umbilicus can then be sutured to a midline abdominal opening at the desired position, and a V-shaped flap of

435

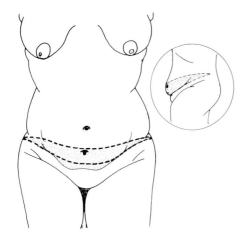

FIG. 27-1. Excision of a small pendulous abdomen. The umbilicus does not require repositioning. In cases requiring minimal tightening, the incision should be below the iliac spine areas laterally, so it is confined to the "Bikini covered" skin.

abdominal skin is fitted into a grooved incision at the bottom of the umbilicus (Figs. 27-2B and 27-3). This prevents a circular umbilical suture line and subsequent contracture

that might cause a limitation of the opening of the umbilicus and difficulty in cleaning. If old scar herniations are present or if an umbilical hernia is found, these should be repaired.

Postoperatively, these wounds should be drained for at least a week, since a tendency for fat necrosis and seroma formation with pocketing has been noted. Sutures should be left in place longer than in the usual abdominal wound.

Prior to surgery, all patients should have daily soap preparation for 3 days. Skin marking should be done in the standing position, and at operation, surgical closure is facilitated by flexing the table. Thromboembolic prophylaxis by early ambulation, isometric exercises, and wrapping the legs is advisable (Fig. 27-5).

Occasionally, the mons pubis will be enlarged, with fat extending into the labial folds. This fat can be removed through the suprapubic incision with great improvement in appearance.

Fat individuals are also plagued with ex-

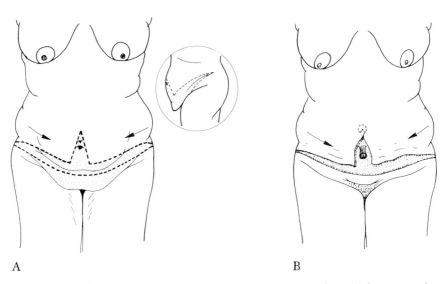

A   B

FIG. 27-2. A and B. Excision of a large pendulous abdomen. The umbilicus must be raised to a new level. The vertical triangular excision is optional, but aids in tightening the flanks.

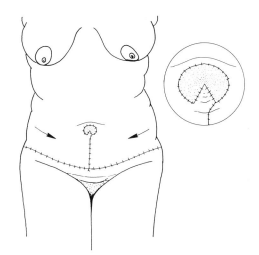

FIG. 27-3. Closure of the umbilicus and abdomen.

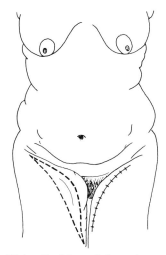

FIG. 27-4. Excision of fatty tissue from the thighs.

cessive tissue of the thighs that is usually situated medially near the genitalia and manifested by folds and masses of tissue high and medial on the upper legs. This can occur in certain lipodystrophies without general body obesity. Abnormal thigh fat causes difficulty in cleaning the skin area around the genitalia and difficulty in walking. It may also cause skin maceration and irritation [3].

Medial skin and fat excisions are of great

help in these cases (Fig. 27-4). Both legs can be corrected at the same operation if the fat is confined to the medial thigh areas; however, if the legs are massive, it may be necessary to do secondary lateral excisions (Fig. 27-6A and B). Occasionally, enlarged buttocks will require excision at the buttock-thigh crease. A large ellipse of skin and fat can be excised here to tighten the "middle-aged spread" seen often in females.

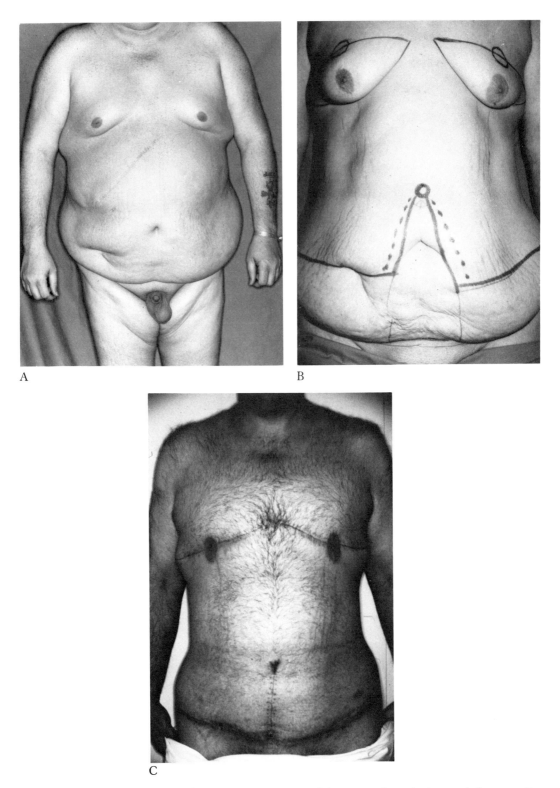

FIG. 27-5. A. Preoperative fatty tissue excess of abdomen, pubis, thighs, and breasts. B. Markings at surgery. C. Postoperative appearance after free nipple transplants and abdominal lipectomy with transposition of the umbilicus.

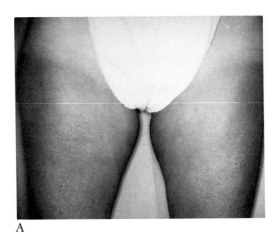
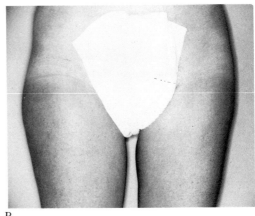

A   B

FIG. 27-6. A. Lax upper thigh and perineal tissue allows medial bulging and skin contact, causing irritation and excoriation. B. Surgical tightening of the perineal and thigh tissue via thigh incisions that are made lateral to the vagina and perineum.

References

1. Castañares, S., and Goethal, J. A. Abdominal lipectomy: A modification of technique. *Plast. Reconstr. Surg.* 40:378, 1967.
2. Lewis, J. R., Jr. Correction of ptosis of thighs: The thigh lift. *Plast. Reconstr. Surg.* 37:494, 1966.
3. Pitanguy, I. Abdominal lipectomy: Analysis of 300 consecutive cases. *Plast. Reconstr. Surg.* 40:384, 1967.

Trauma and Infection of the Genital Area

V

Burns of the Genitalia and Perineum

I. F. K. MUIR
B. D. G. MORGAN

28

BURNS of the external genitalia frequently occur as part of more extensive injuries involving the lower trunk and thighs. Localized burns of the genitalia are less common. During the year March, 1969, to February, 1970, 133 patients were admitted to the burns ward of Mount Vernon Centre for Plastic Surgery, and of these, ten had involvement of the external genitalia.

Burns of the genitalia are commonly caused by scalds, for example, due to a child falling backward into a bath or bucket of hot water, or burns due to clothes catching fire. Particularly severe burns occur when trousers soaked in oil or gasoline catch fire, as sometimes happens to garage workers. Occasionally, more localized burns occur, for example, when a firecracker detonates in a boy's pocket (Fig. 28-1). Burns due to clothes catching fire sometimes show bizarre patterns because of the variation in flammability of garments or even different parts of the same garment; areas of deep burning are mixed with areas where the skin has been partially or completely protected (see Fig. 28-4).

Iatrogenic burns have been recorded as a result of mishaps with diathermy during gynecological treatment or other errors in treatment, such as in chemical treatment of genital warts.

Healing and Infection

The healing of burns of these areas depends on the same principles as the healing of burns of other areas of the body. Regarding depth, the surgeon is concerned with (1) partial thickness or (2) full-thickness skin destruction. If the burns are of only partial thickness and if infection can be prevented, spontaneous healing will take place. On the other hand, if the full thickness of the skin has been destroyed, then any skin loss must be repaired by skin grafting to minimize the subsequent deformity.

The skin of the shaft of the penis is thin, and a burn of any severity is likely to destroy the full thickness of the skin. However, the inner aspect of the prepuce is often viable, even when the skin on the outer side has been destroyed, and this may be very useful in obtaining skin cover for the shaft of the penis.

In still deeper burns, not only the overlying skin of the penile shaft but also the floor of

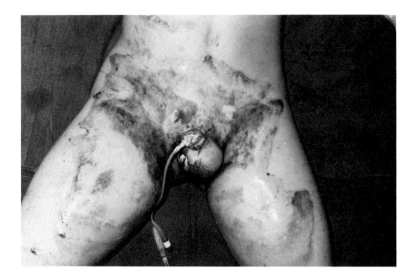

FIG. 28-1.   A firework burn on a 13-year-old boy that needed decompression of the penile shaft. The catheter is smeared with Hibitane cream.

the urethra may be destroyed, thus creating a traumatic hypospadias.

The skin of the scrotum shows great powers of regeneration, and even in burns that appear to be quite deep, epithelial elements may survive and be sufficient to result in healing.

The proximity of the genitalia to the anus makes the likelihood of autoinfection very great; these burns are particularly susceptible to infection with *Pseudomonas aeruginosa* (*pyocyanea*). Sachs [3, 4] has recently designated burns of this area as "pyo-prone burns." Shooter et al. [5] have recently shown that a certain proportion of individuals normally harbor *P. pyocyanea* in the intestine but that after patients have been in the hospital for a comparatively short time, the percentage who carry *P. pyocyanea* rises rapidly. Infection is dangerous not only because it may destroy surviving epithelial cells and convert a partial-thickness defect into a full-thickness defect, but also because it seriously interferes with the take of skin grafts.

Burns of the penis usually show marked edema (Figs. 28-2 and 28-3) and the prepuce may become grossly swollen, causing retention of urine and making it impossible to pass a catheter. In deep circumferential burns of the shaft, the burned skin may form a rigid eschar, with the resulting risks of interruption of blood supply and vascular gangrene.

Treatment of Burns of the Male Genitalia

If the prepuce is very swollen, a dorsal slit should be performed, and if a rigid eschar appears likely to cause a tourniquet effect, then the shaft of the penis should be decompressed by an incision along the entire dorsum (see Fig. 28-1). In cases of full-thickness burns, the skin will be quite insensitive, and it is possible to perform this operation without anesthesia. During the early stages, it

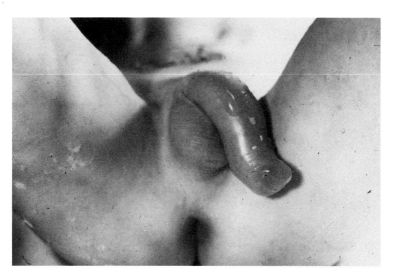

FIG. 28-2. Edema of the penis and prepuce.

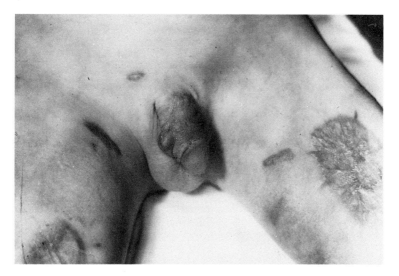

FIG. 28-3. Resolution of the edema with dorsal slit.

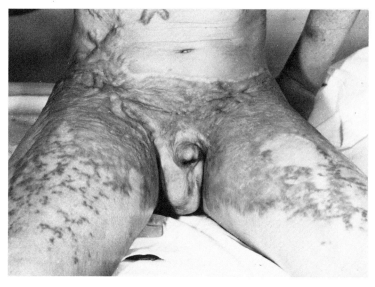

FIG. 28-4. A 13-year-old boy 8 months after an electric and clothing burn that resulted in traumatic hypospadias. This was later repaired using a flap of scrotal skin.

is wise to institute catheter drainage. This can be most conveniently done by a fairly fine Foley catheter.

Any infection of the burn surface readily spreads to the urethra, and urethritis, urethral abscess, and fistula formation may occur. Catheterization will increase the chance of ascending infection, and catheter drainage, therefore, should be used only until the edema has subsided and the patient can urinate with comfort.

LOCAL TREATMENT

Burns of the genital area are not usually suitable for treatment by early excision. Initial treatment should therefore be conservative and directed toward the prevention of infection. After 3 weeks, any areas of partial-thickness damage will have healed spontaneously and the full-thickness skin loss will be demarcated. Attention can then be turned to the removal of sloughs and preparation of the surface for skin grafting.

Burns of the genitalia in children of both sexes can be treated by exposure; a gallows apparatus is employed to give complete and continuous exposure. If the burn dries satisfactorily, then a crust will form which, after some days, will gradually separate from the area of the partial-thickness burn. The crust should be inspected each day, and any part that becomes loose at the edge should be lifted gently and snipped off with scissors. Any crust that is still adherent by the end of 3 weeks almost certainly overlies an area of full-thickness skin loss, and the slough must be removed either by treatment with dressings or by surgical excision (see below).

Treatment of burns of the adult male genitalia by exposure is not suitable, since the greater size and pendulous nature of the parts makes it inevitable that these surfaces will rub together and subsequently become moist and readily infected. Treatment in adults, therefore, is best carried out by antiseptic dressings. In our own experience, Sulfamylon (mafenide) has been most successful for burns of this area. We have used the technique of spreading the Sulfamylon on sheets of gauze that are then applied to the burned areas. No additional packing is placed on the outside of these. In the early stages when there is much exudation, the dressings should be changed every day, and at a later stage, every other day. The dressings are continued either until healing has taken place or until any sloughs of full-thickness destruction are clearly demarcated, which will usually be in about 3 weeks.

Removal of Sloughs of Full-Thickness Skin Destruction

At the end of 3 weeks, the surgeon may continue with treatment by dressings until the sloughs separate spontaneously, or he may surgically excise them. If the area of full-thickness skin destruction is clearly demarcated, surgical excision will save time and is normally the method of choice. If, however, the area of full-thickness destruction is scattered or ill-defined, it will be preferable to continue treatment by dressings until the sloughs have separated spontaneously, thus revealing areas of granulation tissue where the skin has been destroyed. The patient should be bathed or hosed down daily to aid the separation of the sloughs, and any obviously loose tissue should be snipped off with scissors. The dressings may be continued with the original antiseptic preparation (i.e., Sulfamylon), or a change may be made to traditional calcium hypochlorite or sodium hypochlorite dressings. To be effective, calcium hypochlorite dressings should be renewed three times daily.

Resurfacing Areas of Full-Thickness Loss

Occasionally, the inner aspect of the prepuce will survive, and if there has been skin loss on the shaft, the prepuce will be drawn back spontaneously by the healing process and replace the skin of the penile shaft.

Otherwise, any raw areas should be resurfaced with split-thickness skin grafts as soon as the granulations are healthy enough to take grafts (Figs. 28-5 and 28-6). The split skin grafts can be taken from any convenient area and spread on tulle gras to facilitate handling. The grafts can then be treated either by exposure or by dressings, whichever seems most suitable. On the shaft of the penis, it will often be more convenient to apply a light circumferential bandage, but on the scrotum and perineum, the grafts may be laid on and left exposed.

LATE TREATMENT

If a large area has had to be resurfaced by a split-thickness skin graft, particularly if the area of full-thickness loss extends continuously on to the lower abdomen, then it is almost certain that contracture will take place and that there will be insufficient skin for the normal functioning of the penis. Unless there is any particular reason for urgency, it is best to wait until the stage of hypertrophy of the scars has passed (which will usually be in about 9 to 18 months) before carrying out later reconstructive procedures. For the shaft of the penis, division of the contracture and the insertion of a thick split skin graft is a relatively straightforward procedure and often produces good results. If circumferential grafting is necessary, care should be taken to avoid longitudinal scarring by fashioning a zigzag join. In other circumstances, it may be possible to use a flap from the scrotum, and these two methods of repair may be combined.

In cases of traumatic hypospadias due to burns, it will be necessary first to relieve any contractures by the above methods, and then at a later date to reconstruct the urethra either by a modification of the Denis Browne [1] method (perhaps using scrotal flaps to provide external cover) or by implantation of

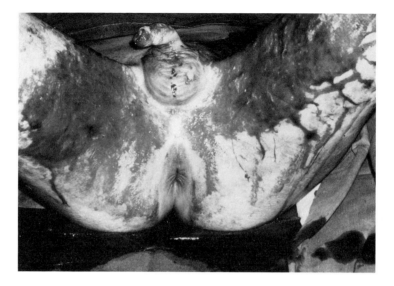

FIG. 28-5.   A gasoline-soaked clothing burn in a 10-year-old 17 days afterward.

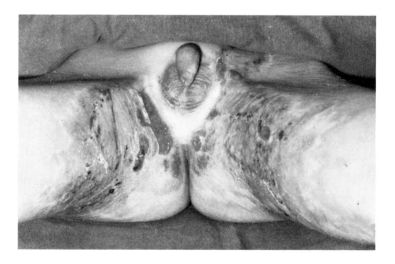

FIG. 28-6.   The same case as shown in Figure 28-5, 3 weeks after grafting.

a Wolfe graft, as described by Horton et al. [2].

Treatment of Burns of the Vulva

Burns of this area are unusual because the area is anatomically well-protected. Burns do occasionally occur, however, as a result of bizarre accidents. A patient came to our attention who had a severe burn in this area due to an accident with a cautery during a gynecological operation.

Treatment of Burns of the Perineum

Burns of the perineum, like burns of the vulva, are rare but do occur as a result of unusual accidents. A man was admitted to our care who had sustained a severe burn of the genitalia and the perineum when the gasoline tank of a motorcycle on which he was riding caught fire. These burns are treated by the same methods as have been outlined above. If full-thickness loss should occur, contractions of this area are troublesome and difficult to treat (Fig. 28-7).

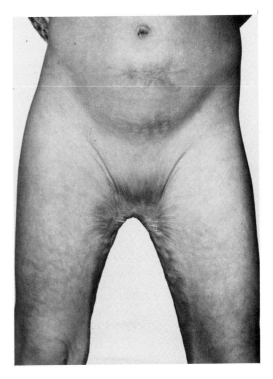

FIG. 28-7. Scarring in a 4-year-old girl 1 year after her pajamas caught fire.

References

1. Browne, D. An operation for hypospadias. *Proc. Roy. Soc. Med.* 42:466, 1949.
2. Horton, C. E., Devine, C. J., Jr., Crawford, H. H., and Adamson, J. E. One Hundred One Stage Hypospadias Repairs. In Sanvenero-Rosselli, G., and Boggio-Robutti, G. (Eds.), *Transactions of the Fourth International Congress on Plastic Surgery,* Rome, 1967. Amsterdam: Excerpta Medica, 1969.
3. Sachs, A. Unpublished paper presented at meeting of British Association of Plastic Surgeons, 1966.
4. Sachs, A. Is the septicaemia/bacteraemia of the disease of burns preventable? In *Report of the First Meeting of the U.K. Section of the International Society for Burn Injuries.* Wembley: Roussel Laboratories, 1968.
5. Shooter, R. A., Gaya, H., Cooke, E. M., Kumar, P., Patel, N., Parker, M. T., Thom, B. T., and France, D. R. Food and medicaments as possible sources of hospital strains of *Pseudomonas aeruginosa. Lancet* 1:1227, 1969.

Avulsion of Penile and Scrotal Skin—I

FRANK W. MASTERS

29

AVULSION of the soft tissue covering of the male genitalia with its accompanying physical and psychological problems poses a complex challenge for the reconstructive surgeon. Although uncommon, this injury in the young male is almost universally accompanied by fear over the potential loss of both sexual potency and reproductive capability. The surgeon must be aware of these associated psychosexual difficulties as well as the multiple problems in the reconstruction of the denuded genitalia.

Avulsion of the skin of the male genitalia may vary from partial loss of penile skin to total denudation of both the shaft of the penis and scrotum. Therapy must be carefully tailored to the individual case not only to provide the necessary soft tissue coverage but also to preserve both reproductive and sexual function if possible. There are, however, general reconstructive principles that serve as a firm foundation for the development of selective therapy.

Anatomical Factors

The characteristic loss of the soft tissue covering of the penis and testes is readily predictable upon a anatomical basis [1, 2]. Unless the entire genital structure is destroyed, separation of the soft tissue covering of the penis occurs in the loose areolar tissue just superficial to Buck's fascia. Because this thick, tough fascial covering protects the underlying urethra and corpora, injury to these structures is uncommon.

The intimate attachment of the dartos muscle to the overlying skin of the scrotum allows avulsion of the scrotal skin between the dartos and the underlying testes. The loose areolar tissue plane beneath the dartos permits loss of scrotal skin without damage to the testis or the spermatic cord. Scrotal loss, however, may be irregular, and often leaves portions of the soft tissue covering behind that may be used to protect the denuded testes. Total loss of the scrotum and its contents is rare.

Avulsion of Penile Skin

Avulsions of the penile shaft may occur singly or in combination with avulsion of varying amounts of scrotal skin. These injuries may be partial or complete, and surgical reconstruction will depend upon the extent of involvement. The skin of the shaft is usually avulsed in a circumferential fashion extending distally to the corona. Proximally, tissue loss is sharply demarcated at the peno-scrotal junction if the scrotum itself is not involved.

Complete avulsion of the penile skin does not pose a difficult reconstructive problem. As with every other soft tissue loss, the ultimate goal of reconstruction is the production of a clean, closed wound with a minimum of scarring; coverage with a split-thickness skin graft is the treatment of choice [2–12].

After thorough cleansing with saline and a mild detergent, an indwelling catheter is inserted and the avulsed penis is carefully debrided, removing all torn and traumatized soft tissue from the base of the shaft to the corona. A small cuff of tissue may be left at the coronal level to be used to anchor the graft. When more than a small cuff is left, however, edema of the distal skin is inevitable. Complete hemostasis is obtained either with fine suture material or pin-point electrocoagulation.

After cleansing and debridement are completed, a split-thickness skin graft is removed from a suitable donor site, usually the anterolateral thigh. The graft is taken as a single sheet between 0.015 and 0.020 inch in thickness, and it is carefully wrapped around the denuded shaft and sutured to itself in a interdigitated fashion to prevent vertical scar contracture. The suture line optimally is placed along the ventrum of the shaft, where the ultimate scar will produce the least functional disturbance (Fig. 29-1).

After the interdigitated edges of the graft are sutured, the proximal end can be carefully sutured to the base of the shaft, and the distal end is sutured to the previously prepared cuff at the level of the corona. These sutures are left long; they can be used to maintain an immobilizing dressing and ensure even pressure upon the underlying graft.

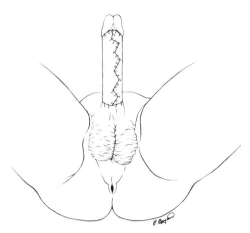

FIG. 29-1. The avulsed penile skin is replaced by a circumferential split-thickness skin graft sutured to itself in an interdigited fashion. The line of closure runs along the ventral surface of the shaft.

Partial avulsions of penile skin present a somewhat more difficult reconstructive problem. The surgeon is tempted to preserve all the remaining uninvolved skin that might be utilized in a definitive repair. This approach, however, may lead to a disastrous result, particularly if the partial avulsion is circular, producing a large distal cuff that will later become edematous.

Utilization of residual penile skin should not be considered unless a very small area of loss exists that can be closed without tension and without the creation of a circumferential scar. A small split-thickness skin graft or preputial full-thickness graft, if available, is most satisfactory for the reconstruction of those avulsions of the dorsum or ventral surface of the shaft that do not extend to the midlateral line nor require closure of the involved soft tissue in a circular fashion.

If the partial loss is more extensive, the defect should be converted to complete denudation that is limited distally by a small cuff of skin at the corona and proximally by the

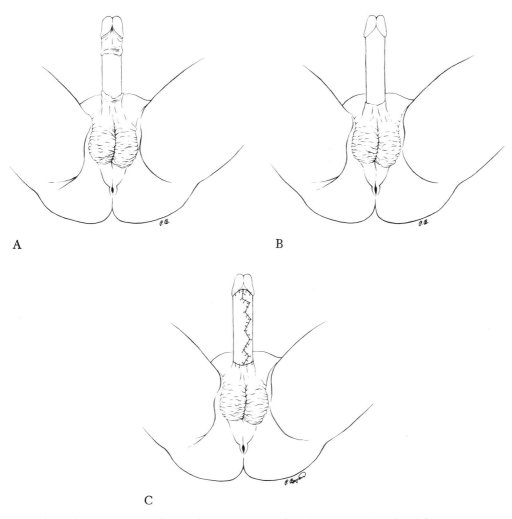

FIG. 29-2. A. Partial circular avulsion of penile skin that cannot be closed by simple suture. B. Complete debridgement to the corona distally and the penoscrotal function proximally is essential. C. Closure is accomplished utilizing an interdigitated split-thickness graft.

penoscrotal junction (Fig. 29-2). Following such debridement, definitive reconstruction can be accomplished by split-thickness skin grafting, as described above.

Although it is tempting to advance the residual redundant penile skin proximally and utilize a split-thickness skin graft to reconstruct that part of the denuded shaft that remains, this is an ill-advised procedure. It

will always produce a thickened edematous distal flap that will persist for months and may never smooth out sufficiently to become the soft pliable covering necessary for erectile function [9] (Fig. 29-3). Even though total denudation may seem to be an unnecessarily radical approach when reliable soft tissue remains attached to the distal shaft, the ultimate result from complete resurfacing of the

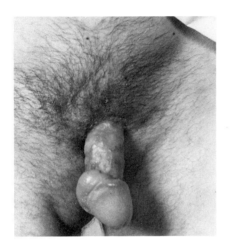

FIG. 29-3. The evident brawny edema of the distal flap persisted for several months after reconstruction. (From F. W. Masters and D. W. Robinson, *J. Trauma* 8:430, 1968. Copyright © 1968, The Williams & Wilkins Co., Baltimore.)

penile shaft with a well-interdigitated split-thickness skin graft remains vastly superior to all other methods of reconstruction.

Avulsion of Scrotal Skin

Avulsion injuries of the scrotum present somewhat different reconstructive problems than those of the penis. Although it is almost always associated with penile injury, the loss of scrotal skin does not follow a particular pattern, nor does the separation of soft tissue occur in a regular fashion because of the underlying dartos attachment. If the scrotum is subjected to a twisting force, the loss may range from a jagged, irregular, partial disruption of the scrotal skin to complete denudation of the testes, and it may even involve the adjacent perineum and upper thigh.

When loss of testicular covering occurs, treatment is designed not only to resurface the soft tissue defect, but also to preserve testicular function. The methods of reconstruction will vary with the extent of soft tissue loss, and the associated care of the denuded testes will determine ultimate reproductive function.

The management of partial loss of scrotal skin is quite different from similar losses of penile soft tissue. In this instance, it is essential to preserve all remaining scrotal skin [9]. Since the scrotum is characteristically capable of stretching, this elasticity may be utilized to produce an adequate functional scrotum. Debridement should be kept to a minimum, in contrast to a similar injury of the penis. Closure is best accomplished by directly suturing the scrotal remnants and then immobilizing the reconstructed scrotum in a supportive dressing until healing is complete (Fig. 29-4). Even though closure is accomplished under some tension, an adequate scrotum will be produced if the testes can be completely covered by residual scrotal skin (Fig. 29-5).

If the entire scrotum or a major portion is lost, preservation of testicular function demands coverage for protection of spermatogenesis. Controlled studies have shown that sperm production is temperature-dependent, and the covered testes cannot be maintained at body temperature and still function [6, 7]. Spermatogenesis can be preserved if the testes are buried in the superficial subcutaneous fat just beneath the skin. If implantation is done at the fascial level, spermatogenesis will be destroyed, since temperature in this region approaches that of the abdominal cavity. Testicular coverage is easily accomplished by immediate implantation of the denuded testes just beneath the skin of the adjacent thigh.

With the patient in the lithotomy position, the perineum, adjacent thighs, and lower abdomen are thoroughly cleansed with saline and a mild detergent, and the avulsed area is irrigated. Sites of implantation can then be marked out on the adjacent thigh at slightly different levels in both the anterioposterior

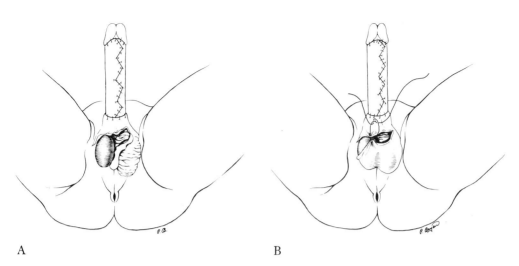

A   B

FIG. 29-4. A. Partial avulsion of the scrotal skin with denudation of one testes. B. Direct suture of the remaining scrotum, even though under some tension, provides adequate soft tissue coverage.

and cephalocaudad directions [6, 7, 9]. It is essential that the testicular implantation take place at an asymmetric level to prevent contact and chronic trauma during ambulation (Fig. 29-6).

The denuded testis and its associated spermatic cord is then buried in a subcutaneous pocket just beneath the skin. Care is taken to place the testis and cord in a relaxed position that can be maintained without tension or torsion, which might interfere with the circulation of the cord [9]. Following implantation, the residual soft tissue defect of the perineum, if any, can be resurfaced with split-thickness skin grafts to complete the immediate soft tissue coverage of the traumatic defect (Fig. 29-7).

After complete healing has occurred, staged reconstruction of the scrotum can be completed if desired, utilizing single pedicle flaps based anteriorly on one thigh and posteriorly on the other and containing the testis and cord (see Figs. 29-6, 8, 9, and 11). After a suitable period of time, these two flaps are elevated, rotated out like the pages of a book,

and sutured one to the other as well as to the perineum at the base of the penis (Fig. 29-9). After circulatory competence of the flaps has been established, the thigh pedicles can be divided and the reconstruction can be completed (Fig. 29-10). All donor sites are resurfaced by split-thickness skin grafts.

Although testicular coverage is essential, thigh flap reconstruction is an elective procedure that permits a more normally appearing scrotum. If the testes are carefully implanted at different levels in the superficial soft tissue of the adjacent thigh (thus allowing mobilization without discomfort and normal testicular function), multiple-staged scrotal reconstruction can be deferred indefinitely if desired.

If the extent of soft tissue destruction prevents the implantation of the testis in the adjacent thigh, the inguinal region may serve as a substitute, and the immediate reconstruction can proceed as previously described. The higher temperatures that result from the proximity to the abdominal cavity, however, may reduce the chances for normal spermato-

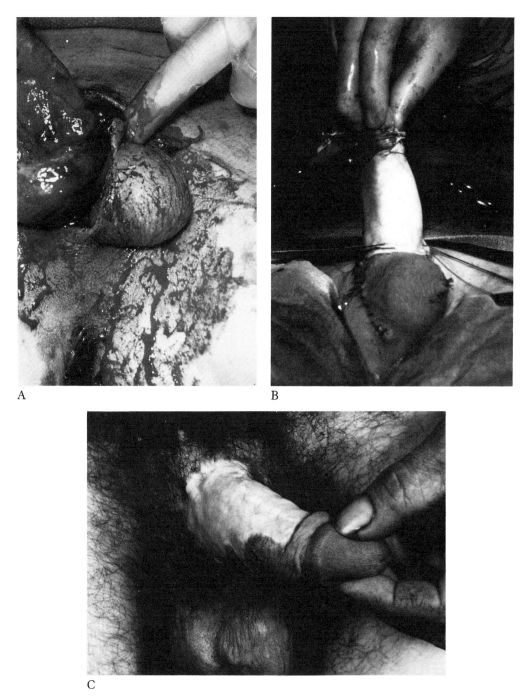

FIG. 29-5. A. Total loss of penile skin and partial scrotal avulsion occurred when clothing was entrapped in mechanized farm machinery. B. The penis was resurfaced with a split-thickness skin graft, and the scrotum was closed by direct suture under tension. C. Postoperatively, a normally functioning penis and scrotum allowed both sexual activity and reproduction. (From F. W. Masters and D. W. Robinson, *J. Trauma* 8:430, 1968. Copyright © 1968, The Williams and Wilkins Co., Baltimore.)

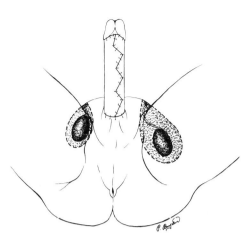

FIG. 29-6. When total loss of scrotal soft tissue occurs, the testes and associated spermatic cords are implanted superficially at different levels in the adjacent thigh without torsion.

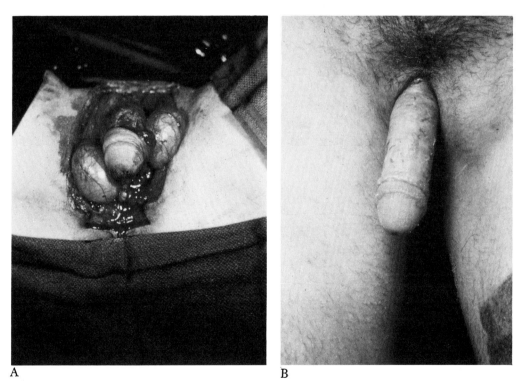

A   B

FIG. 29-7. A. Total avulsion of penile and scrotal skin occurred when the patient's trousers were caught in the power take-off gear of a tractor. B. Immediate reconstruction consisted of an interdigitated split-thickness skin graft for the penile shaft and superficial implantation of the testes beneath the skin of the adjacent thigh. Although no further reconstruction was undertaken, sexual function and reproductive potency remained intact. (From F. W. Masters and D. W. Robinson, *J. Trauma* 8:430, 1968. Copyright © 1968, The Williams & Wilkins Co., Baltimore.)

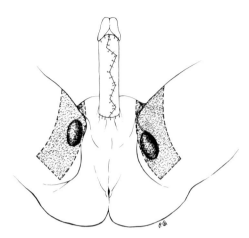

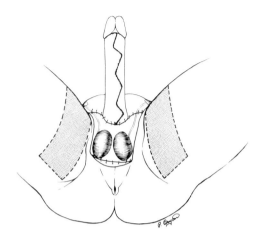

FIG. 29-8. When total scrotal reconstruction is desired, flaps that include the implanted testis and spermatic cord are designed on the adjacent thigh, based in opposite directions.

FIG. 29-9. The flaps containing the testis and spermatic cord are rotated like pages of a book and are sutured to each other and to the perineum at the base of the penis.

genesis. Rarely, the injury is such that implantation beneath either the thigh or inguinal skin is impractical. The entire area is then resurfaced with split-thickness skin grafts. Each testis is covered individually, permitting complete healing of the defect. Unfortunately, testicular function is usually lost by pressure or torsion on the spermatic cord during the contractile phase of the maturing graft.

Postoperative Care

The routine postoperative care of the surgically reconstructed soft-tissue genital envelope does not pose a complex problem. Although the details of such care may vary among surgeons, the care of the grafted penis and reconstructed scrotum is similar to that of any graft or soft tissue wound with the exception of catheter drainage and support. If recurrent erection poses a problem, this can be controlled by the local use of ethyl chloride spray or the oral administration of small

doses of stilbestrol. Amyl nitrite "pearls" may be broken and inhaled to prevent erections. Healing is usually prompt and infection is uncommon, although frequent dressing changes may be needed because of perineal soiling.

A far more complex problem, and one that is often unsuspected, may occur during the immediate postoperative phase due to unexpressed anxiety over the potential loss of sexual function and reproductive capability. These fears may be expressed in a variety of behavioral aberrations that tend to make overall management difficult. Since the loss of sexual capability or sterility are infrequent complications of avulsion of the soft tissue alone, routine reassurance and counseling will tend to allay unnecessary anxiety and allow a more rapid overall recovery. This integral part of postoperative care can be provided by the surgeon in the vast majority of cases. If rehabilitation proceeds slowly and behavioral abnormalities continue to present problems, psychiatric consultation may be of value. Once healing is complete and potency

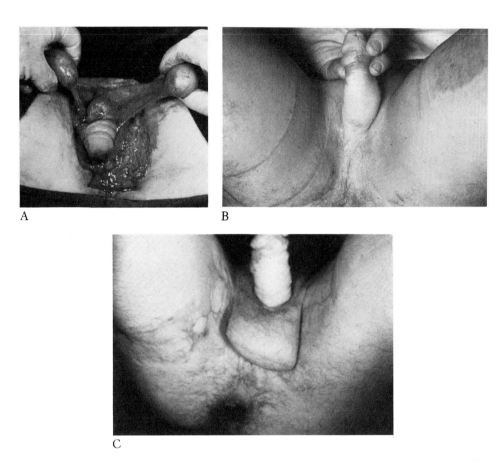

FIG. 29-10. A. Extensive avulsion of the skin of both the penis and scrotum occurred following entrapment in farm machinery. B. The grafted penis is well healed, and the implanted testes are contained within the delayed adjacent thigh flaps. C. Completed scrotal reconstruction containing both testes and spermatic cords. (From F. W. Masters and D. W. Robinson, *J. Trauma* 8:430, 1968. Copyright © 1968, The Williams & Wilkins Co., Baltimore.)

reestablished, however, these inherent fears disappear and social rehabilitation progresses rapidly.*

* *Editor's note:* Our procedure for scrotal avulsion differs slightly from that of Masters. We prefer to assess the blood supply of the denuded testes, and if viability is questionable, then thigh implantation as described by Dr.

Masters is done. If, however, blood supply is good and the tissues around the testes appear adequate, the denuded tissues and testes are sutured together and covered with a split-thickness skin graft. Although this graft will contract considerably, the cuff of scrotal tissue that is usually left at the base will enlarge and stretch, the graft will soften in time, and an adequate scrotum will develop. This will produce a functional and cosmetically acceptable scrotum in one stage.—C. E. H.

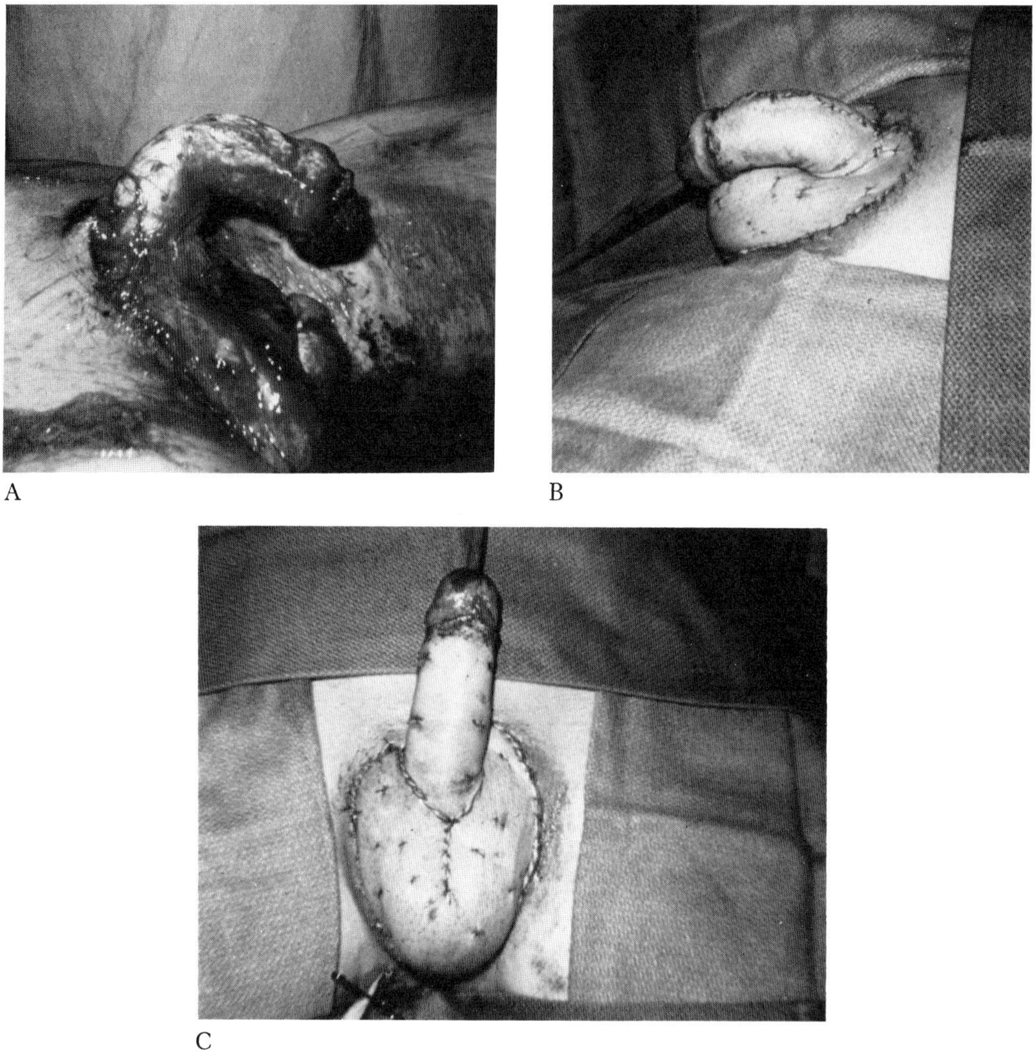

FIG. 29-11. A. Total avulsion of skin of penis and scrotum. B. Split graft, lateral view. C. Split graft, anterior view. (Courtesy of Charles E. Horton and William Tynes, Norfolk General Hospital.)

References

1. Baxter, H., Hoffman, M., Smith, E., and Stern, K. Complete avulsion of the skin of the penis and scrotum: Surgical, endocrinological and psychological treatment. *Plast. Reconstr. Surg.* 4:508, 1949.
2. Byars, L. T. Avulsion of the scrotum and skin of the penis: Techniques of delayed and immediate repair. *Surg. Gynecol. Obstet.* 77:326, 1943.
3. Davis, A. D., and Berner, R. E. Primary repair of total avulsion of the skin from penis and scrotum. *Plast. Reconstr. Surg.* 3:417, 1948.
4. Gillies, H. D., and Millard, D. R. *Principles and Art of Plastic Surgery.* Boston: Little, Brown, 1956. Pp. 368–388.
5. González-Ulloa, M. Severe avulsion of the scrotum in a bullfighter. *Br. J. Plast. Surg.* 16:154, 1963.
6. Huffman, W. C., Clup, D. A., and Flocks, R. H. *Reconstructive Plastic Surgery.* Philadelphia: Saunders, 1964. Pp. 2057–2073.
7. Huffman, W. C., Clup, D. A., Greenleaf, J. S., Flocks, R. H., and Brintnall, E. S. Injuries to the male genitalia. *Plast. Reconstr. Surg.* 18:344, 1956.
8. Malbec, E. F., and Quaife, J. V. Avulsion of scrotum and skin of the penis. *Plast. Reconstr. Surg.* 22:535, 1958.
9. Masters, F. W., and Robinson, D. W. The treatment of avulsions of the male genitalia. *J. Trauma* 8:430, 1968.
10. May, H. Reconstruction of scrotum and skin of penis. *Plast. Reconstr. Surg.* 6:134, 1950.
11. Millard, D. R., Jr. Scrotal construction and reconstruction. *Plast. Reconstr. Surg.* 38:10, 1966.
12. Robinson, D. W., Stephenson, K. L., and Padgett, E. C. Loss of coverage of the penis, scrotum and urethra. *Plast. Reconst. Surg.* 1:58, 1946.

Avulsion of Penile and Scrotal Skin—II

THOMAS GIBSON

30

AVULSION of the skin of the scrotum and penis is often caused by the patient's trousers being caught by a horizontally rotating shaft. The loose folds of material are rolled up, and within them the scrotum is caught. The scrotum is avulsed from back to front, often dragging with it the skin of the penis as far as its attachment at the corona. González-Ulloa [4] has reported a similar injury in a bullfighter who was gored.

There is general agreement that the appropriate technique for resurfacing the penile shaft is split-thickness skin grafting. On the other hand, a wide variety of flaps and grafts, primary or delayed, have been described for scrotal replacement. Many surgeons confronted with the testes dangling freely from the spermatic cords have abandoned any thought of free grafting and have buried the testes in the groin or thigh or fashioned local flaps to cover them.

When I described in 1954 [3] a case in which the testes were free grafted, I was unable to find any previous such case in the literature. The scrotum was still attached to the patient by a thin strip of penile skin. It was completely removed and prepared as a free full-thickness graft. In order to reduce the complexities of the surfaces to be covered, the testes were fixed by catgut sutures to the underlying Colles' fascia and to themselves. The graft, which still retained its typical bag shape, was sutured back in its original position. At first it looked too large for the defect, but by packing acriflavine wool between the stitched edge and the testes, the slack was taken up and the skin over the testes became tense. A certain amount of indirect pressure was thus exerted on the testes, the lower poles of which were left exposed. About two-thirds of the graft survived and healing was complete in 6 weeks.

Balakrishnan [2] reported free grafting of the testes without any previous fixation. He used three split-thickness skin grafts: one to each testis and one passing between them from the root of the penis (which was not avulsed in his case) to the perineum. Many blanket sutures were used to anchor the grafts to the mobile, uneven bed, and an acriflavine wool dressing was employed. Ninety percent of the grafts took. At first, the bifid scrotum had a bizarre appearance, but later, flaps were fashioned from the skin grafts and rearranged to provide a good cosmetic result.

Three cases of split-thickness skin graft replacement of the avulsed scrotum have

463

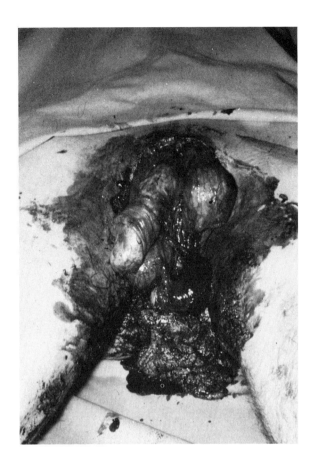

FIG. 30-1.   Avulsion of skin of genitalia. (From Alton [1].)

been described by Alton [1]. He first sutured the testes together but did not fix them to Colles' fascia. The published results are excellent (Figs. 30-1 to 30-2B). By joining the testes to each other, he avoided the bifid appearance of Balakrishnan's case and the need for a secondary operation.

Manchanda et al. [5] reported five cases of free grafting of the testes. They stated that it is the method of choice unless the testes are damaged, in which case temporary insertion in healthy tissue may be worthwhile.

Free skin graft cover not only gives the best cosmetic result, but it would also seem to be the best approach so far as temperature maintenance is concerned. Although the evidence is incomplete, it seems, unfortunately, that testicular atrophy may occur even after free grafting. The only case that has been adequately documented is that of Balakrishnan. Six years after the repair, he recorded low sperm counts with many inactive and abnormal spermatozoa, and a biopsy showed testicular atrophy. So far as I know, there is no record of a patient who suffered this injury having fathered a child.

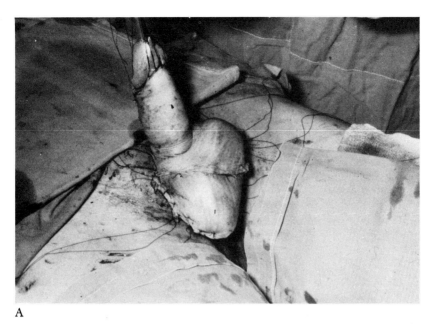

A

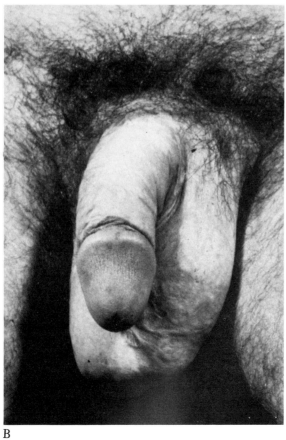

B

FIG. 30-2. A. Full-thickness graft of scrotal skin replaced for coverage. B. Postoperative. (From Alton [1].)

References

1. Alton, J. D. McG.   Complete Avulsion of the Scrotum. In Broadbent, T. R. (Ed.), *Transactions of the Third International Congress of Plastic Surgery*. Amsterdam: Excerpta Medica, 1963. P. 904.

2. Balakrishnan, C. Scrotal avulsion: A new technique of reconstruction by split skin grafts. *Br. J. Plast. Surg.* 9:38, 1956.

3. Gibson, T. Traumatic avulsion of the skin of the scrotum and penis: Use of the avulsed skin as a free graft. *Br. J. Plast. Surg.* 6:283, 1954.

4. González-Ulloa, M.   Severe avulsion of the scrotum in a bullfighter: Reconstructive procedure. *Br. J. Plast. Surg.* 16:154, 1963.

5. Manchanda, B. L., Singh, R., Keswani, R. K., and Sharma, C. G. Traumatic avulsion of scrotum and penile skin. *Br. J. Plast. Surg.* 20:94, 1967.

Reconstruction of the Penis—I

A. J. EVANS

31

THE INDICATIONS for total reconstruction of the penis include traumatic loss by avulsion [9] or gunshot wound [7, 13], amputation for malignancy [4, 6], congenital absence of penis [7], and cases of transexualism [2, 8, 12].

Sir Harold Gillies in 1948 [7] described a method of reconstruction of the penis by means of an abdominal tubed pedicle that contained a urethra formed by turned-in skin flaps. The use of a tubed pedicle flap to form the body of the penis was far from new [1], but attempts at urethral construction by means of free grafts or local scrotal flaps had been disappointing. In many cases, the urethra was simply left to open in the perineum. Gillies considered Frumkin's method [5], in which an abdominal tubed pedicle contained a cartilage graft embedded in the corpora cavernosa, to be sound in principle, but noted the difficulties in forming a urethra and the author's conclusion that no urethra could be incorporated in the body of the new penis.

Gillies himself in previous attempts at penile reconstruction had used an abdominal tubed pedicle containing a free graft on an acrylic rod, and he had also used turned-in abdominal flaps to form a urethra that was then covered with free grafts [7]. These had not been entirely satisfactory, and it seemed reasonable to combine the turned-in flap urethra with the tubed pedicle external cover. In discussing the new method, Gillies stated that it had features in common with a technique suggested by Maltz, although this technique [11] appears impractical since the urethra was to be incorporated within the tubed pedicle in one stage and transferred to the recipient site 2½ to 3 weeks later.

In the Gillies method, the essential steps are:

Stage 1. Formation of the urethra by narrow turned-in skin flaps that are sutured together with the raw surfaces outward. An adjoining double-pedicled skin flap, designed to form the body of the penis, is then moved laterally to cover the urethra.

Stage 2. After 3 weeks, the large flap is tubed in order to contain the previously formed urethra within it.

Stage 3. After a further period of 4 weeks or longer, one end of the pedicle is transferred to the recipient site and urethral anastomosis is performed. It is desirable that the urine be diverted by suprapubic cystostomy or perineal urethrostomy.

Further stages include division of the attached abdominal end of the pedicle, trimming of the free end of the penis and fashioning the new meatus, and the insertion of a cartilage graft to provide rigidity. In the first description of this method, the cartilage was inserted into the fat of the skin flap in the first stage, but it was later recommended [8] that the cartilage graft should be introduced either in the second stage or possibly later, after completion of urethral anastomosis. I am of the opinion, for reasons given later, that the cartilage graft should be deferred until reconstruction has otherwise been completed.

Surgical Technique

STAGE 1

As described by Gillies, the urethra is constructed near the midline of the abdomen, medial to the covering flap, but in a later unpublished case, the position of the flaps was reversed. This location is preferred since the skin near the iliac crest is not hairy and is slightly thinner, which facilitates turning in these narrow flaps.

Two incisions, 6 inches long and 1½ inches apart, are marked out in this area, and ½ inch incisions are made at each end (Fig. 31-1). The two narrow flaps, 6 inches by ½ inch, are carefully undermined, keeping them thin and taking care not to encroach on the central ½ inch strip that provides the blood supply. A rubber catheter is fixed with adhesive along the central strip to facilitate suturing the turned-in flaps. Interrupted fine catgut sutures are used, and care is taken to invert the edges (Fig. 31-2). The covering flap, 8½ inches by 3½ inches, is marked out medially to the urethral flaps; the lateral border is continuous with the medial urethral incision but extends 1¼ inches beyond it at each end. The extremities of the flap may be curved slightly toward the urethra to facilitate its movement in that direction. The double-pedicled flap is now undermined as in preparing an ordinary tubed flap (Fig. 31-3). The usual care is given to hemostasis, particularly to the vessels on the under surface of the flap. The mobilized flap is then moved

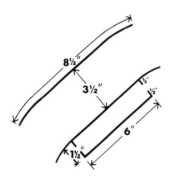

FIG. 31-1. Incisions are marked on the left side of the abdomen for the turned in urethral flaps and bipedicled covering flap.

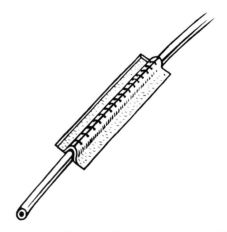

FIG. 31-2. Urethral flaps are sutured with the raw surfaces outward over a rubber catheter.

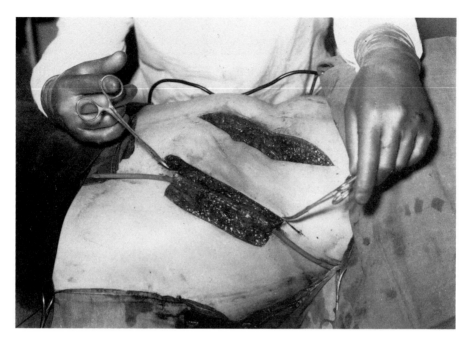

FIG. 31-3. After undermining, the bipedicled flap is to be moved laterally to cover the urethra.

laterally to cover the outer surface of the urethral tube (Fig. 31-4) and is sutured along the outer margins of the urethral incisions. A few fine catgut sutures may be inserted on the under surface of the flap to pin it down on each side of the urethra; they are not essen-

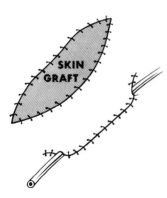

FIG. 31-4. The flap is sutured in position over the urethra.

tial, however, and if there is any risk of producing localized tension, they are best omitted. The free inner margin of the flap is tacked down with interrupted silk sutures, and a split-thickness skin graft is sutured into the remaining defect (Fig. 31-5).

The graft is covered with a firm pressure dressing, but the flap is left exposed and should be inspected frequently in the immediate postoperative period so hematoma can be prevented. The catheter is left within the urethra for 10 to 12 days, and thereafter it is changed every other day.

STAGE 2

Stage 2 is carried out after an interval of 3 weeks. The borders of the flap are incised, and the lateral incision cuts across the previously undivided ends of the urethral floor. Undermining is started from the medial border at the level previously obtained, but is

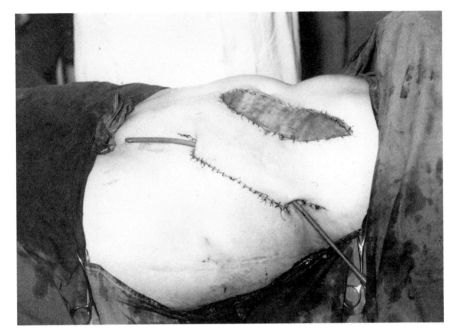

FIG. 31-5. Completion of the first stage.

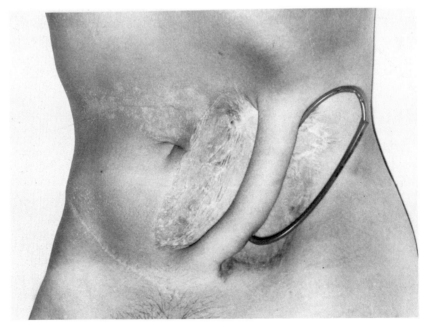

FIG. 31-6. The flap has been formed into a tube containing the new urethra. The rubber catheter is left within the urethra.

deepened as the urethra is approached so that it is raised with the flap. The flap is now tubed in the usual way, but special care is needed in assessing the amount of fat to be retained in order to allow for the incorporation of the urethra. Excess fat must be carefully trimmed away, keeping well clear of the urethra, until it is certain that closure can be obtained without tension. This is a matter of extreme importance, since even a slight amount of postoperative tension within the tube can possibly lead to devitalization of the contained urethra. The catheter is again left as a splint within the urethra, but after healing of the tube has occurred, it is removed daily and the urethra is syringed through to prevent any accumulation of debris (Fig. 31-6).

At this point, if circumstances permit, the patient should be allowed to leave the hospital for several weeks or even months. A period of convalescence not only will benefit the patient's general health, but also will allow the tubed pedicle to mature and soften before the next operative stage.

STAGE 3

After a minimum period of 4 weeks, the upper end of the pedicle is delayed under local anesthesia by an incision across half the width of the attachment. The actual transfer is carried out 1 week later.

The urine is diverted by suprapubic cystostomy or, preferably, by posterior urethrostomy if the local situation permits. The upper end of the pedicle is divided. To provide the further mobility that is particularly necessary for perineal implantation, the lower end of the pedicle may be lengthened by parallel incisions that are carried down toward the pubis. This enables the base to be turned over, and the raw surfaces that are produced are skin grafted (Fig. 31-7). The divided upper end of the pedicle is opened out, and

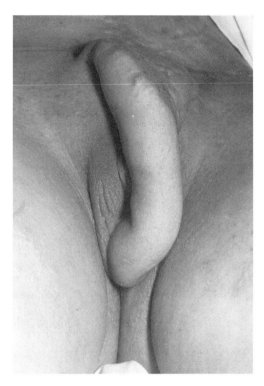

FIG. 31-7. The upper end of the pedicle is attached to the perineum. The base of the pedicle has been turned over and skin grafted to give extra mobility.

the urethra is freed for a distance of about 1 inch. It is then anastomosed obliquely to the urethral stump; good apposition can be obtained with interrupted catgut sutures. The opened end of the pedicle is now let into the surrounding skin. It may sometimes be necessary to sacrifice some of this adjoining skin to ensure a sufficiently wide attachment without bunching of the flap. In perineal implantation, it may be found helpful to splint the lower limbs so the thighs can be kept apart to avoid compression of the pedicle attachment.

The attached end of the pedicle may be divided after 3 weeks. Simple closure is obtained without any attempt at fashioning the tip or rearranging the meatus at this stage,

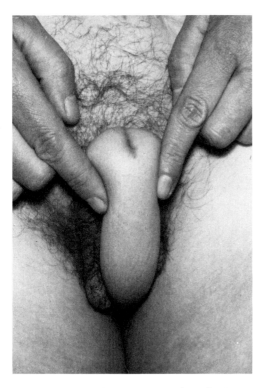

FIG. 31-8. Pedicle transfer and urethral anastomosis have been completed.

since the blood supply is still limited. The final trimming procedure should be postponed for 2 or 3 months (Fig. 31-8).

An alternative method of transferring the pedicle was described by Gillies [7, 8] for cases in which the urethral stump is in the symphyseal region, anterior to the scrotum. After dividing the upper end of the pedicle, the attached base is freed by lengthening the original medial pedicle incision down to the pubis, and the lower end of the tube is rotated medially and downward on a lateral pedicle to permit anastomosis (Fig. 31-9). In cases where this was possible, Gillies considered that it was preferable to somersaulting down the upper end; besides requiring one less stage, it preserved the original superficial epigastric blood supply, and the lymphatic drainage also was not interrupted [8].

To provide rigidity to the new organ, a cartilage graft is later introduced as a separate procedure. Approximately 4 inches of costal cartilage is inserted through an incision at the base of the reconstructed penis to lie in a carefully prepared tunnel in the fat. An attempt may be made to anchor it to the stumps of the corpora cavernosa, as described by Frumkin [5] and recommended by Gil-

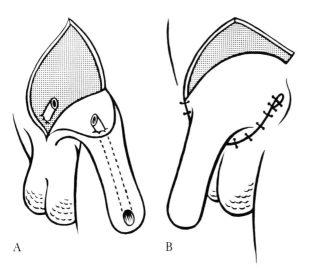

FIG. 31-9. A and B. Alternative method of attaching the lower end of the pedicle by rotating it downward and medially. (After Gillies and Millard [8].)

A   B

that followed inguinal node dissection after amputation of the penis for squamous carcinoma. This necessitates designing the flaps high up near the costal margin and the eventual transfer of the pedicle via the forearm. Their urethral flaps were lateral to the pedicle flap, and they noted the advantage of the hairless skin in this area.

At the second stage, either too short an interval before tubing or excess fat that causes tension within the pedicle may lead to loss of the urethra, a complication that is described below.

The third stage can present difficulties in anastomosing the newly formed urethra to

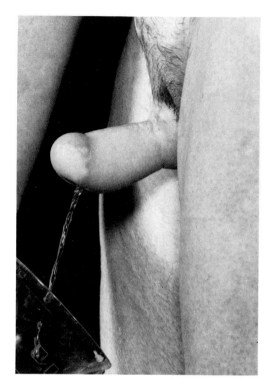

FIG. 31-10. Cartilage has been inserted in the reconstructed penis.

lies, but this is often not practical. Even if a stable attachment of the cartilage at the base is not possible, sexual function can still be achieved. It is probably more important to ensure that there is not too much soft tissue distal to the end of the cartilage, since a "wobbly" tip can be a considerable hindrance to attempted coitus (Fig. 31-10).

Problems in Reconstruction

The first stage of urethral formation and its covering by adjacent skin flaps rarely gives rise to any difficulty. In the Gillies phalloplasty described by Gelb, Malament, and LoVerme [6], planning is complicated by the widespread scarring of the lower abdomen

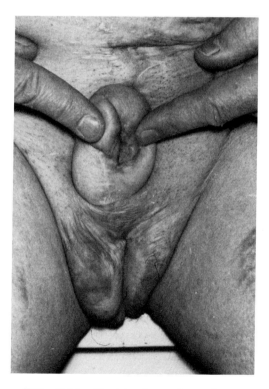

FIG. 31-11. Partial destruction of reconstructed penis was caused by burn from hotwater bottle 7 years after tubed pedicle phalloplasty. (From A. J. Evans, *Br. J. Plast. Surg.* 16:280, 1963.)

the urethral stump, and failure of union with resulting fistula formation is a possible complication. The chance of this occurring is obviously greater if there is a breakdown of the overlying pedicle flap attachment, either because insufficient time has been allowed for the blood supply to develop (accentuated perhaps by delayed healing or hematoma formation after tubing) or because of tension on the suture line. Skin necrosis, with or without urinary leakage, will imperil a cartilage graft, and the presence of such an implant at this stage may itself be a predisposing factor in adding to the tension within the pedicle. For these reasons, it is recommended that cartilage implantation be deferred until later, as noted above.

In some cases, diversion of urine may not have been practical, and urethral suturing over a catheter within the bladder has to be performed. This increases the risk of fistula formation, but fistulization did not occur in the two cases described by Farina and Freire [4] in which anastomosis was performed in this manner. When phalloplasty is performed in female transexuals, the new urethra is joined to a small pouch that is formed by turning in flaps from the labia minora around the existing meatus. In these cases, anastomosis, which has been described by Gillies as "more by juxtaposition than by suture" [8], has been performed over an indwelling catheter. The resulting fistula has had to be closed later in five of the six cases treated in this unit, but there has been no difficulty in obtaining closure and subsequent satisfactory urinary function.

After freeing the attached end from the abdomen, slow healing of the tip of the reconstructed penis may be encountered. This

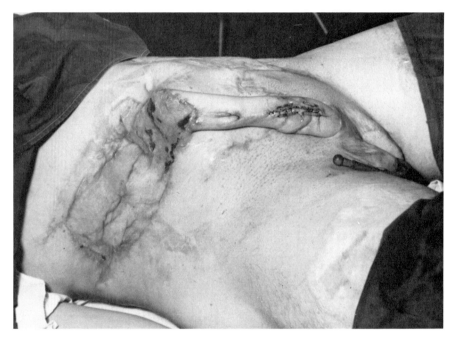

FIG. 31-12. A second pedicle was joined to the stump of the reconstructed penis. Urethral anastomosis was accomplished by a buried skin strip, with tension sutures tied over fine plastic tubing. Urine was diverted by perineal urethrostomy. (From A. J. Evans, *Br. J. Plast. Surg.* 16:280, 1963.)

results from the poor distal circulation that is sometimes seen in a single end-on pedicle attachment. (This also was sometimes found to occur when thumb reconstruction by a tubed pedicle was more in favor than at present.) An indolent stage may be reached in which there is a terminal ulcer with some surrounding induration and a disquieting tendency for the ulcer to increase slowly in size. This occurred in one of our cases, but satisfactory healing followed excision of the ulcer and some of the indurated tissue. Should this not be successful, it would probably be necessary to reattach the end of the pedicle by a small flap to pick up an additional blood supply.

In the following case, which has been more fully described elsewhere [3], poor sensitivity of the pedicle led to its partial loss, 7 years after phalloplasty for traumatic amputation had been performed by Gillies. Although he was aware of the risk, the patient took a hot-water bottle to bed and burned the distal portion of the reconstructed penis, which resulted in the loss of half the length of the organ and the contained urethra (Fig. 31-11). Since he could no longer pass urine without soiling his clothes, a second reconstruction was undertaken in order to lengthen the penis. The pedicle was tubed only 2 weeks after the first stage, and it was also possible that insufficient fat had been removed to permit tension-free closure. The result was that the urethral flap became devitalized and was lost. The pedicle remained healthy, and it was still possible to form a new urethra, using the Denis Browne principle, by burying a strip of pedicled skin that was fortuitously outlined by two parallel scars left after the necrotic urethra had separated. When the pedicle was attached to the penile stump, the urethral ends were left open to form a fistula. This was later closed, again using the buried skin-strip principle (Fig. 31-12) but this time as described by Johanson in his treatment of

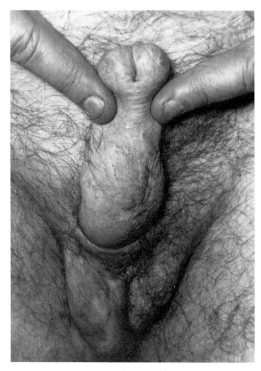

FIG. 31-13. Completion of a second phalloplasty to lengthen the first pedicle that was partly destroyed by the burn injury. (From A. J. Evans, *Br. J. Plast. Surg.* 16:280, 1963.)

stricture [10]. A very satisfactory result was obtained, and the patient was able to pass a good stream of urine through his two-part urethra (Fig. 31-13).

Results

Total reconstruction of the penis by the Gillies method has been performed on nine cases in our unit, five of these being treated by Gillies himself. There were two cases of traumatic loss, one case of congenital absence of the penis, and six cases of transexualism.

Satisfactory urinary function has been achieved in all cases, and it is noteworthy that stricture formation in the new urethra has not occurred in any of these. In one case, intermittent urethral dilatation was necessary, but this was for a stricture in the posterior urethra, which had been damaged in the original avulsion injury.

Cartilage grafts have been inserted in seven cases. Absorption of the cartilage has not been reported, and certainly has not occurred within 5 years of implantation. Sexual function has been possible in five of these cases, was described as unsatisfactory in one, and has not been attempted in the remaining case.

References

1. Borgoras, N. A. Plastic construction of penis (transl.). *Zentralbl. Chir.* 63:1271, 1936.
2. Edgerton, M. T., Knorr, N. J., and Callison, J. R. The surgical treatment of transexual patients. *Plast. Reconstr. Surg.* 45:38, 1970.
3. Evans, A. J. Buried skin-strip urethra in a tube pedicle phalloplasty. *Br. J. Plast. Surg.* 16:280, 1963.
4. Farina, R., and Freire, G. de C. Total reconstruction of the penis. *Plast. Reconstr. Surg.* 14:351, 1954.
5. Frumkin, A. P. Reconstruction of the male genitalia. *Am. Rev. Soviet Med.* 2:14, 1944.
6. Gelb, J., Malament, M., and LoVerme, S. Total reconstruction of the penis. *Plast. Reconstr. Surg.* 24:62, 1959.
7. Gillies, H., and Harrison, R. J. Congenital absence of the penis. *Br. J. Plast. Surg.* 1:8, 1948.
8. Gillies, H., and Millard, D. R. *Principles and Art of Plastic Surgery*. Boston: Little, Brown, 1957.
9. Hoffman, W. C., Culp, D. A., and Flocks, R. H. Injuries of the Male External Genitalia. In Converse, J. M. (Ed.), *Reconstructive Plastic Surgery*. Philadelphia: Saunders, 1964.
10. Johanson, B. Reconstruction of the male urethra in strictures. *Acta Chir. Scand. Suppl.* 176:119, 1953.
11. Maltz, M. *Evolution of Plastic Surgery*. New York: Frobin, 1946.
12. Millard, D. R. Scrotal construction and reconstruction. *Plast. Reconstr. Surg.* 38:10, 1966.
13. Morgan, B. L. Total reconstruction of the penis in an eleven-year old boy. *Plast. Reconstr. Surg.* 32:467, 1963.

Reconstruction
of the Penis—II

VINKO ARNERI

32

BOGORAS [8] in 1936 wrote the first paper cited in the literature on reconstruction of the penis. His first effort at reconstruction was unsuccessful; he tried to use two skin-tubed pedicles from the abdominal wall, one to build the shaft and one to build the urethra. He later reported in 1938 that he had reconstructed 16 cases of absence of the penis, but he had been able to build the urethra in only 10 cases.

Loss of the penis is seen most frequently following injury. Bogoras [8] in 1936, Frumkin [14] in 1944, Maltz [20] in 1946, Gillies and Harrison [16] in 1948, McIndoe [21] in 1948, Majal [19] in 1947, Thorek and Egel [26] in 1949, Kurbanov in 1950, Tagirov in 1958, Morgan [24] in 1963, and Arneri [2] in 1959 have made contributions to the literature. All the above authors used tubed pedicle reconstruction from the abdominal wall. Other surgeons prefer tubed pedicle flaps from the thighs, and Cowan [10] in 1964 and Julian, Klein, and Hubbord [18] in 1969 reported on their techniques with this type of surgery. Goodwin and Scott [17] in 1952 and Morales and colleagues [23] in 1956 advocated reconstruction of the penis from the scrotum.

Loss of the penis may be partial or total. Partial losses are frequently traumatic in origin and may be associated with avulsion of penile and scrotal tissues. Many wartime cases due to gunshot wounds have been reported, occasionally self-mutilation by mentally disturbed patients may occur, and animal bites, thermal injury, and gangrene have also played a part in the etiology of loss of the penis. Radical surgery for cancer of the penis causes extensive loss of tissue, and most cases requiring reconstruction of the penis have occurred in this group.

The penis may have total avulsion or only partial loss of skin or corpora. In cases of partial loss, reconstruction of a new penis is usually not indicated, since sensation and erection are usually possible in the remnants of the corpora. Even a short penis may allow satisfactory coitus and micturition. When the penis is extremely short, however, reconstruction on the penile base may be necessary, even though the reconstructed penis may be lacking in sensation.

Abdominal skin in the form of a tubed pedicle is best suited for a reconstruction of the penis because of its proximity to the genital area and because an ample amount of skin may be obtained in which other material may be incorporated for rigidity and urethroplasty. If abdominal skin is not available, the thigh is the next best donor site, and the scrotum is the least suitable.

Many authors have used various tissues to achieve rigidity of the new penis. Gillies [16], Morgan [24], Bogoras [8], Frumkin [14], Chappell [9], and most Russian authors recommend the use of autogenous cartilage. Goodwin and Scott [17] and Morales and coworkers [23] have used acrylic implants. Periosteal bone grafts have been recommended by Munawar [25]; Lash uses silicone implants. Many authors state that no implant material is necessary, claiming that fibrosis in the tube is sufficient to ensure a rigid penis. The best results in the literature were apparently obtained with the use of autogenous cartilage grafts; acrylic implants have a high rate of failure.

Various techniques have been used to reconstruct the new urethra. The inlay skin graft suggested by McIndoe [21], full-thickness skin grafts, and bladder mucosal grafts have not proved satisfactory in the past. Scrotal skin has been used for urethroplasty; however, the growth of hairs in the new urethra promotes the formation of calcretions and urethritis. Frumkin [14] stated that no urethra could be successfully incorporated in the tube pedicle (quoted by Gillies [16] in 1948). Many authors do not recommend the reconstruction of a new urethral canal, and are satisfied with a new urethral orifice at the penoscrotal junction. Gillies first successfully formed a composite tubed pedicle within a tube, a technique that has been adopted by many authors today. Because the tendency of a buried strip of skin to tube itself has been well-established in hypospadias repair and in esophageal work, it was decided to try this technique in the reconstruction of the penis.

Surgical Technique

It is necessary that the abdominal skin be pliable and free of scars. The remaining external orifice of the urethra should not be stenosed, and the remnant stump of the corpora should be freed of all scar tissue if a functional result is to be expected. It should be carefully explained to the patient that the procedures for reconstruction of the penis are long and fraught with danger, and the patient should be encouraged to cooperate during the entire period of treatment.

FIRST STAGE

A strip of skin 18 cm long and 3 cm wide is formed by two parallel incisions on the thoracoabdominal wall (Fig. 32-1). Two massive sliding flaps on both sides of the original skin strip are then undermined and elevated so they can be sutured together over the strip of buried skin. Two layers of subcutaneous catgut sutures and one layer of nylon sutures in the skin are recommended for the skin. A specially constructed apparatus to prevent skin tension at the suture line is then applied (Fig. 32-2). (This apparatus is also used routinely to reconstruct the esophagus.)

SECOND STAGE

Four or five weeks later, the buried strip of skin has been fully converted into a skin canal, and a No. 24 French catheter should be easily introduced into the channel. A composite tubed pedicle 20 cm long is formed by incisions on each side of the new skin canal (Fig. 32-3). The distance between the two incisions should be 10 to 12 cm. The skin canal for the urethra should be raised intact with the bipedicled flap. A cartilage graft is

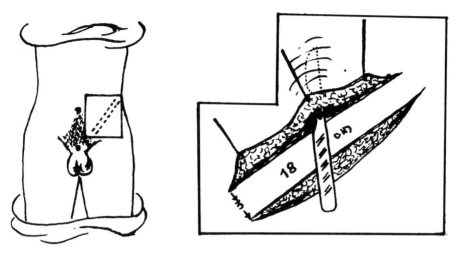

FIG. 32-1.   First stage. The strip of skin 3 cm by 18 cm is outlined by two parallel incisions. Extensive undermining of lateral flaps is performed with a sharp scalpel.

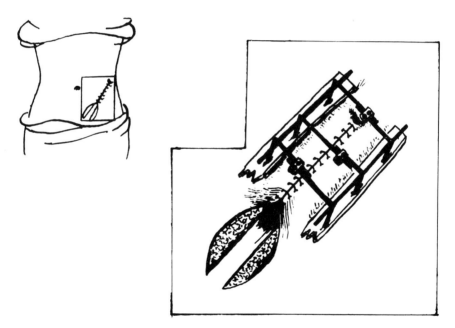

FIG. 32-2.   The edges of the lateral flaps are sutured over the buried strip of skin. A special appliance is fixed over the lateral flaps to keep them in place and to prevent hematoma.

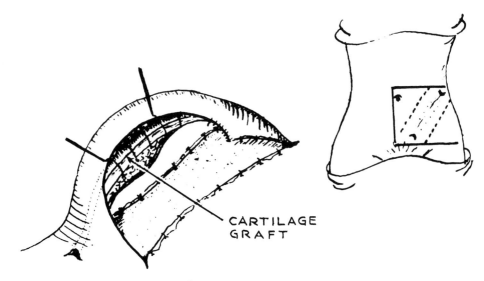

FIG. 32-3. Second stage. The dotted lines in the inset indicate the incisions made to raise the composite tubed pedicle. The tube is raised. The cartilage graft is sutured in position along the outer surface of the skin canal. The tube's bed is covered with a skin dermatome graft.

then taken from the eighth or ninth rib on the right side of the thorax. It is carved in the shape of a rod, and fixed with catgut along the skin canal. This tube, with the cartilage and urethra enclosed, now represents the future penis (Fig. 32-4). The abdominal tube must be free of all tension, and a correct estimate of the size of the tube is of utmost importance. A split-thickness skin graft is used to cover the defect of the abdominal wall.

THIRD STAGE

Five or six weeks after the second stage, a perineal urethrostomy is performed. The abdominal tube is moved to the stump of the penis by cutting the proximal end of the tube (Fig. 32-5) and joining it directly to the base of the penis. If the tube is not pliable enough, the wrist may be used as a carrier for the tube. To perform the anastomosis to the base of the penis, the scars are excised and the

corpora are carefully dissected free. The distal end of the original urethra is mobilized, and an end-to-end anastomosis with the skin urethra is performed (Fig. 32-6). The cartilage graft is inserted between the two corpora and stitched into the interseptum with 4-0 chromic catgut sutures. A direct, end-to-end anastomosis between the skin urethra and the original urethra is performed, using 4-0 chromic catgut sutures (Fig. 32-7). The edges of the skin tube are sutured to the skin edges of the penis.

FOURTH STAGE

The last operation is postponed for 4 to 5 weeks and is done under local anesthesia. At this time, the distal end of the abdominal tubed pedicle is divided, and the terminal end of the skin urethra is sutured to the edges of the skin of the tube. The penis end is shaped by excising redundant skin and fat from the end of the tube.

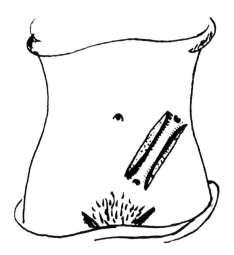

FIG. 32-4. The composite tubed pedicle incorporating the skin canal (new urethra) and the rib cartilage.

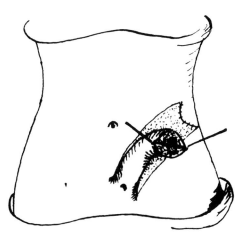

FIG. 32-5. Third stage. The proximal end of the tube is cut. The opening of the skin urethra is freed by 2 cm, while the cartilage graft is freed by 3 cm.

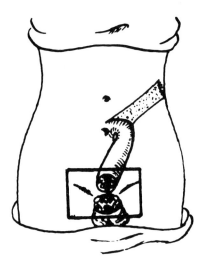

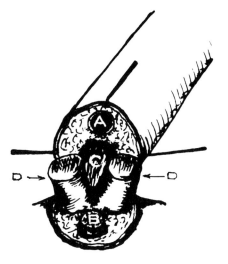

FIG. 32-6. The tube is approximated to the original urethra (*insert*). The cartilage graft (*C*) is implanted in the interseptum of the remnants of the corpora cavernosa (*D*). The opening of the skin urethra (*A*) in the tube will be moved toward the original urethra (*B*).

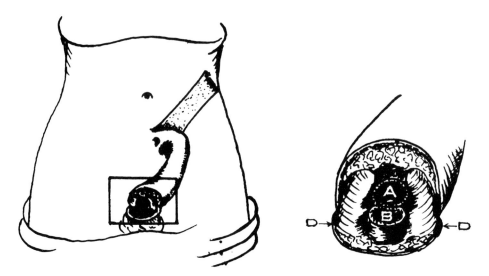

FIG. 32-7. The two openings (*A* and *B*) are anastomosed by subcuticular stitches of chromic catgut.

Results

In seven cases so treated—in which there was loss of the penis due to sexual crime in three, to radical excision for cancer in three, and to a gunshot wound in one—we found that erection was possible in four cases in which remnants of the corpora cavernosa had been preserved. One patient reported that he became the father of a male infant; the patient stated, however, that digital pressure was needed to void sperm on ejaculation (Fig. 32-8).

In cases where the remnants of the corpora cavernosa had not been preserved, a static penis was obtained (Fig. 32-9). The psychological effect of reconstruction, however, was still beneficial. Three patients were able to engage in coitus by introducing the penis manually. No dilatation procedures were necessary in any of these seven reconstructed urethras. Erotic stimulation for the first 2 years postoperatively occurred principally from the corpora or from the pubic area. In

a follow-up study of over 12 years, it was found that the terminal end of the new phallus apparently became more sensitive, although it never reached the normal sensibility of the uninjured penis.

Complications

Most complications involve sloughing strictures and fistula formation. The only fistulas encountered in our series occurred in two of the seven cases. In both cases, they were between the artificial urethra and the original urethral stump. One case healed spontaneously, and in the second case a reanastomosis was performed 16 days after primary surgery, and closure was achieved at that time. A catheter was left indwelling during the secondary operative procedure. No strictures were noted in any of the cases, and the implanted cartilage was retained without rejection.

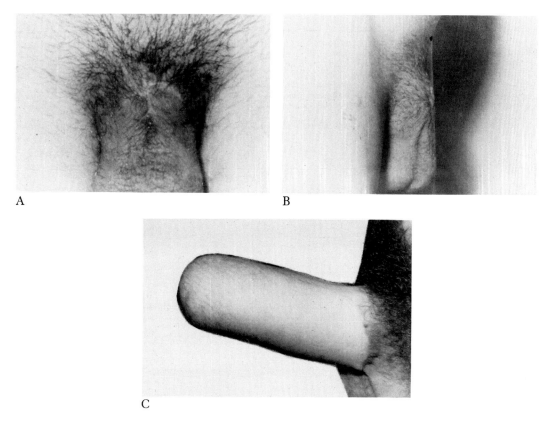

A

B

C

FIG. 32-8. A. Total amputation of the penis for a sexual offense. Corrective urethrostomy was necessary for stricture before the reconstruction was undertaken. B. The remnants of the corpora cavernosa are buried under the scars and can be palpated. C. The condition 10 years after phalloplasty. The penis is shown in erection. This is possible due to the action of the remnants of corpora cavernosa.

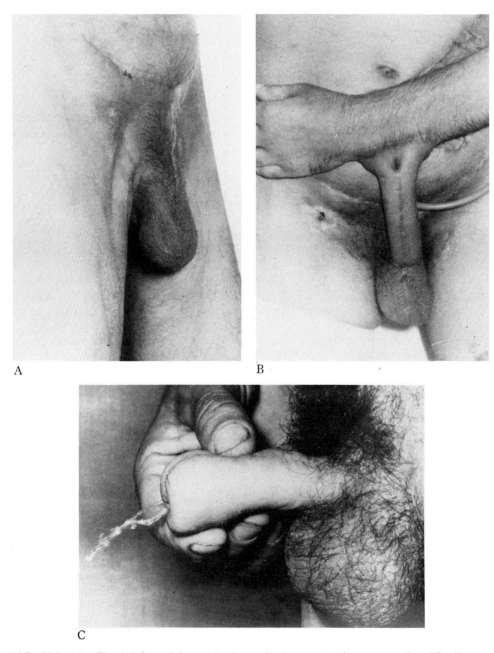

FIG. 32-9. A. Total defect of the penis after radical operation for cancer. B. The "composite" tube has been transferred to the pubic region through the wrist carrier because of the rigid skin of the tube as result of x-ray treatment. The opening of the skin canal on the tube will represent the external orifice of the urethra after the tube is divided from the wrist. C. Erection is not possible because of the radical resection of the corpora cavernosa. Micturition is effected normally.

References

1. Alanis, S. Z. An innovation in total penis reconstruction. *Plast. Reconstr. Surg.*, 1963. Vol. 43.

2. Arneri, V. *Phalloplasty* (film). London: 2nd International Congress of Plastic Surgery, 1959.

3. Arneri, V. Reconstruction of skin oesophagus—a new method. *Br. J. Plast. Surg.* 17:413, 1964.

4. Bergman, R. T., Howard, A. H., and Barnes, R. W. Plastic reconstruction of the penis. *J. Urol.* 59:174, 1948.

5. Best, J. W., Angelo, J. J., and Milligan, B. Complete traumatic amputation of penis. *J. Urol.* 87:134, 1962.

6. Bjalij, M. I. Phalloplastica for impotence. *Urol. Nefrol.* (Moskva), 1962. Vol. 6.

7. Blum, V. A case of plastic restoration of the penis. *J. Mount Sinai Hosp. N.Y.* 4:506, 1938.

8. Bogoras, N. A. Ueber die volle plastische Wiedenherstellung eines zum Koitus fähigen Penis. *Zentralbl. Chir.* 63:1271, 1936.

9. Chappell, B. S. Utilization of the scrotum in reconstruction of the penis. *J. Urol.* 69:703, 1953.

10. Cowan, R. J. Total reconstruction of the penile urethra following a gunshot wound. *Br. J. Plast. Surg.* 17:66, 1964.

11. Evans, A. J. Buried skin-strip urethra in a tube pedicle phalloplasty. *Br. J. Plast. Surg.* 16:280, 1963.

12. Farina, R., and Freire, G. de C. Total reconstruction of the penis. *Plast. Reconstr. Surg.* 14:351, 1954.

13. Fleming, J. P. Reconstruction of the penis. *J. Urol.* 104:213, 1970.

14. Frumkin, A. P. Reconstruction of the male genitalia. *Ann. Rev. Soviet Med.* 2:14, 1944.

15. Gelb, J., Malament, M., and LoVerme, S. Total reconstruction of the penis. *Plast. Reconstr. Surg.* 24:62, 1959.

16. Gillies, H., and Harrison, R. J. Congenital absence of the penis. *Br. J. Plast. Surg.* 1:8, 1948.

17. Goodwin, W. E., and Scott, W. W. Phalloplasty. *J. Urol.* 68:903, 1952.

18. Julian, R., Klein, M., and Hubbord, H. Management of the thermal burn with amputation and reconstruction of the penis. *J. Urol.* 101:580, 1964.

19. Majal, V. S. New principles in the reconstruction of the penis. *Khirurgija* 2:85, 1947.

20. Maltz, M. *Evolution of Plastic Surgery.* New York: Frobin, 1946.

21. McIndoe, A. Deformities of the male urethra. *Br. J. Plast. Surg.* 1:34, 1948.

22. McRoberts, J. W., Chapman, W. H., and Ansell, J. S. Primary anastomosis of the traumatically amputated penis. *J. Urol.* 100:751, 1968.

23. Morales, P. A., O'Connor, J. J., and Hotchkiss, R. S. Plastic reconstructive surgery after total loss of the penis. *Am. J. Surg.* 92:403, 1956.

24. Morgan, B. L. Total reconstruction of the penis in an eleven-year old boy. *Plast. Reconstr. Surg.* 32:467, 1963.

25. Munawar, A. Surgical treatment of the male genitalia. *J. Int. Coll. Surg.* 27:352, 1957.

26. Thorek, P., and Egel, P. Reconstruction of the penis with a split-thickness skin graft. *Plast. Reconstr. Surg.* 4:469, 1949.

War Wounds

JOSEPH R. ZBYLSKI

33

Foreword

With the development of new and more potent weapons for the soldier in land warfare and with the necessity for increased mobility that required discarding fixed or trench warfare, the infantry soldier is more susceptible to multiple wounding, especially in the lower half of the body. The new types of wounds created have stimulated the development of new and better methods of surgical treatment for the soldier. In turn, these new methods also benefit the civilian population, especially automobile accident victims whose self-destruction and mutilation is often due to the use of such weapons as alcohol and drugs.

With the more liberal sexual attitudes and states of undress that abound, it seems fitting that a plastic and reconstructive surgeon, with his specialized training to reestablish function of a part, and also to reestablish the cosmesis of the part, be chosen to write this chapter on war wounds of the external genitalia.

The personal surgical experiences of Dr. Zbylski in the Vietnam War lend added veracity to his words. I should like to emphasize an important point that the author briefly mentions. The triaging of patients necessitates the complete removal of all clothing and careful inspection of all areas to avoid missing a penetrating wound, especially about the folds around the genitalia, perineum, and buttocks. This practice in Vietnam paid magnificent dividends.

—Lt. Gen. H. B. Jennings, Jr., Surgeon General of the Army

WAR WOUNDS of the external genitalia are not a common injury. However, statistics from previous wars show that urological injuries represent 2 to 4 percent of the total casualties. Of these injuries, 50 to 70 percent are of the external genitalia (Table 33-1). In modern mobile warfare, a higher incidence of external genitalia wounds has been noted than in the trench warfare of World War I [6]. Of over 13,500 casualties in the Vietnam War, it was estimated that 2 to 3 percent were wounds of the external genitalia [1].

In Vietnam, a higher proportion of wounds caused by mines and booby traps has been observed than in previous wars. These wounds, caused by high-velocity particles at close range, are characterized by extensive tissue destruction (Fig. 33-1). The vast majority of wounds of the external genitalia are associated with abdominal or lower extremity injury (Fig. 33-2). Tremendous contamination of the wounds is present. This is the result of secondary missiles consisting of clothing, dirt, and vegetation. Associated rectal and bladder injuries add to the contamination.

Adequate wound debridement of these highly contaminated wounds is mandatory. The removal of devitalized tissue and foreign bodies must be done to prevent infection and allow adequate wound healing. A land-mine burst may release fragments at a velocity of 5,000 feet per second (Fig. 33-3). Hand-grenade booby trap fragments may strike an individual 20 feet from the burst at a velocity of 2,000 feet per second. A 150-grain bullet from an AK-47 rifle has a muzzle velocity of 2,800 feet per second and can cause extensive damage.

The great vascularity of the penis and scrotum usually permits conservative soft tissue debridement. However, this excellent vascularity creates problems of hemostasis. If bleeding is not controlled following debridement and adequate drainage is not provided, hematoma formation may later compromise the viability of an injured testis or a previous urethral repair.

Injury to the external genitalia is usually associated with wounds of the perineum, abdomen, or lower extremities. Diagnosis can usually be established by inspection of the wound, palpation of the tissue, rectal examination, and passage of a urethral catheter.

Isolated wounds of the perineum and external genitalia may be easily overlooked when attention is directed initially to the more obvious abdominal or lower extremity wounds. The surgeon triaging large numbers of casualties may initially miss a single fragment wound of the scrotum or penis. However, the routine practice of removing all the patient's clothing during triage and examining the external genitalia and perineum will obviate this. The presence of a penetrating fragment or gunshot wound of the perineum or external genitalia necessitates a rectal examination, insertion of a urethral catheter, and roentgenography to determine the presence of unsuspected upper genitourinary tract injury. Blood at the urethral meatus may mean a urethral injury, and a urethrogram is

TABLE 33-1. Incidence of Wounds of External Genitalia

War and Author	Genitourinary Injury (%)
World War I	
Young [11]	29.4
World War II	
Culp [3]	50.0
Kimbrough [5]	68.1
Korean War	
Schwartz [9]	59.0
Vietnam War	
Busch et al. [2]	66.7
Salvatierra et al. [8]	45.2

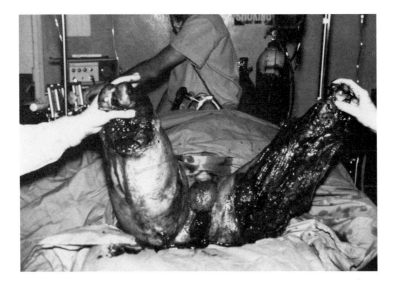

A

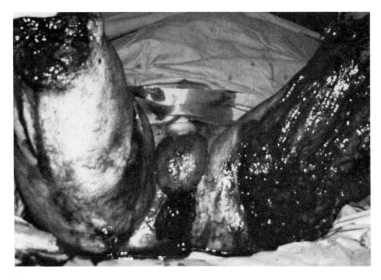

B

FIG. 33-1. A and B. Bilateral high thigh amputation in addition to wounds of the external genitalia.

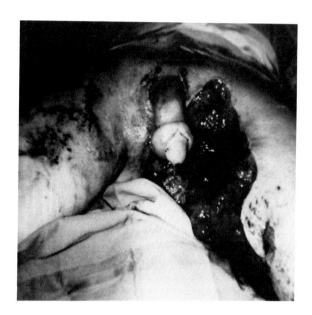

FIG. 33-2. Extensive fragment wounds of the thigh, perineum, rectum, and external genitalia.

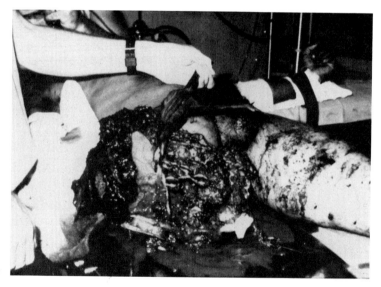

FIG. 33-3. High thigh traumatic amputation and wounds of external genitalia as the result of a land-mine blast.

required to localize the site of injury [4]. Only after intraabdominal injury has been ruled out should attention be directed toward definitive treatment of the external genitalia.

In wounds that are caused by high-velocity missiles and that show extensive damage and skin loss, debridement and hemostasis should be obtained and a delayed primary closure performed. The principle of doing a delayed primary closure of the skin applies to extensive war wounds of the external genitalia as well as other portions of the body. The small, low-velocity fragment wound of the penis or scrotum, however, can usually be closed provided adequate debridement has been performed and the wound in not closed under tension. Extensive reconstruction of high-velocity fragment wounds of the penis and urethra with layer closure of the defects usually results in wound break-down and subsequent increased morbidity [10].

Recognition of injury, diversion of the urinary stream, adequate drainage, control of hemorrhage, and repair of the defect are the principles of early management of genitourinary tract injuries. These principles, as outlined by Patton [7], apply equally well to the management of the external genitalia injury.

Penile Injuries

The major problems in wounds of the penis are urethral injury, maintenance of penile length, prevention of further penile deformity, and control of hemorrhage.

Debridement should be minimal. An anatomical approximation of Buck's fascia is important in preventing later penile deformity. No attempt should be made to remove minute foreign bodies from the corpora cavernosa. With large defects in the corpora cavernosa and Buck's fascia, it may be impossible to do a layer closure without angulation

of the penis. In these cases, the defects should be left open.

Penile skin may be closed loosely with interrupted sutures. With larger skin losses, the skin may be left open, dressed, and later closed with a split-thickness skin graft. Undermining of skin and closure of a wound under tension will result in circumferential constriction or wound breakdown. A light compressive dressing may be applied to splint the penis. In uncircumcised penises, care should be taken to prevent constriction of the glans that may result from latent edema and cause paraphimosis. Such a constriction may necessitate a dorsal slit in the prepuce. Prepuce skin should not be resected, since it may be of value later for possible use in reconstruction, especially in extensive injuries to the penis with associated urethral injury.

If the penis is completely denuded, it may be placed in a scrotal tunnel if there is no associated injury to the scrotum. Otherwise, it should be dressed and later a split-thickness skin graft can be applied. An almost completely severed penis can sometimes survive following meticulous debridement, fine suturing, and postoperative splinting.

Urethral damage is frequently associated with penile injury. Massive destruction and partial amputation of the penis usually results in some urethral injury. Injuries of the penile urethra are managed according to the nature of the missile, size of the wound, extent of soft tissue damage, and continuity of the urethra. Penetrating or perforating wounds of the urethra caused by small, low-velocity missiles may be closed with fine atraumatic chromic catgut sutures over an indwelling catheter stent. A Silastic catheter is preferable. The indwelling catheter should not be so large as to obstruct the periurethral glands. Minimal debridement of urethral and periurethral soft tissue should be done. Some wounds are better managed by diversion of the urinary stream by either a perineal urethrostomy or suprapubic cystostomy. The urethral wound should then be closed over a catheter stent. If desired, this can be removed after the layer closure of the penis, since there is some feeling that the presence of a catheter stent in the area of the repair impairs healing and adds to the incidence of later stricture and fistula formation.

Complete severance of the urethra with small segmental loss can usually be repaired over an indwelling urethral catheter stent. The corpus cavernosum urethra can usually be mobilized a few centimeters for closure or anastomosis. The stent may be removed and proximal urinary diversion can be obtained by either suprapubic cystostomy or perineal urethrostomy. If difficulty is encountered in passing a catheter or in locating a severed proximal end of the penile urethra, interlocking urethral sounds may be passed proximally through the open bladder and distally from the glans. Extensive injuries to the urethra with large segmental loss may best be debrided, and the urethra can then be sutured to the adjacent skin edges as in a first-stage Johanson procedure [4a, 8]. Following wound healing, the patient will void as through a hypospadial penis. Reconstruction of the urethra can be done at a later stage. Attempts at primary urethral repair of extensive injuries result in stricture and fistula formation.

Scrotal and Testicular Injuries

All penetrating injuries of the scrotum should be explored. Frequently, there are associated penetrating intraabdominal injuries with the scrotum as the wound of entrance. Placement of an indwelling catheter is mandatory to assess early the possibility of injury to the upper urogenital tract. Small wounds of entrance of the scrotum should be opened widely with minimal debridement of the scrotal tissue itself. Special care should be taken to control the skin bleeding and any bleeding of the fascial layers. Loss of scrotal tissue due to contractility of the skin is usually more apparent than real. The spermatic cord and structures should be carefully inspected for vascular injury or other possible damage. The testes should be observed for color and bleeding. Herniation of the testes through a torn scrotum frequently occurs (Fig. 33-4). The testes should be cleansed and returned to the scrotal compartment after widely opening the scrotum. Any constricting fascia or tunica vaginalis layers should be resected and hemostasis obtained prior to returning the testes to the sac. The testes should be fixed with a chromic catgut suture to prevent torsion. Completely avulsed scrotal skin with exposure of viable testes necessitates implantation of the testes beneath the skin of the thigh or coverage with split-thickness skin grafts. If the testis is lacerated with extrusion of the seminiferous tubules, minimal debridement of the devitalized tissue may be performed, and the tunica albuginea can be sutured with fine chromic catgut.

Extensive injury to the testes with obvious nonviability (as evidenced by absence of bleeding during debridement) may necessitate orchiectomy. Complete transection of the cord will also necessitate orchiectomy. Every effort, however, should be made to save the testes. Hematoma of the cord should be evacuated and bleeding controlled. Preservation of the internal spermatic artery is important to maintain the viability of the testes. Because of the extensive venous plexus of the cord, viability of the testes may still be present in spite of extensive venous oozing to the cord.

Following debridement and return of the testes to the sac, the scrotum should be drained with a soft rubber Penrose drain,

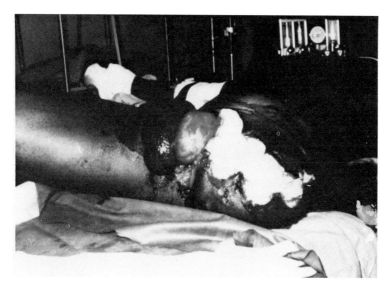

FIG. 33-4. Herniation of the left testis through a scrotal tear as the result of a blast injury with left high thigh amputation.

and the scrotal skin closed loosely with interrupted sutures. A light compressive dressing with scrotal support should be applied.

Antibiotics should be used in injuries of the external genitalia, especially if indwelling catheters are present. Patients with minor injuries and an indwelling catheter may be treated with a sulfonamide or a bacteriostatic agent. The presence of extensive injury to the genitalia or perineum should be treated with broad-spectrum antibiotics.

References

1. Aaby, G. USARV Surgery Consultant's Report, July 1967–June 1968. Pp. 35–40.
2. Busch, F. M., Chenault, O. W., Zinner, N. R., and Clarke, B. G. Urological aspects of Vietnam war injuries. *J. Urol.* 97:763, 1967.
3. Culp, O. S. War wounds of the genitourinary tract. *J. Urol.* 57:1117, 1947.
4. Herwig, K. R. Injuries of the Anterior Urethra. In *Proceedings of the Kimbrough Urological Seminar, Walter Reed General Hospital.* Washington, D.C., October 28–31, 1968.
4a. Johanson, B. Reconstruction of the male urethra in strictures. *Acta Chir. Scand. Suppl.* 176:119, 1953.
5. Kimbrough, J. C. War wounds of the urogenital tract. *J. Urol.* 55:179, 1946.
6. Kimbrough, J. C. Management of genitourinary wounds in the combat zone. *Milit. Surg.* 115:165, 1954.
7. Patton, J. F. Management of Genito-urinary and Perineal Injuries. In *Symposium on Treatment of Trauma in the Armed Forces.* Walter Reed Army Medical Center, XXII–1–8 March 1962.
8. Salvatierra, O., Rigdon, W. O., Norris, D. M., and Brady, T. W. Vietnam experiences with 252 urological war injuries. *J. Urol.* 101:615, 1969.

9. Schwartz, J. W.   The early management of genito-urinary war wounds. Recent advances in medicine and surgery (19–30 April 1954) based on professional medical experiences in Japan and Korea 1950–1953, Army Medical Service Graduate School, Walter Reed Army Medical Center. *Medical Science Publication No. 4,* 458–467.

10. Wettlaufer, J. N.   Experiences with Vietnam GU Tract War Wounds in Japan. In *Proceedings of the Kimbrough Urological Seminar, Walter Reed General Hospital.* Washington, D.C., October 28–31, 1968.

11. Young, H. H.   Wounds of urogenital tract in modern warfare. *J. Urol.* 47:59, 1942.

Vaginal Reconstruction Following Extended Abdominoperineal Resection For Anorectal Tumor

W. M. COCKE

34

I N WOMEN with carcinoma of the ano-rectal canal, it is often necessary to extend the standard abdominoperineal resection to include the entire posterior wall of the vagina, the posterior labia, the contents of the ischiorectal fossa, and a wide amount of skin and subcutaneous tissue [6]. Vaginal reconstruction of this large perineal defect enables these unfortunate women to return to sexual activities, and if they are premenopausal, to use standard techniques to absorb bleeding during menstruation.

Surgical Technique

Gluteal and perineal flaps can be used to replace the tissue that has been resected. These flaps are designed to replace the lining of the posterior vagina and to cover the perineal defect from the vagina to the coccyx (Fig. 34-1).

A spinal or general anesthetic may be used. The patient is placed in the jack-knife position. The skin and subcutaneous tissue surrounding the remaining vaginal vault is raised, folded back, and sutured on itself (Fig. 34-2). This maneuver inverts the skin so that it forms the inner lining of the posterior vagina. A delay of these flaps may be indicated. The large gluteal flap, which also may have been previously delayed, is then rotated over these previously folded-back lining flaps (Fig. 34-3). The skin of the lining flap is sutured to the skin of the covering flap to create the posterior fornix (Figs. 34-5 and 34-7). The donor site of the gluteal flap is closed with a split-thickness skin graft (Figs. 34-4 and 34-6).

The patient is kept in the prone position

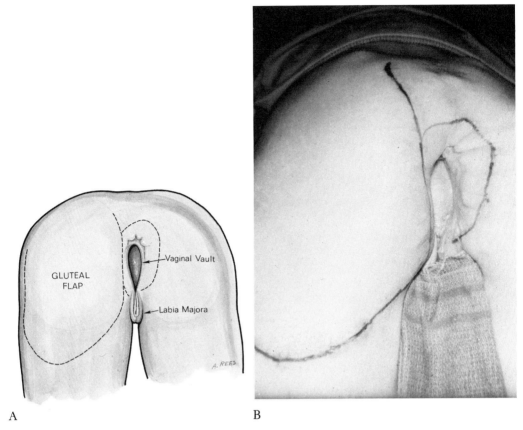

FIG. 34-1. A. Perineal defect. B. Operative view of the perineal defect. (From W. Cocke, B. Bolasny, and J. Sawyers, *Plast. Reconstr. Surg.* 46:372, 1970. Copyright © 1970, The Williams & Wilkins Co., Baltimore.)

with an indwelling catheter for bladder drainage. Packing of the vaginal vault is not necessary. The skin graft to the flap donor site is held in place with a stent dressing. Sutures are removed at the end of a week.

Discussion

This procedure uses well-established techniques and principles to solve a specific problem. Free skin grafts have been used for vaginal reconstruction after irradiation treatment or pelvic exenteration for cancer.

Pratt and Smith [5] reported using the sigmoid loop for vaginal reconstruction following ablative gynecological surgery. Most of their patients had carcinoma of the vagina and cervix. Simmons and Millard [7] and West et al. [8] successfully dissected a new vagina and proceeded with inlay grafting following obliteration due to successful irradiation treatment for cancer.

Delacroix [4] stated that pedicle flap reconstructions of the vagina were difficult, required multiple stages, and left an unsatisfactory cavity. Beare [1] and Conway and Stark [3] used both skin grafts and flaps to

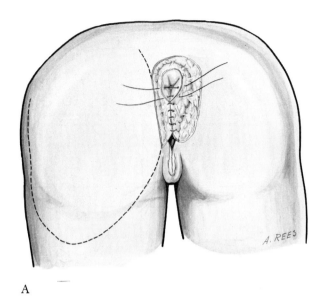

A

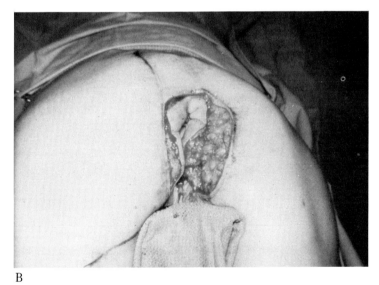

B

FIG. 34-2. A. Perineal skin is turned in as a lining flap of the vaginal vault. B. Operative view. (From W. Cocke, B. Bolasny, and J. Sawyers, *Plast. Reconstr. Surg.* 46:372, 1970. Copyright © 1970, The Williams & Wilkins Co., Baltimore.)

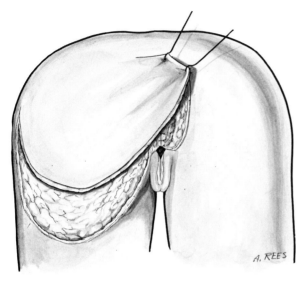

FIG. 34-3. Gluteal flap is rotated over to cover the perineal defect. (From W. Cocke, B. Bolasny, and J. Sawyers, *Plast. Reconstr. Surg.* 46:372, 1970. Copyright © 1970, The Williams & Wilkins Co., Baltimore.)

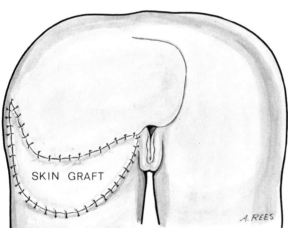

SKIN GRAFT

FIG. 34-4. Completed surgery. (From W. Cocke, B. Bolasny, and J. Sawyers, *Plast. Reconstr. Surg.* 46:372, 1970. Copyright © 1970, The Williams & Wilkins Co., Baltimore.)

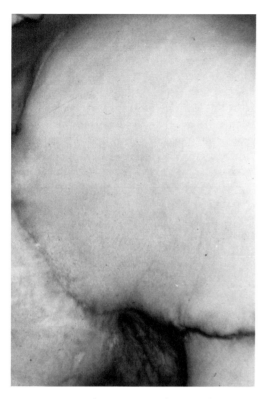

FIG. 34-5. Close-up view showing large gluteal flap in position.

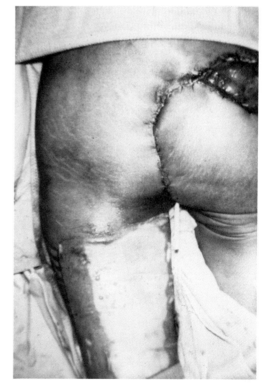

FIG. 34-6. Operative view showing inferiorly based gluteal flap. (From W. Cocke, B. Bolasny, and J. Sawyers, *Plast. Reconstr. Surg.* 46:372, 1970. Copyright © 1970, The Williams & Wilkins Co., Baltimore.)

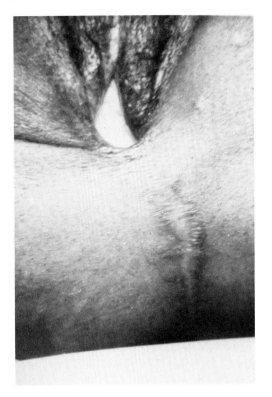

FIG. 34-7. Close-up view showing the posterior fornix of the reconstructed vagina.

repair irradiation injuries of the perineum with good results.

Flaps in this region can be difficult to elevate. They usually require delay in order to rotate them the distance that is required to close a large perineal defect. In spite of these technical considerations, it is believed that pedicle flaps can most adequately replace the tissue that has been lost, and therefore this type of reconstructive procedure can be recommended to help these unfortunate women [2].

Primary reconstruction has not been done, but it would seem logical that initial elevation and flap delay could be accomplished at the time of ablation.

References

1. Beare, R. L. B. Irradiation injuries of the perineum. *Br. J. Plast. Surg.* 15:22, 1962.
2. Cocke, W., Bolasny, B., and Sawyers, J. Vaginal reconstruction following extended abdominoperineal resection. *Plast. Reconstr. Surg.* 46:372, 1970.
3. Conway, H., and Stark, R. Construction and reconstruction of the vagina. *Surg. Gynecol. Obstet.* 97:573, 1953.
4. Delacroix, P. Création d'un nouveau vagin, après amputation abdomino-périnéale du rectum pour cancer. *Ann. Chir.* 91:957, 1965.
5. Pratt, J., and Smith, G. Vaginal reconstruction with a sigmoid loop. *Am. J. Obstet. Gynecol.* 96:40, 1966.
6. Sawyers, J. L. Epidermoid cancer of the perianus and the anal canal. *Surg. Clin. North Am.* 45:1173, 1965.
7. Simmons, R. J., and Millard, D. R. Reconstruction of a functioning vagina following radiation therapy for cancer of the cervix. *Surg. Gynecol. Obstet.* 112:761, 1961.
8. West, J. T., Ketcham, A. S., and Smith, R. R. Vaginal reconstruction following pelvic exenteration for cancer or post irradiation necroses. *Surg. Gynecol. Obstet.* 118:788, 1964.

Irradiation Injury

JEROME E. ADAMSON
CHARLES E. HORTON
RICHARD A. MLADICK
JAMES CARRAWAY

35

WITH THE gradual development of more sophisticated irradiation techniques, especially during the last decade, physicians in the future will encounter fewer and fewer patients who exhibit the effects of irradiation injury. These disorders are still commonly seen in patients who have received irradiation for such malignant conditions as carcinoma of the cervix, rectum, lower colon, bladder, or uterus and ovaries. X-ray treatment of benign disorders, especially pruritis ani, for which at one time the treatment of choice was superficial irradiation, often results in the development of late effects of irradiation injury.

The mechanism of damage from irradiation is not clear. The most likely theory [5] holds that the intracellular formation of ions causes damage to the enzyme systems that function in normal cellular metabolism. Since abnormally functioning cells have enzyme or energy systems that function at a higher rate than normal, such cells appear to be more susceptible to the ionization of their key molecules. The shortest waves in the electromagnetic spectrum, x-rays and gamma rays, are capable of significantly penetrating and actively ionizing (and altering) molecules within living cells. Short wavelength x-rays most easily penetrate body structures and have a much greater therapeutic potential. During recent years, metal filters have been constructed to shield the skin from radiation by longer wavelengths, which will cause some damage to skin at dosage levels that would normally be harmless with short wavelength, or "hard x-rays." Since the ionization effect is cumulative over the lifetime of an individual, the danger to skin and underlying structures increases with each repeated exposure.

Whether the injury is one of acute irradiation damage or chronic irradiation injury, definite destruction of skin and underlying structures occurs. It has been well-established that the ideal treatment for both acute and chronic lesions is appropriate excision of the damaged tissue followed by primary reconstruction, preferably from pedicle flap tissue containing its own blood supply. Occasionally, split-thickness skin grafts will survive in areas in which irradiation injury has produced chronic disease that has resulted in low-grade indolent ulceration. Pedicle flaps from undamaged areas bring in new blood supply and may help heal deeper damage to structures below the skin level.

In chronic irradiation injury, the skin becomes atrophic, and the skin and subcutaneous tissue circulation is considerably compromised by the diminution in size and number of blood vessels. There is a significant increase in fibrous tissue scarring of all structures. The normal skin architecture is destroyed, and a hyalinized collagenous change replaces the epidermis and dermis. The epidermis shows changes of chronic inflammation, with atrophy, hyperkeratosis, and parakeratosis. In the lower dermis and subcutaneous areas, there will be a diminished number of vessels, many thromboses, and much evidence of inflammation as manifested by an intense round-cell infiltrate. In long-standing areas of irradiation injury, the epithelial changes may progress to frank squamous cell or basal cell carcinoma.

Treatment

Conservative attempts to cure chronic irradiation ulcers are usually unsatisfactory, despite ideal wound care, antibiotic ointments, and vigorous general supportive therapy. The tissue, in most instances, has lost its inherent ability to heal as a normal wound. This is probably related to the severe vascular injury that has resulted from the irradiation. Masters and Robinson [5] have reported that many recommend early aggressive excision and reconstruction as the preferred treatment when the diagnosis of irradiation injury is entertained. To wait for the late complications of infection, ulceration, and eventually, malignant degeneration, is not wise. Brown, McDowell, and Fryer [3] have stated that in all areas of skin irradiation injury, if the patient survives long enough, malignant degeneration will finally occur.

In many instances, reconstruction will not be satisfactory—primarily because of the vascular injury—unless tissue as split-thickness skin grafts or full-thickness coverage from pedicle flaps is used to resurface the area. Occasionally, in the perianal and perivulvar

areas, simple excision with advancement of adjacent tissues by undermining can be accomplished, followed by primary wound closure [1]. If the patient is placed in a high lithotomy position with the hips abducted, tension on the skin in the perineum will occur to the extent that primary closure of any wound of this nature may not be possible. If one elects to excise and close small areas of irradiation injury, relaxation of the hips into the normal position will be of great assistance. If simple excision is chosen as the treatment of choice, the excision should extend well beyond the involved area of skin. Radiation damage in neighboring skin is always present, and poor healing may result if damaged skin is used in the closure [2].

Perianal resection that involves the skin around the anal mucous membrane margin may result in rectal strictures. It is unwise to develop mucous membrane darts to prevent contracture at the time of skin grafting or flap closure, since buttock flaps, even those supplied by the inferior gluteal artery, are notoriously unstable, especially when taken from areas adjacent to regions that have received heavy irradiation injury. If a rectal stricture develops postoperatively, second-stage Z-plasties should be performed. If grafts or flaps could be guaranteed survival, interdigitating darts initially placed in the perianal area and interpolating the flap margins with the mucous membrane would be indicated primarily. If a small rim or bridge of normal or nearly normal perianal skin is preserved between the mucous membrane and the area of skin or flap reconstruction, strictures will be avoided. If this is not possible, the patient should be forewarned, and arrangements in anticipation of a second procedure for the stricture should be considered before the initial surgery is performed.

In the male, flaps [6] using the greatly redundant skin of the scrotum are ideal for reconstruction of any portion of the perineum. Not only is the skin of excellent quality with an ideal blood supply, but scrotal skin is present in abundance and can almost completely resurface the perineum, especially in the perianal area. Little deformity to the scrotum and no loss of function will occur.

Large thigh or adjacent buttock flaps may be the only local tissue available in certain cases. These donor areas have usually been exposed to some irradiation and are often unsuitable for use in reconstruction.

In reconstruction of perianal irradiation injury, it is usually not necessary to divert the fecal stream postoperatively. However, if a colostomy is present, reconstruction should be performed prior to closure of the colostomy.

Vaginal stenosis from radiation does not occur as frequently as does rectal stenosis. Radical excision of the vulva accompanied by irradiation for carcinoma of the vulva may lead to severe irradiation damage in this area. However, wide excision of the injured tissue and reconstruction with *delayed* split-thickness skin grafts, which are usually applied 24 to 48 hours after the initial resection, will give satisfactory results in most instances.

Irradiation injury to the lower abdomen, usually resulting from treatment of pelvic carcinoma or lower intestinal malignancies, can often be adequately treated by wide excision and immediate or delayed reconstruction with a superiorly based abdominal flap or skin graft (Fig. 35-1).

Occasionally, osteoradionecrosis of the pubis or a portion of the pelvis will be present in this region. Wide resection of the involved bone is mandatory [4].

Complications

Complications following reconstruction of irradiation injury in these areas are very frequent. Fistulas between the vagina and skin, bladder and skin, rectum and vagina, rectum and skin, and so on, are manifestations of the extensive damage that often occurs from irradiation. Severe infection will involve adjacent normal tissues and, because of the chronicity of this problem, will make normal excision and treatment very difficult. The perineum often develops chronic infection because the considerably diminished blood supply of the region decreases the usual local tissue bacterial resistance that enables continuous exposure to many organisms from the rectum and vagina. Severe, extensive, acute and/or chronic infection, which is similar to hidradenitis suppurativa, may occur. Wide resection of this area in conjunction with delayed primary split-thickness skin grafting is the treatment of choice.

If irradiation injury is not treated promptly by wide excision and reconstruction, the complications will increase in frequency and severity. Excision and reconstruction is highly recommended when irradiation injury is first noted.

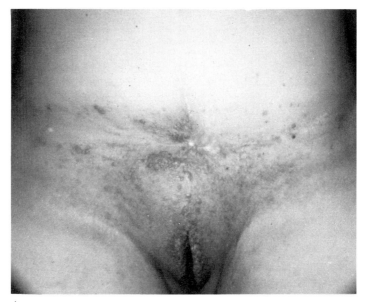

A

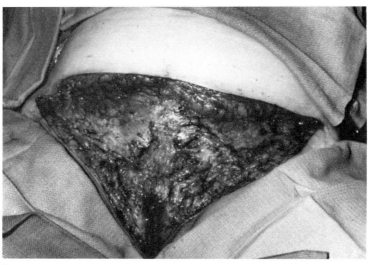

B

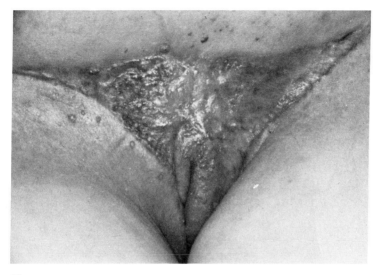

C

FIG. 35-1. A. Radiodermatitis of the pubic area and vulva. (The patient was treated 17 years previously for cancer of the cervix.) B. Surgical excision of radiation injury. C. Skin graft closure.

References

1. Barnes, W. E., Hoffman, G. W., and Pickrell, K. Surgical treatment of irradiation injuries of the perineum. *Surg. Gynecol. Obstet.* 118:1067, 1964.
2. Beare, R. L. B. Irradiation injuries of the perineum. *Br. J. Plast. Surg.* 15:22, 1962.
3. Brown, J. B., McDowell, F. R., and Fryer, M. P. Surgical treatment of radiation burns. *Surg. Gynecol. Obstet.* 88:609, 1949.
4. Dunlap, C. E. Effects of Radiation. In W. A. D. Anderson (Ed.), *Pathology* (5th ed.). St. Louis: Mosby, 1966.
5. Masters, F. W., and Robinson, D. W. Early operation, a conservative approach to the treatment of chronic irradiation injury. *J. Trauma* 1:583, 1961.
6. Pegram, M. W., and Hanno, J. L. Repair of perineal radiation necrosis with a scrotal flap. *J. Int. Coll. Surg.* 30:262, 1958.

Elephantiasis of the Penis and Scrotum

A. MICHAEL WOOD
WILSON J. KERR, JR.

36

CHRONIC lymphedema of the penis and scrotum is a serious condition that causes the patient physical as well as psychological impairment. Patients with this condition lose sexual function. They may also lose family and friends and become social outcasts. This is especially true in young men, several of whom I have seen with no wife, no home, and no employment. Surgical correction of this deformity, therefore, is of a rehabilitative rather than cosmetic nature.

The Lesion

The scrotum, penis, or both assume grotesque proportions when chronically lymphedematous. The limiting factor in terms of size seems to be the rate and degree of involvement of the lymphatics of the cutis. The skin, depending upon the time and amount of lymphatic obstruction, becomes thickened, woody, and may contain warty excrescences. Secondary fungal and bacterial infection in the elephantoid skin is common. Guinea worm infestation has also been reported. When the skin becomes elephantoid (i.e., diffusely thickened due to edema and fibroplasia) early in the disease process, the expansion of the lymphedematous mass is retarded; the skin then acts as the "limiting membrane" with respect to the size of the lesion.

The truly gigantic scrotums (Fig. 36-1), which may weigh 40 lb. or more, have late skin involvement, and, even in some long-standing cases, the skin involvement may be minimal. Penile involvement also appears to differ considerably depending, again, upon the rate and degree of the skin lesion. The penis may literally be "absorbed" into the scrotal mass, or it may assume grotesque proportions itself, being covered with woody elephantoid skin replete with warty excrescences (Fig. 36-2). The latter situation occurs when the cutis of the penis is involved early. When this occurs, the scrotal skin may be similarly involved, and one finds a relatively small scrotal mass.

Since the disease process affects only the cutis and subcutaneous tissue and does not penetrate the deep fascia (Buck's fascia of the penis), on incising this tissue one finds deep to it a layer of areolar tissue that is normal. The uninvolved areolar tissue surrounds the corpora, the cords, and the testes, and it lies deep to the preputial mucosa. The deep lymphatics, deep dorsal nerve, artery, and veins run in this tissue. There is usually an accumulation of lymphatic fluid at the junc-

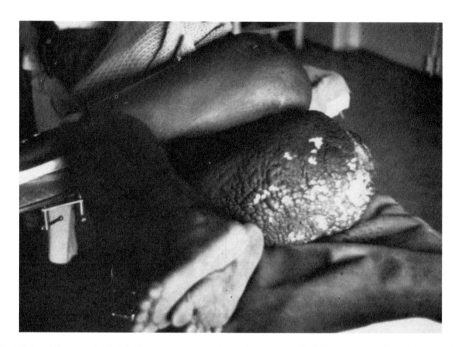

FIG. 36-1. Elephantiasis of the scrotum resulting in severe disability due to the gigantic size.

ture, which further facilitates dissection. This areolar tissue is spared because of its anatomically separate lymphatic drainage. The lymphatics of the skin and subcutaneous tissue of the penis lie superficial to Buck's fascia. They run with the superficial dorsal vein and eventually drain into the subinguinal lymph nodes. In the scrotum, a comparable arrangement is found: those lymphatics superficial to the internal spermatic fascia drain into the regional lymph nodes.

The preservation of this uninvolved areolar tissue deep to Buck's fascia and about the cord and testes is of paramount importance, since our reconstructive procedures are based on its preservation.

Etiology

Elephantiasis of the penis and scrotum may be primary or secondary. Those cases due to

primary causes—aplasia or hypoplasia of the lymphatics—are considered relatively uncommon. However, subclinical hypoplasia coupled with low-grade or repeated infections may account for a significant number of cases. The actual number would be rather difficult to assess, however, without comparative lymphangiography of the state prior to disease.

Secondary etiological factors are thought to be responsible for the majority of cases (Table 36-1).

Genital elephantiasis, as Oomen [4] points out, seems to be related to onchocerciasis in certain endemic areas, whereas in other areas (West Africa, East Africa, and Central America) it is not related. A possible explanation for these findings is that some strains of *Onchocerca volvulus* cause genital elephantiasis and others do not.

In reviewing the findings of many investigators interested in the etiology of elephantia-

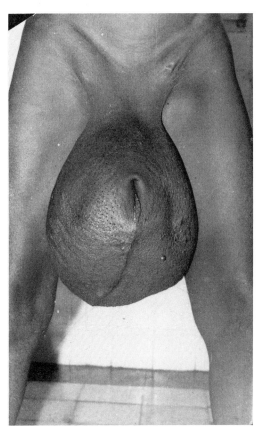

FIG. 36-2. Elephantiasis with "disappearance" of the penis into the enlarged scrotum.

sis, one is struck by the fact that few cases can be shown to be due to filarial disease [1]; the majority of cases are due to either tuberculosis or repeated nonspecific bacterial infections. One must wonder, then, why we do not see more cases of elephantiasis than we do, since both these disease states are quite common in East Africa [2]. The answer probably depends on two factors: (1) the increased tendency to fibroblastic reaction to injury in certain individuals and (2) subclinical anomalous variations of the affected individual's lymphatics.

TABLE 36-1. Classification of Secondary Causes of Lymphedema

Inflammatory	Tuberculosis
	Nonspecific bacterial infections
	Lymphogranuloma venereum
	Secondary to urethral fistulas; either urethral trauma with chronic infection or urethral infection alone
Parasitic	*Onchocerca volvulus*
	Wuchereria bancrofti
	Schistosoma
Noninflammatory	Malignant obstruction
	Radiation therapy

Pathogenesis

Elephantiasis is thought to be due to lymphatic obstruction regardless of the etiological factors involved [3]. When the lymphatic channels are damaged, their valvular function is destroyed, and backflow and accumulation of lymphatic fluid occurs. The destructive process must also involve the regional lymph nodes to such an extent that collaterals are unable to develop and drain the affected areas sufficiently to prevent edema. This is especially true in several young patients that I have treated who had received x-ray therapy in large doses for such disorders as Hodgkin's disease and testicular neoplasms in the pelvic and periaortic areas. Once the major lymphatic channels and regional lymph nodes are damaged, the superficial lymphatic plexuses are secondarily involved. This leads first to edema of the subcutis and later to edema of the cutis, which results in elephantiasis of the involved parts. In those cases shown to be due to filariasis, the pathogenesis is rather clear. One finds adult dead worms and filaria in the larger lymph vessels and lymph nodes, and a surrounding granulomatous foreign-body reaction leads to complete lymph stasis due to the mechanical blockage of the worm itself and the attendant inflammatory reaction.

This simplified version leaves many questions unanswered. The most pertinent of these is: What is the role of fibrous protein synthesis? It has been shown in tissue culture that with proper oxygen tensions and motions, fibroblasts can form bone, cartilage, or large quantities of collagen. Perhaps the right combination is found in the lymph-soaked penis and scrotum, which brings about increased deposition of fibrous tissue and further choking off of the lymphatic venous and arterial systems.

Other factors of importance in the production of fibroplasia are the high concentration of albumin present in stagnant lymphatic fluid, the increased number of mast cells present in lymphedematous tissue, and the increased tendency to fibroplasia that is found in dark-skinned races and that seems to be correlated with higher cutaneous mast cell counts.

The exact physical chemistry of the fibroplasia that is present in lymphedematous tissue is unknown. However, one can surmise that with increased fibroblastic activity and the right "stimulus" present in the ground substance, considerable procollagen is excreted and fibrous protein deposition occurs.

In summary, it is the combination of lymph stasis and enhanced fibroblastic activity that leads to elephantiasis.

Diagnosis and Investigation

Rational treatment of elephantiasis of the penis and scrotum requires the establishment of the cause in each case. In Table 36-1, one can see that the etiological factors are quite variable, and one must remember that elephantiasis or lymphedema are symptoms and not diseases per se.

In any disease state, a detailed history and physical examination is mandatory before contemplating therapy for the disease. With elephantiasis, this survey should include a careful family history and a knowledge of the problems with different parasites or tuberculosis in the area in which the patient resides.

Clinical Features

Of the different causes of lymphedema encountered, the history is usually quite revealing in determining the etiology.

In cases of tuberculous lymphedema, the patients are usually adults with a long history of lymphadenitis involving the inguinal, cervical, and axillary nodes. As in most cases of tuberculosis in the early stages of the disease, fever, anemia, fatigue, and generalized wasting are quite common.

When lymphedema is due to chronic infection—whether it be venereal (i.e., gonococcal), lymphogranuloma venereum, or other bacterial infections—the history usually contains recurrent attacks of lymphangitis, fever, pain, and swelling in the involved areas, leading eventually to lymphedema.

This is especially relevant when one considers the sequence of events following urethral stricture, whether it be due to venereal disease or due to trauma. There is usually a chronic infection present in these cases, and, with the development of urinary fistulas from the urethra, a suffusion of contaminated urine into the subcutaneous tissue and a chronic process of continuing inflammation lead to lymphatic blockage and lymphedema of the involved parts.

In cases that are secondary to irradiation therapy, there is usually a period of a year or so following irradiation in which the patient is essentially free of lymphedema. However, the irradiation process damages endothelium of both the venous arteriolar and lymphatic systems, and it eventually leads to a fibrosis in and about the lymph vessels, causing lymphatic blockage. Soon edema begins to appear and shortly thereafter fibrosis occurs, producing the classic findings of lymphedema followed by elephantiasis of the skin of the involved parts. The radiation damage is irreversible. One might think of this tissue as being prematurely aged by the irradiation process, and, unfortunately, as the patient grows older, the irradiated tissue seems to age at an accelerated rate. Thus, following intensive radiation in and about the pelvic and periaortic areas, lymphedema is almost an invariable sequel.

Physical Examination

Careful examination for lymphadenopathy or lymphadenitis in other areas of the body is of extreme importance, especially when one is concerned with the possibility of a tuberculous cause.

The following investigations are carried out: (1) lymphangiography, if possible; (2) biopsy examination of regional lymph nodes and culture tests of regional lymph nodes, if possible; (3) night blood smears for microfilaria; (4) skin tests for filarial antigens; and (5) tuberculin skin tests.

Preoperative Preparation of the Patient

If a satisfactory surgical result is to be obtained, the patient must be carefully prepared prior to operation. Many of these patients are anemic, most of them have malaria, and they may have other blood diseases as well, such as sickle cell anemia or sickle cell traits. Careful attention to the patient's blood condition is essential. He should receive transfusions, if necessary, prior to operation and should definitely receive specific treatment for malaria with antimalarials, starting several days prior to surgery.

In those patients with tuberculosis, the tuberculosis obviously needs to be treated intensively prior to any surgical attempts aimed at reconstruction of the elephantoid parts.

Patients with chronic urinary tract fistulas may still be infected with gonococci or a mixture of organisms by this time; therefore, they need careful culture tests and specific antibiotic therapy prior to any operative intervention. In these cases, one must plan to divert the urinary stream and to reconstruct a suitable urethra during the resection of the elephantoid penis or scrotum.

In the case of patients suffering from lymphedema following irradiation for malignant disease, one must be absolutely certain that the disease process itself is well controlled. This requires a careful survey of the chest by bronchography, a battery of liver function tests, and perhaps a bone survey. Obviously, it makes little sense to proceed with a large reconstructive procedure in a patient who has uncontrolled metastatic disease and is doomed to die from his malignancy long before he would reap any harvest from the surgical reconstruction of lymphedematous parts.

We have found a most useful technique in preoperative preparation to be as follows:

1. Careful and prolonged scrubbing of the patient is done the night before surgery with surgical soap and a scrub-brush. This should probably be done in the bathtub,

with the aid of a medical assistant to ensure that the job is done properly. Many of our patients come in from the bush immediately prior to surgery, and they often are in a disastrous state of personal hygiene. Cleansing is of paramount importance prior to any surgical intervention in this lymphedematous tissue.

2. Early in the morning prior to surgery, rewash of the perineal area is warranted.

3. Careful sterile preparation in the operating room must also be carried out. Our current routine is to wash the parts carefully for a period of 5 minutes, followed by scrubbing for a minute and a half or so with an alcohol (spirit) preparation.

Surgical Technique

Some of the finest surgical efforts are destroyed by postoperative infection and hematoma. Since there is a large area to be operated on and postoperative hematoma seems to be one of the most common problems encountered, the use of careful hemostasis must be emphasized. Hemostasis can be attained either by use of electrocautery or by careful clamping and tying off of all vessels. We maintain that prior to the actual reconstruction of the area, all that remains of the scrotal or penile tissue following resection should be carefully rinsed with saline to ensure that all the bleeding points have been accounted for.

RESECTION OF THE INVOLVED SKIN

When the scrotum itself is involved, the abdominal skin that has been drawn down by the great weight of the scrotum brings essentially uninvolved anterior abdominal wall skin into the area; we believe that incision should be made in this skin, and all the involved skin of the scrotum can be dispensed with in this fashion. Isolation of the cords themselves can be done by an incision above the inguinal rings, isolating the cords at this point and dissecting them down through the inguinal canal into the enlarged scrotal mass. Great care must be taken to preserve the areolar tissue around the cords. I think that once the cords and testes have been isolated, they should immediately be wrapped in saline-soaked gauze sponges and kept adequately moist throughout the rest of the procedure.

Having developed an apron of skin from the stretched anterior abdominal wall skin, there may be sufficient skin present to reconstruct a scrotum of sorts. The testes are placed within this, and closure without tension can then be achieved. However, if there is insufficient skin at this point, it has been shown that burying the testes in subcutaneous pockets that have been developed in the thighs has essentially no effect on spermatogenesis and provides good results. The subcutaneous pockets should be placed as posteriorly as possible, and they should be developed at different levels so that when the patient places his thighs together, the testes are not brought into approximation to cause the usual abdominal pain one experiences from testicular trauma.

As far as the penis is concerned, we advocate that as much of the involved skin be removed as possible. We have no qualms whatsoever about removing all the penile skin and replacing it with a fairly thick split-thickness skin graft. However, in the uncircumcised patient, the cuff of skin about the corona may provide sufficient tissue to be rolled back to cover the majority of the shaft of the penis. The normal preputial mucosa, because of its anatomically different lymphatic drainage, is usually spared from disease. When there is insufficient tissue present, this may be used in conjunction with a split-thickness skin graft to cover the entire penile shaft. Our results with split-thickness skin grafts of the penis have been excellent, as has been the experience of many others. The suture line in a penile graft should be placed dorsally so if any contracture occurs, there will not be a resultant chordee. Closure without tension should be done with mattress sutures.

Postoperative Management

Adequate postoperative support of the operative area with a light pressure dressing and some kind of suspension apparatus for the testes in their new location are mandatory. One can either construct a new scrotum or bury the testes in thigh pockets. The penis, if it has been involved and its skin has been resected, must be splinted with a catheter and rigged to a traction apparatus above the patient's abdomen so the skin graft is not allowed to slide and fold upon itself during healing.

In resecting this massive amount of tissue, even if hemostasis has been carefully maintained, the lymphatic drainage has obviously been impaired, and there is a tendency for formation of postoperative seroma and hematoma. Several small rubber drains placed in the operative field are worthwhile. The use of drains is not without hazard, since they are a route of entrance of infection. We recommend, therefore, that the drain should be removed within 24 to 48 hours after surgery.

Skin Grafts

Skin grafting in this condition, especially of the penile shaft, has been performed with great success. The areolar tissue in and around Buck's fascia accepts grafts readily. The graft size should be of considerable thickness, i.e., 0.018 to 0.022 inch, with a dorsal suture line to prevent contracture. The graft should be loose fitting to allow for some future erectile tissue expansion. The splinting of the urethra with an indwelling catheter—which is suspended, especially when the penis has been grafted, to overhead traction—is important. The catheter should be placed as soon as possible during the operative procedure to help avoid urethral trauma; it should be left in place for at least 7 to 10 days.

Prophylactic Antibiotics

Although we do not necessarily advocate the use of an empirical antibiotic, we believe that since a large area of undermining is necessary to close the resected area, and especially if skin grafts are used, penicillin should be given prophylactically in doses of about 1,000,000 units of crystalline penicillin every 6 hours intramuscularly for 5 days. This dosage will prevent the disastrous complications of streptococcal infection, which will destroy grafts in a matter of hours. Antibiotics can usually be discontinued after 5 days. If infection or excess drainage occurs at this time, culture tests should be carefully performed. If sensitivity tests are available, these should be done on the cultured material, and an appropriate antibiotic is then started.

References

1. Cohen, B., Nelson, C., Wood, A. M., Manson-Bahr, P. E. C., and Bowen, B. C. Lymphangiography in filarial elephantiasis. *Am. J. Trop. Med. Hyg.,* 1961.
2. Davey, W. W. *A Companion to Surgery in Africa.* Edinburgh: Livingstone, 1968.
3. Fogh-Anderson, P. and Sorensen, B. Surgical treatment of genital elephantiasis. *Acta Chir. Scand.* 124:539, 1962.
4. Oomen, A. P. *Studies on Onchocerciasis and Elephantiasis in Ethiopia.* Haarlem: De Erven F. Bohn, 1969.

Hidradenitis Suppurativa of the Perineum

RICHARD A. MLADICK
CHARLES E. HORTON
JEROME E. ADAMSON
JAMES CARRAWAY

37

HIDRADENITIS suppurativa (HS) is a chronic, recurrent infection of the apocrine sweat glands. The late stages of this disease are characterized by extensive involvement of the skin and subcutaneous tissues, with multiple abscesses, sinus tracts, and a cicatrization that makes it an irreversible problem requiring surgical therapy. Because the apocrine glands are vestigial in man and are located only in the axillary, perianal, genital, inguinal, posterior neck, areolar, eyelid, and periumbilical areas, the disease is limited to these regions.

History

HS was known as "Verneuil's disease" from 1854 to 1865, since Verneuil wrote many papers in which he related the disease to the apocrine sweat glands purely on a clinical suspicion [11]. Prior to Verneuil's observation, Purkinje in 1833 discovered sweat glands in the skin, and in 1839 Velpeau actually described HS as we know it. In 1922 Schiefferdecker [18], on the basis of micropathological descriptions, classified and named the sweat glands "apocrine and eccrine," and positively related HS to the apocrine glands. In 1929 Cole and Driver [9] reported a case of HS. In 1933 Lane [14] wrote the first article in English on HS, which was a review of foreign literature. Major credit should be given to Brunsting [4], who in 1939 wrote the second article in English, providing an extensive review of the problem and a report on 22 cases. Brunsting's article helped make physicians aware of the entity of "hidradenitis suppurativa."

Incidence

Although the age limits are not sharply defined, the disease is generally found in adults between 20 and 40 years of age [1, 4]. The age dependence is believed to be related to endocrine function, since the apocrine glands are inactive until puberty and decrease in activity in advanced years. Some have stated that the disease is more prevalent in women [2, 15], others have maintained that the sex incidence is equal after puberty [11, 17], and still others have stated that perianal involvement is more common in men than in women [1]. There is agreement that blacks are more commonly affected than whites and that Oriental persons are rarely afflicted with this problem [11]. The axilla is the most commonly involved region, and the perianal and genital regions are second in frequency. One in six patients with axillary HS has perianal involvement, and one in 13 has only perianal disease [17]. The disease has been reported as part of an "occlusive triad," a syndrome in which the patient has HS, acne conglobata, and dissecting cellulitis of the scalp [17].

Pathological Anatomy

MACROSCOPIC

The apocrine glands are derived from the hair follicles, whereas the exocrine glands are derived from the epidermis [4]. The apocrine glands are regionally distributed, macroscopic, compound, tubular glands that open into hair follicles, as opposed to the microscopic, simple, tubular exocrine glands that are distributed over the entire body. The only parts of the body without sweat glands are the cornea, sclera, nails, hairshafts, lips, clitoris, glans penis, and inner surface of the prepuce. The apocrine glands are located deep in the corium and subcutaneous tissue. They have tortuous ducts with a muscular coat and a narrowed meatus that opens into the cavity of the hair sheath. This ductile structure provides relatively poor drainage and has been implicated as a causative factor in this disease [10]. The severity of the disease in the axilla, groin, scrotum, or perineum is directly related to the high concen-

tration of aprocrine glands in these areas. A peculiar clump of apocrine glands in the region of the anal orifice has been termed the *anal organ,* and in dogs is partially responsible for the sexually stimulating odors produced during their heat period [12].

HS does not ordinarily spread deep to the subcutaneous tissues, since the process is usually limited by the deep fascial barrier. This results, however, in wide, extensive involvement in the late stages that can mean confluent disease over the entire perineum, groin, and suprapubic areas [17]. Penetration through the fascia into the rectum, bladder, or peritoneum is extremely rare, but it has been reported [17].

MICROSCOPIC

Microscopically, the earliest cell reaction is in the subcutis, primarily within the lumen of the apocrine gland and in the neighboring periglandular tissue [4]. The many distended lymph channels can be seen containing inflammatory cells and cocci. As the chronicity of the disease develops, perivascular infiltration is common, with plasma cells, lymphocytes, and giant cells appearing. In the late stages, the upper parts of the cutis and the deep subcutaneous tissues are involved by multiple abscesses and sinus tracts, which may be either lined by granulation tissue or epithelized. The infection may be so destructive in the late stages as to destroy all apocrine glands, thus making histological diagnosis difficult. The fibrotic changes can be so extensive as to appear almost neoplastic.

Etiology and Pathophysiology

The apocrine gland functions by rupturing its cell membrane and discharging its cellular protoplasm to form a thick secretion. The thick secretion (as opposed to the exocrine gland's thin, watery secretion), when coupled with a tortuous ductile system that has an apparent meatal narrowing, predisposes these glands to excretory stasis. In addition to being thick, milky, and odoriferous, the apocrine secretion is relatively low in volume (exocrine glands have a high volume). The activity of the apocrine glands begins at puberty and then runs in a definite functional cycle, which, in some cases, may be related to the menstrual cycle [10]. HS has been reported to have menstrual and premenstrual exacerbations [7]. There are three times as many apocrine glands in blacks as in whites, which helps explain the higher incidence of HS in that race. The apocrine glands are under adrenergic stimulation, and they respond to emotional stimuli and hormones such as epinephrine and oxytocin.

In spite of the rather clear relationship of the pathophysiology of the apocrine glands to the extent and severity of the disease, the etiology remains obscure. Many contributing factors are known, e.g., mechanical irritation, poor hygiene, chemical depilatories and deodorants, shaving, tight garments, seborrheic skin, hyperhidrosis, acne, moist contiguous surfaces, and hair plucking. Seven out of ten cases are reported to have active acne or acne scars, and mechanical plugging of the ductile system must be considered as one of the most important causative factors in the disease [10]. Although most authorities agree that the infection is exogenous, some disagree as to whether the apocrine glands are primarily or secondarily infected [1]. In almost all cases, the bacteria responsible will be found, on culture, to be hemolytic *Staphylococcus aureus,* both coagulase positive and negative, and *Aerobacter aerogenes.* In long-standing cases, however, there will be many other contaminants, such as *Streptococci* and coliform and anaerobic microorganisms; thus no single organism is completely responsible [15]. Some

believe there is a genetic predisposition that is important in the etiology of this disease.

Clinical Findings

The onset of HS is quite insidious, with the most common symptom being a slight burning or itching in a localized area that progresses to a mobile subcutaneous nodule. This nodule, over 3 or 4 days, slowly becomes tender and painful; it soon attaches to the overlying skin, which becomes reddened and inflamed. This early lesion may sometimes resolve with conservative treatment, but more often it progresses until it drains spontaneously or requires an incision and drainage. Usually, it produces only a drop or two of purulence.

Whether the early lesion clears spontaneously or by incision and drainage, the resultant scarring pulls the skin in a stellate fashion around a central enlarged pore. The indurated area typically remains static for a while before a series of recurrences and remissions begin. Following each exacerbation of the infection, which develops in small foci that are usually close to the original lesion, the discomfort and pain increase, and soon subcutaneous fibrotic cords can be felt beneath the skin connecting the small abscesses. With increasing discomfort, the patient with groin and genital involvement has a tendency to abduct the thighs to decrease motion and splint the involved tissues, further hindering proper cleansing and leading to an increase in the moist, contiguous, opposing surfaces. Eventually the multiple areas of involvement coalesce, forming a very definite indurated shelf that is easily palpated, as well as forming fibrous, cord-like bands. Soon the fluctuation of numerous superficial small abscesses is palpable. Many begin to drain spontaneously through the small pores. In spite of the use of antibiotics, soaks, and other conservative measures, the involvement of these sinus tracts steadily increases over a wider area. Thick, creamy pus is discharged whenever motion or pressure is applied to the involved area. With severe perianal involvement, patients may complain of discomfort on defecation and may not be able to sit down.

With more extensive involvement of the perineum and groins, the patients may become bedridden, being unable to walk without pain, and the legs are usually in a characteristic, abducted, semiflexed position. It is extremely difficult in this late stage to abduct the thighs to carry out a proper examination, and in most cases general anesthesia will be necessary for adequate pelvic and rectal palpation. Coitus is obviously not possible in these advanced cases, and even in the early cases it may be accompanied by so much pain as to be avoided. If the disease is not interrupted in this late stage, scattered areas of skin may begin to break down, producing numerous superficial ulcerations. Undermining and burrowing into adjacent areas can be extensive. The entire buttocks may become involved. Advanced lesions about the anus penetrate into the rectum and complicate the condition and treatment [4].

Differential Diagnosis

The early lesion may resemble a furuncle, a carbuncle, or a localized area of cellulitis. The lesion may easily be confused with a Bartholin abscess, dermoid cyst, pilonidal cyst, lymphadenitis, perirectal abscesses, or anal fistulas. The lesion closely resembles an anal fistula, and the existence of an internal opening into the rectum should be ruled out by anoscopic, proctoscopic, and routine rectal examination. If an internal opening cannot be found, HS must be considered the problem. Generally a fistula has a well-defined

tract lined by granulation tissue that connects with one of the crypts, whereas in HS, the sinus tract leads to a superficial cavity [12]. An ischiorectal abscess may develop multiple draining sinuses, but internal induration on rectal examination will reveal this problem. Other infectious processes to consider are tuberculosis, actinomycosis, cat-scratch fever, lymphogranuloma venereum, granuloma inguinale, regional ileitis, and ulcerative colitis. Other disorders to consider in the differential diagnosis are carcinoma and urethral fistulas. HS can masquerade as a perineal urethral fistula, but it can rarely produce this lesion.

Careful questioning may help uncover the proper diagnosis for perineal infections by pinpointing a genetic disposition toward HS or by uncovering a history of venereal disease, previous rectal problems, anal fistulas, and so on. In severe cases, a complete workup must include a genitourinary examination, lower proctoscopic examination, intravenous pyelography, cystography, and voiding urethrography, as well as the complement-fixation tests for the various venereal diseases. In most cases, however, the diagnosis is obvious and such an extensive work-up is not necessary. It is important that in all cases a thorough evaluation of the patient's condition be made to rule out the known complications of this disease, such as anemia, reversed albumin-globulin ratios, renal disease, and amyloidosis [3]. Other less common complications of advanced HS include interstitial keratitis [3], fistulas to the peritoneal cavity [17], and squamous cell carcinoma [17]

Treatment

For the early cases that are seen prior to the formation of abscess cavities and sinus tracts, conservative local therapy is frequently successful, bringing about a resolution of the inflammatory process. Unfortunately, this control is frequently only a temporary success, since sooner or later the process starts over again. Applying local wet heat, local and systemic antibiotics, x-ray treatment, vaccines, ointments, lotions, ultraviolet lights, and incision and drainage have all been reported successful for clearing early cases. Ideally, once the early lesion is under control, the attention should be directed toward preventing a recurrence by discussing proper hygienic measures with the patient, advising the patient on types of garments and clothing and the use of deodorants, and so forth. In many cases, however, no matter how conscientious the patient may be and no matter what measures are taken, there is a relentless progression of the problem.

Once the disease has reached the chronic stage, nothing short of complete surgical excision is helpful. For a small perianal involvement, the wound may be left open to heal by epithelization after the excision. Frequent sitz baths help speed the healing process. For more major perineal excisions, skin grafting will decrease the morbidity and produce the best result. Excision must be complete, going deep enough (usually down to the fascia) and wide enough to get a rim of normal tissue. Hemostasis should be ensured by cauterization, since it is inadvisable to place any catgut or other suture material beneath the skin grafts. The patients must be operated on under general anesthesia, usually in the lithotomy position.

Postoperatively, the lithotomy position should be maintained, using plaster splints and a crossbar at the knee. In some cases, traction may also be helpful to lift the legs off the bed and provide proper aeration to the surgical wounds.

In the past, excision and delayed skin grafting was advocated, but Conway [10] found that immediate skin grafting decreased morbidity. Multiple, small abscesses frequently develop under the skin grafts, so grafts must be inspected within 48 to 72 hours after surgery. If a bolus dressing is used, it is taken off on the second or third day postoperatively. A helpful adjunct in the skin grafting of these wounds is the use of the mesh dermatome. Mesh skin grafts allow superior drainage from these wounds and give excellent results. The grafts may be laid on without stitches if the patient's legs are properly immobilized, but scattered peripheral sutures help protect the graft from slipping. The skin graft is best made about 0.010 to 0.012 inch thick (Fig. 37-1).

Helpful preoperative adjuncts include a thorough mechanical preparation of the colon, the administration of preoperative systemic antibiotics selected according to the sensitivities of the sinus tract drainage, and, in rare cases, a diverting colostomy. The colostomy is reserved only for cases with the most extensive perianal and perineal involvement. In most cases, the colostomy is unnecessary, because the patient can be prepared with a clear liquid diet 3 to 4 days prior to surgery, followed by thorough preoperative mechanical cleansing. Postoperatively, a constipating regime can be used for 5 to 7 days, which is long enough for the split-thickness grafts to become well attached. An indwelling urinary catheter is usually necessary, since the patients have difficulty voiding because of the prolonged anesthetic, pain, and being in the prone position.

If the skin grafts are well attached but are being destroyed by multiple small infections (abscesses), it is useful to begin silver nitrate compresses on a regular schedule. Antibiotics are, of course, used postoperatively. Whirlpool baths can be started as early as the fourth or fifth postoperative day. Constant and close attention is necessary for the success of large split-thickness skin grafts.

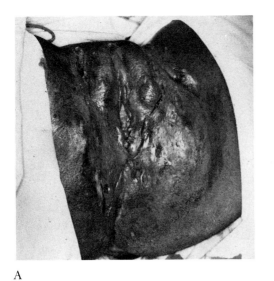

A

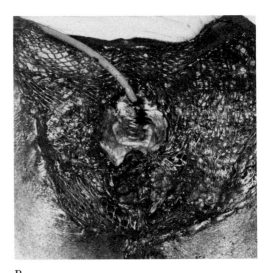

B

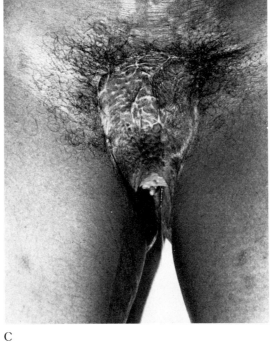

C

FIG. 37-1. A. Extensive perineal hidradenitis suppurativa in a 38-year-old female. The advanced state of the disease has produced multiple sinus tracts, fistulas, and extensive brawny edema of the entire perineal region. The disease at this stage can only be treated by surgical excision and skin grafting. B. After the resection (which had to include the labia), the defect is grafted with a meshed split-thickness skin graft. A catheter is in the urethra. C. Postoperative view 3 months later shows that the skin graft is well healed with no evidence of any residual disease.

Flap closure is rarely applicable in the advanced cases because of the large defects involved and the frequent postoperative infections.

References

1. Anderson, M. J., and Dockerty, M. B. Perianal hidradenitis suppurativa: A clinical and pathologic study. *Dis. Colon Rectum* 1:23, 1958.
2. Armstrong, D. P., Pickrell, K. L., Giblin, T. R., and Miller, F. Axillary hidradenitis suppurativa. *Plast. Reconstr. Surg.* 36:200, 1965.
3. Bergeron, J. R., and Stone, O. J. Interstitial xeratitis associated with hidradenitis suppurativa. *Arch. Dermatol.* 95:473, 1967.
4. Brunsting, H. A. Hidradenitis suppurativa: Abscess of apocrine sweat glands. *Arch. Dermatol.* 39:108, 1939.
5. Carter, A. E. Hidradenitis suppurativa masquerading as perineal urinary fistulas. *Br. J. Surg.* 49:686, 1962.
6. Ching, C. C., and Stahlgren, L. H. Clinical review of hidradenitis suppurativa. Management of cases with severe perianal involvement. *Dis. Colon Rectum* 8:349, 1965.
7. Christensen, J. B. Hidradenitis suppurativa involving the perianal region. *Am. J. Surg.* 79:61, 1950.
8. Cocke, W. M., Jr. Surgery of hidradenitis suppurativa of perineum. *Plast. Reconstr. Surg.* 39:178, 1967.
9. Cole, H. N., and Driver, J. R. Hidradenitis suppurativa. *Arch. Dermatol. Syph.* 19:10285, 1929.
10. Conway, H., Stark, R. B., Climo, S., Weeter, J. C., and Garcia, F. A. The surgical treatment of chronic hidradenitis suppurativa. *Surg. Gynecol. Obstet.* 95:455, 1952.
11. Donsky, H. J. Squamous cell carcinoma as a complication of hidradenitis suppurativa. *Arch. Dermatol.* 90:488, 1964.
12. Hughes, E. S. R. Inflammation and Infections of the Anus. In Turrell, R. (Ed.), *Diseases of the Colon and Ano-Rectum*. Philadelphia: Saunders, 1959.
13. Hurley, H. J., and Shelly, W. B. *The Human Apocrine Sweat Gland in Health and Disease*. Springfield, Ill.: Thomas, 1960.
14. Lane, J. E. Hidradenitis axillaris of Verneuil. *Arch. Dermatol. Syph.* 28:609, 1933.
15. Masson, J. K. Surgical treatment for hidradenitis suppurativa. *Surg. Clin. North Am.* 49:1043, 1969.
16. McAnally, A. K., and Dockerty, M. B. Carcinoma developing in chronic draining cutaneous sinuses and fistulas. *Surg. Gynecol. Obstet.* 88:87, 1949.
17. Moschella, S. L. Hidradenitis suppurativa: Complications resulting in death. *J.A.M.A.* 198:83, 1966.
18. Schiefferdecker, P. Über morphologische Sekretionserscheinungen in der ekkrinen Hautdrusen des Menschen. *Arch. Dermatol. Syph.* 132:130, 1921.
19. Snyder, C. C., and Farell, J. J. Hidradenitis suppurativa. *Plast. Reconstr. Surg.* 19:502, 1957.
20. Tennant, F., Bergeron, J. R., Stone, O. J., and Mullins, J. F. Anemia associated with hidradenitis suppurativa. *Arch. Dermatol.* 98:138, 1968.
21. Woolard, H. H. The cutaneous glands of man. *J. Anat.* 64:415, 1930.

Strictures of the Male Urethra

PATRICK C. DEVINE

38

A URETHRAL stricture is an abnormal narrowing of the urethra, and it is either the result of a congenitally decreased lumen size or of a constriction secondary to the scar tissue of inflammation or trauma. The external meatus is the most common site of stricture in the male. Because of the terminal location and easy accessibility, meatal strictures are easily treated. Urethral meatal strictures are often considered congenital, but since they are more frequent in the infant who has been circumcised, they are probably the result of ulceration of the urethral meatus due to irritation by the diaper. Strictures of the deep urethra, on the other hand, are either congenital or secondary to inflammation or trauma. The scarring associated with gonococcal urethritis was probably due in part to the vigorous local treatment that was necessary before specific antibiotics were available, as well as to the urethritis itself.

Anatomically, the urethra is made up of four major segments: (1) the prostatic urethra, which is lined by transitional epithelium; (2) the membranous urethra, which is lined by stratified columnar epithelium; (3) the bulbous urethra with its stratified columnar epithelium; and (4) the pendulous urethra with its epithelium changing distally from stratified columnar epithelium to stratified squamous epithelium in the fossa navicularis and terminal urethra (Fig. 38-1B). The urethra is surrounded by the erectile tissue of the corpus spongiosum and its covering tunica albuginea. This in turn is surrounded by Buck's fascia and the deep layers of Colles' fascia (Fig. 38-1A), distally by the dartos fascia, and proximally by the bulbocavernous muscle.

The pathology of urethral stricture depends, of course, on its cause and extent. In a case of congenital stricture, the anatomy might well be normal except that the cross section of the urethral lumen itself is small. On the other hand, the inflammatory or traumatic stricture is accompanied by scarring of the urethra itself or, more often, of the urethral and periurethral tissues (Fig. 38-2).

Signs and Symptoms

The signs of urethral stricture are those of back pressure: first there is hypertrophy of the detrusor muscle (pubovesical muscles), and later, as the detrusor decompensates, it becomes thin-walled and inefficient. Early in the disease, starting with the initial hyper-

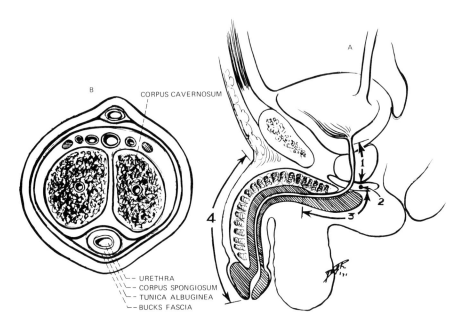

FIG. 38-1. A. Sagittal section of the penis. *1.* Prostatic urethra. *2.* Membranous urethra. *3.* Bulbous urethra. *4.* Pendulous urethra. B. Cross section of penis.

trophy of the detrusor muscle, the ureters can be partially obstructed and proximal dilatation of the upper collecting system can develop. Local inflammation, abscess formation, and urinary extravasation at the stricture site can result in further periurethral scarring and fistulous tracts to the skin of the perineum.

The presence of a urethral stricture is suspected from the patient's history, but definite diagnosis begins with calibration of the urethra, generally with a soft catheter, to establish the presence and distal limits of the stricture. Following this, a retrograde urethrogram should be made by the injection of 20 ml of any radiopaque medium suitable for intravenous injection. It is important that the medium be suitable for intravenous injection,

since occasionally the periurethral veins are found to be opacified when the urethrogram is taken. A voiding cystourethrogram should be made with the same medium, and by the combination of these x-ray films, the length and caliber of the urethra, as well as the distal and proximal margins of the stricture, can be ascertained.

Treatment

The treatment of the strictured male urethra depends on the location and severity of the stricture present. For the urethral meatal stricture, simple urethral meatotomy is usually sufficient. This is most easily done after

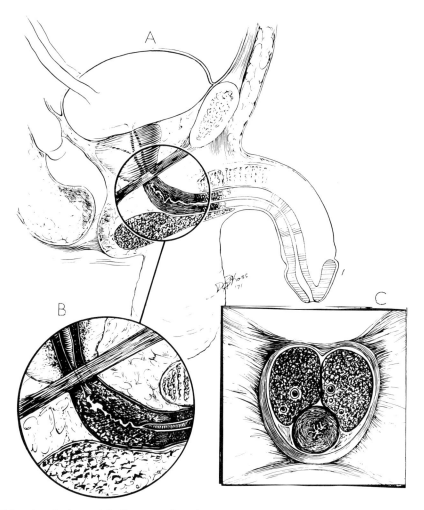

FIG. 38-2. A. Strictured bulbous urethra (sagittal section). B. Close-up of strictured bulbous urethra (sagittal section). C. Close-up of urethral stricture (cross section).

the ventral margin of the distal urethra at the glans penis has been infiltrated with a local anesthetic agent. A clamp is applied to the ventral lip of the urethral meatus and left for approximately 5 minutes, and an incision is made through the tissue that is crushed by the clamp as far as necessary to open the urethra adequately (Fig. 38-3).

The treatment of a stricture of the urethra proximal to the fossa navicularis can consist of simple dilatation if the stricture is soft and pliable and will remain open following dilatation. Dilatation must be done without force, since trauma results in further scarring and subsequent increase in the length or density of the stricture. Prior to instrumentation, the urethral meatus and surrounding tissues are carefully prepared, and the instruments are lubricated with a sterile, anesthetic lubricating jelly. The urethra is gently cali-

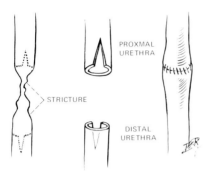

FIG. 38-3. Stricture is excised and the normal urethra is mobilized and anastomosed.

brated with a soft catheter to locate the distal limits of the stricture. Properly sterilized filiforms and Phillips woven urethral bougie followers provide the most satisfactory combination of instruments for safe, gentle dilatation of the urethra. When it is difficult to introduce the filiform, a spiral-tipped filiform can usually be manipulated into the proper passage and passed into the bladder. The filiform is then used to guide firmly attached bougies into the bladder. Dilatation should be gradual and should be done at intervals, if necessary, until adequate dilatation can be obtained. After dilatation, 15 ml of nitrofurazone (Furacin) solution, diluted 1 to 10, can be instilled into the bladder to inhibit the growth of bacteria introduced at the time of instrumentation. When the urinary tract is grossly infected, it is wise to start appropriate antibacterial therapy prior to the introduction of instruments to reduce the risk of bacteremia.

Internal urethrotomy may be sufficient to open the urethra if the scar tissue is limited to the mucosa and submucosa of the urethra itself. The technique of internal urethrotomy requires gentle dilatation of the urethra until the urethrotome can be inserted in the closed position. The stricture is then incised with multiple incisions in the same plane until the

entire thickness of the urethra and periurethral scar has been incised. A urethral catheter, No. 24 French in caliber, with a nonreactive coating is passed into the bladder and left inlying for a 6-week period to allow the urethra to heal with this larger lumen.

Patients who fail to respond to simple dilatation or internal urethrotomy can be treated by one of several methods of open surgical urethroplasty. Operative techniques that have been recommended include:

1. The use of a stent catheter [11]
2. Excision of the stricture and primary anastomosis [1, 18]
3. Excision of the stricture and replacement by homograft [2]
4. Excision of the stricture and replacement by a silicone tube [3]
5. Excision of the stricture and replacement by a split-thickness skin graft [12]
6. Excision of the stricture and replacement by a bladder mucosal graft [10, 15]
7. Excision of the stricture and replacement with a full-thickness skin graft [5, 13]
8. Excision of the stricture with replacement by a strip of buried skin that forms a urethra around a stent catheter [7, 14, 16]
9. Incision of the stricture with marsupialization of the strictured *urethra* and secondary closure [6, 8, 9, 17]

The patient who has a short segment of stricture with a normal urethra proximal and distal to the stricture can best be treated by mobilization of the urethra, excision of the stricture, and proximal anastomosis of the urethra; a fish-mouth incision is made ventrally in the distal urethra and dorsally in the proximal urethra to avoid a circular scar (see Fig. 38-3). The dense stricture of greater length can best be treated by incision of the strictured urethra and patch-graft urethroplasty using a full-thickness skin graft of hairless skin [4] (Fig. 38-4). When the stric-

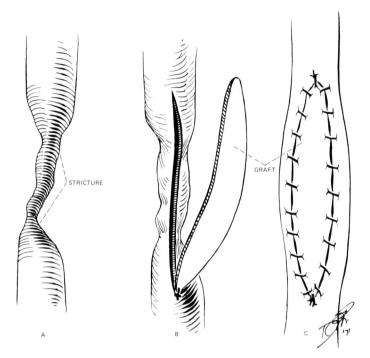

FIG. 38-4. Devine-Horton urethroplasty, type I. A. Urethra with stricture. B. Stricture is incised with grafting. C. Free full-thickness skin graft is in place.

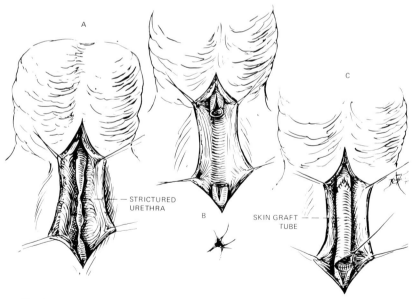

FIG. 38-5. Devine-Horton urethroplasty, type II. A. Strictured bulbous urethra is exposed. B. Strictured urethra is then excised. C. Free full-thickness skin graft being applied.

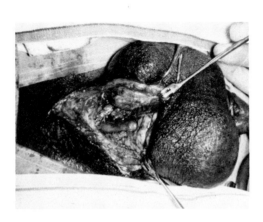

FIG. 38-6.   Full-thickness preputial skin graft is used to replace urethral stricture.

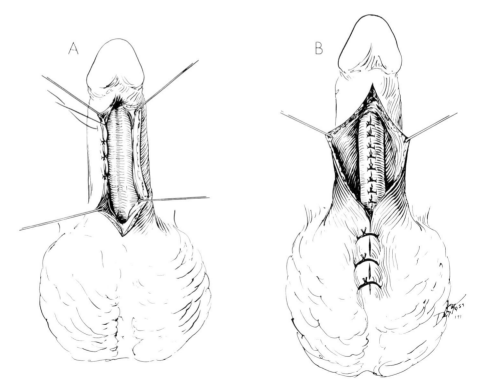

FIG. 38-7. Two-stage urethroplasty. A. Marsupialization. B. Closure (urethra has been closed separately). Modification of Johnson urethroplasty.

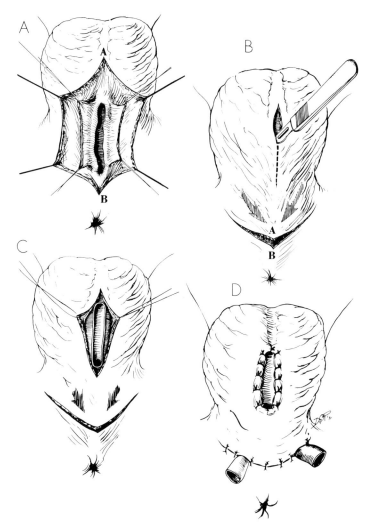

FIG. 38-8. Turner-Warwick urethroplasty (first stage). A. Stricture is exposed and incised. B. Initial incision is approximated and the scrotum is incised. C. Stricture is exposed through the scrotal incision. D. Urethra is marsupialized and the perineum closed.

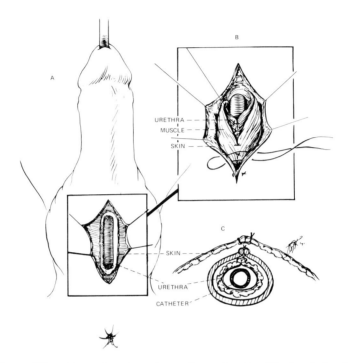

FIG. 38-9. Turner-Warwick urethroplasty (second stage). A. Urethra is freed from the skin of the scrotum. B. Urethra, muscles, and skin are closed. C. Cross section of the closure.

ture is long and so dense that none of the urethral wall is satisfactory for reconstruction, complete excision of the urethra and replacement with a full-thickness skin graft tube is the treatment of choice [4] (Figs. 38-5, 38-9). When the periurethral tissues are densely scarred and when urethrocutaneous fistulas have to be excised, one of the two-stage procedures, which consist of marsupialization and secondary closure of the urethra,

is the procedure of choice [8, 9, 17] (Figs. 38-6 to 38-8).

In surgical treatment of urethral stricture, the simplest procedure that will correct the constricted lumen of the urethra should be applied. It is important to remember, however, that a successful postoperative result is one in which the lumen size of the urethra is restored and no additional urethral dilatations are necessary.

References

1. Badenoch, A. W. Pull-through operation for impassable traumatic stricture of urethra. *Br. J. Urol.* 22:404, 1950.
2. Bourque, J. P. New surgical procedure for cure of scrotal hypospadias: Grafting of male human urethra taken from fresh cadaver. *J. Urol.* 67:608, 1952.
3. diNicola, R. R. Permanent artificial (silicone) urethra. *J. Urol.* 63:168, 1950.
4. Devine, P. C., Horton, C. E., Devine, C. J.,

Sr., Devine, C. J., Jr., Crawford, H. H., and Adamson, J. E. Use of full-thickness skin grafts in repair of urethral strictures. *J. Urol.* 90:67, 1963.

5. Devine, P. C., Sakati, I. A., Poutasse, E. F., and Devine, C. J., Jr. One-stage urethroplasty: Repair of urethral strictures with a free full-thickness patch of skin. *J. Urol.* 99:191, 1968.

6. Gil-Vernet, J. M. Un traitement des sténoses traumatiques et inflammatoires de l'urètre postérieur: Nouvelle méthode d'uréthroplastie. *J. Urol. Nephrol. (Paris)* 72:97, 1966.

7. Hand, J. R. Surgery of the Penis and Urethra. In Campbell, M. F., and Harrison, J. H., (Eds.), *Urology* (3rd ed.), Vol. III. Philadelphia: Saunders, 1970.

8. Johanson, B. Reconstruction of the male urethra in strictures. *Acta Chir. Scand.* Suppl. 176, 1953.

9. Leadbetter, G. W., Jr. A simplified urethroplasty for strictures of the bulbous urethra. *J. Urol.* 83:54, 1960.

10. Marshall, V. F., and Spellman, R. M. Construction of urethra in hypospadias using vesical mucosal grafts. *J. Urol.* 73:335, 1955.

11. Mettauer, J. P. Practical observations on those malformations of the male urethra and penis, termed hypospadias and epispadias, with an anomalous case. *Am. J. Med. Sci.* 4:43, 1842.

12. Peyton, A. B., and Headstream, J. W. Construction of perineal urethra by split-thickness skin graft. *J. Urol.* 76:90, 1956.

13. Presman, D., and Greenfield, D. L. Reconstruction of perineal urethra with free full-thickness skin graft from prepuce. *J. Urol.* 69:677, 1953.

14. Russell, R. H. The treatment of urethral stricture of excision. *Br. J. Surg.* 2:375, 1915.

15. Stevenson, A. J., and Mackey, J. R., Jr. Urethroplasty: Use of bladder mucosa. *J. Missouri Med. Assoc.* 48:990, 1951

16. Swinney, J. Reconstruction of urethra in male. *Br. J. Urol.* 24:229, 1952.

17. Turner-Warwick, R. T. A technique for posterior urethroplasty. *J. Urol.* 83:416, 1960.

18. Villanueva, A. Invagination technique for urethral reconstruction. *Arch. Surg.* 70:253, 1955.

Rupture of
the Urethra

JOSEPH M. MALIN, JR.
JAMES F. GLENN

39

THE FEMALE urethra is well protected by the bony pelvis, but birth trauma and urethral instrumentation will occasionally cause injuries. Serious injury to the male urethra is a more common occurrence; the external location, tortuous course, and lack of protection by the pelvis expose the male urethra to trauma more frequently. This chapter will therefore be limited to a discussion of diagnosis and treatment of male urethral injuries.

The male urethra is divided into two anatomical parts: the anterior and posterior urethra. The anterior urethra is that portion which lies below the urogenital diaphragm and is surrounded by the corpus spongiosum with its investing layer of Buck's fascia (Fig. 39-1). The dartos fascia lies beneath the penile and scrotal skin and is continuous with Scarpa's fascia, the deep layer of superficial fascia of the anterior abdominal wall. These fascial compartments are extremely important in that they limit the extent of urinary extravasation at the time of urethral injury.

Variable degrees of urethral injury occur (Fig. 39-2). Mucosal lacerations and simple contusions may produce edema and bleeding, but they are not associated with extravasation of urine. Full-thickness tears or complete transection of the urethra may produce urinary extravasation. If Buck's fascia remains intact, the extravasation of urine is limited to the penis in all anterior urethral lacerations. If Buck's fascia is also disrupted, then the extent of urinary extravasation is limited only by dartos and Scarpa's fascia. Urine may extend to the perineum and the anterior abdominal wall (Fig. 39-3). In posterior urethral tears and transection, urine will extrude into the perivesical retroperitoneal space (Fig. 39-4). Urine will not enter the peritoneal cavity unless there is also a defect in the peritoneal membrane.

Two types of force, internal and external, produce urethral injuries. Iatrogenic injuries are not uncommon and are the result of excessive force during instrumentation. Contusions, lacerations, tears, and occasional complete avulsion of the urethra may result from forceful passage of instruments through the normal urethra, but these occur most often when a strictured or inflamed urethra is being instrumented. Injuries occur most often at three sites: the external urethral meatus, the bulbous portion of the anterior urethra,

533

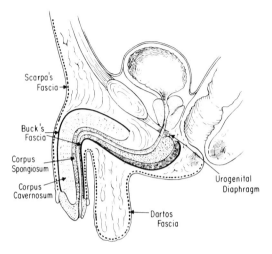

FIG. 39-1. Normal anatomy of the male pelvis.

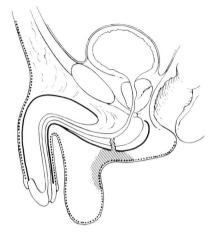

FIG. 39-3. Laceration of the urethra and Buck's fascia, with extravasation of urine.

and at the bladder neck. Urethral instruments are occasionally passed into the rectum by inadequately trained personnel.

One of the most common urethral injuries involves the anterior bulbous urethra and

occurs when a blunt force is applied to the perineum, as in falling astride an object. The bulbous urethra is crushed between the external object and the inferior pubic arch. The degree of injury may vary from a simple contusion to complete urethral transection.

Most posterior urethral injuries are associated with pelvic fractures. The incidence of

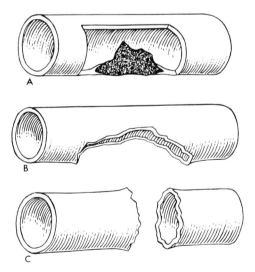

FIG. 39-2. Types of urethral injury. A. Urethral contusion. B. Urethral laceration. C. Urethral transection.

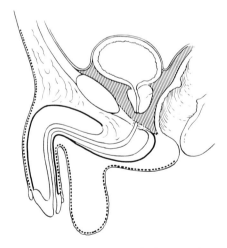

FIG. 39-4. Transection of the membranous urethra with retroperitoneal extravasation of urine.

lower urinary tract injury, including rupture of the bladder, associated with fracture of the pelvis has been reported to be 9.8 to 25 percent [6, 7, 12, 15]. The incidence of urethral injury alone in pelvic fractures is 5 percent [5]. Automobile accidents are by far the leading cause of pelvic fractures, and therefore urethral injuries are seen most often in the younger group, 16 to 25 years of age [10].

The membranous portion of the urethra is firmly fixed within the rigid urogenital diaphragm, and the puboprostatic ligaments fix the apex of the prostate to the pubic symphysis. The shearing forces that occur during fracture of the pelvis move the symphysis and prostatic apex away from the urogenital diaphragm. The prostate is avulsed from the membranous urethra, and urine extrudes into the perivesical space.

Avulsion injuries of the penis and scrotum are usually associated with industrial and farm accidents, and penetrating injuries such as knife and gunshot wounds occasionally account for urethral trauma, especially in wartime.

Diagnosis

History of the injury, physical examination, diagnostic catheterization, and radiographic evaluation of the urethra are important in evaluating patients with suspected injury to the lower urinary tract. It is essential to determine the time when the patient last voided, and whether there was a sensation of bladder fullness immediately preceding or following the injury. Further, it should be determined whether the patient voided following injury, whether there was suprapubic or rectal discomfort, or if blood was noted in the urine. Patients with urethral injury may present with blood at the external meatus or gross hematuria, inability to void, a palpable suprapubic mass due to urinary

retention, a swelling of the penis, scrotum, perineum, or anterior abdominal wall, or any combination of these symptoms or physical findings. Avulsion of the prostate can often be diagnosed upon rectal examination. The prostate cannot be palpated in its normal location, but occasionally a posterior urethral tear will produce enough extravasation of urine or blood to make the prostate indistinguishable even though it remains in its normal location.

The amount of bleeding from the urethra cannot be correlated with the severity of injury. A small contusion may produce large amounts of blood at the external meatus; on the other hand, complete separation of the urethra may produce very little obvious bleeding. Patients with small contusions may be unable to void because of edema or sphincter spasm, and yet patients with urethral lacerations may void with an almost normal urinary stream.

Diagnostic catheterization has been both advocated and condemned [2, 3, 8, 13, 15]. There are the obvious dangers of introducing infection, increasing the amount of damage to the urethra, and obtaining false information by introducing a catheter. A catheter may easily pass into the urinary bladder when there is significant urethral damage. In cases of complete avulsion, a catheter may pass into the retroperitoneal space, draining extravasated urine and producing a false sense of security.

The information that is usually gained from catheterization exceeds the risks of increased damage and infection. A small catheter should be passed gently, employing strictly sterile technique. When a catheter readily passes into the urinary bladder and several ounces of clear urine are obtained, the probability that complete disruption of the urethra exists is negligible. This does not, however, indicate a lack of other significant urethral injury. The catheter is then used to

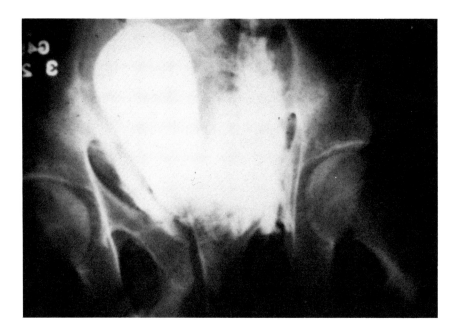

FIG. 39-5. Cystogram demonstrating retroperitoneal extravasation of contrast material and laceration of the membranous urethra.

obtain a cystogram, which is mandatory for all patients who have had significant pelvic trauma (Fig. 39-5). To overlook the possibility of a ruptured urinary bladder would be disastrous. An intravenous urogram is also indicated in order to evaluate the upper urinary tracts in all patients with hematuria following abdominal or pelvic trauma. Significant renal or ureteral injury should not be overlooked.

If a small catheter will not pass easily or if it passes and urine is not obtained, then the physician should be alerted to the possibility of a ruptured bladder or complete disruption of the urethra with the catheter tip lying in the retroperitoneal or intraperitoneal space. Injection of a small amount of contrast material into the catheter or a retrograde urethrogram will usually provide evidence to verify the diagnosis.

Urethral lacerations or complete avulsion of the urethra may prevent the passage of a catheter. Of extreme value in this group of patients is retrograde urethrography. This technique was first introduced by McCrea in 1940 [9] and has since been both recommended and condemned [2, 14]. There is a risk of introducing infection and increasing urethral damage by this diagnostic technique. However, if the retrograde urethrogram is performed using strictly sterile technique and if water-soluble contrast material is injected without excessive force, the information gained far outweighs the risks entailed in the procedure (Fig. 39-6). It is most valuable in patients who cannot be successfully catheterized and in patients with multiple additional injuries that necessitate immediate evaluation prior to moving the patient to the operating room.

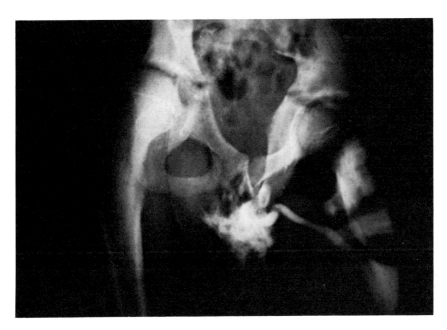

FIG. 39-6. Retrograde urethrogram showing laceration of the bulbous urethra with extravasation of contrast material.

Treatment

The principles of treatment of urethral injury are: (1) adequate urinary diversion and, occasionally, fecal diversion; (2) drainage of extravasated urine; (3) control of infection; and (4) repair of the injured portion of the urethra.

Urethral contusions and partial urethral tears are best treated conservatively. Urethral catheter drainage alone is often adequate and excellent results are usually obtained. If a urethral catheter can be passed into the urinary bladder, if clear urine is obtained, and if the cystogram and intravenous urogram are normal, then nothing else need be done except to provide 7 to 10 days of urethral catheter drainage and the administration of antibiotics to prevent infection.

If it is not possible to introduce a catheter easily through the penile urethra and a urethrogram demonstrates extravasation of contrast material, then more extensive open surgery is often necessary. The simplest procedure for reestablishing continuity is by the antegrade insertion of a urethral catheter. Often a small catheter can be successfully passed from the bladder neck through the urethra to the urethral meatus at suprapubic cystotomy. A Foley catheter is then attached to the tip of the antegrade catheter with a silk suture, and the Foley catheter is drawn into the urinary bladder. When a small catheter cannot be successfully passed from above, then interlocking sounds are often useful. Two meatal sounds, one with a convex and the other with a concave tip, are used. The sound with the convex tip is passed retrograde to the region of the injury while the second sound is passed through the bladder neck to the site of injury. By gentle manipulation of the tips of the sounds, they can be

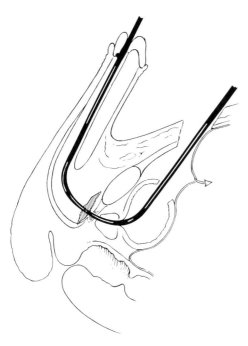

FIG. 39-7. Interlocking sounds in apposition; bulbous urethral transection.

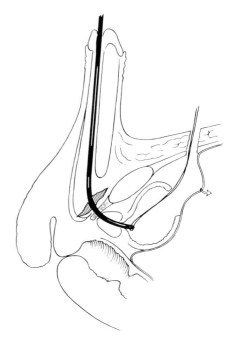

FIG. 39-8. Retrograde interlocking sound with a suture attached.

brought into approximation and interlocked. The retrograde sound can be then guided into the bladder by the sound passed from above (Fig. 39-7). A long silk suture is tied to the eye of the retrograde sound, and the sound is withdrawn. A Foley catheter is attached to this guide suture, and the suture is used to draw a Foley catheter into the urinary bladder (Fig. 39-8). If urinary extravasation has occurred, then incision and drainage are indicated. Accessory suprapubic catheter drainage is essential.

Occasionally, in partial and complete anterior urethral tears, it is impossible to pass any instrument antegrade or retrograde. An incision over the site of injury will expose the underlying urethra. A vertical incision along the ventral surface of the penis will expose the pendulous urethra, or an inverted

U-shaped incision in the perineum will expose the bulbous urethra. The bulbocavernosus muscle is incised and retracted to expose the underlying injured urethra. Blood and urine are evacuated and the edges of the injured urethra freshened by sharp dissection. A catheter is then passed from the urethral meatus to the site of injury, and it then can be easily directed into the proximal urethra and urinary bladder. The injured urethra is then closed with interrupted sutures of fine chromic catgut (Fig. 39-9). The wound is closed and drained, and catheter drainage is maintained for at least 7 to 10 days and possibly as long as one month, depending upon the extent of injury.

Many authors advocate routine exploration of bulbous urethral injuries with excision of injured tissue and direct repair of all urethral lacerations. It is difficult to assess the pub-

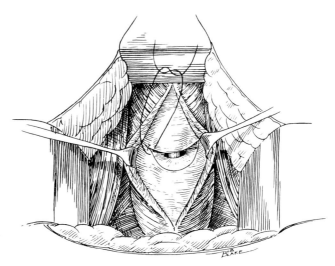

FIG. 39-9. Direct repair of a bulbous urethral laceration.

lished results of direct repair because of the small number of cases reported. Often, immediate postoperative results are excellent. Adequate follow-up to assess posttreatment complications, especially strictures, takes a minimum of 5 years.

Complete separation of the urethra at the prostatic apex results in retroperitoneal extravasation of urine and blood. The prostate is found to be elevated from its normal position on rectal examination, or it may not be at all palpable if the amount of extravasated urine and retroperitoneal blood is great. A number of surgical approaches have been advocated [1].

The retropubic space may be explored through a transverse or vertical suprapubic incision, and extravasated urine and blood is removed from the wound. Not infrequently, the torn edge of the membranous urethra cannot be identified because of retraction into the urogenital diaphragm. The simplest method of repair consists of passing a Foley catheter through the penile urethra to the site of injury. The catheter is then inserted through the torn prostatic apex into the urinary bladder, and the balloon is inflated.

Traction is applied to the catheter for 10 to 14 days in order to reapproximate the injured parts (Fig. 39-10).

Another method of reapproximation by traction can be accomplished by heavy silk traction sutures (Alcock) (Fig. 39-11). A heavy silk mattress suture is placed blindly through the urogenital diaphragm to the perineum, where traction is applied and the sutures are tied over buttons.

Direct anastomosis of the prostatic apex to the membranous urethra can be accomplished with interrupted sutures of chromic catgut if the torn edge of the membranous urethra can be identified (Fig. 39-12). Additional exposure of the membranous urethra can be obtained by surgical excision of the crest of the pubis and the underlying anterior portion of the urogenital diaphragm [4]. The sutures are placed after freshening the edges of the injured membranous urethra. A Foley catheter is used for urinary diversion for 7 to 10 days, and, as in all cases of urinary tract injury, it is important to adequately drain the wound.

Complete separation of the membranous urethra at the prostatic apex can also be sur-

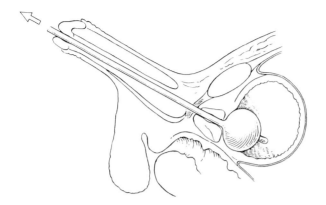

FIG. 39-10. Catheter traction in membranous urethral transection.

gically corrected through the perineum. Direct anastomosis of the injured parts or repair by traction sutures can be accomplished easily by a surgeon with experience in perineal surgery. An inverted U perineal skin incision is made with the patient in the exaggerated lithotomy position. The central tendon of the perineum is divided, and the area of injury is entered. Dissection of the rectum from the posterior prostatic capsule usually has already been accomplished by the extravasation of blood and urine. Evacuation of blood and urine exposes the prostatic apex

for introduction of a Foley catheter and direct repair.

The complications of urethral injury are urinary extravasation, infection, and postoperative urethral strictures [11]. Local infection and urinary extravasation will contribute to the formation of severe postoperative strictures if not adequately treated. Adequate

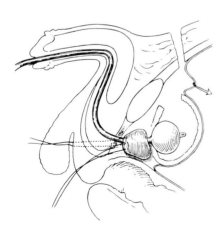

FIG. 39-11. Perineal traction sutures in membranous urethral transection.

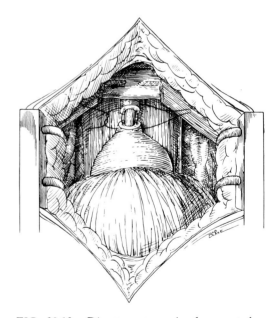

FIG. 39-12. Direct anastomosis of transected membranous urethra.

drainage of the site of injury will decrease the incidence of severe postoperative strictures. Strictures also result from incomplete approximation of the injured urethra, and this has led many authors to advocate direct repair of the injured parts. Treatment of the most common postoperative complications—urethral strictures and fistulas—is discussed in Chapters 22 and 28.

References

1. Carswell, W. R. Primary and secondary repair of the posterior urethra. *Aust. N. Z. J. Surg.* 36:252, 1966–67.
2. Culp, O. S. Treatment of ruptured bladder and urethral analysis of 86 cases of urinary extravasation. *J. Urol.* 48:266, 1942.
3. Culp, O. S. War wounds of the genitourinary tract: Early results observed in 160 patients treated in the European theater of operations. *J. Urol.* 57:1117, 1947.
4. Dees, J. E. Transsymphyseal approach to the urethra. *J. Urol.* 81:440, 1959.
5. Holdsworth, F. W. Injury to the genitourinary tract associated with fractures of the pelvis. *Proc. R. Soc. Med.* 56:1044, 1963.
6. Kisner, C. D. Injuries of the urethra: With special reference to those occurring in fracture of the pelvis. *S. Afr. Med. J.* 32:1105, 1958.
7. Kusmierski, S., and Tobik, S. Some problems in surgical management of ruptured urethra in fracture of pelvis. *J. Urol.* 93:604, 1965.
8. McCague, E. J., and Semans, J. H. The management of traumatic rupture of the urethra and bladder complicating fracture of the pelvis. *J. Urol.* 52:36, 1944.
9. McCrea, E. D'A. *Diseases of the Urethra and Penis.* Bristol: Wright, 1940. P. 67.
10. Mitchell, J. P. Injuries to the urethra. *Br. J. Urol.* 40:649, 1968.
11. Mulholland, S. W., and Madonna, H. M. Urethral rupture: Early and late posterior complications. *J. Urol.* 68:489, 1952.
12. Peacock, A. H., and Hain, R. S. Injuries of the urethra and bladder. *J. Urol.* 93:604, 1965.
13. Smith, G. G., and Mintz, E. R. Traumatic rupture of the urethra. *Trans. Am. Assoc. Genitourin. Surg.* 24:241, 1931.
14. Veiga-Pires, J. A., and Elebute, E. A. Urethrocystography in the male. *Br. J. Urol.* 39:194, 1967.
15. Vermooten, V. Rupture of the urethra, a new diagnostic sign. *J. Urol.* 56:228, 1946.

Tumors

VI

Tumors
of the Vulva

ROBIN ANDERSON
LESTER A. BALLARD, JR.

40

THE SURGICAL treatment of tumors of the vulva is, in most instances, relatively straightforward. Most vulvar tumors can be totally excised unless they are unusually extensive or invade vital structures. The reconstruction of the surgically created defect may be either simple, consisting of no more than primary closure of the wound, or complicated, involving the use of skin grafts or pedicle flaps from the abdomen or thigh. Occasionally, it may be necessary to reconstruct the urethra or vagina. Normally, there is considerably more vulvar skin and soft tissue available for reconstructive purposes than one might suspect on first viewing a given lesion, and it is surprising how rarely one must resort to the use of grafts and flaps.

Pathology

Tumors of the vulva can be divided into three groups: benign tumors, vulvar dystrophies (which may or may not be true tumors), and malignant tumors. The diagnosis of most of these is obvious to the trained observer. It cannot be emphasized too strongly, however, that biopsy, with or without frozen section, must precede definitive treatment unless the benign nature of the lesion is obvious.

BENIGN TUMORS

This group consists of a number of frequently encountered tumors whose diagnosis is rarely difficult. Biopsy is usually not needed. *Fibroma*, the most common of the solid benign tumors of the vulva, occurs rarely. The soft variant, usually called *fibroma molle*, may become very large and will occasionally interfere with sitting or walking (Fig. 40-1).

Lipomas and *hidradenomas* are extremely rare. Lipomas are slow growing, usually lobulated, and softer than fibromas. Hidradenomas tend to be small and asymptomatic, and they present problems only when their diagnosis is difficult to establish. Although a benign lesion, the appearance of hidradenoma under the microscope may allow it to be mistakenly interpreted as adenocarcinoma.

Papillomas may appear in the simple form that can be found anywhere on the skin, or as *condylomata acuminata*, which are found only in the vulva and associated moist areas. The latter have a characteristic appearance,

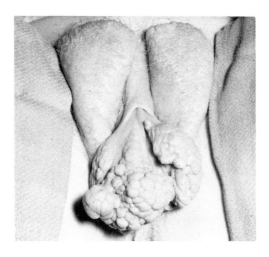

FIG. 40-1. Typical fibroma molle (soft fibroma) producing symptoms sufficient to require excision.

with prominent masses of hypertrophied squamous epithelium. Papillomas are usually excised with ease. Condylomata, when small, may respond to chemical treatment with podophyllin, but extensive lesions may require electrocauterization or surgical excision.

Two types of *vulvar cysts* are encountered: those arising from Bartholin's duct and those of sebaceous gland origin. Their diagnosis is usually obvious. If these cysts display symptoms or become infected, simple surgery usually suffices, and, as in other parts of the body, this may consist of either marsupialization or total excision. In most instances, such cysts are of little consequence to the patient and require no treatment.

VULVAR DYSTROPHY

This group includes three lesions that may be considered less benign than the above and, in this sense, are potentially malignant.

The three lesions are *kraurosis vulvae, lichen sclerosus et atrophicus,* and *leukoplakia.* These lesions may be red or white in color. Diagnosis can be established with certainty only by biopsy. Bowen's disease (or carcinoma in situ), Paget's disease, and early invasive squamous cell carcinoma of the vulva may be indistinguishable from dystrophic lesions until examined microscopically.

Kraurosis and *lichen sclerosus et atrophicus* are clinically identical (Fig. 40-2). They appear as chronic inflammatory lesions with induration, atrophy, and, occasionally, ulceration. They are most commonly found in postmenopausal women and require no more than local topical treatment once the diagnosis is established. Patients with symptoms that are resistant to medical therapy may occasionally require simple vulvectomy.

Kraurosis is usually not considered to be a premalignant lesion. However, the presence of any inflammatory change requires careful histological control and a long period of observation during and after treatment, be it

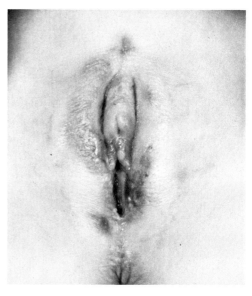

FIG. 40-2. *Lichen sclerosus et atrophicus* is indistinguishable on gross examination from kraurosis.

surgical or medical. After the diagnosis has been established by means of biopsy, any subsequent change, such as ulceration or new induration, should be regarded with suspicion. Skin biopsies may be carried out as office procedures under local anesthesia; a dermatologist's skin punch is excellent for this purpose.

Leukoplakia of the vulva is as pathologically confusing as is leukoplakia elsewhere (Fig. 40-3). The word *leukoplakia* simply means "white plaque," and many benign lesions fall into this category. We employ the word to describe a specific pathological entity with characteristic changes on microscopic examination and with definite premalignant implications. It is identical to the lesion found on the lips and within the oral cavity. It is characterized in its early stages by a superficial, white hyperkeratatic lesion that is easily scraped off and, in its more advanced form, by thicker, indurated plaques within which cancer may already exist. In the past, a number of reports have suggested that serial sections will show unsuspected malignancy in as many as 25 percent of the lesions. Current thought is that such malignant change is not that common, probably being more in the range of 5 to 10 percent. The diagnosis can be made only by multiple biopsies. Even if no malignancy is found, these vulvae require careful periodic examinations for an indefinite period.

The treatment of leukoplakia is based on the extent of the patient's symptoms. If the patient is asymptomatic, no more than periodic examination is required. If the leukoplakia produces symptoms, the symptoms are treated using topical agents, such as steroid ointments. These lesions tend to have intermittent exacerbations and regressions. If leukoplakia is persistently symptomatic, unrelieved by medication, or develops worrisome changes grossly and microscopically, treatment should consist of total, though not radical, excision. The procedure utilized is commonly termed *simple vulvectomy,* but it probably should be merely called total excision of involved tissues.

MALIGNANT TUMORS

Basal cell carcinoma of the vulva is similar in behavior and pathology to basal cell carcinoma elsewhere and has a characteristic clinical and microscopic appearance. Again, preoperative biopsy is essential. The lesion may become an invasive tumor when long established. It virtually never metastasizes. Local excision with reasonable margins of normal tissue is usually sufficient for cure.

Paget's disease of the vulva is probably identical to that found in the breast and must be considered to be a true adenocarcinoma of somewhat doubtful origin (Fig. 40-4). It is discussed in detail elsewhere in this book (see Part VI, Chap. 41).

Carcinoma in situ (Fig. 40-5), originally

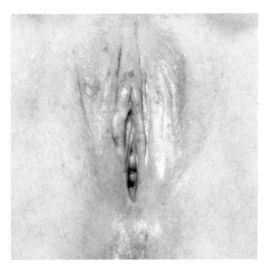

FIG. 40-3. This lesion, which clinically may be any vulvar dystrophy or carcinoma in situ, is found to be leukoplakia on microscopic study.

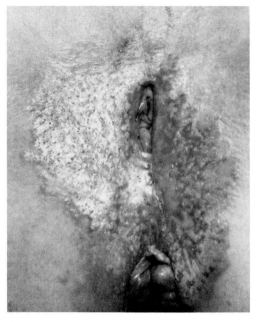
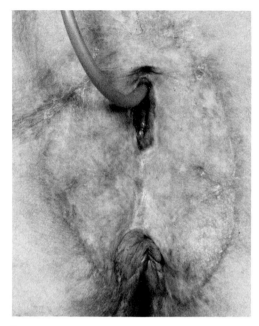

A   B

FIG. 40-4.   A.   Large, mottled, red and white lesion is clinically suggestive of Paget's disease. Diagnosis was established by biopsy.   B.   Lesion is excised and the large defect is covered with a split-thickness skin graft from the adjacent thigh.

described by Bowen as intraepithelial carcinoma and now frequently termed Bowen's disease, is also discussed in detail elsewhere (see Part VI, Chap. 41).

Invasive carcinoma of the vulva may occur as either squamous cell carcinoma or adenocarcinoma, with the squamous lesions predomianting by approximately twenty to one. The lesion is ubiquitous in appearance, and it may be preceded by leukoplakia or other vulvar dystrophies. Biopsy remains the only method of establishing a definitive preoperative diagnosis. Metastasis does not usually occur early in the course of the disease, but it is difficult to find when it has done so. Since the lymphatic drainage of the vulva is generally into the inguinal nodes, the treatment of choice is en bloc excision of the primary lesion in continuity with the regional drain-age area. Since the lymphatics of the labia minora may also drain into the femoral lymphatics, a proper continuity node dissection must include the lymph node-bearing tissue of the femoral triangle as well as the inguinal area. Radical vulvectomy with regional node dissection is the operation of choice (Fig. 40-6).

Melanoma of the vulva is very rare and, because of its poor prognosis, should be viewed as distinct from invasive carcinoma. As with melanoma elsewhere, the early lesion, particularly if it has invaded only moderately into the dermis, is probably quite benign. Unfortunately, such tumors of the vulva usually are seen by the surgeon late in their course and have both invaded through the dermis and possibly already metastasized. They then behave quixotically, with early

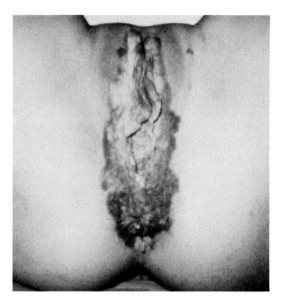

FIG. 40-5. Extensive lesion on biopsy examination showed carcinoma in situ. Excision was staged to avoid anal stricture. A skin graft was necessary for repair.

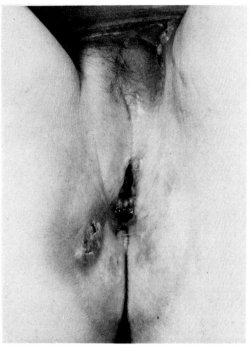

FIG. 40-6. Advanced squamous carcinoma with ulcerated inguinal metastasis requiring radical vulvectomy and regional node dissection.

distant metastasis, and the chance of cure drops precipitously. Unless preoperative biopsy examination establishes the diagnosis of a superficial melanoma, the treatment of choice includes regional node dissection in continuity with the primary dissection.

Treatment

EXCISION OF A SMALL PRIMARY TUMOR

These cases do not require extensive reconstruction. Since vulvar skin is plentiful, there is little difficulty in closing any surgical wound that involves one side of the vulva without encroachment upon midline structures such as the urethra and vagina. Vertical incisions are always to be preferred. If a transverse incision must be used, it may be converted to a more vertical one by means of

the commonly employed maneuver of planning the incision initially in an S shape. Hemostasis is rarely a problem, but good subcutaneous closure with fine catgut should be employed to eliminate dead space. Skin closure may be carried out with nonabsorbable sutures, but catgut is just as satisfactory and eliminates the necessity of removing skin sutures that often disappear in the moist and edematous skin of the area. In the absence of tension across the wound, 3-0 or 4-0 chromic catgut will suffice.

EXCISION OF A LARGE PRIMARY TUMOR

This often requires extensive reconstruction. If the surgical wound resulting from the excision of a benign vulvar lesion is of such a size that simple closure cannot be carried out without tension or distortion of vital structures, the covering material of choice is a split-thickness skin graft. A graft of thin to moderate thickness, usually about 0.015 to 0.020 inch, ensures satisfactory coverage.

SIMPLE VULVECTOMY

Simple or conservative vulvectomy implies total excision of the labia, with the dissection being carried down only into the underlying fat (Fig. 40-7). As mentioned above, this procedure is particularly useful for carcinoma in situ in which the entire vulva is involved and when the carcinoma is not invasive.

The proposed incision is marked on the lateral aspects of the labia; it extends anteriorly to encompass the disease process and posteriorly to a point well anterior to the anus. The inner incision is made in vulvar

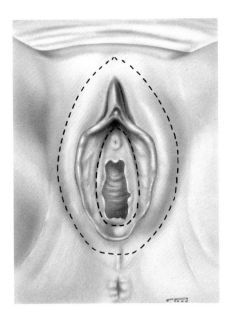

FIG. 40-7.   Extent of simple vulvectomy. The operative wound can be closed primarily with ease.

mucous membrane. The intervening tissue, including skin and fat, is excised. Underlying muscles are not disturbed. Closure is carried out by simple approximation of skin and mucosa using interrupted 3-0 chromic catgut in both subcutaneous tissue and skin. During the immediate postoperative period, modest pressure is applied by means of a T-binder to prevent local edema and the accumulation of fluid within the wound. This is discontinued after 24 hours.

RADICAL VULVECTOMY

The term *radical vulvectomy* is applied to the en bloc resection of the vulva down to the fascia, including the superficial muscles of the perineum. Most radical vulvectomies include bilateral groin dissections to remove the lymph-bearing soft tissue of the inguinal and femoral regions in continuity with the primary tumor. It is primarily used for the treatment of invasive carcinoma of the vulva, with or without metastasis. In view of the well-known difficulty of detecting the presence of metastatic cancer in these regional zones, the continuity dissection is carried out whether nodes are palpable or not.

The incision is planned to provide wide excision of the primary vulvar lesion. It is not necessary to excise large areas of uninvolved skin except in the perineal area, where lymphatic pathways are known to be closely adjacent to the skin surface. The incision is marked out with methylene blue, and care is taken to ensure an adequate margin beyond all involved tissue, including leukoplakia if present. The incision is made and carried down to the fascia of the external oblique and anterior rectus muscles superiorly. The portions of the incision from the anterior iliac spines to the perineum pass directly through fat to the fascia lata femoris. The dissection is started superiorly and carried downward on the surface of the fascia until the femoral areas are reached. The femoral sheath is opened along the medial border of the sartorius muscle, and the femoral triangle contents are removed, including the sheath of the artery as well as all tissue surrounding the femoral vein and nerve. The inguinal canal is then opened and the contents of the canal removed, starting laterally so they remain in continuity with the primary specimen. Unless a more extensive extraperitoneal node dissection is to be performed, the vulva is then excised along with the fascia and muscles of the urogenital diaphragm. The mucosal incision is in close proximity to the urethra and vaginal orifices. If the tumor involves the urethra or rectum, a pelvic exenteration may be necessary to encompass the disease.

Closure is carried out primarily if possible. It is useful to undermine the superior abdominal flap for a short distance, taking care to leave an adequate fat layer beneath the skin. The remaining posterior vaginal mucosa is undermined and brought out over the perineum to prevent contracture of the vaginal orifice. Closure is accomplished with 3-0 chromic catgut. The skin of the abdominal portion of the wound is closed with interrupted silk sutures.

If an extraperitoneal node dissection is to be carried out because of involvement of the so-called Cloquet node that lies just beneath the inguinal ligament, the dissection must be continued superiorly, with removal of all node-bearing tissue around the iliac, hypogastric, and obturator vessels (Fig. 40-8). This procedure is more extensive than the standard radical vulvectomy, but it has increased the survival rate by approximately 20 percent in most series. Extreme care must be used to maintain viable skin and soft tissue flaps for closure, since any wound breakdown will result in exposure of the femoral vessels. In some instances, it is useful to transpose the upper portion of the sartorius muscle

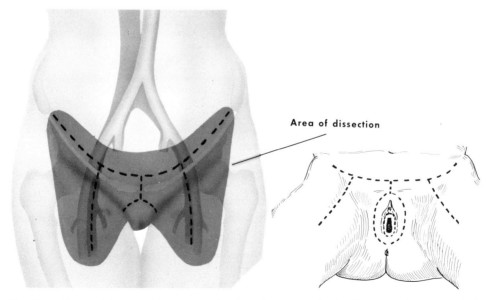

Area of dissection

FIG. 40-8. A. Incisions and limit of node dissection for radical vulvectomy. The area of dissection may be extended superiorly to include the hypogastric, obturator, external, and common iliac nodes. B. Perivulvar incision for radical vulvectomy.

medially and tack it in place to protect the vessels in the event of such breakdown.

The wound is drained by large suction catheters bilaterally, and pressure dressing is applied using gauze fluffs or mechanics' waste in conjunction with a T-binder. A Foley catheter is left in place.

RECONSTRUCTIVE PROCEDURES

The simplest and most commonly used reconstructive procedure is the application of a split-thickness skin graft. This covering material can be used without hesitation to cover any defect of an area for which primary closure will produce undue tension or distortion of other structures.

The donor site for a skin graft is the adjacent medial thigh or buttock, which has been previously prepared and draped into the field.

There are rare occasions when the removal of large amounts of tissue, particularly with the exposure of bone, larger nerves, or arteries, makes a skin graft inadequate for coverage. Under these circumstances, pedicle flaps are the covering material of choice. They can be brought into the area from the abdominal wall, thigh, or buttock, depending on the size and location of the defect to be covered. They are best planned so that the length of the flap never exceeds the width of its base, and it is essential that the flaps be raised with meticulous care to avoid damaging their blood supply. This requires the use of fine skin hooks, little or no clamping or cauterizing of vessels on the flap itself, and the transfer of the pedicle into the defect without major distortion or any tension whatsoever. The flaps are sutured in position in the usual manner. The donor site, if it does not close with ease, must be covered with a skin graft. Mild to moderate pressure in the postoperative period is essential to prevent edema of the transferred flap, and it should be maintained for at least 4 or 5 days.

References

1. Rutledge, F. N., Smith, J. P., and Franklin, E. W. Carcinoma of the vulva. *Am. J. Obstet. Gynecol.* 106:1117, 1970.

2. Te Linde, R. W., and Mattingly, R. F. *Operative Gynecology* (4th ed.). Philadelphia: Lippincott, 1970. P. 665.

Intraepithelial Tumors of the Perineum

FREDERIC RUECKERT
CHARLES E. HORTON
FORST E. BROWN

41

INTRAEPITHELIAL carcinoma is a specific pathological entity and is identical to carcinoma in situ. It encompasses the following clinical diseases and pathological variants: extramammary Paget's disease (when confined to the epidermis), Bowen's disease, erythroplasia of Queyrat, and papillary carcinoma in situ. The first two will be discussed in detail below. Erythroplasia of Queyrat appears to be a variant of Bowen's disease. Papillary carcinoma in situ differs from Bowen's disease in having a gross papillary or granular appearance; however, it overlaps with Bowen's disease and histologically requires comparable clinical management.

Extramammary Paget's Disease

HISTORY

In 1874 Sir James Paget, in his original report [30] describing 15 cases of the unique breast tumor that bears his name, also mentioned another patient with "a persistent *rawness* of the glans penis like a long endur-ing balanitis followed after more than a year's duration by cancer of the substance of the glans." This is probably the first reported case of extramammary Paget's disease. The epidermal manifestations of the mammary and the extramammary forms of these two skin tumors are very similar, and typical large, mucin-producing Paget cells are present in both.

ETIOLOGY

Although it is generally agreed that Paget's disease of the nipple is almost always associated with an underlying ductal adenocarcinoma of the mammary gland [3, 7], such a relationship is not always present in extramammary Paget's disease with respect to the underlying apocrine sweat glands. This disease can be limited to the epidermis, or it can occur with an associated underlying carcinoma of the dermal appendages. A number of authors [16, 17, 24, 35, 41] have noted adenocarcinomas in tissues other than skin—such as the breast, the gastrointestinal tract, and the genitourinary tract—that occur simultaneously with Paget's disease. This would suggest an unknown carcinogenic stimulus to these various glandular organs, possibly of a hormonal or endocrine nature. In any event, a careful search for other primary tumors in patients with Paget's disease during the preoperative work-up is certainly indicated.

Helwig and Graham [17] have concluded that extramammary Paget's disease in the skin is most likely of multicentric origin, arising from both the epidermis and the dermal appendages, rather than being caused by a migration of cancer cells into the epidermis from the dermal structures. These authors believe that the tumor may occur in the epidermis and remain superficial without involvement of the apocrine glands and without metastasis for many years. In such cases, the tumor behaves much like a superficial case of Bowen's disease. They maintain, however, that there is a second variety of the disease that involves the glandular skin appendages in the dermis; in this variety, there is regional lymph node and even distant metastasis in a high percentage of cases.

When an underlying adenocarcinoma of the apocrine glands is present along with Paget's disease in the epidermis, the tumor behaves similarly to adenocarcinoma elsewhere. The majority of authors [2, 9, 13, 23, 28, 38, 39] writing on the subject now agree in principle with these concepts and do not insist on the presence of an adenocarcinoma in the deeper layers of the skin to verify the diagnosis of extramammary Paget's disease.

DIAGNOSIS

Extramammary Paget's disease is a relatively rare and confusing malignant tumor of the skin which few surgeons see or treat with sufficient frequency to become proficient in its management. It is most often present as a chronic, itching, weeping, red, eczematous

lesion in the anogenital region (Figs. 41-1 and 41-2), where apocrine glands are numerous [1, 18, 20, 27, 29]. Much less frequently the tumor is seen in the axilla. It is a slowly progressive disease that does not improve with the measures used to treat chronic dermatitis, and the lesions may persist for months or even years before a biopsy examination establishes the correct diagnosis and proper definitive surgical treatment is undertaken [45]. The possibility of a skin malignancy should always be considered when a chronic eczematoid lesion is seen in the perineal area.

The various other forms of intraepithelial carcinoma (Bowen's disease, erythroplasia of Queyrat, papillary carcinoma in situ) and amelanotic melanoma are the tumors most apt to be confused grossly and histologically with Paget's disease. Grossly, there is no sure

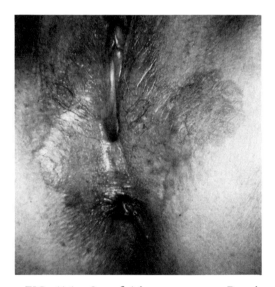

FIG. 41-1. Superficial extramammary Paget's disease of the perineum in a 71-year-old woman, which was treated by wide local excision and closure with bilateral thigh pedicle flaps (see Figure 2-9). There was no recurrence after 5 years.

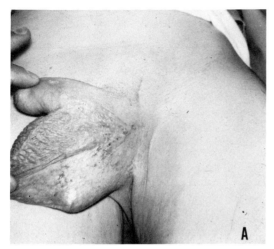 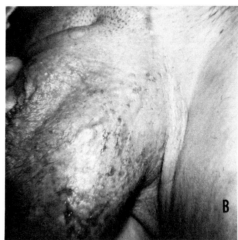

FIG. 41-2. A. A 60-year-old man with extramammary Paget's disease of the scrotum and groin. B. Close-up view. There was involvement of the dermal appendages and metastasis to several left iliac lymph nodes. The case was treated by wide local excision and bilateral radical groin dissections. The patient was alive and well 4 years postoperatively, although local superficial recurrence has occurred twice.

way to make a differential diagnosis consistently [28], and a biopsy is almost always necessary. Histologically, the diagnosis is made by the presence of characteristic large, pale vacuolated Paget cells in the epidermis (Figs. 41-3 and 41-4). The characteristic cells are also present when the dermal appendages are involved and in lymph node metastasis. The Paget cells are mucin producing, so the presence of mucin, as determined by differential staining techniques such as those using PAS (periodic acid, Schiff), mucicarmine, or aldehyde fuchsin [2, 14, 17, 27], will establish the diagnosis of Paget's disease and exclude the presence of non-mucin-producing epidermoid tumors and melanoma.

LYMPHOGRAPHY

Preoperative lymphography can be helpful in diagnosis and in planning treatment for regional lymph node involvement [4, 6, 8, 19, 26, 32, 36, 40]. Metastatic nodes, when present, are often demonstrated (Fig. 41-5). However, a negative finding does not rule out the possibility of metastatic disease (Fig. 41-6).

A lymphogram allows one to study the lymph node pattern preoperatively and alter the plan of operation if an unusual pattern exists. It also permits immediate checking of the completeness of the dissection by x-ray before wound closure is undertaken.

TREATMENT

Surgical excision is the treatment of choice. Most reports in the literature indicate that either this tumor does not respond to radiation, cauterization, or curettage or it recurs in a high percentage of cases following such treatment [15, 17, 38]. Very little is to be found in the literature on topical chemotherapy for the treatment of the superficial form [42] of extramammary Paget's disease.

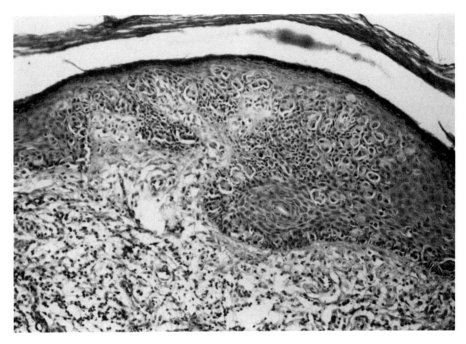

FIG. 41-3. Typical large Paget cells in the epidermis (low power).

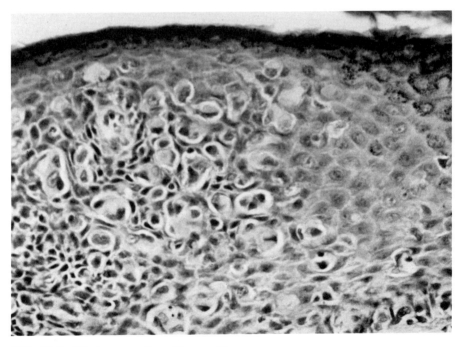

FIG. 41-4. High power view of Paget cells.

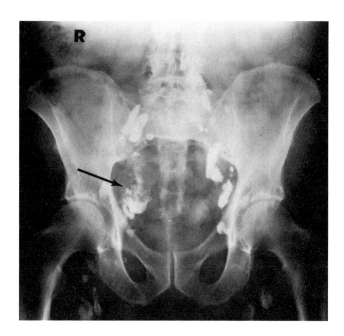

FIG. 41-5. Preoperative lymphogram showing metastatic tumor in the right iliac lymph node (*arrow*).

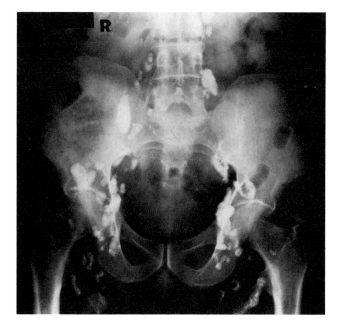

FIG. 41-6. Negative lymphographic finding in a patient who was found to have left iliac lymph node metastasis at operation.

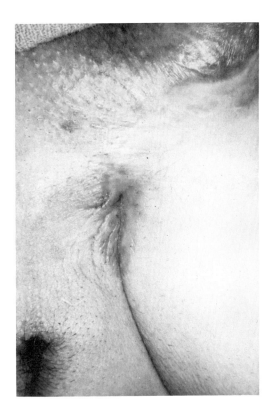

FIG. 41-7. Recurrent superficial Paget's disease in the left groin before treatment with topical 5-fluorouracil.

The use of topical 5-fluorouracil has been mentioned briefly, and good short-term follow-up results were reported [42]. One of our patients with local superficial recurrent disease (Fig. 41-7) has responded well to topical 5-fluorouracil; local control of the disease was demonstrated by negative biopsy findings for more than 1 year. Topical 5-fluorouracil is not recommended at this time as a primary, definitive form of treatment for Paget's disease. Its general use should probably be deferred until more has been learned about the long-term results of its use in cutaneous Paget's disease.

For noninvasive superficial tumors limited to the epidermis, wide local excision is indicated. Resurfacing by direct suture, free skin grafts (Fig. 41-8), or local pedicle flaps (Fig. 41-9) can be performed as necessary. For invasive tumors involving the deeper structures of the skin and for frank adenocarcinoma of the apocrine glands, a radical ileoinguinal lymph node dissection should also be carried out because of the high incidence of metastasis to the regional lymph nodes in this form of the disease. A bilateral lymph node dissection is indicated for lesions at or near the midline and when positive nodes are found on the side of the unilateral tumor [33].

Epidermoid carcinoma of the vulva is fre-

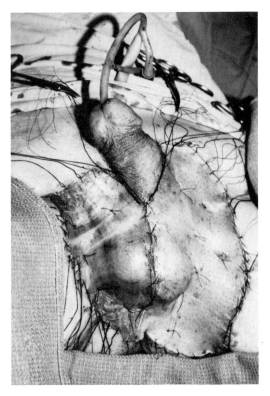

FIG. 41-8. A 68-year-old man who had wide local excision of superficial Paget's disease of the scrotum and perineum. Closure was with split-thickness skin grafts.

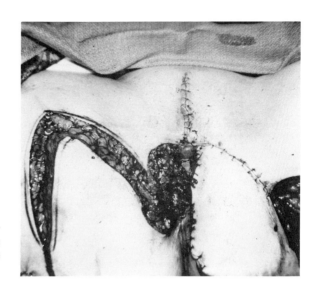

FIG. 41-9. After excision of the perineal lesion shown in Figure 2-1, closure was effected with bilateral thigh pedicle flaps.

quently associated with extramammary Paget's disease in the perineum [11, 12]. Up to one-third of these lesions (including both small and well-differentiated tumors) will metastasize to regional lymph nodes. Bilateral and contralateral spread is common. This association of Paget's disease with epidermoid carcinoma requires aggressive surgical therapy, and a bilateral groin dissection is routinely recommended when invasive epidermoid carcinoma exists.

PROGNOSIS

The prognosis is good for the noninvasive tumors involving only the epidermis. These tumors are prone to recur locally in the face of what appear to be adequate gross and microscopic margins [16, 31, 44]. However, various reports have indicated long-term survival in patients having multiple recurrences as long as the tumor remains superficial and not invasive [7, 16, 44].

If the tumor is invasive and the deep glandular structures of the dermis are involved, lymph node metastasis and even distant metastasis are common; the prognosis

for cure is then relatively poor. One series [17] reported 13 of 38 patients with extramammary Paget's disease who had glandular involvement of the skin. Of these 13 patients, 11 had regional or widespread metastasis. All 11 patients died, but the two patients without metastasis have survived. In another series [44], two of eight patients with this disease died from metastases. Another author [7] reported four of ten patients who died with metastatic disease. In yet another series [16], there were five patients with perianal Paget's disease, four of whom had underlying adenocarcinoma (three from the apocrine glands and one from the anorectal mucous membrane). One of these four died from tumor, and one was alive $2\frac{1}{2}$ years after operation but still had a tumor.

Bowen's Disease

In 1912 Bowen reported two cases of precancerous dermatoses. The atypical proliferation that he described is characteristic of squamous cell carcinoma in situ. Although some clinicians and pathologists differentiate

Bowen's disease as a specific entity, we shall consider it to be the same as carcinoma in situ.

Bowen's disease originates in the epithelium. In contrast to Paget's disease, it does not involve the deep, dermal appendages. It is not precancerous, but is actually cancer restricted to the epidermis. In the perineal region, it is commonly of multicentric origin. It has been estimated [34] that after a period of time 25 percent of these lesions become invasive. On the other hand, only 2 of 100 cases on file at the Armed Forces Institute of Pathology developed invasive carcinoma [18]. The average age for occurrence of Bowen's disease of the vulva precedes that for invasive carcinoma by 5 to 7 years. It is frequently associated with other lesions of the female genitalia. Moreover, carcinoma in situ is reported as occurring occasionally after irradiation therapy for carcinoma of the cervix [43].

DIAGNOSIS

The patient with Bowen's disease of the perineum usually complains of burning or itching that does not respond to symptomatic treatment. On examination, the lesions appear as slightly raised plaques that are dull red to reddish-brown in color with crusted or eroded surfaces (Fig. 41-10). The outline of these is sharp but irregular. The lesions spread by peripheral extension. When multicentric, the lesions tend to coalesce. The variant described by Clark [18] presents a more papillary appearance, varying from small granular areas to large plaques with rough papillary surfaces (Fig. 41-11). A lesion of the groin with extensive pigmentation that resembles those of Bowen's disease has also been reported [25].

Histologically, the epidermis is thickened with hyperkeratoses, parakeratoses, and acanthosis (Fig. 41-12). The rete pegs are thickened and elongated. The basal layer of

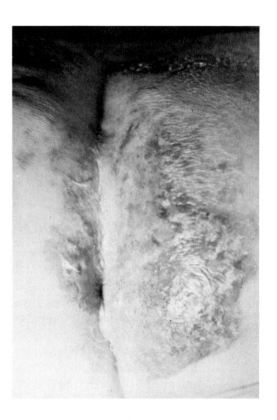

FIG. 41-10. Bowen's disease of the perineum showing crusted, plaque-like surface.

cells is intact. The size and shape of the cells are highly irregular, and giant, multinucleated, and vacuolated cells are found (Fig. 41-13). Mitotic figures are numerous. The dermis usually shows chronic inflammatory changes such as abundant lymphocytes and plasma cells.

Diagnosis is definitively established by histological examination of the biopsy specimen. Because of its similarity to other lesions and the multicentric nature of the disease, techniques to aid in the determination of sites for biopsy are valuable. Toluidine blue is a vital nuclear stain that appears to stain certain malignant and dysplastic skin lesions differentially; the precise mechanism for this

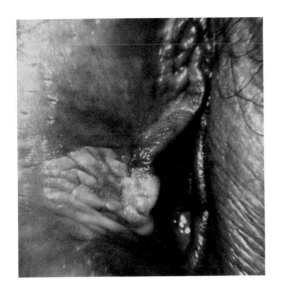

FIG. 41-11. Papillary variant of carcinoma in situ.

is unknown. In one study [5], all 19 patients with carcinoma of the vulva had a positive stain; there were no false negative results. Seventeen patients with inflammatory ulcers or excoriations had a false positive stain. In another study [37], 11 out of 12 patients with carcinoma in situ displayed a positive stain with toluidine blue. On the basis of these studies, the routine use of 1 percent toluidine blue staining prior to biopsy is recommended.

TREATMENT

Surgery is accepted as the proper treatment for intraepithelial carcinoma of the external genitalia. A high cure rate following surgery has been reported [43, 34]. In contrast, a recurrence of 72 percent after curettage and desiccation and 87 percent after irradiation therapy has also been reported [10]. Topical

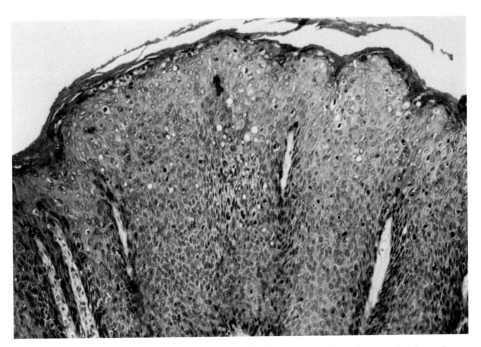

FIG. 41-12. Photomicrograph of a case of Bowen's disease showing elongated, blunted rete pegs, cellular atypism, hyperkeratosis and parakeratosis, and vacuolated cells.

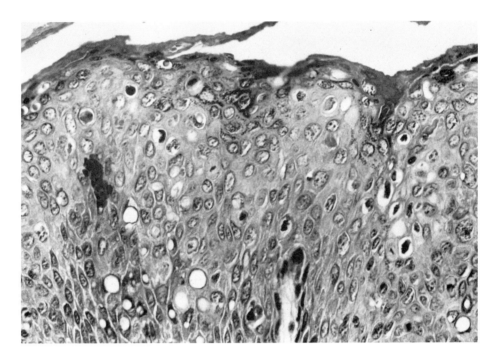

FIG. 41-13. High power view emphasizes cellular atypism, mitosis, and vacuolated cells.

chemotherapy using neoarsphenamine, methotrexate, and mechlorethamine has been tried in the treatment of these superficial lesions. In recent years, topical 5-fluorouracil has been introduced in the treatment of actinic keratoses and superficial skin tumors. Jansen [21] reported primary treatment of two vulvar and two penile lesions with 5-fluorouracil. Vulvectomy was subsequently required in one case, and another course of topical 5-fluorouracil was necessary for control of the two penile lesions.

Surgical therapy for carcinoma in situ of the external genitalia should be tailored for the lesion, location, and patient. Where surgery would be deforming, for example, for penile lesions, 5-fluorouracil could be employed first. In small lesions that are unicentric, as shown by toluidine blue stain, simple excision and closure is the treatment of choice. Speaking of vulvar lesions, Woodruff [42] stated "We have encountered no demonstrable lesion which could not be removed and closure effected without skin graft." In multicentric vulvar lesions or in lesions confined to the vulva but associated with other diseases of the perineum, simple vulvectomy is the preferred treatment. The less functionally disabling (but more technically demanding) superficial skin excision and split-thickness grafting technique should be considered for younger patients [34].

RESULTS

Anything less than complete cure of Bowen's disease should be unacceptable. Intraepithelial carcinoma does not metastasize until it becomes invasive. Its multicentric nature, however, demands total excision and close follow-up.

References

1. Allen, A. C. *The Skin: A Clinicopathological Treatise.* New York: Grune and Stratton, 1967.
2. Becker, S. W., Jr., Brennan, B., and Weichselbaum, P. K. Genital Paget's disease. *Arch. Dermatol.* 82:857, 1960.
3. Bennet, W. A. Pathologic study of Paget's disease of the nipple. Master's thesis, University of Minnesota, 1943.
4. Bruce, P. T., and Hare, W. S. C. Failure of metastatic nodes to fill during lymphography. *Clin. Radiol.* 18:88, 1967.
5. Collins, C. G., Hanson, L. H., and Theriot, E. A clinical stain for use in selecting biopsy sites in patients with vulvar disease. *Obstet. Gynecol.* 28:158, 1966.
6. Cox, K. R., Hare, W. S., and Bruce, P. T. Lymphography in melanoma: Correlation of radiology with pathology. *Cancer* 19:637, 1966.
7. Fardal, R. W., Kierland, R. R., Clagett, O. T., et al. Prognosis in cutaneous Paget's disease. *Postgrad. Med.* 36:584, 1964.
8. Farrell, W. J. Lymphography in the diagnosis and management of lymphoma and metastatic disease. *Surg. Clin. North Am.* 47:565, 1967.
9. Fisher, E. R., and Beyer, F. D., Jr. Extramammary Paget's disease. *Am. J. Surg.* 94:493, 1957.
10. Graham, J. H., and Helwig, E. B. Precancerous Skin Lesions and Systemic Cancer. In *Tumors of the Skin: A Collection of Papers* (Clinical Conference on Cancer, M. D. Anderson Hospital and Tumor Institute, Houston, Texas, 7th, 1962). Chicago: Yearbook, 1964. Pp. 209–222.
11. Green, T. H., Jr. Discussion in Rueckert, F., and Durham, C. Extramammary Paget's disease of the groin. *Trans. N. Engl. Surg. Soc.* 48:41, 1967.
12. Green, T. H., Jr. Personal communication, 1970.
13. Grimes, O. F. Extramammary Paget's disease. *Surgery* 45:569, 1959.
14. Gupta, R. K. Extramammary Paget's disease: Report of two cases. *Obstet. Gynecol.* 28:663, 1966.
15. Hambrick, G. W., Jr., Whelan, S. T., and Wood, M. G. Extramammary Paget's disease. *Arch. Dermatol.* 97:598, 1968.
16. Harrison, E. G., Jr., Beahrs, O. H., and Hill, J. R. Anal and peranal malignant neoplasms: Pathology and treatment. *Dis. Colon Rectum* 9:255, 1966.
17. Helwig, E. B., and Graham, J. H. Anogenital extramammary Paget's disease: A clinicopathological study. *Cancer* 16:387, 1963.
18. Hertig, A. T., and Gore, H. Tumors of Female Sex Organs—Part I. In *Atlas of Tumor Pathology* (Section IX, Fascicle 33). Washington, D.C.: Armed Forces Institute of Pathology, 1960, 1968.
19. Hodari, A. A., and Hodgkinson, C. P. Lymphography as a diagnostic aid in female genital malignancy. *Obstet. Gynecol.* 29:34, 1967.
20. Holleran, W. M., and Schmutzer, K. J. Paget's disease of the groin. *J.A.M.A.* 193:965, 1965.
21. Jansen, G. T., Dillaha, C. J., and Honeycutt, W. M. Bowenoid conditions of the skin: Treatment with topical 5FU. *South. Med.* 60:185, 1967.
22. Jeffcoat, T. N. A., Davis, T. B., and Harrison, C. U. Intraepidermal carcinoma of vulva. *J. Obstet. Gynecol. Brit. Emp.* 51:377, 1944.
23. Koss, L. G., Ladinsky, S., and Brockunier, A. Paget's disease of the vulva: Report of ten cases. *Obstet. Gynecol.* 31:513, 1968.
24. Linder, J. H., and Myers, R. T. Perianal Paget's disease. *Am. Surg.* 36:342, 1970.
25. Lloyd, K. M. Multicentric pigmented Bowen's disease of the groin. *Arch. Dermatol.* 101:48, 1970.
26. Love, L., and Kim, S. E. Clinical aspects of lymphangiography. *Med. Clin. North Am.* 51:227, 1967.
27. Lund, H. Z. Tumors of the skin. In *Atlas of Tumor Pathology* (Section 1, Fascicle 2). Washington, D.C.: Armed Forces Institute of Pathology, 1957.

28. Montgomery, H. *Dermatopathology*. New York: Hoeber Med. Div., Harper & Row, 1967.

29. Novak, E. R., and Woodruff, J. D. *Novak's Gynecologic and Obstetric Pathology*. Philadelphia: Saunders, 1967.

30. Paget, J. On disease of the mammary areola preceding cancer of the mammary gland. *St. Bartholomew's Hosp. Rep.* 10:87, 1874.

31. Parks, T. G. Paget's disease of perianal skin. *Proc. R. Soc. Med.* 61:445, 1968.

32. Rigos, A., Chrysanthakopoulos, S., and Tsardakas, E. Diagnostic and therapeutic applications of lymphography in clinical medicine. *Am. J. Surg.* 120:66, 1970.

33. Rueckert, F., and Durham, C. Extramammary Paget's disease of the groin. *Trans. N. Engl. Surg. Soc.* 48:41, 1967.

34. Rutledge, F., and Sinclair, M. Treatment of intraepithelial carcinoma of the vulva by skin excision and grafting. *Am. J. Obstet. Gynecol.* 102:806, 1968.

35. Salazar, G., and Frable, W. J. Extramammary Paget's disease: A case involving the prostatic urethra. *Am. J. Clin. Pathol.* 52:607, 1969.

36. Spratt, J. S., Shieber, W., and Dillard, B. M. *Anatomy and Surgical Techniques of Groin Dissection*. St. Louis: Mosby, 1965.

37. Sugerman, H. J., Hamilton, R., Graham, W. P., and Randall, P. Diagnostic staining of neoplastic skin lesions with toluidine blue. *Arch. Surg.* 100:240, 1970.

38. Taki, I., and Janovski, N. A. Paget's disease of vulva: Presentation and histochemical studies: 4 cases. *Obstet. Gynecol.* 18:385, 1961.

39. Vogel, E. W., and Ayers, M. A. Primary epidermal Paget's disease of the vulva. *Obstet. Gynecol.* 36:284, 1970.

40. Wallace, S. Lymphangiography: Diagnosis of nodal metastases from testicular malignancies. *J.A.M.A.* 213:94, 1970.

41. Weilburg, R. D., Miller, G. V., and Von Pohle, K. C. Paget's disease of the vulva associated with adenocarcinoma developing in a hidradenoma papilliferum. *Am. J. Obstet. Gynecol.* 98:284, 1967.

42. Woodruff, J. D. Discussion in Rutledge, F., and Sinclair, M. Treatment of intraepithelial carcinoma of the vulva by skin excision and grafting. *Am. J. Obstet. Gynecol.* 102:806, 1968.

43. Woodruff, J. D., and Hildebrandt, E. E. Carcinoma-in-situ of the vulva. *Obstet. Gynecol.* 12:414, 1958.

44. Woodruff, J. D., and Pauerstein, C. J. Differential metabolic activity in Paget's cells and associated epithelia of the vulva. *Obstet. Gynecol.* 28:663, 1966.

45. Zimmerman, M. C. Tinea rubrum. 1) Tinea pedis and cruris. 2) Verrucous dermatitis perianal: Extramammary Paget's disease. *Arch. Dermatol.* 98:322, 1968.

Common Birthmarks and Keloids

CHARLES E. HORTON
JEROME E. ADAMSON
RICHARD A. MLADICK
JAMES CARRAWAY

42

Birthmarks

Benign birthmarks are seen frequently in the genital area [5]. Small juvenile hemangiomas may be present at birth or appear soon after. These usually are red in color, nonpainful, and compressible. Over a period of time, they tend to regress and disappear, usually by 4 to 5 years of age. Occasionally, larger, more diffuse hemangiomas occur which, because of the anatomical site, pose peculiar problems [1]. The skin covering the larger hemangioma is usually thin and easily macerated. Moisture caused by urine or feces retained in soiled diapers may cause early ulceration with surface infection and pain. Bleeding usually occurs from ulcerated lesions, and parents may become distraught at the pain and bleeding evidenced. It has long been our policy to allow uncomplicated hemangiomas to resolve spontaneously (Fig. 42-1). Once pain and bleeding occur in a large tumor, however, we usually prefer to excise the lesion and employ grafts. Even if conservative therapy is continued, the resolution time may be prolonged to a degree that is intolerable [6]. Ulceration and infection cause thrombosis within the hemangioma, and, in this area, healing is slow (Fig. 42-2). Thin split-thickness grafts take well and convert a difficult problem into a simple case in most instances. Intralesional injection of cortisone has been advocated to hasten involution.

Arteriovenous fistulas and hemangiomas of mature vascular tissue will not disappear spontaneously. These should be removed electively when the child is 3 to 4 years of age to prevent psychological disturbances as well as physical complications [2].

The pigmented nevus is another common benign tumor of the genital area (Fig. 42-3). We routinely recommend removal of all nevi of this area because of the high frequency of junctional activity noted in the lesions. Most small nevi can be treated by excision of a simple ellipse of tissue and primary closure. We prefer skin closure with 5-0 chromic catgut sutures, and the patients are allowed to continue bathing. The sutures dissolve spontaneously, and scarring is minimal.

Occasionally, a giant pigmented birthmark may occur. This may involve large areas and be hairy, nodular, or both. Malignant degeneration later in life frequently occurs, and

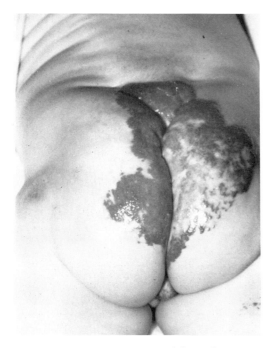

FIG. 42-1. Hemangioma of buttocks, anus, and scrotum. This tumor resolved spontaneously.

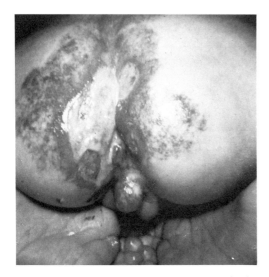

FIG. 42-2. Ulcerated hemangioma of the buttocks, anus, and scrotum. This hemangioma caused so much pain that it was necessary to excise it and to use a graft to promote healing.

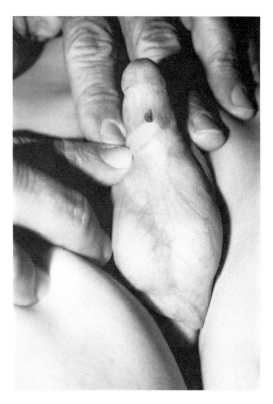

FIG. 42-3.   Junctional nevus of the penis.

this, as well as the cosmetic disfigurement, makes surgical excision desirable. We prefer to excise the lesion and close this area primarily whenever possible. Frequently, large defects can be covered by undermining to allow wide mobilization of the skin edges (Fig. 42-4).

In cases where primary closure is not feasible, two alternatives are possible. The surgeon may elect to excise a portion of the tumor to allow approximation of the defect edges without undue tension. This requires cutting through tumor, but since these lesions are benign, no harm ensues if later stages are planned for total excision of the birthmark. At least a 6 to 12 month period between stages is desirable to allow stretching of the adjacent skin. If necessary, two or three staged

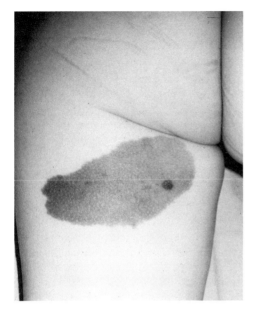

A

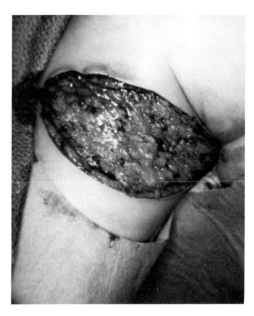

B

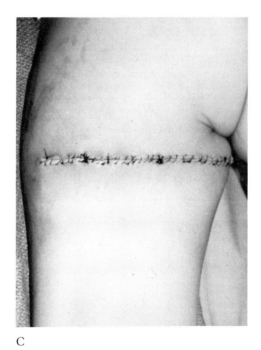

C

FIG. 42-4. A. Birthmark of buttocks and leg. B. Wide excision is performed. C. Primary closure after undermining.

excisions can be done to remove a large affected area. This type of surgery eventually results in only a single scar, and it is therefore desirable from a cosmetic standpoint.

In certain large lesions, the surgeon may also elect to excise the entire tumor at one operation. Primary closure in such instances is not feasible, and the wound must be covered with a flap or graft. Usually a graft will provide sufficient coverage for the genital area. Such a graft can be obtained from the adjacent buttocks, where little concern need be given to the resulting minor donor site scar. An additional advantage of graft closure results when contracture of the graft site reaches its maximum extent, causing the original skin defect to shrink as much as one-third to one-half. Subsequent excision of the graft may become feasible, and eventually a better cosmetic result can be achieved.

Because large pigmented birthmarks grow at the same rate as normal skin, it is highly desirable to excise them early while they are small. The resulting small scar will not grow appreciably, much less scarring will be present, and the scar will remain inconspicuous while the adjacent areas grow normally. We prefer to operate on most large birthmarks when the patient is 1 to 2 years of age if no contraindicating circumstances exist.

The true juvenile malignant melanoma is a rare tumor that will infrequently occur prior to puberty. All specimens should be carefully examined histologically, and if malignancy is present, extensive surgery is indicated.

Keloids

Keloids of the genital area are rare. Most plastic surgeons have commented on the fact that they have never seen a keloid in an episiotomy scar, even in patients who have a keloidal tendency. Keloids from hemorrhoid-ectomies or from flap incisions on the buttocks have never been reported.

Only in two places in the genital area are keloids likely to occur. One is located at the base of the penis, where the shaft skin meets the pubic skin [7]. If an incision is carried over this junction, a contracture of the scar will usually occur, and, due to the irritation, a keloid or hypertrophic scar may result. A keloid will grow beyond the original scar area, whereas a hypertrophied scar will enlarge within the original scar area.

If a scar must be carried from the shaft to the pubic area, it should be broken with a Z-plasty or with staggered incisions. Once such a scar has occurred, it should be excised, and Z-plasties or flaps are used to correct the defect. X-ray therapy or the injection of cortisone intralesionally will have little effect until the mechanical irritation of the scar is corrected.

The second place in the genital area where keloids are common is at the pubic-abdominal skin junction (Fig. 42-5). An incision

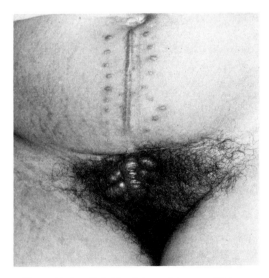

FIG. 42-5. Keloid of the pubic area. This was brought about by the straight entension of an abdominal incision inferiorly.

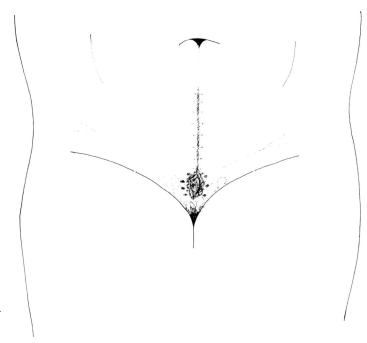

FIG. 42-6. A keloid occurring in a vertical pubic scar.

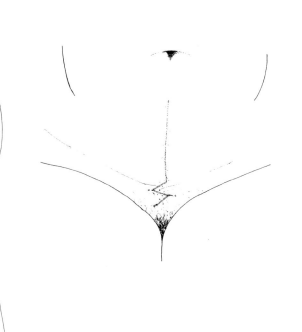

FIG. 42-7. Extension of a vertical scar in a zig-zag fashion to prevent a scar line against the skin planes.

that is carried along the pubic skin lines in a transverse fashion will usually heal well. However, if a vertical abdominal incision is extended inferiorly onto the pubic skin, the lower portion may enlarge and become hypertrophic or keloidal (Fig. 42-6). The scar will enlarge, and it may cause itching and burning to the extent that the patient will be unable to sleep.

If a vertical incision must be extended inferiorly, a zig-zag extension should always be done to prevent later contracture (Fig. 42-7).

Once the keloid has occurred, it should be excised and Z-plasties should be performed to correct the abnormal scar pull across the pubic crease line. If the keloid is too large for primary closure, a skin graft can be used if absolutely necessary. Postoperative cortisone injections and x-ray treatment may be indicated in extensive cases, in which the skin cannot be closed without excess tension and in the proper skin lines [3, 4].

References

1. Blackfield, H. M., Torry, F. A., Norres, W. J., and Low Boor, B. V. A. Management of hemangiomas. *Plast. Reconstr. Surg.* 20:38, 1957.
2. Figi, F. A. Treatment of hemangioma. *Plast. Reconstr. Surg.* 3:1, 1948.
3. Griffith, B. H., Monroe, C. W., and McKinney, P. Follow-up study of treatment of keloids with triamcinolone acetonide. *Plast. Reconstr. Surg.* 46:145, 1970.
4. Ketchum, L. D., Smith, J., Robinson, D. W., et al. The treatment of hypertrophic scar, keloid and scar contracture by triamcinolone. *Plast. Reconstr. Surg.* 38:209, 1966.
5. Lewis, J. R. J. Treatment of hemangiomas. *Plast. Reconstr. Surg.* 19:201, 1957.
6. Matthews, D. N. Hemangiomata. *Plast. Reconstr. Surg.* 41:528, 1968.
7. Parsons, R. W. A case of keloid of penis. *Plast. Reconstr. Surg.* 37:431, 1966

Tumors of the Penis

PETER L. SCARDINO
SAMUEL TORRES

43

THE PENIS is frequently inspected and should be an ideal site for early detection of abnormalities. However, failure to circumcise the newborn, fear, slow lesion progression, and persistent Victorian attitudes often permit a disease with an otherwise good prognosis to advance far beyond control before medical advice is sought. The disease may progress insidiously under the shielding foreskin until it has become incurable.

Incidence

Since it is a disease of the uncircumcised, penile cancer is uncommon in Europe and the Western hemisphere. Of cancers in the male population, penile neoplasms account for less than 3 percent of cancer deaths in the United States, almost 5 percent of cancer deaths in Europe, but more than 18 percent of such deaths in China. Excision of the prepuce in newborns could irradicate the disease. Penile cancer is essentially unknown in Jewish populations, but it occurs among Mohammedans, who circumcise their youths later in life. Except for penile cancer, there is an equal prevalence of all malignancies among the noncircumcised Hindus and Moslems and the circumcised Mohammedans. The disease is five times more common in black men than in white. The peak incidence occurs at the age range of 40 to 70 years, but cases have been reported in children and octogenarians.

Etiology

Chronic irritation by smegma, a product of Tyson's glands, may be related to the development of penile cancer. A source of the irritant may be the epithelial prominences of noncornified glandular cells that undergo fat dystrophy and desquamation. Smegma might be converted to a carcinogenic agent by *Mycobacterium smegmatis*. Most lesions begin within the preputial cavity; this fact supports the theory that smegma is involved in the cause, as does the suggestion that early circumcision precludes development of the disease. A plethora of theories have emerged over the years. Among the most plausible of the proposed agents are associated viruses, venereal diseases, late circumcision, venereal warts, burns, trauma, and coitus with one having carcinoma of the cervix.

Benign Lesions

CYSTS

Penile skin is thin, elastic, and abundant in smooth muscle, but hair follicles, fat, and sebaceous glands are absent in the glans of the penis. The penis is vulnerable to lesions that range from simple benign cysts to a variety of malignancies.

Congenital cysts and acquired *traumatic inclusion and retention cysts* are rarely observed on the penis. Large *hemangiomas* are seldom seen; the smaller and relatively common lesions are purplish macules or papules on the coronal aspect of the glans and are of little significance. *Nevi* of the skin of the penis must be distinguished from serious penile lesions.

Hirsutoid papillomas of the corona—the small, grayish-white or reddish-gray projections that are usually found arranged in irregular rows along the corona of the glans penis—are seen in young adults whether circumcised or not. The lesions are asymptomatic, and no treatment is indicated.

Condylomata acuminata—venereal or genital warts—are common lesions caused by a filterable virus. The disease is transmissible and autoinoculable, but it responds to treatment by circumcision and fulguration.

Buschke-Lowenstein tumor—a giant condyloma acuminatum or carcinoma-like papilloma—is a large papillary lesion that is frequently associated with ulceration, infection, local extension, and destruction of adjacent tissue. It is not malignant. Pathogenesis of the lesion has not been determined. The lesion is mutilating and poorly controlled, and it often justifies amputation.

Penile horn is a wart of excessive hypertrophy and cornification of the epithelium in which malignant changes may occur.

Keloids, neurofibroma, and *myoma* of the penis are rare conditions.

PRECANCEROUS LESIONS

Balanitis xerotica obliterans may occur in the circumcised or uncircumcised patient at any age. This interesting lesion usually involves the meatus, where it appears as a white, swollen induration that obstructs urinary flow. Characteristically, the lesion has a thin atrophic epidermis with loss of rete pegs, homogenization of the collagen in the epidermis, and variable changes. Superficial ulcerations and fissures may develop. When treatment is necessary, meatotomy, urethral dilatation, and the injection of hydrocortisone acetate may be helpful.

Leukoplakia (or leukokeratosis) occurs as white or grayish-white plaques that may be rough or smooth and atrophic. The generally sharply defined raised areas usually measure a few centimeters or less in diameter. Removal of the irritant may be all the treatment necessary for cure of the disease. Local excision is recommended. Leukoplakia may coexist with or antecede development of penile cancer, but the precise relationship is uncertain. After removal of the lesion, regular annual examination for at least 5 years is mandatory.

Erythroplasia of Queyrat usually appears as a velvety red plaque, occurring either singly or multiply, with a smooth but slightly elevated surface. Malignant transformation is noted by the development of ulceration or papillomatous proliferation. The lesions are usually found on the dorsal aspect of the glans, but they have also been found on the inner preputial surface. There is very little change in the epithelium. A moderate hyperplasia occurs, along with thickening of the rete pegs and superficial abrasion. Cell separation by inflammatory cells and edema is commonly noted. The capillaries are increased in number and engorged with red blood cells. Neither the clinical appearance nor the microscopic picture is characteristic of malignancy. Infiltration within the lesion may make treatment with ointments or local excision useless. Whatever the treatment, annual examination after local excision is essential since the disease may represent carcinoma in situ of the penis.

Paget's disease and *Bowen's disease* of the penis and perineum are discussed elsewhere in this book (see Part VI, Chap. 41).

Malignant Lesions

Epidermoid carcinoma is the most common of the malignant penile lesions, whereas *basal cell carcinoma* is the most rare. Supportive tissue tumors—such as fibrosarcoma, endothelioma, and various carcinomas—rarely occur on the penis. *Melanoma* may occur on the skin of the shaft, the glans, the coronal sulcus, or in the fossa navicularis, but this must be distinguished from *angiomatous lesions* of a similar distribution. *Metastatic tumors* on the penis are rare and represent a late manifestation of carcinoma elsewhere in the body.

Symptomatology

The stage of the disease determines the presenting symptoms. An early lesion is painless. Unsuccessful local treatment results in bleeding and purulent discharge from a superimposed infection. Only in advanced cases is the urethra involved, causing urinary frequency, urgency, dysuria, decrease in stream size, and poor trajectory; these often occur in conjunction with urinary tract infection. Inguinal lymphadenopathy may be secondary to infection and tumor extension from the primary focus. The prepuce may become fused with the glans by the new growth beneath the unretractable foreskin. Ignorance coupled with poor hygiene permits the development of a tumor that is neither seen nor felt until enlargement and infection cause pain or discharge from the ulceration. Some lesions advance incredibly before medical consultation is requested (Fig. 43-1). Often the glans penis is destroyed and the

urethral lumen is obstructed before the patient presents with acute urinary retention. Tumor cords or nodules may extend along the penile shaft as the lymphatics become involved.

Pathology

The lesion has usually been present for at least 6 months prior to examination by a physician. Eighty percent of patients have not seen a physician for more than a year after first noting the sore, ulcer, or growth. Four stages of development of the tumor are seen: (1) diffuse, irregular epithelial hyperplasia, (2) nodular proliferation, (3) papilloma; and (4) cancer. One-half of the neoplastic lesions start on the glans and the rest on the prepuce or the coronal sulcus. One-fifth of the lesions have extended into the corpora cavernosa when first examined by the physician.

The tumor may begin as a malignancy on the glans in an area of leukoplakia, erythroplasia, or Bowen's disease that may have existed for years beneath a shielding phimosis. Insidiously, malignant changes take place. Most cancers of the penis present as papillary excrescences or as an ulcerated induration. The papillary lesions appear on the glans, proliferate, and blossom to a foul-smelling, fungating, cauliflower-like mass. The ulcerated lesion often begins on the corona or in the sulcus and may resemble a syphilitic chancre.

Whatever the stimulating agent, the lining epithelium undergoes hyperplasia and squamous cell metaplasia. As the epithelium thickens, projections reach deep into the glans as local resistance is overcome. Large cells in the subepithelium accumulate, of which some undergo central degeneration and hyalinization. In the stroma, there is a luxuriant cellular reaction of mast cells and polymorphonuclear leukocytes. Inflammation develops as the ulceration breaks through to

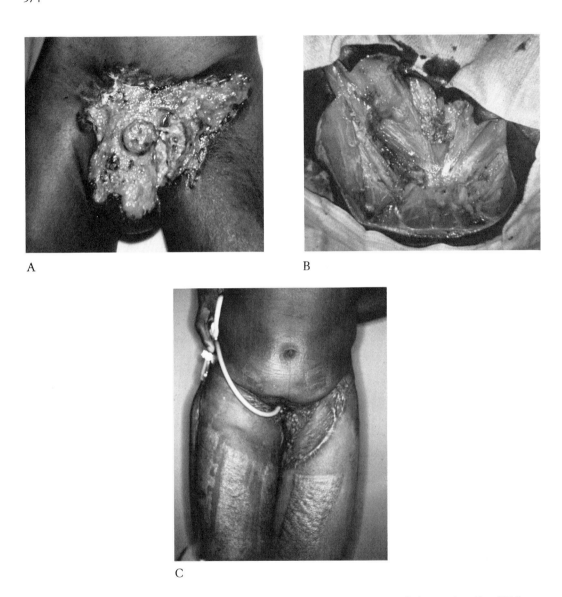

FIG. 43-1. A. Highly advanced primary squamous cell carcinoma of the penis. B. Wide excision and groin dissections were performed. C. Postoperative result. Split-thickness skin graft coverage was used. The patient was alive and well 5 years after surgery. (Case of C. E. Horton, J. E. Adamson, and R. A. Mladick.)

manifest both tumor and infection. Penetration of the urethra produces fistulous tracts. Cancer cells invade the lymphatics and extend to the inguinal lymph field by contiguous growth or embolic propulsion.

The lesions, graded histologically from 1 to 4, range from well-differentiated through moderately differentiated to poorly differentiated tumors. Grading is of prognostic significance. A 60 percent 5-year survival rate for patients with well-differentiated tumors can be expected, whereas less than 40 percent of patients with grade 2 lesions and only 25 percent of those with grade 3 tumors survive 5 years. Grade 2 and 3 lesions metastasize with equal frequency, each having 40 percent positive findings on node biopsy examination for cancer when first observed.

Staging is required for treatment as well as prognosis. *Stage I* tumors are limited to the glans penis, coronal sulcus, or prepuce. *Stage II* lesions are Stage I tumors with invasion of the corpora cavernosa but without lymph node involvement. *Stage III* tumors include Stages I and II plus lymph node extension. *Stage IV* embraces the previous three stages but with inoperable lymph nodes, distant metastases, or both. When staged and graded, the well-differentiated tumors limited to the glans penis or prepuce (stage I) result in an 85 percent 5-year survival rate when surgically excised, whereas lesions of comparable grade and stage when treated with radiotherapy result in a 5-year survival of 46 percent.

The result of treatment of cancer of the penis depends on the role of the lymphatics that drain the anatomical sites involved. Tumor embolization by direct extension beyond the initial site usually travels via rich lymphatics to both inguinal areas through three sets of lymphatics. One network leads to the femoral canal, the superior inguinal nodes, and the node of Cloquet. The second network branches to the inguinal canal,

passes alongside the spermatic cord, and terminates in the external retrofemoral nodes. The third set of lymphatics from the corpora cavernosa terminates in superficial and deep inguinal nodes and in the retrofemoral nodes. The superficial and deep inguinal nodes have anatomical connections. Lymphatics of the penile shaft anastomose extensively. Penile lesions of the right side may develop left inguinal lymphadenopathy. Scrotal and perineal lymphatic extension is rarely seen. Enlargement of the inguinal glands may be due to both infection and metastatic disease; however, at least one-half of enlarged lymph glands contain malignant cells. The absence of palpable lymph nodes does not preclude metastic involvement. Extension may proceed via the venous system from the dorsal vein of the penis with extension to the central nervous system, bony pelvis, prostate, lungs, spleen, skull, or mediastinal glands.

Diagnosis

Biopsies must be performed on all penile lesions, whether of the prepuce, glans, or coronal sulcus. Ideally, frozen-section biopsy examination followed by definitive therapy is the course of choice. Little delay should occur between biopsy and surgery. Aspiration biopsy of the inguinal lymph nodes is recommended, and if the results are positive, lymphadenectomy is performed.

Inguinal lymphadenopathy may be the first sign or symptom noted by the patient with an unretractable foreskin. Examination of the penis may be difficult. Adjunctive studies to staging and grading the penile lesion should include intravenous pyelography and lymphangiography. Involved retroperitoneal lymph nodes may cause renal or ureteral displacement. A test for syphilis is obtained, and the lesion is differentiated from papillomas, condyloma acuminatum, syphilis, soft chancre, and the premalignant lesions of erythroplasia, leukoplakia, and Bowen's disease. Primary carcinoma of the urethra seldom appears in the anterior location. Metastatic carcinoma to the penis, malignant melanomas, and sarcomas are rarely observed.

Treatment

The value of radiotherapy in the treatment of penile cancer is uncertain. The surgery required for the treatment of penile cancer does not demand special skills, equipment, or sophisticated management. Tumor grading and staging (see above), when followed by universally accepted surgical techniques, provide results that are superior to any other treatment method now available.

The first step in treatment is an adequate biopsy of the penile lesion and enlarged lymph nodes. The second is classification. Biopsy examination provides a differential diagnosis and tumor grade. Tumors are staged as described above.

Lesions of the prepuce may be treated by simple circumcision. Tumors limited to the glans or coronal sulcus are locally excised; these require careful follow-up. If the biopsy finding shows definite malignancy all such lesions are treated similarly: the glans penis is excised by amputation 2 cm proximal to any visible or palpable neoplasm. Lack of extension is confirmed by careful surgical histological examination.

Local control by appropriate amputation provides excellent results. The adverse cosmetic, sexual, and urinary effects are minimal. Subsequent lymphadenopathy may develop, and subsequent biannual examination of the inguinal area is as necessary as biopsy and amputation. Since only 3 percent of nonpalpable nodes are involved with cancer, lymphadenectomy is not advocated if the nodes are not palpable. Histologically proven penile cancer of the glans, corona or sulcus, and inguinal lymph glands demands wide amputation of the lesion and bilateral inguinal, femoral, and iliac lymphadenectomy. Some surgeons delay lymphadenectomy 4 to 6 weeks after penile amputation to allow resolution of inflamed lymph nodes. Combined bilateral groin dissection and penile amputation, however, is preferable. Intensive administration of antimicrobials during the brief presurgical period and during convalescence eliminates an otherwise undesirable waiting period.

Radical inguinal, femoral, and iliac dissection may require the transfer of superficial muscles of the thigh for protection of exposed blood vessels. Reconstruction of the divided urethra is painstakingly performed. Sufficient urethral length is provided distal to the amputated corpora cavernosa. The urethra and corpus spongiosum are seldom involved in penile cancer. Insufficient urethral length permits retraction, fibrosis, and stenosis of the urethral meatus. Careful anastomosis of an excessively long urethra and corpus spongiosum to the skin of the penile shaft, which is free of tumor, provides a satisfactory urethra for both micturition and ejaculation. The urethral meatus should be spatulated and positioned ventrally beneath the penile stump, and the corpus spongiosum is anchored to the fascia of the corpora cavernosa with fine catgut sutures. The urethral edges are anastomosed to the penile skin to provide a normal voiding trajectory. An indwelling, nonreactive urethral catheter usually must be maintained for 1 week after reconstruction of the meatus. Both closed system catheter drainage and urethral meatal care with antiinflammatory, antimicrobial agents reduce secondary infection and stenosis.

Total penile amputation requires either urinary diversion (i.e., ureteroileostomy) or perineal urethrostomy. The penis is removed along with the ischiocavernous muscle to its bony insertion. Emasculation is seldom necessary. Sufficient urethra is retained for construction of a perineal urethrostomy utilizing the previously described technique, which will reduce urethral retraction and fibrosis. In stage III tumors wherein unilaterally involved lymph nodes are attached to adjacent structures, hemipelvectomy has prolonged the patient's survival.

Radiotherapy

The radiotherapist views carcinoma of the penis as a radiocurable disease. If properly administered, local control by irradiation provides preservation of function. The therapist views amputation as traumatic, mutilating, and emotionally distressing and suggests that surgery should be reserved for radiation treatment failures in spite of evidence of the stimulation of tumor growth following irradiation. The results of irradiation in the treatment of penile cancer depend on the skill, training, knowledge, and experience of the therapist. Techniques are available for isolating the penile lesion during therapy to provide protection of adjacent organs. When careful shielding is used and dose-time relationships are properly calculated, then edema, mutilation, and disturbance of micturition or sexual potency seldom occur. Nonetheless, when complications of irradiation do occur, they may be as disastrous as any surgical complication. Sepsis and necrosis may require penile amputation. The significant incidence of leg edema, urethral stricture, and pulmonary embolus reduces the survival rates to less than those achieved with surgery. Treatment complications occur with equal frequency in early and late lesions to preclude the "advantage" of radiotherapy. Irradiation is most effective in the treatment of superficial, exophytic lesions. The phimotic patient

must be circumcised to expose the lesion to therapy and to permit resolution of infection if irradiation is to be effective. Radiation is probably effective in the control of metastatic lymph node deposits, but most clinicians prefer surgical removal of the nodes. Occasionally, irradiation of inoperable inguinal involvement produces beneficial results.

Combined Therapy

Patients with penile cancer who are treated with a combination of surgery and irradiation may have a possible advantage over those who are treated by either method alone. The primary lesion in selected cases may be irradiated, and any subsequent recurrence is surgically excised without increasing the risk of metastasis. The primary lesion may be excised and tumoricidal doses of radiation given to the inguinal and femoral lymph nodes. No series of penile cancer in the literature is sufficiently large to permit dogmatic statements regarding the superiority of methods, but the 5-year survival rates for surgically treated cancer lesions are better than those for radiation treated cancer. The clinician must select a method that he can best apply after careful grading and staging of the disease under his supervision. In the United States, surgery takes precedence over radiation therapy.

Summary of Treatment Methods

1. Lesions of the prepuce require circumcision.
2. Nonmalignant lesions of the glans or coronal sulcus require elimination of irritants, treatment of medical conditions, or local excision.
3. Malignant tumors of the glans, coronal sulcus, or prepuce without lymphadenopathy

require partial penile amputation without groin dissection.

4. Malignant tumors of the glans penis, coronal sulcus, or prepuce with corpora cavernosa involvement require appropriate amputation and radical groin dissection whether or not the lymph nodes are palpably enlarged.

5. Malignant tumors of the glans penis, coronal sulcus, or prepuce with lymphadenopathy require appropriate amputation and radical groin dissection.

6. Insufficient evidence is available to justify irradiation as the initial treatment in an otherwise operable lesion. Palliative irradiation may be considered in selected cases.

7. The combination of surgery and irradiation is not a treatment of choice. Primary penile lesions that recur after irradiation may be surgically removed without decreasing survival rates. Simple amputation may be accompanied by irradiation of the lymph nodes, but most clinicians prefer groin dissection.

8. The antitumor antibiotic Bleomycin has shown promising results in the treatment of penile cancer. Fatal pulmonary fibrosis, however, may result from the use of the drug.

Case Report

A 60-year-old white man noted swelling beneath an unretractable prepuce 2 years prior to seeking medical advice. The case points up the ignorance associated with this potentially lethal disease. Frequent and difficult urination as well as pain and swelling of the distal penile shaft occurred in mid-1969. The urinary stream was severely compromised by meatal obstruction resulting from extension of the tumor through the glans to the distal urethra. Palpable extension into the corpora cavernosa and right inguinal lymph nodes was observed when the patient was first examined. He was febrile, with infection in the penile lesion, inguinal lymph glands, and upper urinary tract.

A dorsal slit, urethral meatotomy, and penile biopsy were performed in mid-1969. The ulcerative lesion (squamous cell carcinoma) beneath the prepuce was excised by partial amputation 2 cm proximal to the demonstrable tumor cells that were determined by frozen-section biopsy examination. The urethra and corpus spongiosum were positioned beneath the reconstructed amputation site in the manner described above. Pyelonephritis and the infected lymph glands were treated with appropriate antibiotics. While we were awaiting resolution of the inflamed lymph glands, tumor recurred at the incision site.

Total penile amputation was performed 2 months after partial amputation. Perineal urethrostomy, right inguinal, femoral, and iliac lymphadenectomy, and transposition of the sartorius muscle to cover the exposed femoral vessels were performed at the same time. Microscopic malignant cells were found deep in the ischiocavernous muscle and the iliac, inguinal, and femoral lymph nodes. Administration of the antitumor antibiotic Bleomycin was begun 3 weeks after surgery. The patient suffered from significant nausea and vomiting. Six weeks after completion of the fourth course of therapy, early signs of pulmonary fibrosis were seen on the chest x-rays.

Within 8 weeks after total penile amputation, radical lymphadenectomy, and the initiation of Bleomycin therapy, cancer recurred in the perineum, scrotum, and inguinal skin edges. Multiple scrotal and perineal urinary fistulas developed. Irradiation of the area was ineffective. Death occurred 2 years after the first medical consultation.

This case report is included to point up certain obvious needs in the treatment of penile cancer: (1) circumcision of the newborn, with an active attack against those who have in recent years exploited the emotional aspects of the retained prepuce, (2) education of the adult male population regarding self-examination and prompt medical attention for any penile lesion, (3) knowledge of treatment methods—the treatment of choice is surgical, (4) performing inguinal, femoral, and iliac lymphadenectomy with partial amputation without a waiting period for infected lymph gland resolution, and (5) administration of antimicrobials as soon as the patient comes under observation, which is continued during the postoperative period (lymphadenectomy should not be prolonged), the value of chemotherapy for penile cancer is, at present, uncertain.

References

1. Bassett, J. W. Carcinoma of the penis. *Cancer* 5:530, 1952.
2. Beggs, J. H., and Spratt, J. S., Jr. Epidermoid carcinoma of the penis. *J. Urol.* 91:166, 1964.
3. Buddington, W. T., Kickham, C. B. J., and Smith, W. An assessment of malignant disease of the penis. *J. Urol.* 89:442, 1963.
4. Ekstrom, T., and Edsmyr, F. Cancer of the penis. A clinical study of 229 cases. *Acta Chir. Scand.* 115:25, 1958.
5. Hanash, K. A., Furlow, N. L., Utz, D., and Harrison, E., Jr. Carcinoma of the penis: A clinical pathologic study. *J. Urol.* 104:291, 1970.
6. Hudson, P. B., Cason, J. F., and Scott, W. W. The value of radical operation for carcinoma of the penis. *South. Med. J.* 41:761, 1948.
7. Ichikawa, T., Nakano, I., and Hirokawa, I. Bleomycin treatment of the tumors of the penis and scrotum. *J. Urol.* 102:699, 1969.
8. Jackson, S. M. Treatment of carcinoma of the penis. *Br. J. Surg.* 53:33, 1966.
9. Lenowitz, H., and Granam, A. P. Carcinoma of the penis. *J. Urol.* 56:458, 1946.
10. Marcial, V. A., Figuerda-Colon, J., Marcial-Rojas, R., and Colon, J. E. Carcinoma of the penis. *Radiology* 79:209, 1962.
11. Melicow, M. M., and Ganem, F. J. Cancerous and precancerous lesions of the penis. A clinical and pathological study based on twenty-three cases *J. Urol.* 56:486, 1946.
12. Murrell, D. S., and Williams, J. L. Radiotherapy in the treatment of carcinoma of the penis. *Br. J. Urol.* 37:211, 1965.
13. Paymaster, J. C., and Ganbadhakan, P. Cancer of the penis in India. *J. Urol.* 97:110, 1967.
14. Rivenos, M., and Gokdstiaca, R. Cancer of the penis. *Arch. Surg.* 85:377, 1962.
15. Shabad, A. L. Some aspects of the etiology and prevention of penile cancer. *J. Urol.* 92:696, 1964.
16. Vaeth, J. M., Green, J. P., and Lowy, R. Radiation therapy of carcinoma of the penis. *Am. J. Roentgenol. Radium Ther. Nucl. Med.* 108:130, 1970.

Groin Dissection
for Tumors

LUIS O. VASCONEZ
M. J. JURKIEWICZ

44

GROIN DISSECTION for metastatic malignancy can be either superficial or radical. Superficial groin dissection entails excision of the areolar tissue, the superficial and deep fascia, and the lymph nodes of the femoral triangle and inguinal region. In a radical groin dissection, the operation is extended superiorly to include the lymph nodes of the obturator fossa, the adjacent areolar tissue, and the retroperitoneal lymphatic chain along the external iliac vessels to the level of the aortic bifurcation and formation of the inferior vena cava. Such operations are commonly performed as an integral part of the surgical therapy for metastatic epithelial malignancy involving (1) the skin of the trunk below the level of the umbilicus, perineum, or lower extremities; (2) the anus below the dentate line; (3) the genitalia; or (4) the urethra.

The operative technique of groin dissection is reasonably straightforward, and there have been appreciable advances in surgical technique since Basset first described the operation in 1912 [2]. However, immediate convalescence is often marred by skin necrosis, infection, wound breakdown, and lymphatic fistula formation. Moreover, lymph-edema of the extremities may persist as a most bothersome long-term complication.

Gross precipitous surgery with little regard to the admonition of Moynihan [14] for attention to detail might not necessarily be followed by failure of wound healing, but if failure does not occur, such is luck, not skill.

Every detail in every operation is of importance, and should be conceived, practised, and tested with unwearying patience by the operator himself, and by him in conjunction with all his assistants. Was it not Michael Angelo who first said that success depends upon details, but success is no detail? In surgery, at least, success may well depend upon the scrupulous, exacting, and unceasing supervision and close scrutiny of every smallest incident of procedure. In respect of surgical work there may be some truth in Blake's assertion that all excellence is in minute particulars. . . .

In all the movements of the surgeon there should be neither haste nor waste. It matters less how quickly an operation is done than how accurately it is done. Speed should result from the method and the practised facility of the operator, and should not be his first and formal intention. It should be an accomplishment, not an aim. And every movement should tell, every action should achieve something. A manipulation, if it requires to be carried out, should not be half-done and hesitatingly done. It should be deliberate, firm, intentional, and final. Infinite gentleness, scrupulous care, light handling, and purposeful, effective quiet movements which are no more than a caress, are all necessary if the operation is to be the work of an artist, and not merely of a hewer of flesh [14].

In order to minimize postoperative problems, there must be a strict adherence to time-tested surgical principles: atraumatic technique, meticulous control of blood and lymph channels, closure of the wound either with well-vascularized flaps without tension or primarily with skin grafts, prevention of hematoma and seroma formation by the use of suction catheters, protection of the femoral vessels by transposition of the origin of the sartorius muscle, and prevention of inguinal herniation by utilizing a Cooper's ligament type reconstruction.

As in all cancer surgery, one must aim to remove the primary tumor, the intervening lymphatics, and the regional nodes in continuity when possible. Bilateral dissections are frequently indicated when neoplasms involve midline structures, since the lymphatic channels that drain the area decussate, and the spread of tumor is often to both groins.

Anatomy of the Inguinal Region

The anatomical basis for inguinal lymph node dissection was established by the masterful work of Daseler, Anson, and Reineman [4]. They studied 450 dissections of the groin in both fresh and preserved specimens, and published a remarkably detailed description of the lymphatics of the area. It was shown that all lymph nodes in the groin lie within the confines of a quadrilateral area that is bounded above by a 12 cm line drawn just over the pubic tubercle

(parallel to and 1 cm above the inguinal ligament), medially by a 15 cm line caudal from the pubic tubercle, laterally by a 20 cm line caudal from the superior boundary, and inferiorly by a line circumferentially across

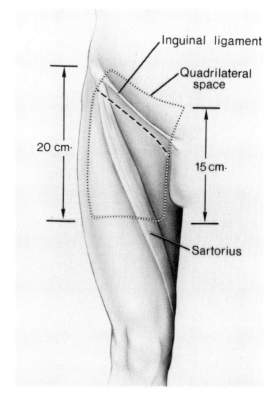

FIG. 44-1. The dotted line indicates the boundaries of the quadrilateral space. It contains all the lymph-node bearing tissue of the superficial inguinal node. The superior border extends from the anterior-superior iliac spine to a point cephalad to the pubic tubercle at the level of the upper margin of the external inguinal ring. The lateral border is a 20 cm line caudal up from the anterior-superior iliac spine. The medial border extends 15 cm from the pubic tubercle and the inferior border connects the two lines on the side. The skin incision (dashed line) is placed approximately 4 cm below the inguinal ligament and parallel to it. Skin flaps are elevated to the margins of this block.

the anterior thigh joining the two vertical lines. These, therefore, constitute the boundaries for a groin dissection (Fig. 44-1).

The inguinal lymph nodes are described as superficial or deep. The superficial inguinal nodes are the most important and are imbedded in the adipose tissue superficial to the fascia lata. They are arranged in zones: the central one is at the saphenous-femoral junction, and the remaining zones correspond to the regions drained by the four superficial veins of the inguinal region, namely the superficial circumflex iliac, the superficial epigastric, the superficial external pudendal, and the accessory lateral saphenous veins (Fig. 44-2) [15].

One lymph node of importance, the prepubic node, should be considered with the superficial inguinal group. Such a node is occasionally found in the subcutaneous tissue anterior to the pubic symphysis. It receives lymphatic channels from the penis or the clitoris and drains into the superficial inguinal nodes. Occasionally, metastatic carcinoma that arises in the penis or vulva may be found in this node, and recurrence in the presymphyseal region might occur if this node is left behind at the time of groin dissection [20].

The deep inguinal lymphatics are situated deep to the fascia lata of the thigh and superficial to the connective tissue sheaths of the individual muscles; they are intimately covered by the femoral sheath. In the pelvis, the iliac and hypogastric groups of lymphatics are between the iliac and endopelvic fascia on one side and the retroperitoneal subserous tissue on the other [4].

Surgical Technique

PREOPERATIVE CONSIDERATIONS

A systematic preoperative assessment of the patient's condition should be completed and the possibility of distant metastases reasonably excluded. Roentgenographic examination of the chest and of any localized skeletal pain are essential preliminary steps. We agree with Spratt, Shiever, and Dillard [17] that if

FIG. 44-2. Structures of the femoral triangle. The inguinal lymph nodes are distributed along the course of the superficial veins: the superficial circumflex iliac, the superficial epigastric, the superficial external pudendal, and the accessory lateral saphenous veins.

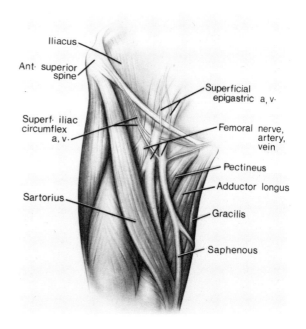

cancerous nodes are palpable in the groin and the presence of distant metastases is uncertain, it is better to proceed with a groin dissection to ensure local control of the cancer.

POSITION

Positioning of the patient on the operating table requires thought and care. The following points should be kept in mind when planning the extent of the skin preparation: (1) Is a unilateral or bilateral ilioinguinal lymphatic dissection needed? (2) Will skin grafting be necessary? (3) Is the primary tumor to be included in the en bloc dissection? (4) Will the procedure be performed by one team or with two teams of surgeons?

A satisfactory method has been to place the patient on the operating table in the supine position with orthopedic attachments for abduction of the lower extremities. The thigh is flexed, abducted, and externally rotated. In patients with carcinoma of the vulva, the lithotomy position is perhaps best with the legs abducted, thus allowing access to both groins and the perineum simultaneously.

INCISION

The area of the quadrilateral block that is to encompass the dissection is marked with methylene blue. It should extend from the anterior-superior iliac spine toward the pubic tubercle approximately 3 or 4 cm above the inguinal ligament and parallel to it. Perpendicular lines are then drawn from the anterior-superior iliac spine and the pubic tubercle for 20 and 15 cm respectively, and a transverse line is made to join them inferiorly (see Fig. 44-1).

An oblique incision, 15 cm long, is made approximately 4 cm below the inguinal ligament and parallel to it. One should not hesitate either in leaving an island of skin on the specimen if there is any suspicion of involvement of skin lymphatics or in excising an ellipse of skin to prevent necrosis at the edges and facilitate exposure. Skin flaps 3 to 4 cm thick are then carefully dissected with the knife. Skin edges are handled with minimal trauma by the application of skin hooks. A most difficult area to expose is the inferior extent of the lower flap. A medium-sized Deaver retractor has been helpful for this purpose.

DISSECTION

The first field of dissection is the lower quadrant of the abdominal wall. The upper skin flap is retracted with skin hooks, and the subcutaneous tissues are swept from above downward from the surface of the external oblique aponeurosis. At the inguinal region, care is taken to go below and slightly under the inguinal ligament. This can be accomplished easily because Scarpa's fascia (i.e., the fibrae intercrurales) is attached below the inguinal ligament to the fascia lata of the thigh at a transverse line [18]. The risk of damage to the femoral vessels is minimized if the ligament is first identified at the medial end close to the pubic tubercle and near the femoral canal [13]. As the dissection proceeds laterally along the inguinal ligament, the blue color of the femoral vein is perceived more easily than the femoral artery. The femoral nerve lying behind the fascia lata cannot be seen at this stage.

The second field of dissection is in the anterior part of the thigh. It begins laterally by the division of the deep fascia over the insertion of the sartorius muscle, and medially at the medial border of the adductor magnus. These vertical limbs extend as far down as the borders of the quadrilateral block marked on the skin surface.

The deep fascia of the thigh separates easily from the sartorius, leaving the muscle fibers bare. Small branches from the lateral circumflex artery and vein are encountered and ligated.

The incision is carried along the transverse inferior margin, again down to bare muscle. The saphenous vein will be encountered at this point and should be carefully divided and ligated. Any open lymphatic channels should be carefully clamped and ligated. One method to ensure ligation of all lymphatic channels and prevent postoperative lymph collection or seroma is to place a continuous suture of chromic catgut along the fibroadi-

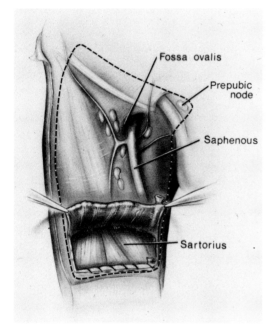

FIG. 44-3. The margins of the dissection have been marked along the quadrilateral area. The dissection is shown beginning inferiorly. All the fibroadipose tissue and fascia lata are removed, leaving the underlying muscle bare. The saphenous vein has been divided and ligated. The fibroadipose tissue at the inferior margin is ligated with a continuous catgut suture to ensure ligation of all lymphatic channels and prevent lymph collection under the flap. The dissection continues cephalad, removing the lymph-node bearing tissue and adventitia from all surfaces of the femoral vessels.

pose tissue inferiorly, as suggested by Woodhall [19] (Fig. 44-3).

Next the tissues are dissected in a cephalad direction along the femoral vessels and underneath the lower flap. The sartorius muscle is retracted, exposing the neurovascular bundle in the upper part of Hunter's canal. The femoral nerve is identified and exposed. It is best found by following one of its muscular branches proximally. All the loose adipose tissue outside the femoral sheath, as well as all the gland-bearing tissue covered by the femoral sheath, should be removed along with the adventitia of the blood vessels. As this meticulous dissection is carried cephalad, muscular vessels from the femoral artery and vein are cut and ligated. At the fossa ovalis, the greater saphenous vein is ligated and divided at its junction with the femoral vein (Fig. 44-4). Similarly, the smaller branches of the femoral artery in the groin are secured and ligated. Following completion of the dissection, the field of operation presents the bared muscular bed and the femoral vessels and nerve.

The femoral lymphatics join the iliac lymphatics through the femoral canal. Here also lies the major deep inguinal lymph node, Cloquet's node. It has been suggested that this be excised separately and submitted to frozen-section examination, especially in malignancies of the vulva. If there is nodal involvement, deep inguinal node dissection is indicated. The prognosis, at least for vulvar carcinoma, decreases significantly when there is metastatic tumor in Cloquet's node. On the other hand, if this node is normal, some advocate not doing a parailiac dissection, since the chances of encountering metastases in the iliac nodes are very slight [10, 16].

The third field of dissection is the retroperitoneal pelvic lymphatic bed. Several approaches have been proposed for this part of the dissection. Hovnanian frees up the inguinal ligament by an osteotomy through the

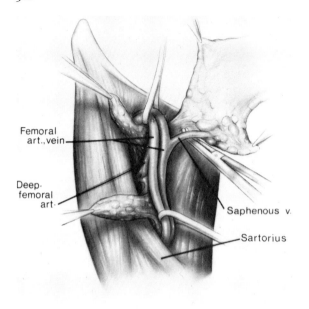

Femoral
art., vein

Deep-
femoral
art.

Saphenous v.

Sartorius

FIG. 44-4. Division of the saphenous vein. The specimen is shown hanging by the saphenous vein, which is finally divided at its junction with the femoral vein. Additional lymph-node bearing tissue is removed from the posterior surface of the femoral vessels.

anterior-superior iliac spine and raising it toward the midline as a hinge [6, 7]. This offers excellent exposure and has the advantage of maintaining the specimen en bloc while doing the deep node dissection. Others advocate division of the inguinal ligament, which is to be followed by resuturing at the end of the procedure. DasGupta begins the retroperitoneal dissection by an incision that starts in the flank, extends vertically and anteriorly to the anterior-superior iliac spine, and curves below the inguinal ligament into the thigh [5].

We prefer to do this part of the dissection by dividing the external oblique aponeurosis in the direction of its fibers, proceeding from the subcutaneous inguinal ring to a point approximately 4 cm lateral to the abdominal inguinal ring. The internal oblique muscle and transverse fascia are freed from their attachments to the inguinal ligament and the subjacent iliopsoas muscle and pectineal fascia (Fig. 44-5). To facilitate this exposure, it is necessary to doubly ligate and sever the inferior epigastric artery and the deep circumflex iliac branches of the external iliac artery

and the corresponding veins. By blunt dissection, the peritoneum is raised from the lateral wall and floor of the pelvis and retracted cephalad to expose the common iliac vessels to a point well above their bifurcation. There, the ureter will be seen and should remain adherent to the peritoneum. The obturator nerve and the vessels of the lateral pelvic wall are also clearly exposed. The spermatic cord and its contents should be retracted medially by means of a Penrose drain.

Dissection starts superiorly and lateral to the vessels near the bifurcation of the aorta; the fat and fascia are divided from the iliac fossa and reflected toward the main vessels (Fig. 44-6). The femoral branch of the genitofemoral nerve is identified and divided. The femoral nerve, which is identified in the femoral area, is followed superiorly, and its position is noted. It lies behind the plane of the dissection posterior to the fascia iliaca. This nerve, which has a somewhat variable position, may be 2.5 cm lateral to the femoral artery and partly concealed in a fold of the iliopsoas muscle, or it may be almost behind the femoral artery.

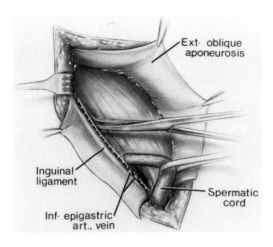

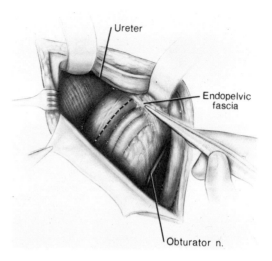

FIG. 44-5. Division of the internal oblique muscle to enter the retroperitoneal space. The external oblique aponeurosis has been divided at the upper margins of the subcutaneous inguinal ring for the length of the oblique incision. The fibers of the internal oblique and transverse abdominal muscles are separated from the inguinal ligaments. The inferior epigastric and deep circumflex iliac vessels are ligated and divided.

FIG. 44-6. Beginning deep dissection. The peritoneum has been raised from the lateral pelvic wall and retracted cephalad, exposing the common iliac vessels. The ureter should be seen and protected since it remains adherent to the peritoneum. The dissection starts lateral to the vessels by incising the endopelvic fascia, overlying the psoas muscle. The fascia and the circumferential sheath of the iliac vessels are swept down from near the bifurcation of the aorta to the inguinal ligament. The nodes of the true pelvis are also removed by blunt dissection, clearing the obturator nerve.

Once the femoral nerve has been identified, the dissection of the lateral aspect of the vessels is completed safely. The adventitia of the iliac artery and vein is then freed together with the lymphatic channels and nodes on all aspects of the vessels. It should be noted that the lymph channels lie very close to the main blood vessels and that when the outer layers of the adventitia are removed, major lymph trunks will be divided. The lymph nodes may even lie between or behind the vessels. It is therefore important to strip those vessels of adventitia on all surfaces.

To reach the nodes within the true pelvis, the position of the broad Deaver retractors should be altered. One holds the peritoneum medially, and the second one holds it upward. If there is a branch from the medial aspect of the external iliac vein that crosses the pelvic brim to enter the obturator fora-

men, it is divided between ligatures. Next, starting as posteriorly as possible, one separates the fat, fascia, and contained lymph nodes from the medial pelvic wall by blunt dissection.

Frequently, a lymph node is close to the obturator nerve near the obturator foramen. This node is often long and thin, resembling a tubular structure. Careful dissection around it will demonstrate its true nature and avoid confusion. The obturator nerve will be seen to be clear of the pelvic wall and free of surrounding tissue.

There may be some bleeding from the superior vesical vessels; this is usually venous

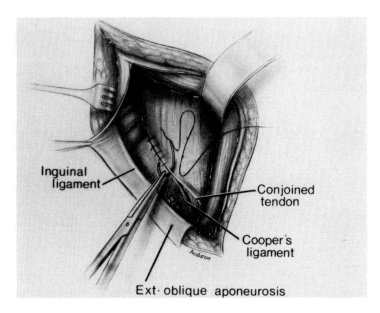

FIG. 44-7. Closure of Cooper's ligament. The conjoined tendon and transverse fascia are sutured to Cooper's ligament from the pubic tubercle up to the femoral vein. This will prevent a direct inguinal herniation.

and is easily controlled with a pack or well-placed vascular sutures.

The dissected tissue is then removed by delivering it under the inguinal ligament, thus completing the radical groin dissection. This deep dissection is rather tedious since the nodes in the retroperitoneal area are held together by thin, filmy, areolar tissue; the fragile nature of this tissue makes it difficult to keep the specimen in one block.

CLOSURE

The deep part of the dissection is closed first by utilizing the technique for hernia repair devised by McVay and Anson [12]. Improper, hasty closure of this area can lead to the formation of postoperative hernias (Fig. 44-7).

The conjoined portions of the internal oblique muscle, the transverse muscle of the abdomen, and the underlying transverse fascia are approximated to the superior pubic ligament (Cooper's ligament) by means of nonabsorbable sutures. This approximation is carried laterally from the pubic tubercle to the medial edge of the external iliac vein. More laterally, the abdominal layers are approximated to the inguinal ligament. The external oblique aponeurosis is then sutured above the spermatic cord in order to reconstruct the subcutaneous inguinal ring at a point just medial to the pubic tubercle (Fig. 44-8).

TRANSPLANTATION OF THE SARTORIUS MUSCLE

A most important and critical step is the transfer of the sartorius muscle to cover the femoral vessels (Fig. 44-9). This muscle is divided at its origin from the anterior superior iliac spine and is transposed to cover the vessels. The cut end of the sartorius is then

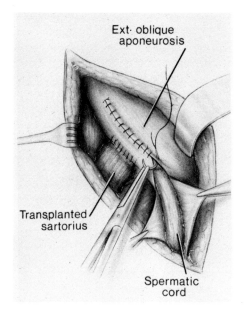

FIG. 44-8. The external oblique aponeurosis is closed over the spermatic cord. The transplanted sartorius muscle covers the femoral vessels (see Fig. 44-9).

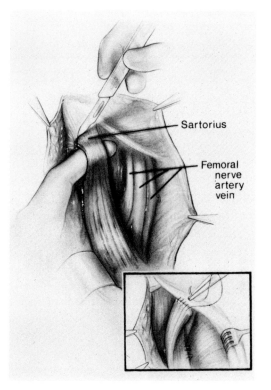

FIG. 44-9. The origin of the sartorius muscle is divided from the anterior superior iliac spine and is transposed directly to cover the femoral vessels, or it is rotated 180 degrees (as shown in the inset), whichever way can be done with less tension on the neurovascular bundle. It is then sutured to the inguinal ligament.

sutured with horizontal mattress sutures to the inguinal ligament and medially to the adductor muscle. By this technique, the femoral artery is protected if postoperative skin breakdown or infection occurs. This maneuver apparently was first performed by Wangensteen and Baronofsky [1].

SKIN CLOSURE

The wound is then thoroughly irrigated with saline, and the skin flaps are objectively evaluated for vascularity. If they appear mottled or if there is no blanching on slight pressure, they should be excised and the wound covered with split-thickness skin grafts at this time. Fluorescein dye and ultraviolet scanning has been used with some success to evaluate the vascularity of the skin edges. Others routinely excise a portion of the skin margins prior to closure [3]. If vascularity seems to be adequate, the skin should be carefully sutured with fine interrupted nylon sutures. Two large, soft rubber suction catheters with extra openings (size French 24) are placed; one is located along the inguinal ligament and the second along the medial margins of the incision. The suction catheters are brought out through separate stab wounds laterally and inferiorly to the distal extent of the dissection. The catheters are connected to a low wall suction to keep the skin flaps in close apposition with the underlying musculature; they are not removed before the fifth day postoperatively. A light dressing is applied, and the leg is immobilized with a posterior plaster splint.

Postoperative Management and Complications

NECROSIS

Skin necrosis is one of the most common complications following groin dissection. The reasons for this are clear. Thin flaps are elevated extensively, thus devascularizing a large segment of skin. This is minimized by the routine use of an oblique incision that parallels the inguinal ligament and is in the direction of the vessels supplying the skin of the groin [1, 19]. A vertical incision on the thigh is certain to divide the vessels and devascularize a portion of skin. Should an area of necrotic skin become apparent postoperatively, it should be excised back to vascularized skin, and the wound is then grafted promptly before gross sepsis intervenes.

The approach suggested by Johanson and others for carcinoma of the vulva, which employs wide excision of skin and primary coverage with split-thickness skin grafts, has resulted in less morbidity and faster healing of the wound, and it should therefore be practiced [8, 9, 11].

LYMPHATIC FISTULAS

Lymph drainage from groin wounds is common, and an effective suction drainage system is essential. Postoperative lymph discharge is from 500 to 1,000 ml, primarily occurring during the first 5 days and decreasing rapidly thereafter. Suction catheters should not be removed until drainage has ceased completely for at least 24 to 48 hours.

The use of transfixion and an interlocking U suture of the divided lymphatics along the inferior edge of the dissection aids in decreasing the amount of postoperative drainage.

If lymph collects after the suction catheters are removed, the treatment consists of daily aspiration, a light, even pressure dressing, Ace bandages to the entire leg, elevation of the extremity, and bed rest. If lymph is not aspirated, drainage will occur through the suture line and effectively delay healing.

AMBULATION

Bed rest with elevation of the leg is essential for at least 5 days postoperatively, since ambulation increases the lymphatic flow from the extremity and predisposes to fluid collection. If bed rest is necessary for wound healing, it in turn predisposes to thrombophlebitis. Therefore, anticoagulation with heparin is suggested until ambulation has been restored [8]. If heparin is contraindicated, 500 ml of low molecular weight dextran should be administered daily for approximately 5 days [16].

INFECTION

Infection other than that secondary to skin necrosis is relatively rare. However, obstruction of the lymphatic flow provides a fertile field for streptococcal infection. Therefore, penicillin therapy is given throughout the hospitalization.

POSTOPERATIVE LYMPHEDEMA

This occurs in a significant number of patients and can be minimized by the continuous use of a well-fitted elastic stocking. Byron [3] points out that the edema of the leg usually diminishes in the months following operation, an observation that is in accord with our experience.

References

1. Baronofsky, I. D. Technique of inguinal node dissection. *Surgery* 24:555, 1948.
2. Basset, A. Traitement chirurgical opérative de l'épithélium primitif du clitoris. *Rev. Chir. Paris* 46:546, 1912.
3. Byron, R. L., Jr., Lamb, E. J., Yonemoto, R. H., and Kase, S. Radical inguinal node dissection in the treatment of cancer. *Surg. Gynecol. Obstet.* 114:401, 1962.
4. Daseler, E. H., Anson, B. J., and Reineman, A. C. Radical excision of the inguinal and iliac lymph glands (A study based upon 450 anatomical dissections and upon supportive clinical observation). *Surg. Gynecol. Obstet.* 87:679, 1948.
5. DasGupta, T. K. Radical groin dissection. *Surg. Gynecol. Obstet.* 129:1275, 1969.
6. Hovnanian, A. P. Radical ilio-inguinal lymphatic excision. *Ann. Surg.* 135:520, 1952.
7. Hovnanian, A. P. Ilio-inguinal lymphatic excision. *Surgery* 54:592, 1963.
8. Johanson, B., and Lewin, E. Cancer of the vulva. Vulvectomy, primary skin grafting and regional gland excision. *Acta Chir. Scand.* 126:483, 1963.
9. Lees, D. H. Treatment of carcinoma of the vulva with an assessment of results. *J. Obstet. Gynecol.* 68:730, 1961.
10. Luddwall, F. Cancer of the vulva. A clinical review. *Acta Radiol. (Stockh.)* Suppl. 208, 1961.
11. McGregor, I. A. Delayed exposed grafting following radical vulvectomy. *Br. J. Plast. Surg.* 15:293, 1962.
12. McVay, C. B., and Anson, B. J. Inguinal and femoral hernioplasty. *Surg. Gynecol. Obstet.* 88:473, 1949.
13. Milton, G. W., Williams, A. E. J., and Bryant, D. H. Radical dissection of the inguinal and iliac lymph nodes for malignant melanoma of the leg. *Br. J. Surg.* 55:G41, 1968.
14. Moynihan, B. *Abdominal Operations.* Vol. I. Philadelphia and London: Saunders, 1928. Pp. 43–44.
15. Rouviere, H. *Anatomy of the Human Lymphatic System.* Translated by M. J. Tobias. Ann Arbor: Edwards Brothers, 1938.
16. Rutledge, F., Smith, J. P., and Franklin, E. W. Carcinoma of the vulva. *Am. J. Obstet. Gynecol.* 106:1117, 1970.
17. Spratt, J. S., Shiever, W., and Dillard, B. M. *Anatomy and Surgical Technique of Groin Dissections.* St. Louis: Mosby, 1964.
18. Treves, F. *Surgical Applied Anatomy* (11th ed.). London: Cassel, 1947.
19. Woodhall, J. P. Radical groin surgery with particular reference to post-operative healing. *Surgery* 33:886, 1953.
20. Young, H. H. A radical operation for the cure of cancer of the pelvis. *J. Urol.* 26:285, 1931.

Modified Incisions for Radical Groin Dissections*

FREDERIC RUECKERT
FORST E. BROWN

45

A COMMON and potentially serious complication of radical groin dissection is ischemic necrosis of the skin flaps, as shown in Figure 45-1. When this complication occurs, it leads to an increased incidence of postoperative wound infection and danger to the underlying femoral vessels.

It has been pointed out that the blood supply to the flaps in the groin area is derived primarily from the superficial external pudenal, superficial circumflex iliac, and inferior epigastric arteries. These vessels are usually divided during the course of the dissection, and the flaps rely on anastomotic circulation. This blood supply lies within the fatty layer of superficial fascia (Camper's fascia), and the branches tend to parallel the natural skin creases, which in turn parallel the inguinal ligament. The safest skin incisions would seem to be those that parallel these skin folds [1, 3, 4].

A single oblique incision over the inguinal ligament has been described [3] that has minimized postoperative wound healing problems in radical groin dissection. Possible

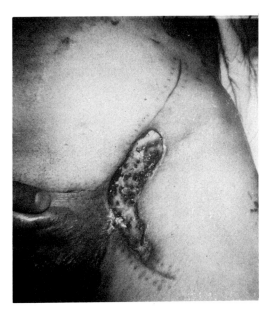

FIG. 45-1. Ischemic necrosis in the skin flap after radical groin dissection.

* Since this chapter was submitted for publication, an article by Walker et al., "A New Approach to Radical Retroperitoneal Ileac and Femoral Node Dissection (*Arch. Surg.* 103:681, 1971), independently arrived at the same concept that is outlined here.

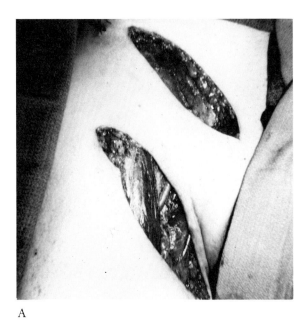

A

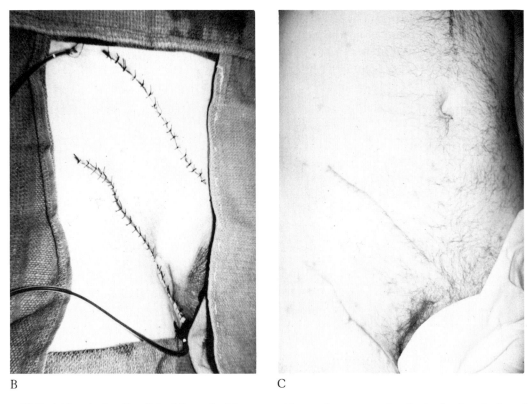

B   C

FIG. 45-2. A–C. Parallel oblique incisions provide good exposure for both the inguinal and pelvic portions of the dissection. Suction drainage catheters are used.

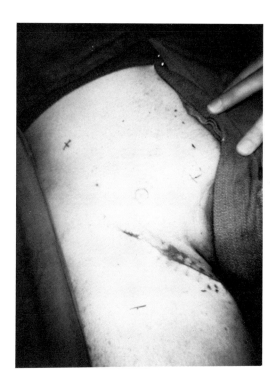

FIG. 45-3. A preexisting groin scar that makes modification of other radical dissection incisions necessary can often be excised and readily incorporated into the two parallel oblique incisions.

disadvantages of this incision are the somewhat limited exposure for extensive dissection and the amount of retraction necessary at the inferior and superior limits of dissection.

After considerable gratifying experience with the two parallel transverse incisions described by MacFee [2] for radical neck dissection, we have used two similar oblique incisions paralleling the inguinal ligament (Fig. 45-2) for radical groin dissection. This technique has resulted in good exposure for both the inguinal and pelvis portions of the operation, uncomplicated wound healing, and protection of the femoral vessels under an intact bipedicle skin flap.

Occasionally, there will be a preexisting biopsy incision or scar in the groin area (Fig. 45-3) that makes modification of other radical dissection incisions necessary. Often the excision of the existing scar can be readily incorporated into the two parallel oblique incisions without compromising exposure or wound healing.

References

1. Baronsky, I. D. Technique of inguinal node dissection. *Surgery* 24:555, 1948.
2. MacFee, W. F. Transverse incisions for neck dissection. *Ann. Surg.* 151:279, 1960.
3. Spratt, J. S., Shieber, W., and Dillard, B. M. *Anatomy and Surgical Technique of Groin Dissection.* St. Louis: Mosby, 1965.
4. Woodhall, J. P. Radical groin surgery with particular reference to post-operative healing. *Surgery* 33:886, 1953.

Resurfacing the Genital Area

VII

Resurfacing the Perineum

LESTER M. CRAMER
J. KENNETH CHONG

46

THE PERINEUM is one of the most difficult parts of the body to resurface. Adverse factors—such as the proximity of the anus, fecal soiling, heat, moisture, intertrigo, unavoidable movement of the buttocks or extremities, and difficulty in applying immobilizing dressings—contribute to the technical difficulties of successful coverage. Some of the problems posed by these factors are surmountable in part. Local and general measures in the preoperative management of the patient if carried out stringently and intelligently, will help to obtain a successful outcome.

Preoperative Management

NUTRITION AND DIET

A patient about to undergo elective wound coverage of the perineum should be in a good nutritive state. Chronic low-grade sepsis with purulent discharge leads to hypovolemia, hypoproteinemia and negative nitrogen balance, gluconeogenesis, vitamin deficiencies (especially of vitamin C), and a hypochromic, microcytic anemia. Correction of these is accomplished by a high calorie, high protein diet with high dosages of vitamins, particularly of ascorbic acid. Blood transfusions are given if needed, and anabolic steroids occasionally may be useful. Appetite stimulants of either medicinal or alcoholic content can also be helpful. Five days prior to surgery the diet is changed to a low residue type and is maintained as closely as possible to its high nutritious state.

BOWEL STERILIZATION

It has not been our routine to "sterilize" the alimentary tract by means of preoperative oral administration of neomycin or one of the nonabsorbable sulfonamides. However, should fecal diversion be indicated preoperatively, bowel sterilization is advocated over performing a defunctioning colostomy. We have not found it necessary to divert the fecal stream for the less complicated wounds of the perineum. Granulomatous lesions of the bowel—such as regional ileitis, regional colitis, tuberculosis, and even diverticulitis—may be complicated by perineal and perirectal fistula formation. Treatment is specific and should be directed toward the underlying pathology by appropriate measures. The most important preoperative bowel preparation is the use of enemas. It has been our practice to

599

600 RESURFACING THE GENITAL AREA

begin evacuating the large bowel at least 5 days prior to surgery. Lukewarm soap suds enemas, up to 20 fluid ounces at a time, are utilized once daily in order to facilitate the expulsion of fecal pellets. These are supplemented twice daily by water colonic washouts, each measuring up to 20 fluid ounces in volume. A minimum of three daily enemas for the 5 preoperative days is required for an efficient bowel preparation. Prothrombin time is determined, and vitamin K is given as needed.

LOCAL CARE TO THE PERINEUM

Inpatients soon learn how well they can keep themselves clean by a daily regimen of sitz baths every 3 hours during their waking hours. For the more extensive wounds involving not only the perineum but also the lower portions of the trunk (pubic, inguinal, and gluteal regions), twice daily cleansing in either a whirlpool or a Hubbard tank proves to be a valuable adjunct. The use of either Telfa or Vaseline dressings is mentioned only to be condemned, because their water impermeability serves to prevent the drainage of exudate. Following the cleansing, the wounds may be covered with gauze soaked in the appropriate antibiotic as determined by culture and sensitivity testing. Bacitracin, neomycin, polymyxin, and Gentamycin are the common antibiotic solutions employed. Creams of either Sulfamylon (mafenide) or silver sulfadiazine in a water-soluble base have, when buttered on the wound and covered with gauze sponges, also proved effective. Because it is usually not possible to eradicate completely the resident flora of the bowel and perineum, the use of systemic antibiotics preoperatively has not been a routine with us. However, if such pathogens as beta-hemolytic streptococci can be cultured from a sample taken by perineal swab, appropriate systemic antibiotics must be insti-

tuted prior to any consideration of skin grafting. In the few situations requiring the closure of a contaminated defect by means of a local pedicle flap, we have found that using a closed irrigation system with drop-by-drop instillation of the appropriate antibiotic solution beneath the flap helps to obviate wound infection.

PREPARATION OF THE GRAFT BED

Cooperation between the surgeon, nursing staff, and patient is essential in the preparation of the graft bed for split-thickness skin grafting. Meticulous wound care is directed by the surgeon, and is conducted by the surgeon, the house staff, and the nursing staff. It requires frequent and thorough attention to detail. Most patients will tolerate some discomfort encountered in the physical debridement of the perineal wounds, and if they are told beforehand that they can expect some discomfort, they will cooperate and will not require multiple general anesthetics for debridement. Gentleness on the part of the medical attendant and rapport with the patient provide the key to a successful result.

Nonviable tissues are debrided with sharp instruments at least once a day by the physician. "No-touch technique" is utilized in employing sterile instruments. Dressing changes should be carried out once every 3 hours during the waking hours and are preceded by sitz baths, whirlpool, or Hubbard tank treatments. In addition to the sharp debridement, the physical act of removing the dry gauze dressings that are laid directly on the wound further helps to accomplish the desired debridement.

The Graft Bed

In the majority of cases, a granulating graft bed will be obtained by a combination of surgical debridement and meticulous wound care by frequent dressings. The criteria for favorable conditions prevailing in the granulation tissue that are necessary for optimal take of skin grafts are (1) a salmon-pink color, (2) a fine, granular texture, (3) the absence of a yellow or gray "pannus," (4) the absence of odor, (5) evidence of "creeping in" of the peripheral epithelium with indistinctness or fuzziness between the advancing edge and the granulation tissue, and (6) a minimum of clear exudate. Not infrequently, however, in spite of all exhaustive general and local measures to secure optimal wound conditions, the bed of granulation tissue will either be overluxuriant, be pale, or assume a "cobblestone" appearance. Split-thickness skin grafts applied to such a graft bed are doomed to failure. The recipient site for skin grafting has to be prepared surgically in such cases. Either the granulation bed can be avulsed, or the wound can be formally excised. The word "avulsion" is inaccurate inasmuch as it implies violence; the technique of avulsion of the granulation bed involves a meticulous, gentle, surgical excision of the granulation tissue, which must not be ripped off, filed down, or erased. The sharp scalpel blade should be carried down around the edges of the granulating surface to the connective tissue base (yellow scar base) that lies beneath it. Sharp dissection is continued just superficial to this connective tissue base and only as deep as the capillary loops of the overluxuriant granulation tissue. Dissection carried out at this plane is a relatively bloodless procedure.

The connective tissue base that is uncovered must be evaluated from the point of view of vascularity, viability, and bacterial contamination. Depending on these factors, one can either graft directly upon the base or apply wet dressings upon it and secondarily graft it 3 to 5 days later. Whenever delayed grafting is decided upon, it is imperative that

the graft bed be kept moistened by continuous wet dressings before the application of skin; this prevents the formation of a coagulum of exudate on the wound. When a perineal wound exhibits indolency, a decision will usually have to be made to proceed with formal excision. Excision of the wound differs from avulsion of granulation tissue in that it involves a larger and deeper wound, with the attendant drawbacks of great blood loss and trauma to a patient who may already be sick. However, even though one might have contemplated the wound avulsion technique as the method of choice initially, one should not hesitate to perform a formal wound excision if, at operation, the avulsion technique reveals an unfavorable connective tissue base with poor healing capabilities.

Choice of Skin Grafts

Since thin split-thickness grafts have a higher probability of successful take and since the perineum is one of the most difficult areas of the body to be grafted successfully, it is reasonable to use thin split-thickness skin grafts for the perineum [1]. Split-thickness grafts of approximately 0.010 to 0.012 inch thickness are ideal. They may be laid on as intact sheets or in the meshed form. If they are used in the form of sheets, they should be well fixed to the underlying bed by multiple basting sutures of 5-0 chromic catgut. Anchorage to the periphery of the bed is also important.

Mesh Grafts

Mesh grafts are generally indicated (1) when there is a paucity of donor sites, e.g., in small children, in cases of extensive burns, and in sick patients with large raw areas for skin cover, (2) when there is questionable bacteriological control with a need to secure skin cover earlier than is allowable by local wound conditions, (3) when complete immobilization of the skin graft is difficult to obtain, and (4) when the recipient bed presents a complicated contour.

The last three conditions apply to perineal wounds, and therefore meshed skin grafts are very frequently indicated in this area (Fig. 46-1).

Immobilization

The use of tie-over bolster dressings in the perineum has many drawbacks. Because of the complicated contour, tie-over bolster dressings cannot conform well and may, by virtue of bulk, prevent drainage in an area that requires drainage.

We believe that immobilization, which is necessary for a successful take of the skin graft, is best accomplished by the immobilization of the patient with the hips kept in 30 degrees flexion and 30 degrees thigh abduction. A well-padded posterior plaster shell is

constructed preoperatively for the patient to lie upon; this extends to support the lower limbs. It is used to maintain the postoperative position (Fig. 46-2) to facilitate immobilization, cleanliness, comfort, and wound care.

Local Care of the Grafted Area in the Perineum

Wet dressings applied to the grafted areas in the perineum are kept continuously moistened and are changed at least twice daily. This ensures local wound cleansing and the clearance of any exudative discharge. Collections of serosanguineous fluid from beneath the graft can also be gently rolled out by the use of applicator sticks.

Care of the Bowels

Postoperatively, the patient is given a preparation of one of the opium alkaloids, such as paregoric, morphine, or codeine, for

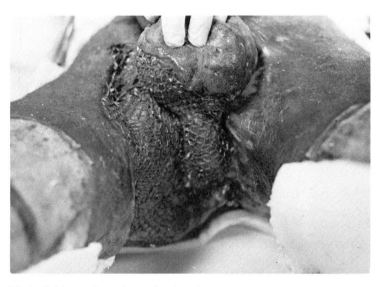

FIG. 46-1. Meshed skin grafts to the perineal region.

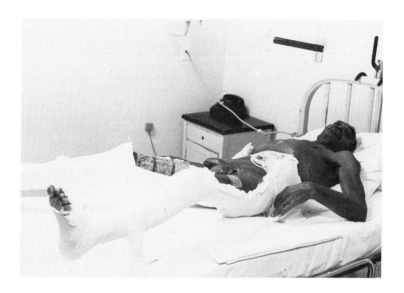

FIG. 46-2. A padded plaster of Paris shell for immobilization of the patient after mesh grafting of the perineum is well tolerated.

its analgesic and constipative effects. Paregoric is administered for a minimum of 3 days following surgery. Abdominal gaseous distention is seldom troublesome, and it may be alleviated by the passage of a flatus tube. It is quite easy to ensure that no bowel movement will take place for at least a week following surgery if the bowel preparations are efficiently performed preoperatively and a low residue diet at least 5 days before and after surgery is maintained.

Hidradenitis suppurativa chronica is the most common cause of these wounds. If it has caused multiple fistulas with intricate ramifications, it may be necessary for all the tracts to be laid open and for pockets of suppuration to be uncovered to allow drainage and encourage granulation. In this period of relative quiescence, the granulating surface may then be grafted, or it may be handled by masterful inactivity, avulsion of the granulation bed, or formal wound excision [2].

In contrast to most other parts of the body where wound closure is frequently accomplished by flap replacement cover, whether local or distant, wound closure in the perineum is best managed by split-thickness skin grafting, either immediate or delayed.

References

1. Rosenberg, I. L., et al. The relative significance of preoperative bowel preparation, phthalylsulphathiazole and neomycin, and the avoidance of sepsis after radical large-bowel surgery. *Br. J. Surg.* 57:389, 1970.

2. Brown, J. B., and McDowell, F. *Skin Grafting* (3rd ed.). Philadelphia: Lippincott, 1958.

Skin Grafts
to the Vulva

IAN A. McGREGOR

47

THE definitive treatment for carcinoma of the vulva is by extended radical vulvectomy [6]; excision of the vulvar lesion with continuity clearance of the inguinal nodes yields an overall 61 percent 5-year survival rate [8]. The extensive excision of the skin overlying the inguinal lymph nodes, which is required by the procedure, leaves a large skin defect. This is the least satisfactory aspect of the procedure, since the resulting raw surface takes a very long time to heal. The possible methods of expediting healing by covering the defect involve the use either of a flap or a graft.

Skin Flaps

Flaps of various kinds, both local and distant, have been tried, and, in general, they have not proved satisfactory. Experienced plastic surgeons avoid local flaps in the perineum if at all possible [1, 5]. Nursing is difficult, complications are common, and failure leaves the patient in a worse condition than if nothing at all had been done. A distant flap in the form of a tubed pedicle has been described [9], but for several reasons it is seldom feasible. The technique of tubed

pedicle transfer is long, staged, and tedious; it is technically difficult and out of the question in the majority of patients who are in the older age group. It has been stated that this technique makes subsequent childbearing feasible. In light of this, the method might be considered in the younger age group, although it is our experience that the use of simple grafting does not preclude subsequent pregnancy and normal parturition.

Skin Grafts

Split-thickness skin grafting is a much more feasible method; the main difficulty is to devise a technique that fits in with the other aspects of the problem.

PRIMARY GRAFTING

Primary grafting carried out immediately following the vulvectomy, though undoubtedly possible, has certain disadvantages, both general and local.

The most obvious of the general disadvantages are:

1. The patient is frequently old and frail and is being made to undergo what are in

605

effect two operations in one: the excisional procedure and the reconstructive procedure. The excision itself is an operation of some magnitude, and the cutting of the split-thickness skin graft, the suturing of it in position, and the provision of postoperative fixation add considerably to the operating time and trauma.

2. The postoperative course for the patient is made much more uncomfortable, since she must remain immobilized, with an indwelling catheter, for 5 days while the graft is in process of taking. Immobilization of the elderly in this way is well recognized to be undesirable and would be expected to add to the immediate mortality of the procedure.

3. If take of the graft is poor, and this must be expected in some patients because of the technical difficulties of grafting, the eventual healing time will not have been reduced significantly by the use of a primary graft unless a subsequent graft can be made to take.

The local disadvantages similarly are not inconsiderable:

1. The usual mode of fixation of a graft used primarily is by a pressure dressing. In this, the sutures that are used to fix the margins of the graft are left long and tied over a bolus dressing, which when thus held tightly against the graft, exerts uniform pressure. It is hoped this will provide fixation of the graft during the process of taking. After radical vulvectomy, however, such uniform pressure is virtually impossible to achieve. The raw area includes both the perineal and inguinal regions, and the bolus must consequently be applied partly with the patient in the lithotomy position and partly lying flat. It is a practical impossibility to get both pressures correct simultaneously.

2. It is recognized that it is essential to avoid any sliding movements of the graft while the graft is taking, since this prevents the capillary link-up which is necessary for vascularization of the graft. The graft which slides on its bed will not take. Such sliding is virtually impossible to prevent in the perineum when pressure is used in this region.

3. When a graft fails to take, a common cause is the occurrence of hematoma under the graft, which separates it from its bed. Absolute hemostasis after vulvectomy is not easily achieved, and hematoma might consequently be expected to take its toll of the graft.

It is not difficult to see why the plastic surgeon views the possibility of successful primary grafting after radical vulvectomy with extreme pessimism, and the results reported have been poor [5]. The occasional success has only tended to highlight the much more frequent failures.

DELAYED EXPOSED GRAFTING

Grafting in certain areas of the body has always been regarded as technically difficult when the conventional methods of fixation with a tie-over bolus are used. Recognition of the reasons for failure in those situations has allowed more successful methods of grafting to be developed. Failure, it is now recognized, is due to the inability to immobilize the area and prevent the graft from sliding on its bed [4]. The development of exposed grafting has solved this problem. The graft is laid on the area to be grafted and left without any dressings; it is merely protected from the bed clothes. Reliance is placed first on the natural fibrin adhesion between the graft and the surface on which it is being placed. This is followed by ingrowth, first of capillaries and then by fibroblasts to provide the final fixation by fibrous tissue [3]. The adhesion that this provides from the outset is enough to allow the graft to move with any minor movements of the patient, although naturally such movements are confined to an absolute minimum.

Exposed grafting can be used either primarily or delayed, but there are obvious advantages in delaying it. Hematoma is a well recognized hazard to graft take, and, since hemostasis in vulvectomy is a problem, there are advantages in waiting for a few days until hemostasis is assured or even in waiting longer until good granulations have developed.

The use of delayed exposed grafting clearly eliminates all the local disadvantages cited above. The general disadvantages are also largely eliminated, since the magnitude of the excisional procedure is not increased and early ambulation, which is desirable for the older patient, is not interfered with.

Surgical Technique

Radical vulvectomy is carried out in the usual way, but there are a few points of technique that should be stressed—points which in no way compromise the radical nature of the procedure, but which, nonetheless, if scrupulously observed, make grafting easier.

1. Part of the raw area left following excision lies over the pubic symphysis and inguinal region. There is a strong temptation to reduce the size of this area by suturing together the margins of the defect at the apex in each inguinal region in the mistaken belief that this will make grafting easier. In this area, it makes no significant difference whether the plastic surgeon has 5 or 50 sq cm to graft, and attempts to reduce the area by suturing may hold up grafting if they in any way interfere with the development of granulations by the occurrence of slough, by the cutting-in of sutures, or by minor infection (Fig. 47-1).

No attempt should be made to mobilize the abdominal or thigh skin to allow further suturing and reduction of the raw surface (Fig. 47-2), since this is likely to cause bleed-

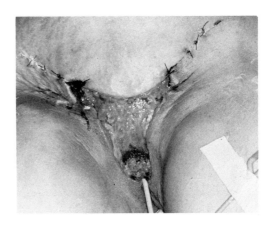

FIG. 47-1. The occurrence of slough and minor local infection following ill-advised attempts to reduce the postvulvectomy raw surface by suturing the apex of the wound on each side.

ing under the flap with resulting infection.

2. Fine ligature materials should be used. It is depressing to see how often a slowly separating slough over a coarse ligature on the saphenous vein holds up granulations and unnecessarily delays grafting.

3. The sartorius muscle should be used to protect the femoral vessels [7]. The muscle can be detached from its upper attachment, mobilized, and swung over to cover the vessels. Its vascular supply is segmental from a series of small vessels, and as few as possible of these should be divided so that its vascularity and consequent capacity to granulate quickly is reduced as little as possible.

4. These patients are frequently overweight, and fat should be removed as far as possible as part of the specimen and not left on the groin or abdomen. Fat granulates poorly, and its presence slows down the development of good granulations. As a corollary, the abdominal and thigh incisions should be vertical [2], since this reduces the fat exposed on the wound margin to a minimum (see Fig. 47-2). On the abdomen, the

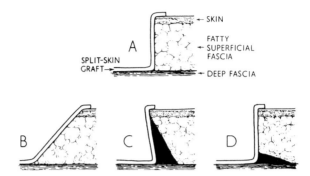

FIG. 47-2. A. Correct technique using vertical incisions. B and C. Oblique cut either increases the area of poorly granulating exposed fat or leaves an overhang with "dead space" leading to grafting difficulty. D. Undercutting leaves overhang with "dead space" and grafting difficulty. (From I. A. McGregor, *Br. J. Plast. Surg.* 15:302, 1962.)

plane of dissection should leave the fine areolar tissue over the aponeurosis but nothing else. On the thigh, the muscles should be laid bare. Dissection in these planes leaves a surface that granulates fast and well.

Following the vulvectomy, the aim of treatment is to produce clean and relatively sterile granulations in preparation for grafting. For this purpose, frequent baths are used and suitable antiseptic wet local dressings are applied. For the first few days, an indwelling catheter is used, but it can be removed as soon as possible to allow early ambulation.

Grafting itself must await the development of clinically healthy granulations, and bacteriological samples, collected with a swab, should be free of *Streptococcus pyogenes* and *Pseudomonas aeruginosa,* both of which are recognized graft destroyers. The time taken to achieve this state is variable, 10 to 26 days having been our extremes, and nothing is gained by rushing to graft before the surface is really ready.

METHOD OF GRAFTING

The requirements for successful exposed grafting are good granulations, cooperation from the patient in lying immobile, and protection of the graft from being dislodged.

Cooperation is most likely to be lacking during recovery from a general anesthetic. Of course, depending on the general condition of the patient and the local circumstances, it may be considered advisable to use local anesthesia. If hyaluronidase is added to the local anesthetic agent [4], large grafts can be cut successfully. In either case, movement while the patient is being moved on and off the table is likely to dislodge the graft. Consequently, it is best to store the graft overnight in the refrigerator and apply it when the patient is back in bed, awake, and cooperative. Since the patient is going to be immobile on her back for 5 days, the surgeon should avoid using donor areas on which the patient will be lying during that time.

The next stage involves maintaining the patient as immobile as possible for the 5 days or so following application of the graft, and a tranquilizer may help to make this period more tolerable for the patient. An indwelling catheter must be inserted. Unnecessary movement can be avoided if an enema is given before the graft is applied and a low-residue diet is given thereafter. The legs are held

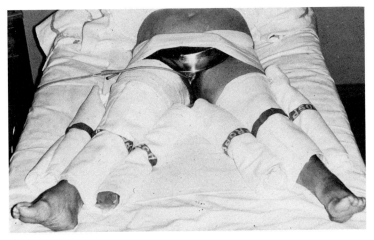

A

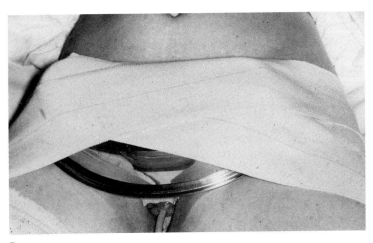

B

FIG. 47-3. A. Method of immobilization of the legs in abduction using sandbags. B. Method of protection of the graft using a kidney dish.

immobile with sandbags in a reasonably abducted position (Fig. 47-3A).

The graft is applied to the raw area as either large sheets or stamps (Fig. 47-4), depending on the experience and confidence of the surgeon. The whole area should be covered carefully, with the graft slightly overlapping the skin edges. The surgeon should press out all air bubbles between the graft and its bed. No dressings of any kind are applied directly on top of the graft; protection is provided very simply and effectively by a kidney dish strapped across the pubic area (see Fig. 47-3B).

The position and protection of the patient are maintained for 5 days; the graft is then

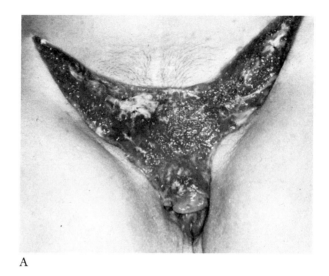

A

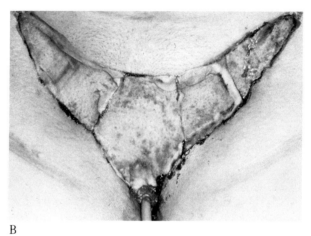

B

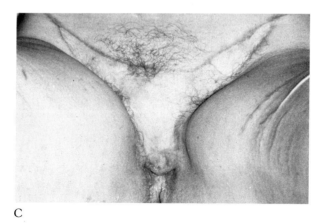

C

FIG. 47-4. Grafting of the postvulvectomy defect. A. The granulations are virtually ready for grafting. B. The appearance 5 days after grafting. C. The end result.

inspected. A good take appears as healthy-looking pink skin. At this stage, an odd blister may need to be snipped; and the graft overlapping onto the surrounding skin is carefully trimmed. The patient is now encouraged to move more freely in bed, the catheter is removed, and a regime of regular baths instituted. If a good take has occurred, the patient is allowed to walk in 7 to 10 days.

Results

Take of the graft is generally excellent and the patient walks well. In the 70 to 80-year-old age group, ambulation is liable to be slow, but this is only to be expected and the grafting per se is not responsible. Very occasionally, the area directly over the pubis is slow to granulate. In such circumstances, there is no need to postpone grafting; this area can be allowed to heal spontaneously without affecting the convalescence of the patient. The graft usually shrinks to about 75 percent of its original area, and in so doing, softens slowly.

One would expect contraction of the circular scar around the vaginal opening to produce a degree of stricture of the introitus. This has been clinically significant in only two patients, both in the younger age group, in whom the stricture prevented coitus. In both instances, a multiple Z-plasty relieved the stricture and removed the disability. One patient subsequently became pregnant and had a successful vaginal delivery.

Malignant tumor of the vulva is a disease of the elderly, and subsequent pregnancy is an unlikely eventuality. Three of our patients, however, were in the child-bearing age when vulvectomy was carried out, and they later became pregnant. Of the three, two had successful vaginal deliveries that required only episiotomies. The third, more because of the wish to sterilize the patient than because of dire obstetric need, was delivered by cesarean section. It would appear that a patient of child-bearing age can be reassured regarding subsequent pregnancy.

No patient considered fit for vulvectomy was turned down as unfit for delayed grafting. Not the least of the merits of the method is that failure of the graft to take does not add materially to the patient's overall disability, since, in such a case, management can then be along the lines of a fresh attempt to graft or of simply allowing spontaneous healing. In either event, the method of repair increases neither the morbidity nor the mortality.

References

1. Beare, R. L. B. Irradiation injuries of the perineum. *Br. J. Plast. Surg.* 15:22, 1962.
2. McGregor, I. A. Delayed exposed grafting after radical vulvectomy. *Br. J. Plast. Surg.* 15:302, 1962.
3. McGregor, I. A. Skin grafting after radical vulvectomy. *J. Obstet. Gynaecol. Br. Commonw.* 73:599, 1966.
4. McGregor, I. A. *Fundamental Techniques of Plastic Surgery* (4th ed.). Edinburgh: Livingstone, 1968. Pp. 94–96.
5. Robinson, F. Repair after vulvectomy. *Br. J. Plast. Surg.* 15:293, 1962.
6. Way, S. The anatomy of the lymphatic drainage of the vulva and its influence on the radical operation for carcinoma. *Ann. R. Coll. Surg. Engl.* 3:187, 1948.
7. Way, S. Carcinoma of the vulva. In Miegs,

J. V., and Sturgis, S. H. (Eds.), *Progress in Gynaecology,* Vol. 3. New York: Grune & Stratton, 1957. P. 489.

8. Way, S., and Hennigan, M. The late results of extended radical vulvectomy for carcinoma of the vulva. *J. Obstet. Gynaecol. Br. Commonw.* 73:594, 1966.

9. Williams, S. B. Reconstruction of the vulva —a new approach. *Br. J. Plast. Surg.* 22:4, 1969.

CHARLES E. HORTON
JEROME E. ADAMSON
RICHARD A. MLADICK
JAMES CARRAWAY

48

IN MOST INSTANCES, skin grafts are the treatment of choice to cover skin defects of the genital area. There are, however, a few problems that can best be solved by the use of skin flaps or tubes (Table 48-1). Two factors limit flap usage: one, flaps should not contain hair if they are to be used in intravaginal or intraanal areas, and two, many donor sites for flaps in this area do have profuse hair growth. Thus, donor areas for flaps are somewhat limited, even though many thigh and gluteal flaps can be moved without delay to the perineum. Flaps heal without contraction and prolonged splinting, and they carry vascularity with healing potential into areas with decreased circulation and scarring that might otherwise not support a free graft. Grafts do not ordinarily take in the presence of infection, and in certain instances, flaps can be used after debridement of infected areas where grafts might otherwise be compromised. Flaps can be drained, or they can be brought in from a distance. Certain flaps retain sensation if the nerves are not divided in their pedicle base. On the other hand, if the flap is completely severed from its nerve source, it may be less sensitive than a split

graft and may mask, by bulky tissue, any sensation from underlying normal tissue.

In male patients, flaps have been used for scrotal and penile reconstruction. Pollock has recently reported the use of a flap around the anus to correct scarring and incontinence. Unless tissue bulk in the perineum is lost, grafts would seem to be more reasonable for most other circumstances. In cases of bulky perineal body skin loss with irregular scarring and recession of the perineum that causes uncleanliness and irritation, a gluteal or thigh flap is indicated to smooth the area and remove scarring. This method can be used for cases of watering-can perineum (Fig. 48-1). Scrotal flaps are easy to elevate and can cover a vast area without compromising the primary use of the scrotum (Fig. 48-2).

In female patients, wide excision of tissue of the vulva can be done with primary closure. If more radical excision is done, the hairy skin surrounding the vagina should not be pulled into the vagina, and the defect should be closed with either flaps or grafts. Laterally, grafts can be used with great success; however, posteriorly, if wide excision is done, the posterior vaginal wall is moved too

TABLE 48-1. The Use of Skin Grafts versus Flaps for Resurfacing the Genital Area

Skin Grafts	Flaps
Advantages:	*Advantages:*
1. Easily procured	1. Local tissue available
2. Donor site heals primarily	2. Carries own blood supply
3. Easy to fit to defect	3. Does not contract
4. Large amounts can be obtained	4. Retains sensation (partial)
5. Adjusts to new environment	5. Retains bulk of perineum
6. Regains minimal amount of sensation	6. Can be drained
7. Resists trauma (tough)	7. Immobilization not essential
	8. Provides padding to bony areas
Disadvantages:	*Disadvantages:*
1. Donor site scar	1. Limited donor areas
2. Contracts considerably	2. Hair growth in donor areas
3. Must be immobilized to heal	3. Large flaps require grafts to donor areas
4. Never gains total sensation	
5. Cannot be used in infected areas	
6. Cannot be used in avascular area	
7. Bleeding must be controlled (hematoma will cause loss of graft)	

close to the anus. In this case, it is best to use local flaps to rebuild the perineal body to keep a normal distance between the vagina and the rectum. Gluteal or thigh flaps can be used either as a double rotation flap or as a single flap rotated into the area (Fig. 48-3).

When excessive vulvar tissue is destroyed and skin grafting reconstruction will not allow a normal depth and aperture to the vagina, distant tissue in the form of tubes can be used to rebuild the labia and to produce a functioning vagina.

In selective cases, discrete scarring or pathology within the vagina must be excised. Primary closure may compromise the size of the vagina. Split grafts will contract unless splinted for prolonged periods; therefore, a local rotation flap of hairless labial tissue may

be best utilized (Fig. 48-4A). This flap of tissue, when unfolded, will cover defects measuring up to 4 by 6 cm without compromising the blood supply to the flap (Fig. 48-4B).

The competent surgeon should be aware of the advantages and disadvantages of graft versus flap coverage for the perineal area and, by evaluation and planning, should be able to use the most desirable reconstructive methods to suit the individual problem (Figs. 48-5B and 48-6).

If major vessels are exposed after postoperative skin sloughs, flaps should be used to resurface the exposed arteries, veins, and nerves before infection and rupture of the vessels occurs.

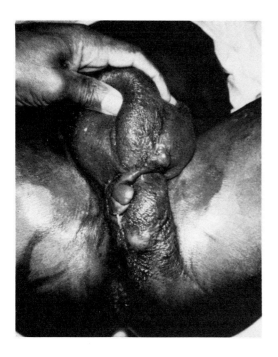

FIG. 48-1. Multiple fistulas involving the scrotum and perineum.

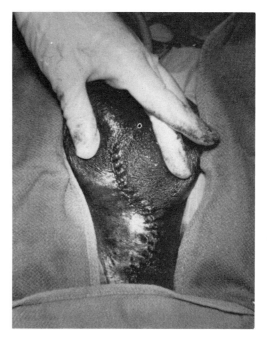

FIG. 48-2. Same case as in Figure 48-1 after excision and closure with scrotal flaps. The urethral repair has been completed.

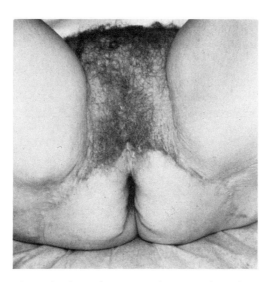

FIG. 48-3. Flaps taken from the buttocks are used to resurface the posterior vaginal wall and perineal body.

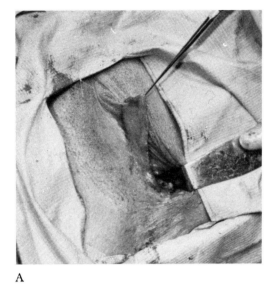

A

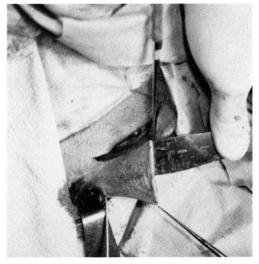

B

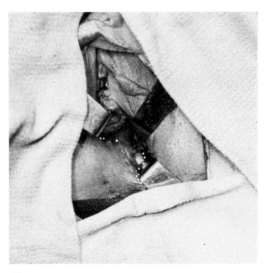

C

FIG. 48-4. A. Labial flap prepared for transfer to release intravaginal scarring. B. Hairless labial flap is elevated and unfolded. C. The labial flap used to resurface one-quarter of the circumference of the vagina (the white dots show the extent of the flap).

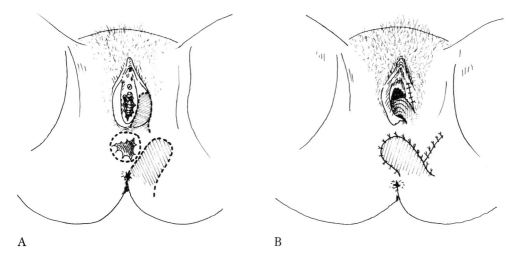

FIG. 48-5. Two useful flaps for vaginal and perineal resurfacing. A. The vaginal flap from the labia minora will supply a surprisingly large amount of hairless skin where the labia is unfolded. B. The lower flap is useful to retain space between the vagina and the anus.

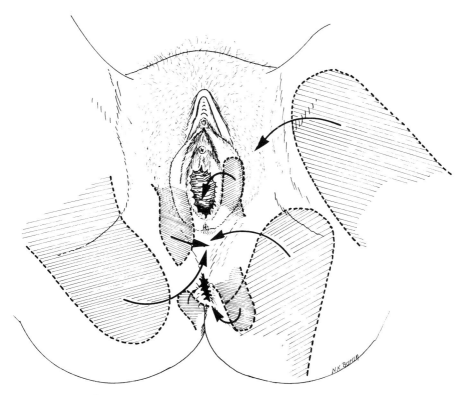

FIG. 48-6. Possible flap designs around the genital areas. Larger flap donor sites would require grafting for closure. Smaller flap donor sites could be closed primarily.

References

1. Converse, J. M. (Ed.) *Reconstructive Plastic Surgery: Principles and Procedures in Correction, Reconstruction and Transplantation.* Philadelphia: Saunders, 1964.
2. Grabb, W. C., and Smith, J. W. (Eds.) *Plastic Surgery: A Concise Guide to Clinical Practice* (2nd ed.) Boston: Little, Brown, 1973.
3. Pollock, W. J., and Litwin, M. S. Hemianoplasty. *Plast. Reconstr. Surg.* 47:568, 1971.

Erectile Disorders

VIII

Peyronie's Disease

EUGENE F. POUTASSE

49

I N 1743 François Peyronie, a French surgeon, described a fibrous induration of the penis that produced a painful curvature and delayed ejaculation. Many cases have been reported since that time, mostly regarding the clinical aspects of the disease. Until recently, very little had been written on the pathology or specific treatment of this disabling deformity. Peyronie's disease is more common in the middle decades in life, but it can occur at any age.

Pathology

In the normal penis the following fascia layers can be demonstrated (Fig. 49-1): (1) a superficial layer, *dartos fascia,* underlies the skin of the penis; (2) a stronger fascial layer, *Buck's fascia,* wraps around the corpora cavernosa and corpus spongiosum; (3) surrounding the corpora cavernosa and the corpus spongiosum is the tough *tunica albuginea;* and (4) underlying this is a thin layer of vascular, loose connective tissue that separates the tunica from the erectile tissue. The main penile vessels and nerves run under Buck's fascia on the dorsal surface of the penis. A superficial vein lies outside dartos fascia.

Peyronie's disease is most commonly found midway between the corpora cavernosa on the dorsal side of the penis. It may, however, occur in various parts of the penis, for example, near the coronal sulcus or deep within the corpora cavernosa. It may even occur in multiple sites simultaneously. The length of the fibrotic plaque varies considerably, ranging from only one to several centimeters. It may extend from the coronal sulcus back to the ligament of the penis, with the average plaque being about 2 cm in length. It may vary in width from 0.5 to 1.5 cm. Smith [5], in a careful study of the pathology of Peyronie's disease in necropsy specimens, showed that the earliest site of involvement was the areolar connective tissue between the tunica albuginea and the corpora cavernosa. He noted that in cases of short duration, there was a predominance of an inflammatory cellular infiltrate, consisting of lymphocytes and plasmocytes, that was located chiefly around the vessels. More advanced or older cases showed a thickened fibrous connective tissue plaque separating the tunica albuginea and corpora cavernosa; ultimately this plaque extended into the tunica albuginea and the corpora cavernosa, destroying smooth muscle bundles in the intercavernous septa. Three cases in Smith's series showed ossification between the corpora cavernosa and the tunica albuginea. It was his

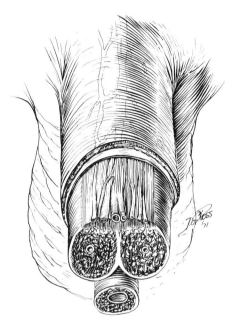

FIG. 49-1. Cross section of the penis showing dartos fascia and the superficial dorsal vein. Buck's fascia (broad line), and the tunica albuginea surrounding the corpora cavernosa and corpus spongiosum. Peyronie's disease characteristically involves the connective tissue layer between tunica and corpus, and it extends into both structures to form a fibrotic plaque, as shown by the cross-hatched area.

conclusion that Peyronie's disease begins as a vasculitis in the areolar connective tissue beneath the tunica albuginea, later extends into adjacent structures, and is followed finally by fibrosis and production of useless elastic fibers.

In support of this conclusion, it has been found impossible at surgery to strip the fibrous plaque off the corpora cavernosa: it has to be removed by sharp dissection. The fibrotic plaque also includes the adjacent tunica albuginea. Frequently a fibrotic, inelastic dorsal vein of the penis has to be removed to allow maximum correction of chordee. Further support of Smith's conclu-sion may be derived from the fact that some cases of Peyronie's disease spontaneously remit with complete disappearance of all evidence of disease or chordee. It is possible that in these instances, vasculitis subsided and the disease did not progress to fibrosis with production of inelastic fibers.

Symptoms

The first symptoms usually noted are that the erect penis bends to one side and erection is painful. The patient may detect a hard, tender knot in his penis. Painful erections may continue for several months, when finally the pain disappears and the man is left with an embarrassing curvature of the penis on erection. A thick fibrous plaque can be felt, usually on the dorsal surface of the penis. When the penis is stretched, a relatively thin cord extends from either side of the plaque along the dorsum of the penis from the glans back to the suspensory ligament. The curvature may be mild, or it may be so severe that the patient is unable to use the penis for sexual relations. The erect penis usually arcs backward toward the abdomen, as shown in Figure 49-2. In some cases, however, it may bend laterally or, rarely, downward, depending on location of the fibrous plaque.

Treatment

Various types of treatment have been used in the past—vitamin E, x-ray therapy, applications of radium, and various types of physical therapy—with improvement being noted in some patients. A few cases of Peyronie's disease will show spontaneous remission of the fibrosis with complete disappearance of the fibrotic plaque. Steroid injections into or around the plaque have been utilized with

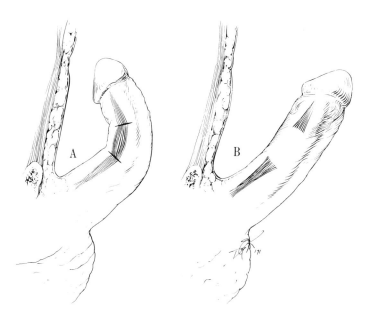

FIG. 49-2.   A.   An erect penis with a disabling dorsal chordee. Lines indicate the area of proposed resection in the thickest part of the plaque.   B.   Erect penis after excision of the plaque, showing dorsal lengthening and less chordee.

varying degrees of success. This is now regarded as an adjunct to therapy [1, 2]. In my experience, steroid injections are helpful in the early stages of the disease when erections are painful, insofar as they help diminish the amount of pain experienced by the patient. It is not easy to inject the steroid into the fibrotic induration; hence the material is frequently mixed with hyaluronidase to help dissipate the medication in the area of the fibrosis.

Surgical treatment of Peyronie's disease has not been popular. An operation was described in 1947 by Lowsley and Gentile [4]. Lowsley and Boyce [3] in 1950 reported their operation for correction of Peyronie's disease. After applying a tourniquet to the base of the penis, a midline incision was utilized to expose the induration. The fibrous plaque was dissected from the corpora cavernosa as completely as possible, and a block of fat was

fitted into the defect. Care was taken not to approximate the deep fascial layers but to allow the fat to interpose between them. Their last report included 50 cases operated on between 1935 and February, 1949. Of 17 operated upon without the use of fat, nine were cured of the curvature, four improved, one slightly improved, one did not improve, and two could not be followed. Of the 33 patients in whom a fat graft was interposed between the fascial layers, 20 were cured, six improved, four slightly improved, one improved, and two were not followed up. Seven patients required reoperation because of the formation of scar tissue that reproduced the original deformity. It was their conclusion that Peyronie's disease was curable by surgery if the plaque formation was not too extensive. They preferred to operate on those cases in which the plaque was limited to the dorsal cleavage line betdween the corpora cavernosa,

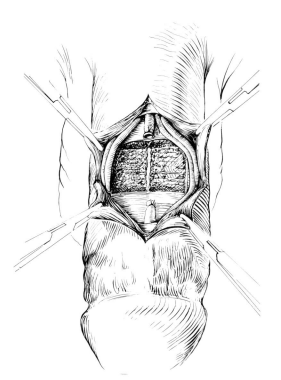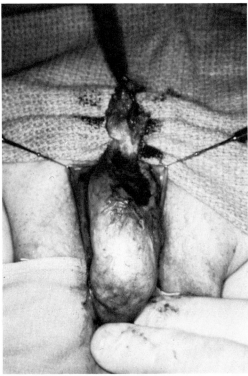

FIG. 49-3.   Surgical exposure demonstrating the divided deep dorsal vein and excision of fibrotic, inelastic tissue and tunica to expose 2 to 3 cm of normal corpus.

and they avoided operating on those in which the plaque extended laterally over the surface of the corpora cavernosa.

During the last 15 years, I have selected about 36 cases for surgical treatment (about two-thirds in Cleveland and one-third in Norfolk). None of these was operated on in the early stages of the disease when erections were painful. The patients were followed for many months, usually for a year or longer, to make sure that the disease had reached a stable point and that the curvature was truly a handicap or obstacle to sexual relations. The fibrotic plaque must be well defined and so located that, when the penis is stretched, it can be shown to limit stretchability of the dorsal surface of the penis. If a section of the fibrous plaque can be removed to allow

lengthening of the dorsal surface of the penis by a centimeter, the curvature can be decreased from a disabling 75 to 90 degrees to a usable 15 to 25 degrees (Fig. 49-3).

Surgical Technique

A transverse incision is made on the top of the penis. No tourniquet is used; the skin may be moved back and forth sufficiently to give exposure (see Fig. 49-3). The superficial vein can be retracted readily. Buck's fascia is opened, exposing the deep dorsal vein and the paired dorsal arteries and nerves. If the dorsal vein is inelastic and fibrotic, a segment must be removed to permit lengthening of the penis. The arteries and nerves must be protected and are retracted laterally to give exposure. The fibrotic plaque is opened with an incision going just deep enough to enter the normal cavernous tissue. The plaque is cut away in small chips, gradually exposing more of the normal corpus. The fibrosis is usually deepest in the median sulcus between the two corpora, thinning out as it spreads laterally over the surfaces of the corpora. A block of this white fibrous tissue is removed with the scalpel until a length of about 2 to 3 cm of normal cavernous tissue is exposed. The penis is stretched periodically to note how much lengthening occurs as the fibrous plaque is removed. The finger can detect any residual inelastic tissue that must be removed to permit correction of chordee. Bleeding is controlled by the application of sponges soaked with dilute topical adrenalin. No attempt is made to close the tunica albuginea. The fascial layers, Buck's and dartos, are drawn together with fine sutures of chromic gut, and the skin is closed with subcuticular sutures. A pressure dressing of Elastoplast is applied for 3 days. Patients have noted no difficulty in voiding after the procedure.

Results and Complications

For the first 2 weeks, a soft induration and edema are noted in the operative site. Erections are usually fairly straight at this time.

As this soft induration disappears, the patient is encouraged to have sexual relations. In most cases, patients have been able to accomplish coitus satisfactorily and are delighted to be able to function again sexually. They usually still have some degree of curvature, since it is rarely possible to straighten the penis completely.

A few words of caution should be stressed. The sensory nerves in the penis must be protected; one patient had a distressing numbness on one side of the glans that eventually improved. One should avoid cutting deeply into the corpora cavernosa and removing too much of the tissue because the penis may then become flail, i.e., erections occur on either end with a weak, thin point in the middle. This has occurred in a few patients. Careful selection of the patient with a relatively thin but restrictive fibrosis and selection of the operative site to avoid cutting deeply into the corpora are important. Surgery should be avoided in the early stage of the disease, when there is usually an infiltration of inflammatory cells, because of the possibility of inciting a worse fibrotic reaction than was present beforehand.*

* Ed. note: Encouraging results with the use of dermal grafts to replace the diseased tunica albuginea have been reported by Horton and Devine. At the Educational Foundation Symposium on Hypospodias held at Virginia Beach in 1972, the authors reported success in several cases which were otherwise refractory to treatment. A complete report on this technique will be published in *Plast. Reconstr. Surg.*—C. E. H.

References

1. Chesney, J. Plastic induration of the penis: Peyronie's disease. *Br. J. Urol.* 35:61, 1963.
2. Furey, C. A., Jr. Peyronie's disease: Treatment by the local injections of meticortelone and hydrocortisone. *J. Urol.* 77:251, 1957.
3. Lowsley, O. S., and Boyce, W. H. Further experiences with an operation for the cure of Peyronie's disease. *J. Urol.* 63:888, 1950.
4. Lowsley, O. S., and Gentile, A. An operation for cure of certain cases of plastic induration (Peyronie's disease) of the penis. *J. Urol.* 57:552, 1947.
5. Smith, B. H. Peyronie's disease. *Am. J. Clin. Pathol.* 45:670, 1966.

Priapism

WILLIAM V. TYNES, II

50

THE TERM *priapism* is derived from ancient Greek mythology and takes its origin from the Greek god, Priapus, the symbol of fertility. Priapism defines a condition in which a prolonged erection of the penis occurs, usually unaccompanied by sexual stimulation or excitation. In most cases it becomes very painful and leads the patient to the physician (Fig. 50-1).

Priapism has been classified broadly into two groups: idiopathic and secondary. Primary or idiopathic priapism generally refers to an erection that is unaccompanied by a disease process. There are cases in which sexual activity is thought to be the only cause. Secondary priapism, on the other hand, is that condition which is caused by factors directly related to a pathological process. In all cases of priapism, tumescence continues and the erect penis does not return to a flaccid state.

Pathology

Penile erection is initiated by physical or psychic stimuli traveling through the lumbar and sacral nerve centers. Sympathetic inhibition of vasoconstriction occurs, and direct vasodilatation results from sacral parasympathetic activity. Thus, the corpora cavernosa fill with large amounts of blood. In 1952 Conte showed that penile erection is controlled primarily by a series of muscular pillars extending into the lumens of the arterioles, venules, and arteriovenous anastomotic channels of the corpora cavernosa. These pillars are under nerve control and serve to open and close the vessels. In the normal flaccid state, these arterioles are partially closed, and the venules and the arteriovenous anastomoses remain open. In the erect state, the arterioles are fully open while the venules and arteriovenous shunts are partially closed. Prolonged erection by psychic or local stimulating factors may cause venous stasis, which in turn results in an increased viscosity of the blood from an increased carbon dioxide tension. This produces relative venous occlusion at the junction of the cavernous spaces with the collecting veins. Edema of the corporal trabeculae occurs, and a mechanical resistance to venous drainage is present. Eventually occlusion of the arterioles occurs, and finally fibrosis develops [4].

Etiology

The diagnosis of priapism is made by the physical examination. A complete medical history of the patient should indicate whether

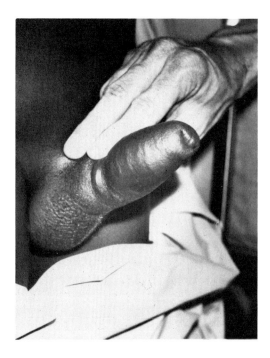

FIG. 50-1. Typical case of priapism seen in association with sickle-cell anemia disease.

this is a primary or secondary disorder. In patients who have priapism secondary to a disease process, a careful history and physical examination must be made in order to discover what the cause might be. Although priapism may be secondary to a specific condition, the correction of that abnormality should not be expected to correct the priapism that exists.

The following is a classification modified from that of Becker and Mitchell [1]:

I. Primary or idiopathic priapism. In this condition there is no specific pathological cause for the priapic state. Primary priapism is generally thought to be secondary to a prolonged period of sexual activity; however, this is not always true. The latter condition has been termed *idiopathic priapism*

II. Secondary priapism
   A. Neurogenic
      1. Direct central nervous system stimulation such as seen in multiple sclerosis, tabes dorsalis, or injuries to the spinal cord of cerebral hemispheres
   B. Infectious or inflammatory conditions
      1. Congenital syphilis
      2. Complications of mumps
      3. Drug poisoning
      4. Bacteremias causing pelvic thrombophlebitis and focal suppuration
   C. Mechanical
      1. Reflex from local stimuli
         a. Phimosis
         b. Benign tumors of the urethra
         c. Urethral polyps
         d. Urethral or vesical calculi
         e. Prostatitis or urethritis
      2. Hemorrhage resulting from straddle injury to the perineum or rupture of the urethra
      3. Metastatic tumors of the prostate, bladder, testis, rectum, kidney, or liver that invade the corpora
   D. Hematological
      1. Chronic myelogenous leukemia, chronic lymphocytic leukemia, and chronic granulocytic leukemia
      2. Sickle cell anemia

Treatment

On the basis of the previous classification of priapism, whether or not the condition is primary or secondary is of no great importance when a physician is faced with a patient in this condition. This is a surgical emergency; time is a critical factor. Two objectives must be reached. The first is to restore venous drainage to the corpora cavernosa. The second is to eliminate damage to the local erectile mechanism. The embarrassed patient often delays his visit to the physician, and this may cause permanent damage to the erectile mechanism.

The medical management of priapism has usually been unsuccessful because of a failure to attain these two goals. Attempts have been made to reduce the erect phallus by administering a spinal anesthetic, sedatives, hormones, or other agents. Proteolytic enzymes fractionated from the venom of a pit viper have been used to cause a rapid reduction in the plasma fibrinogen to reduce clotting in the corpora cavernosa [2]. Other enzymes have been used to lyse thrombosed blood vessels. In 1959 Ulm [10] reported the use of Arfonad (trimethaphan) to create a hypotensive state and allow venous engorgement of the penis to subside. Grace and Winter [4] mention a variety of other measures, consisting of local treatment with bed rest, analgesics, ice packs, pressure dressings, and massage of the corpora cavernosa. None of these methods has withstood the test of time, and they offer little relief to the patient.

Surgical management of priapism has been somewhat more effective in the attempts to restore venous drainage and lessen damage to the erectile tissue. If the patient reaches the physician in time and if fibrosis has not occurred in the corpora cavernosa, a simple technique of needle aspiration may be employed [6, 8]. This utilizes a large-bore hollow needle inserted at the base of the corpora on each side of the penis. An attempt is made to remove all of the dark venous sludge until the penis is flaccid and bright red bleeding occurs. This is accomplished by manual massage of the corpora as well as by needle aspiration. Irrigation of the corpora with

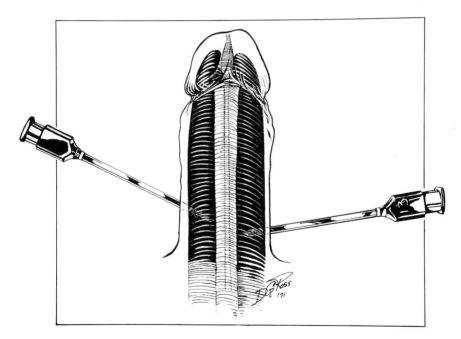

FIG. 50-2. Large bore 13 gauge needles are inserted in the base or proximal portion of the corpus cavernosum. The venous blood and clotted material is aspirated, and a heparinized solution may be used to irrigate the erectile bodies. Manual massage of the penis is advantageous and facilitates aspiration.

heparinized saline can be used to speed up this process and inhibit the clotting mechanism (Fig. 50-2).

Another surgical procedure that has been employed in the treatment of this disease is ligation of one internal pudendal artery [3]. It was reasoned that the erect state is maintained by a high input of arterial blood. This technique is rarely used today.

In 1964 Grayhack and associates [5] described an operation in which a venous bypass is used to control the priapism. In his operation, Grayhack utilizes the saphenous vein, which is exposed through a vertical incision in the groin (Fig. 50-3). The vein is mobilized and divided about 8 to 10 cm from its junction with the femoral vein. The free end of the distal portion of the divided saphenous vein is led through a subcutaneous tunnel to the area of the right corpus cavernosum. The right corpus cavernosum may be opened by excising a 1 cm elliptical segment of Buck's fascia and tunica albuginea near the base of the penis on its dorsolateral aspect. When this is done, the blood clots and venous sludge should be evacuated by irrigation with a dilute heparin solution. The distention of both corpora diminishes considerably, as occurs in a needle aspiration. The end of the vein is cut obliquely and anastomosed to the elliptical opening in Buck's fascia and the tunica albuginea. Postoperatively, local measures should be used to maintain an adequate flow through the venous

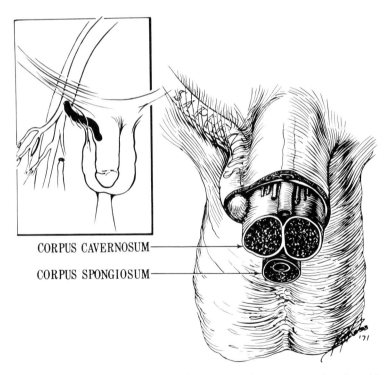

CORPUS CAVERNOSUM

CORPUS SPONGIOSUM

FIG. 50-3. Cavernosaphenous shunt. The saphenous vein is anastomosed end-to-side to the corpus cavernosum. The relationship of the saphenous vein to the skin, fascia, corpus cavernosum, and dorsal nerve, artery, and vein of the penis is shown. The course of the saphenous vein through its tunnel is shown in the inset at the upper left.

shunt. These consist of aqueous subcutaneous heparin injections and distal compression of the penis with a blood pressure cuff. These shunts will generally thrombose after several weeks when priapism is no longer a problem. This shunt may be done bilaterally if both corpora are not reduced in size by aspiration of one erectile body.

The corpus spongiosum is generally not involved in priapism. Because of this finding,

Quackels [9] described a cavernospongiosum anastomosis in 1964 (Fig. 50-4). The patient is placed in the lithotomy position, and exposure is made through the perineum. A midline vertical incision extends from the base of the scrotum to the perianal area. The skin and subcutaneous tissues are divided and the bulbous urethra is identified. Parallel and lateral to the bulbous urethra are found the proximal portions of the corpora cavernosa.

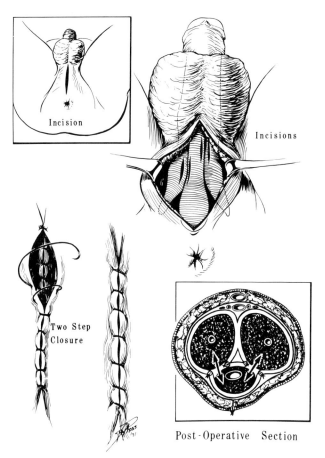

FIG. 50-4. Cavernospongiosum shunt. The inset at the upper left outlines the surgical approach. The incisions into the corpora cavernosa and corpus spongiosum are shown in a bilateral procedure. The bulbous urethra is seen as an expanded area of the corpus spongiosum lying between the proximal ends of the corpora cavernosa. A postoperative cross section of the penis shows the pathway for the blood flow from the corpora cavernosa into the corpus spongiosum that surrounds the urethra. The two-step closure at the lower left illustrates the deep and superficial margins of the shunt being approximated with continuous suture material.

A linear 1 to 2 cm incision is made into the corpus cavernosum on one side, and the clots and venous sludge are evacuated by standard methods previously described. A corresponding incision in the lateral margin of the corpus spongiosum is made, and these two openings are closed side to side with continuous sutures of 3-0 chromic catgut or a similar dissolvable suture material, thus creating a shunt. Communications are known to exist between the corpora cavernosa through the fascia. If these are blocked and both corpora cavernosa do not soften, a bilateral procedure should be employed. The placement of the incisions is shown in Figure 50-3 as well as a cross section of the penis after bilateral shunts have been constructed. This procedure has been favorably accepted, since it does not interfere with a subsequent cavernosaphenous shunt should this become necessary.

Discussion

It must be emphasizd that this condition is truly a surgical emergency. In all cases of priapism, time is of the essence. In most cases, however, the patient does not immediately come to the physician with his complaint. The diagnosis is made by the history and physical examination, and immediate measures to reduce venous engorgement and restore blood flow should be started. If the patient is late in seeking medical attention, pathophysiological changes may have already occurred, and fibrosis and permanent damage

will be present. As little as 3 days may be enough time for these changes to occur.

The treatment outlined in this chapter is for priapism, whether it be primary or secondary. The classification and etiology of secondary priapism should make us aware that an underlying disease process may exist. Regardless of the causes, surgical intervention is likely necessary. Occasionally, the patient's general medical condition is a contraindication to major surgery. In these cases, vigorous medical management and simple needle aspiration under local anesthesia may be the treatment of choice. It is generally well known, however, that an elderly patient responds less favorably to these measures. The loss of sexual potency in patients with priapism is not a predictable conclusion but it occurs in a large percentage of cases.

Complications

No surgical procedure is without complications. A recent case of pulmonary embolism following a cavernospongiosum shunt has been reported [7]. The authors believed this represented thrombosis of a shunt with extension of the thrombus into the saphenofemoral junction. Anticoagulation measures should be employed in patients who have undergone surgery for priapism. It is interesting, however, that in a large series of patients reported by Grace and Winter [4], three patients with priapism were already receiving anticoagulants for cardiovascular disease.

References

1. Becker, L. E., and Mitchell, A. D. Priapism. *Surg. Clin. North Am.* 45:1523, 1965.
2. Bell, W. R., and Pitney, W. R. Management of priapism by therapeutic defibrination. (Medical Intelligence Brief Recordings). *N. Engl. J. Med.* 280:649, 1969
3. Burt, F. B., Shirmer, H. K., and Scott, W. W. A new concept in the management of priapism. *J. Urol.* 83:60, 1960.
4. Grace, D. A., and Winter, C. C. Priapism: An appraisal of management of twenty-three patients. *J. Urol.* 99:301, 1968.

5. Grayhack, J. T., McCullough, W., O'Connor, V. J., Jr., and Trippel, O. Venous bypass to control priapism. *Invest. Urol.* 1:509, 1964.

6. Harrow, B. R. Simple technique for treating priapism. *J. Urol.* 101:71, 1969.

7. Kandel, G. L., Bender, L. I., and Grove, J. S. Pulmonary embolism: A complication of corpus-saphenous shunt for priapism. *J. Urol.* 99:196, 1968.

8. Krauss, L., and Fitzpatrick, T. The treatment of priapism by penile aspiration under controlled hypotension. *J. Urol.* 85:595, 1961.

9. Quackels, R. Cure of a patient suffering from priapism by cavernospongiosa anastomosis. *Acta Urol. Belg.* 32:5, 1964.

10. Ulm, A. H. Treatment of primary priapism with Arfonad. *J. Urol.* 81:291, 1959.

Surgical Treatment
of Impotence
in the Male

ROBERT A. LOEFFLER

51

IMPOTENCE may be defined in many ways. This discussion will be confined to the inability to obtain or maintain an adequate penile erection in order to have successful coitus. This obviates the complex discussion of the various roles that frustration, guilt, homosexual tendencies, and inadequate personalities play in the many variations of impotence in those patients who may present for consideration of surgical treatment. Freud has written voluminously in an attempt to explain the differences in love and sex and the biological, psychological, physical, and spiritual causes of impotence.

A complete physical examination, an adequate history, and indicated laboratory testing should precede any form of treatment. Such factors as infections or other abnormalities of the genitourinary tract, gross endocrine abnormalities, pelvic vascular insufficiency, diabetes, cirrhosis [17], psychoneurosis, or true psychosis must be weighed in the decision of whether to use medical treatment or a surgical procedure consisting of an arterial bypass. Neuropsychiatric consultation is often advisable for the patient in whom the cause of the disease is obscure. Frequently, however, impotence is evident following trauma or a surgical procedure that has interrupted the neuropathways mediating the function of erection or ejaculation.

The neurophysiological system [7] that controls sexual functions is a part of the autonomic nervous system and is composed of two parts. The *parasympathetic fibers* from sacral nerves 2, 3, and 4 originate in the intermediolateral cells of the spinal cord segments and pass via the pelvic nerves to form the perivesicular prostatic and cavernous plexuses. The ischiocavernous and bulbocavernous muscles of the urethra, which are concerned with erection and ejaculation, are supplied by these parasympathetic fibers through the pudendal nerves. Parasympathetic stimulation results in erection by engorgement of the corpora cavernosa. The *sympathetic fibers* descend through the hypogastric plexus from the lumbar spinal cord. The dorsal nerve of the penis is believed to carry the sympathetic fibers that cause vasoconstriction of the corpora cavernosa, resulting in relaxation of the penis following ejaculation.

Ejaculation involves reflex patterns originating in the glans penis by way of the dorsal nerve and the common pudendal nerves. These reflexes enter by the sacral spinal cord and by the upper lumbar spinal cord via the hypogastric nerves to the unstriated muscles of the bladder, seminal vesicles, prostate, and ductus deferens. Soon after the activation of the upper lumbar reflex mechanisms, the sacral spinal cord stimulation activates muscle fibers of the sphincter muscle of the urethra (compressor urethrae) and the bulbocavernous and ischiocavernous muscles, leading to the clonic contractions of ejaculation. Orgasm is made up of the associated reactions and sensations occurring with ejaculation of semen in men and with the rhythmic contraction of the muscles of the distended vagina in women. The vessels that penetrate both the ischiocavernous and bulbocavernous portions of the erectile tissue in the male are separately controlled branches of the terminal branches of the pudendal artery.

In the pathological erection known as priapism, only the corpora cavernosa are involved. The erection of the corpus spongiosum and glans penis is not involved in this state. Similarly, loss of the ability of erection may be separate from the loss of the ability of ejaculation. The ability of erection may be lost following a sympathectomy involving lumbar nerves 1 and 2 on both sides, yet the ability to ejaculate may not be lost. Almost complete loss of ability to have erections may be associated with almost complete ability to have an ejaculation and orgasm, as evidenced by patients who have had a perineal total prostatectomy.

Priapism may result in a nonfunctioning corpora cavernosa, because the organization of coagulated blood in the corpora cavernosa can lead to complete fibrosis of these structures. This condition responds readily to the insertion of a rod in the shaft of the penis to assist the thin and weak erectile tissue that remains (Fig. 51-1). Insertion of the rod is

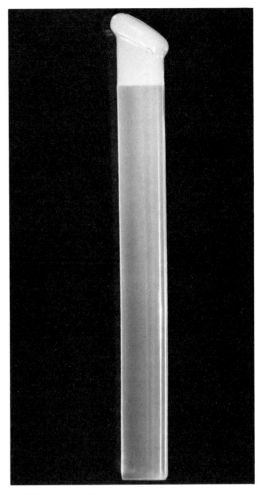

FIG. 51-1. Silastic penile implant; Lash-Loeffler design. (Courtesy of Dow-Corning Corporation, Midland, Michigan.)

difficult in these cases, however, because of the dense fibrous tissue that has replaced the normally spongy corpora cavernosa.

In Peyronie's disease, when considerable contracture and deviation of the penis occurs or when pain prohibits coitus, surgical intervention may be indicated. Removal of large plaques results in flaccid areas that can be bridged by well-placed rods [16] or a splint made out of plastic material. Diffuse involvement of the entire investing fascia or tunica albuginea of the corpora cavernosa results in a small sclerotic penis that cannot be managed well by any method.

Ventral curvature of the penis on erection without evidence of hypospadias has been called "short urethra" and is associated with chordee caused by fibrous tissue. Repeated unsuccessful attempts to correct this condition, even when the urethra has been lengthened by a graft or other reconstructive procedure, may occasionally be aided by the insertion of a penile rod. If the penis is large and powerful in erection, a Silastic rod may not be rigid enough and an acrylic [11] or polyethylene rod may be required. These have been well tolerated and their rigidity has not been a problem; the Silastic rod, however, is apparently more comfortable.

Impotence frequently follows injuries that cause temporary paraplegia. Surgical repair of the bladder neck following fractures of the pelvis, prostatectomy, abdominoperineal resection, excision of the urinary bladder and urethra, lumbar sympathectomy involving lumbar nerves 1 and 2 on each side, and aortic resection or bypass in which considerable dissection is involved are the most common types of surgery that result in postoperative impotence. The incidence of impotence does not seem to be related to the extent of the dissection but more to the location of the dissection.

Impotence resulting from industrial injury [13] is awarded the same compensation as is given for loss of the penis. This value is comparable to the compensation for losing a thumb: 10 percent of the body as a whole.

The restoration of potency by the use of a penile rod is worthy of consideration, especially if the patient is anxious to recover. The prognosis for improving potency by the insertion of a penile rod is inversely proportional to the degree of lost ability to obtain an erec-

tion and proportional to the ability, understanding, and cooperation of the patient's mate.

The impotence associated with multiple sclerosis may display great variations in libido and performance. The latter may be improved by the insertion of a penile rod, but since the nature of the disease is progressive, eventually coitus becomes impossible. Such a patient is often grateful for any assistance prior to the onset of paraplegia. The indications for inserting a penile rod in an already paraplegic patient are, in my opinion, indefinite. The patient who has no sensation will have a high incidence of complications. Failure of healing of the operative wound may require removing the rod. Complete anesthesia of the genitalia is one of the few contraindications to this operation.

On the other hand, if the patient has normal sensation in the penis and there are no serious psychiatric contraindications to the operation, I believe that the insertion of a penile rod is a safe and dependable aid to the patient with impotence, whether psychic or organic in cause. The rod is not easily detected, and the rod, when in place, merely makes the shaft of the penis relatively rigid. It does not cause an erection, but it does assist in initiating vaginal penetration. It may be desirable in the future to design a rod with extensions that pass along the crura of the corpora cavernosa, such as the two rods employed by Beheri [3]. Such a prosthesis has not as yet been perfected. The use of a penile rod to enlarge the size of the penis is not indicated, since the size of the penis has little or nothing to do with satisfactory coitus.

The anatomy of the penis lends itself to the insertion of a rod because of the anterior fusion of the corpora cavernosa. The urethra, with its surrounding corpus spongiosum, and the glans penis have a separate vascular and nerve supply. The corpora cavernosa are paired structures which are composed of spongy erectile sinusoids that arise from beneath the ascending rami of the ischia and pubis. The corpora are fused anteriorly into a single structure that extends just above the urethra and tapers into a recess behind the glans. They are covered by a dense fibrous investment, the tunica albuginea, which limits the size of the penile shaft. The suspensory ligament of the penis arises from the pubic symphysis and becomes part of Buck's fascia, which invests the tunica albuginea and may be separated from the tunica on the dorsum [14]. Pearman originally described a pocket in Buck's fascia for which he fashioned a specific rod, but he now places this rod within the corpora cavernosa [15].

Bone occurs in the penis in many animals [4–12]. The first attempts to make the impotent human male capable of coitus were performed in reconstruction of the amputated penis [1, 8]. Periosteal rib and bone grafts, which were originally used in reconstructions of the penis, were found to be eventually absorbed. Alloplastic materials, such as acrylic or polyethylene rods, were then tried, but did not prove reliable. We now prefer the use of Silastic (silicone rubber) rods. These have been tolerated without extrusion or other difficulties when they have been placed within the fused corpora cavernosa. Any rod that is placed outside of this dense, investing fascia will likely extrude. Beheri [3] described the use of twin polyethylene rods with thin tails that extend along the pubic rami attachments of the corpora cavernosa. There are two benefits of this design: first, additional erectile assistance is provided by virtue of the longer rod, and second, when the size of the penis is extremely short, cutting the suspensory ligament and inserting a longer rod than otherwise gives a forward projection of the penis and increases the length.

Surgical Technique

The operation starts with placing a suture through the glans for slight traction. A tourniquet is used around the base of the penis for hemostasis. A 1-inch incision is made in the middle of the dorsum of the shaft of the penis in a longitudinal fashion to avoid injury to the dorsal nerve and vessels. The incision is carried in the midline to and through the tunica albuginea of the corpora cavernosa. The dissection is carried anteriorly to the limit of the anatomical end of the corpora cavernosa. Blunt dissection proximally through the tourniquet is completed. The rod is then placed with the bulbous end beneath the glans (Figs. 51-2 to 51-9). The untapered rod extends proximally to beneath the edge of the pubic symphysis. The bifurcation of the corpora along the ramus of the pubis should not be entered by this procedure. The obvious small veins that have been cut are ligated with 5-0 plain ligature or are controlled with the coagulation current. The tunica albuginea is approximated with interrupted 5-0 Dacron sutures. The remainder of the fascial layers are approximated with interrupted small catgut sutures, and the skin is closed with a subcuticular nylon suture tied over a gauze stent. The stent is allowed to remain in place for about 2 weeks.

Only in cases of postpriapism will the entire length of the bed that is to receive the rod have to be opened and cut by sharp dissection; this is necessary because of the dense fibrous tissue that is found in such cases. Great care must be exercised not to penetrate the investing fascia or enter the urethra, since the rod will then extrude. The most likely location for entering the urethra is anteriorly, where the fossa navicularis is close to the distal portion of the corpora cavernosa. Blood may be noted in the urethra should injury to the urethra occur. No urethral catheter is

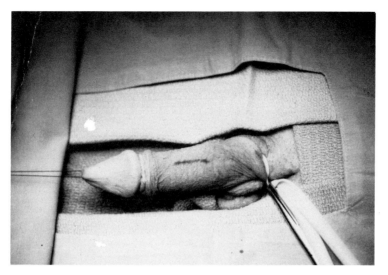

FIG. 51-2. Tourniquet is placed at the base of the penis, and a traction suture is inserted through the glans penis. The incision is outlined.

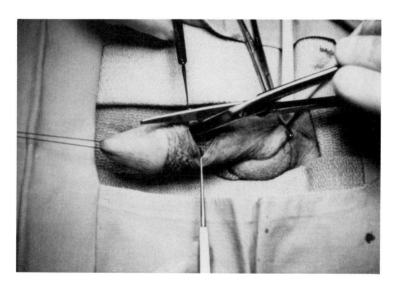

FIG. 51-3. Distal extent of dissection is carried to the end of the corpora.

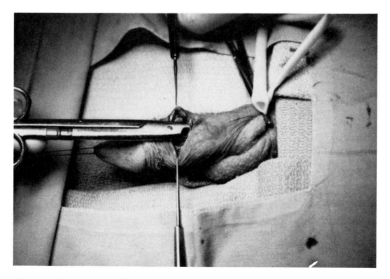

FIG. 51-4. Proximal extent of dissection is carried past the tourniquet.

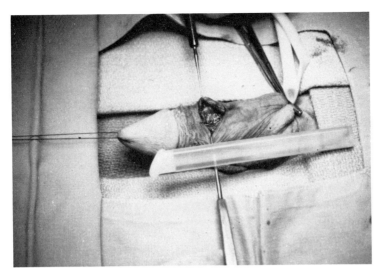

FIG. 51-5. The Silastic rod is trimmed to 10 cm; the soft expanded end is placed distally.

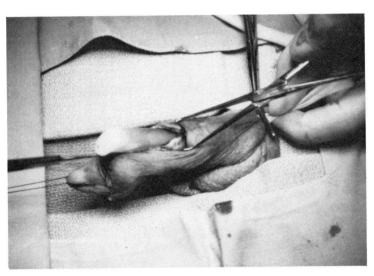

FIG. 51-6. The rod is first placed proximally after trial of the dissected rod bed distally under glans.

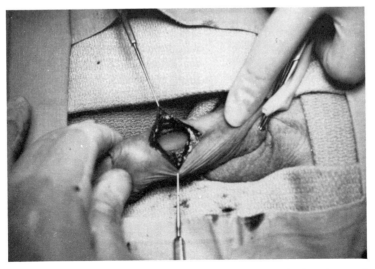

FIG. 51-7. The rod is inserted. The superficial fascia is lifted to locate the tunica albuginea for closure over the rod.

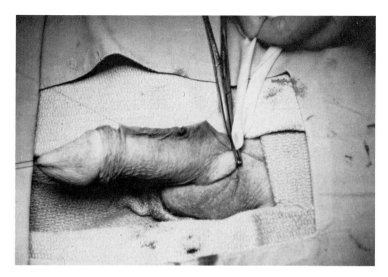

FIG. 51-8. The skin is closed with subcuticular nylon sutures and tied over a stent of 2 by 2 gauze pads.

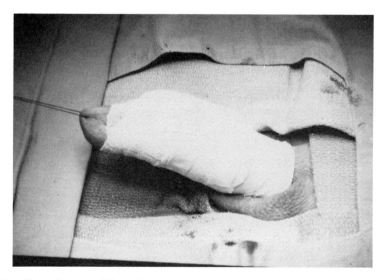

FIG. 51-9. Final dressing. Then the tourniquet is released and the traction suture is removed.

used postoperatively unless the patient has urinary retention resulting from postspinal or general anesthesia. Destruction of the corpora cavernosa from priapism that requires a difficult dissection may dictate the use of a catheter for better orientation of the urethra. The subcuticular nylon suture is left in place for 2 weeks, and the wound is supported for 1 week with tape. Coitus is postponed for 6 weeks.

Results

In the past 15 years, the author, and surgeons directly corresponding with the author (such as E. Sayegh [16], H. Lash, R. Pearman, E. Blakey [5], and many others) have used over 200 penile implants. Extrusions of the rod have occurred in five cases, and three of these cases were paraplegic patients with anesthesia of the tissues. In two cases, the rod was not placed within the corpora cavernosa.

The vast majority of the organically impotent males who were treated had postoperative or posttraumatic problems, and these patients have responded very successfully. The degree of success, however, is variable. A few patients have poor sexual cooperation at home, and they do not blame the prosthesis for their less than successful result. Two psychically impotent physicians have reported excellent personal results with the implants.

The journal *Medical Aspects of Human Sexuality* has covered most of the medical aspects of the causes of impotence but has paid little attention to surgical therapy [2]. More than 20 years ago, Kinsey [9] exposed many facets about sex that were heretofore unknown and gave interesting statistics regarding the incidence of impotence. He found that less than 0.4 percent of males under 25 years of age, less than 1 percent under age 35, 20 percent at age 60, and up to 80 percent of 80-year-old males suffer from impotency. Kinsey states that the desire for sexual activity in the aging male outlives his ability by about 10 years. There is no medical reason to withhold assistance from a man in his years of declining sexual abilities.

References

1. Ali, M. Surgical treatment of the male genitalia. *J. Int. Coll. Surg.* 27:352, 1957.
2. Bartone, F. Roundtable: Recognition and management of impotence. *Med. Aspects Hum. Sexual.* 1:76, 1967.
3. Beheri, G. E. Surgical treatment of impotence. *Plast. Reconstr. Surg.* 38:92, 1966.
4. Bett, W. R. The os penis in man and beast. *Proc. R. Soc. Med.* 44:433, 1951.
5. Blakey, E. Personal communication, 1969.
6. Blocksma, R., and Braley, S. The silicones in plastic surgery. *Plast. Reconstr. Surg.* 35:366, 1965.
7. Chusid, J. G., and McDonald, J. J. *Correlative Neuroanatomy and Functional Neurology* (13th ed.). Los Altos, Calif.: Lange Med. Publications, 1967.
8. Goodwin, W. E., and Scott, W. W. Phalloplasty. *J. Urol.* 68:903, 1952.
9. Kinsey, A. C., Pomeroy, W. B., and Martin, C. E. *Sexual Behavior in the Human Male.* Philadelphia: Saunders, 1948.
10. Lash, H., Zimmerman, D. C., and Loeffler, R. A. Silicone implantation: Inlay method. *Plast. Reconstr. Surg.* 34:75, 1964.
11. Loeffler, R. A., and Sayegh, E. S. Perforated acrylic implants in management of organic impotence. *J. Urol.* 84:559, 1960.
12. Loeffler, R. A., Sayegh, E. S., and Lash, H. The artificial os penis. *Plast. Reconstr. Surg.* 34:71, 1964.
13. McBride, E. D. *Disability Evaluation & Principles of Treatment of Compensable Injuries.* Philadelphia: Lippincott, 1963.
14. Pearman, R. Treatment of organic impotence by implantation of a penile prosthesis. *J. Urol.* 97:715, 1967.
15. Pearman, R. Treatment of organic impotence by implantation of silastic penile prosthesis: Further evaluation. *Dow Corning Bull.* 9:4, 1967.
16. Sayegh, E. S. Personal communication, 1969.
17. Scheig, R. Sexual sequelae of liver disease. *Med. Aspects Hum. Sexual.* 3:10, 1969.

Correction of Curvatures of the Penis

CHARLES E. HORTON
CHARLES J. DEVINE, JR.

52

THE MOST common curvature of the penis is associated with hypospadias. Here, the penis turns downward due to abnormal fibrous tissue which extends from the abnormally placed urethral meatus to the glans penis. This fibrous tissue lies external to the tunica albuginea. Abnormal bending of the penis can also be produced by external scarring due to trauma. Such scarring usually remains superficial to the tunica albuginea. Fortunately, this type of scarring is usually quite easily corrected by excising either the congenital bands associated with hypospadias (or the scars created by trauma) and resurfacing the penis with either flaps or skin grafts [1].

Certain types of trauma or congenital maldevelopment may affect the tunica albuginea, which as an envelope or restraining membrane against which the corporal vascular spaces expand, causing increased internal pressure. This produces a turgid, firm erection of the penis. When one side of the tunica is shortened excessively, the longer side ex-

pands more than the shortened side, and therefore a curvature of the penis results. Peyronie's disease is a typical example of a developmental anomaly involving the tunica albuginea in which a painful abnormal curvature is encountered. Other examples of penile curvature due to tunica albugineal maldevelopment include cases of trauma, in which the penis is "fractured" or the tunica albuginea ruptured, which leads to formation of scar tissue in the tunica. This scar tissue, being inelastic, prevents expansion of one side of the tunica as compared to the opposite, normal side. Hypospadias may also restrict development of the ventral side of the tunica albuginea, allowing the normal dorsal side to elongate while the ventral surface remains in a restricted, shortened condition. In a few rare cases, usually in older individuals, when the fibrous tissue bands causing chordee are removed for correction of hypospadias, if the tunica albuginea on the ventral surface has not developed appropriately, a disproportion develops, and chordee persists [1, 3, 4].

643

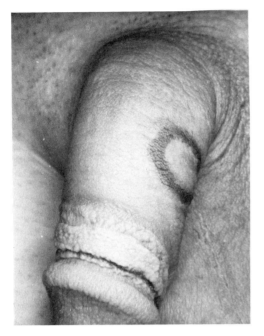

FIG. 52-1. Site of desired shortening of tunica albuginea.

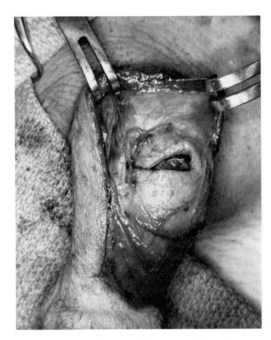

FIG. 52-2. The incision is made and shortening of the normal tunica is begun.

Treatment

When a discrepancy in length occurs between opposite sides of the tunica albuginea causing the penis to curve on erection, excision of the excess length on the normal side will correct this discrepancy and thereby improve the curvature (Fig. 52-1) [5]. As an alternative, plicating the tunica on the normal side of the penis also reduces the length of the normal side. This procedure necessarily shortens the penis; however, a shorter and more normal penis is more efficient from a functional standpoint than a longer abnormal one. There are no measurements available to help the operator determine how much tunica albuginea to remove, or how much to plicate or to excise the elongated side. Usually, if curvature is severe, the tunica on the normal side should be shortened 2 to 4 mm. Excessive bleeding is usually not a problem,

and the vascular spaces within the corpora can be dissected with ease from beneath the tunica albuginea (Fig. 52-2). This produces a ledge of tunica suitable for plication or direct closure. The use of nonabsorbable sutures is preferable. A pressure bandage is kept in place for 3 days, and unless the urethra is inadvertently damaged, no catheter drainage is necessary. Sexual intercourse is not advisable for 6 weeks after the operation.

Results

We have operated on six cases with this complex problem. These cases consisted of congenital malformations of the ventral surface of the tunica albuginea, as well as of so-called "fractures" due to trauma to the tunica albuginea. In each case, the condition has been greatly improved with this technique.

The minor shortening of the penis has not adversely affected the patient.

This operation has been recommended to correct the acute angulation of the glans on the penile shaft in hypospadias. A section of tunica on the dorsal surface just posterior to the glans is excised in order to place the glans on the immediate center of the shaft. Careful attention must be given to avoid cutting into the dorsal artery vein and the nerve which supplies sensation to the glans in this area. While this procedure is effective in the usual hypospadias case, we prefer to release the chordee by excision from the ventral surface of the glans rather than to shorten the dorsal surface of the tunica.

References

1. Farkas, L. G. *Hypospadias*. Prague: Academia, 1967.
2. Horton, C. E., and Devine, C. J., Jr. A one stage repair for hypospadias cripples. *Plastic and Reconstr. Surg.* 45:425, 1970.
3. Horton, C. E., and Devine, C. J., Jr. Hypospadias Repair for Television Demonstration. In *Transactions of the Fifth International Congress of Plastic and Reconstructive Surgery*. Melbourne: Butterworth, 1971. Pp. 333–342.
4. Horton, C. E., and Devine, C. J., Jr. *Hypospadias and Epispadias. Clin. Symp.* Vol. 24. Number 3, 1972.
5. Nesbit, R. M. Congenital curvature of the phallus: Report of three cases with description of corrective operation. *J. Urol.* 93:230, 1965.

Intrascrotal Reconstruction

IX

Testicular Prosthesis

ROBERT J. PRENTISS
MARK B SORENSEN

53

THE ABSENCE of one or both testes in males of any age may, and often does, cause psychological difficulty [1]. Children may be subjected to embarrassment if their contemporaries notice an empty scrotum. Only very sensitive adults would be bothered in this manner. However, adults sometimes have profound psychological problems relative to their sexual profile and ability. A unilaterally or totally empty scrotum has been shown, in some men, to produce psychological sexual dysfunction [2]. The only indication for placement of a testicular prosthesis is to prevent or remedy a psychological difficulty.

The causes of an empty scrotum include agenesis or torsion of a testis; injury, primary tumors, or infections may require removal of the testes; and endocrine therapy for carcinoma of the prostate may include bilateral orchiectomy.

The problem of placement of testicular prostheses has engaged the interest of many clinicians. Gelpi [6], in a 1917 publication, referred to the performance of the first successful introduction of an artificial testes by E. M. Hermance in 1885. Since then, many different materials have been used including silver, paraffin, petroleum jelly, silk, celluloid, vulcanite, rubber, plaster, marble, Vitallium, Lucite and Plexiglas (which are

methacrylates), Gelfoam, polyethylene, Dacron, glass, and ivory. The wide variety of materials and unsatisfactory results with many of them led the authors to investigate these materials in 1961 [11]. The results of this study indicated that Silastic (silicone rubber) is the best material [3, 4] (Table 53-1 and Fig. 53-1). However, even Silastic could be improved by creating a material with softer consistency than what is commercially available at present.

Our experience for 10 years has involved 66 patients and 115 prostheses. Most of our experience was obtained experimentally between 1961 and 1963. Our subsequent implacements of prostheses in the scrotum have been for ordinary indications in routine clinical and hospital practice.

Prosthetic Materials

The materials selected must be inexpensive, easy to shape, simple to sterilize without changing the appearance or consistency, nonreactive to tissue, and relatively nonconductive of heat. The weight or specific gravity of the prosthesis must be unnoticed by the patient. We have used Gelfoam, Vitallium,

TABLE 53-1. Physical Characteristics of Testicular Prostheses

Material	Weight (Grams)	Method of Sterilization	Texture	Heat Conduction	Method of Manufacture
Silicone	15.0	Autoclave	Resilient	Minimal	Molded
Plexiglas	15.0	Autoclave	Hard	Minimal	Lathe
Polyethylene	11.5	Chemical	Hard	Minimal	Lathe
Vitallium	13.0	Autoclave	Hard, hollow	Rapid?	Casting
Dacron	0.5	Autoclave	Pliable, hollow	Minimal	Fashion graft
Gelfoam	2.5	Dry heat	Pliable, absorbable	Minimal	Hand-molded

Dacron, Silastic medical-grade silicone rubber, polyethylene, and Plexiglas.

Gelfoam and Dacron are shaped manually. Dacron is obtained in the desired size by excising and compressing a segment of an arterial graft. Gelfoam is wrapped to size and secured with a suture. Both of these are makeshift. Plexiglas and polyethylene are machined to the proper size. Silastic 370 silicone rubber is molded.

Sterilization of any prosthesis is best achieved by autoclaving. Silicone, Plexiglas, Vitallium, and Dacron tolerate autoclaving (15 lb for 10 minutes), but polyethylene loses shape with excess heat, and it must be chemically sterilized. Gelfoam is sterilized by dry heat (290°F for 4 hours) and is available in any operating room.

Silicone is resilient, whereas Plexiglas, polyethylene, and Vitallium are hard. Dacron and Gelfoam are pliable; Gelfoam is also absorbable. Heat conduction is minimal in all six of these materials. Vitallium is very expensive, but the costs of other materials are relative and reasonable.

We concluded from our study that silastic medical-grade silicone rubber is the most desirable of all prosthetic materials because it

FIG. 53-1. Prosthetic materials.

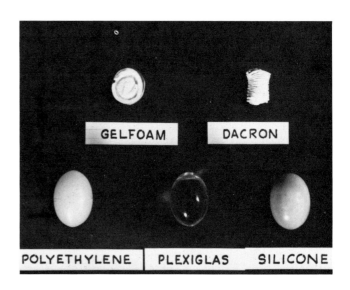

can be autoclaved, is of reasonable specific gravity, is resilient, is nonreactive in tissue, is simple to sterilize without change, and is thermally nonconductive. Polyethylene is unsatisfactory because of its hardness and the difficulty in sterilizing it. Plexiglas is unacceptable because it is too hard [10, 12]. Vitallium is unacceptable because of its hardness and great expense [8]. Dacron and Gelfoam are really makeshift and should not be used electively [13]. Dacron can be used in an emergency [9].

Another modification of the testicular prostheses of Silastic medical-grade silicone rubber is being manufactured on special order. These are based on the same methods and techniques as the Silastic mammary prostheses used in thousands of women [6]. This type is equally safe and much more life-like than the solid Silastic testicular prostheses, though more expensive [11].

Of equal importance to sterilization of the prostheses is the special cleansing that is necessary. The prosthesis is made chemically clean and free of foreign material by thorough brush scrubbing with green soap, followed by rinsing with copious amounts of water. The prosthesis must then be placed in a lint-free plastic sac, using instruments for the transfer. The plastic sac must be autoclavable. After autoclaving the prosthesis in the sac, it is placed on the operating instrument table.

On the basis of our experience and study of the literature, we arbitrarily chose the size of 3.5 by 2.5 by 2.5 cm for adult testes and 2.5 by 2.0 by 2.0 cm for those for children. Children at puberty may have an adult prosthesis placed, but children 5 and 6 years old should have the juvenile size because they appear grotesque with an adult size [7]. We have yet to have a child return after puberty requesting an adult-size testis. Since the size of testes often varies, apparently these boys can accept one testis smaller than the other [14].

Surgical Technique

The prostheses must be prepared as described above. Extreme cleanliness and complete sterility are of greatest importance. When the prosthesis is delivered to the nurses's table in the operating room, it must be handled by lint-free and powder-free instruments. The prosthesis must be protected from the chance of being dropped; reserve sterile prostheses should be on hand in case such an accident occurs.

An oblique incision is made about 2 to 3 cm in length distal to the external inguinal ring (Fig. 53-2). The incision is not made through the scrotum. The scrotal pouch is developed and widely spread digitally. (In the past we have developed dartos pockets for the prostheses, but this technique has been abandoned. Creation of a dartos pocket will hold the prosthesis in the position in which it is placed, but the technique is difficult, time-consuming, and increases com-

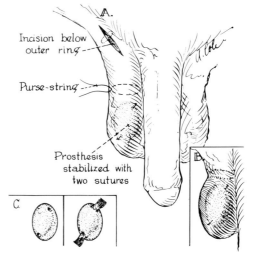

FIG. 53-2. A. Overall view with the incision location shown. B. Interval purse-string suture. C. Slots or mesh used to obtain vertical fixation.

plications. Ischemic necrosis or actual button-holing of the skin in the preparation of the pocket occasionally occurs.)

Bleeding points are controlled by fulguration or ligation. When the scrotal pouch is dry, it is thoroughly irrigated with sterile distilled water so that all fragments of fat, lint, or powder are removed. The surgeon's hands and the instruments are thoroughly rinsed with lint-free water.

Using a sterile sponge clamp, the prosthesis is extracted from the plastic container. It is wise to have the assistant hold his hands under the prosthesis as the surgeon carries it from the container to the opening in the scrotum. The opening is retracted and the

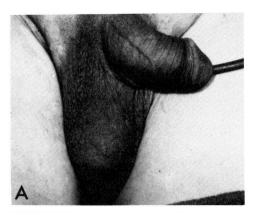
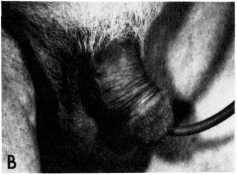

FIG. 53-3. A. Preoperative state. B. Post-operative view with prostheses in place.

prosthesis is placed in the depth in a vertical position. The prosthesis is never touched by hand.

Visualization is maintained, and a purse-string suture is then placed circumferentially above the prosthesis to trap it in the vertical position in the depths of the scrotum. The prosthesis can be modified to include superior and inferior surface slots to permit suture fixation of the prosthesis in the vertical position. Dacron mesh can be glued to each pole of the implant with Silastic Adhesive Type A. Sutures through the mesh will hold the implant properly while the fibrous tissue invades the mesh. Sutures through the prosthesis itself can tear out and are not recommended.

The subcutaneous wound is closed with running 3-0 or 4-0 catgut sutures; camelback clips are used to close the skin. A drain should not be used, and an ordinary dressing is placed. The patient is allowed to be up and around and can leave the hospital the next day (Fig. 53-3). Since infection is so much of a hazard to any prosthesis, broad-spectrum antibiotics are given before, during, and after the procedure. The operation should not be performed if there is presence of local infection.

Complications

Complications and morbidity in the young have been practically nonexistent in our series. In elderly patients with malignancies of the prostate, subsequent removal of the prosthesis due to infection that is secondary to the poor condition of the patient is occasionally necessary.

In 10 years of experience, we have had no problems with delayed reactions to Silastic prostheses.

Meticulous attention to avoiding foreign

material (lint and powder), combined with careful preparation of the prosthesis and the skin, will produce results that are satisfactory to both the patient and the surgeon.

References

1. Ajamil, L. F. Prosthesis for Testicle in Prostatic Cancer. *American Urological Association Southeast Section Transactions, 1954–60.* Pp. 132–133.
2. Baumrucker, G. O. Testicular prosthesis for an intracapsular orchiectomy. *J. Urol.* 77:756, 1957.
3. Blocksma, R., and Braley, S. The silicones in plastic surgery. *Plast. Reconstr. Surg.* 35:366, 1965.
4. Braley, S. A. Acceptable Plastic Implants. In Simpson, D. C. (Ed.), *Modern Trends in Biomechanics.* London: Butterworth, 1970.
5. Cronin, T. D., and Greenberg, R. L. Our experiences with the Silastic gel breast prosthesis. *Plast. Reconstr. Surg.* 46:1, 1970.
6. Gelpi, P. J. The tolerance of the scrotum for foreign bodies. *New Orleans Med. Surg. J.* 1917.
7. Gilbert, M., and Mencia, L. Artificial testicles in children. *South. Med. J.* 62:611, 1969.
8. Girsdansky, J., and Newman, H. F. Use of a vitallium testicular implant. *Am. J. Surg.* 53:514, 1941.
9. Hazzard, C. T. The development of a new testicular prosthesis. *J. Urol.* 70:959, 1953.
10. McCrea, L. E. Lucite: A new synthetic material suitable for testicular prosthesis. *Urol. Cutan. Rev.* 42:732, 1938.
11. Prentiss, R. J., Boatwright, D. C., Pennington, R. D., Hohn, W. F., and Schwartz, M. H. Testicular prosthesis: Materials, methods and results. *J. Urol.* 90:208, 1963.
12. Rea, C. E. The use of a testicular prosthesis made of lucite with a note concerning the size of the testis at different ages. *J. Urol.* 49:727, 1943.
13. Wright, B. W. Testicular prosthesis. *Urol. Cutan. Rev.* 42:491, 1938.
14. Wulff, H., and Sand, K. Sur la prosthèse testiculaire après la castration legale. *Acta Chir. Scand.* 92–93:476, 1945–1946.

Reconstructive
Surgery for
Male Infertility

P. FOGH-ANDERSEN

54

IN A WORLD where one of the biggest problems of the future is the surplus population and enormous amounts of money are invested in attempts to effectively control birth rates, research in sterility and the treatment of infertility might seem of minor social importance. Yet for a particular married couple, it might be very important, and therefore it is still a challenge to the medical profession to help in cases of involuntary childlessness [5].

The data for unintentional sterility vary considerably from country to country, but we roughly estimate that 10 to 15 percent of marriages are unintentionally childless. In 30 to 50 percent of the cases, it is probably only the female partner who is responsible, and in 30 to 40 percent the male is alone responsible. In 20 to 30 percent of the cases, there is most likely a combined male-female responsibility. Although the male partner is responsible, alone or in part, in at least half of the cases, female sterility so far has elicited the greatest interest in the scientific literature, as well as in therapeutic practice. This is probably due in part to the fact that childless married couples are mostly dealt with by gynecologists and in part because the therapeutic pos-

sibilities in cases of male infertility have, until recently, been regarded as poor in comparison with those for cases of female sterility.

Surgical treatment of male sterility and subfertility comprises a series of operations which, with present improved techniques, produces far better results than in the past. The majority of the operations fall into the following three categories:

1. Correction of deformities of the urethra or penis that have rendered coitus impossible or prevented normal deposition of otherwise normal semen.
2. Anastomosis operations in patients with azoospermia that is associated with normally functioning testes.
3. Varicocele operations for cases of subfertility caused by oligospermia.

Deformities of the Urethra or Penis

This group includes various conditions, chiefly phimosis and hypospadias. Phimosis does not need particular discussion; in severe cases it may give rise to impotence, and surgical treatment has long been a gratefully accepted intervention.

Hypospadias is a frequent congenital malformation. Severe hypospadias with significant chordee will often cause impotence if untreated, and childlessness for this reason was not unknown in the past. With modern techniques of operation, satisfactory results are usually obtained (see Part IV Chap. 18). The same applies to the more unusual condition, congenital shortness of the urethra (Part IV, Chap. 19). Also, plastic induration of the penis (Peyronie's disease) will, in selected cases, be amenable to surgical correction (Part VIII, Chap. 49), as will penile elephantiasis (Part V, Chap. 36).

Azoospermia Due to Blockage

Azoospermia—i.e., total absence of spermatozoa in the ejaculated semen—may be caused by an affliction of the testes with resulting failure of spermiogenesis, and in such cases no surgical treatment is possible. Azoospermia might also be due, however, to a blockage in the epididymis or the ductus deferens. In some of these patients, it is possible to perform an anastomosis operation, i.e., a vasoepididymostomy, but only if the blockage is located in the lower part of the epididymis or the adjacent part of the duct. This condition is certainly the finding in cases following gonorrheal epididymitis and also apparently in some cases of congenital strictures. Another requirement for the performance of the operation is that a preceding testicular biopsy examination has shown normal spermatogenesis.

The technique of vasoepididymostomy has been known for a long time; it was originally described by American surgeons and is simple in principle. The published results of the operation, however, have been so varying—and often so poor—that it has been discredited by many authors. The intricate nature of the reconstructive surgery for azoospermia demands a meticulous and delicate atraumatic technique. Equally important, however, is the close team-work that is required among four specialists: a gynecologist with interest in sterility research, a trained pathologist to interpret testicular biopsies, an experienced spermatologist to analyze the samples of semen, and last—but not least—the reconstructive surgeon.

The indications for a reconstructive procedure are: (1) unintentional sterility of more than one year's duration, (2) a gynecologically normal female partner, and (3) total azoospermia in the male on repeated samples of semen that is associated with normal spermatogenesis as proved by testicular biopsy on one or both sides.

The operation involves an anastomosis between the head or, preferably, the body of the epididymis and the ductus deferens (i.e., a side-to-side shunt) after having made sure that mobile spermatozoa are present in the epididymis and that the duct is patent distally [3]. In some published methods [11], the established fistula has been kept open temporarily by means of one or more wires of silver, stainless steel, or nylon as a pull-out wire. It is preferable, however, to omit this wire [1], because foreign material in the lumen may cause irritation and secondary stricture formation after the removal.

The first step of the operation is isolation of the ductus deferens, which is opened longitudinally. A fine, blunt cannula is inserted, and saline solution is injected. It is easy to determine whether there is free passage distally or a block. An oval-shaped opening is then made in the epididymis, preferably in the body or the adjacent part of the head, and the secretion is examined immediately under the microscope. If motile spermatozoa are present, an anastomosis between the epididymis and the duct is performed with the finest atraumatic silk or nylon; for this procedure, magnifying spectacles or an operation microscope are useful. Postoperative administration of hormones has been recommended [8], but this seems to be unnecessary.

In cases of azoospermia after vasectomy or unintentional ligation or division of the duct, it will usually be possible to isolate a proximal and a distal end, which should be carefully cut obliquely and then united with the finest atraumatic sutures.

The results of shunt operations and recanalizations vary considerably from clinic to clinic, but apparently they are far more successful now than previously. In about 50 percent or more of the cases, it has been possible to demonstrate spermatozoa in the ejaculated semen sometime after the operation, and a subsequent conception is no longer a rare occurrence. The largest series of patients and best results so far have been reported by Bayle [1] in Paris, who has more than 20 years' experience in this field.

Varicocele and Subfertility

This type of case is very interesting from both a theoretical and practical point of view.

A relation between varicocele and male subfertility was apparently first demonstrated in 1944 [6], and Tulloch [12] seems to be the first who reported on the restoration of fertility after a varicocele operation in a previously sterile man. Since then, several publications have shown a clear correlation between the occurrence of varicocele and oligospermia (low sperm count) or asthenospermia (poor sperm motility), and a series of reports have demonstrated considerable improvement of the spermiogram after operation on the varicocele, which in the majority of the patients is located on the left side [9].

The operation consists in high ligation or division of the spermatic vein in or just above the inguinal canal. Approach to the vein can be either through an inguinal incision, as in a hernia operation, or from above, by means of laparotomy [7]. In at least 50 percent of the cases, an improvement of the sperm density and sperm motility can be expected; the conception rate after operation varies, but an incidence of about 25 percent is not unusual.

The explanation of the surprisingly good effect of the operation is still under discussion: the factors involved are the decrease of intrascrotal temperature, a change of venous blood pressure, or, possibly, the prevention of reflux of blood containing adrenal hormones down the left spermatic vein [13].

References

1. Bayle, H. Stérilité masculine, résultats opératoires du traitement des azoospermies excrétoires. *Presse Méd.* 68:760, 1960.
2. Fogh-Andersen, P. Hypospadias. Thirty-four completed cases operated on according to Denis Browne. *Acta Chir. Scand.* 104:414, 1953.

3. Fogh-Andersen, P., and Hammen, R. Reconstructive Surgery in Azoospermia. *Transactions of the Fourth International Congress on Plastic Surgery, Rome 1967.* Amsterdam: Excerpta Medica, 1969. P. 999.

4. Fritjofsson, Å., and Åhren, C. Studies on varicocele and subfertility. *Scand. J. Urol. Nephrol.* 1:55, 1967.

5. Hagner, F. R. Operative treatment of sterility in male. *J.A.M.A.* 107:1851, 1936.

6. Hammen, R. Studies on Impaired Fertility in Man with special reference to the male. Thesis. Copenhagen and London: Munksgaard, 1944.

7. Hanley, H. G., and Harrison, R. G. The nature and surgical treatment of varicocele. *Br. J. Surg.* 50:64, 1962.

8. Lane-Roberts, C., Sharman, A., Walker, N., and Wiesner, B. P. *Sterility and Impaired Fertility.* London: Hamish Hamilton, 1939. P. 169.

9. MacLeod, J. Seminal cytology in the presence of varicocele. *Fertil. Steril.* 16:375, 1965.

10. Martin, E., Carnett, J. B., Levi, J. V., and Pennington, M. E. The surgical treatment of sterility due to obstruction at the epididymis. *Univ. Penn. Med. Bull.* 15:2, 1902.

11. Michelson, L. Vasoepididymal anastomosis by reproduction of permanent fistula with use of stainless steel wire. *Surg. Gynecol. Obstet.* 82:327, 1948.

12. Tulloch, W. S. A consideration of sterility factors in the light of subsequent pregnancies. II. Subfertility in the male. *Edinburgh Med. J.* 59:29, 1952.

13. Tulloch, W. S. Varicocele in subfertility. Results of treatment. *Br. Med. J.* 2:426, 1955.

Unusual Cases

X

Thirteen
Unusual Cases

COMPILED BY
CHARLES E. HORTON

55

Introduction

The field of genital plastic surgery deals with many unusual and perplexing problems. For this reason, several unusual cases are presented in this section. Even though these cases are seen infrequently, their consideration should be a part of the general knowledge of this anatomical area. Many of these problems are "one of a kind" or represent facets of virtually unpublished patient condition complexities. They are presented in this chapter to familiarize the reconstructive surgeon with "unusual problem cases."

The authors kindly allowed the publication of these unusual problems and provided the photographs.

Lymphogranuloma Venereum

CHARLES E. HORTON
JAMES H. CARRAWAY
STANLEY HIRSCHBERG

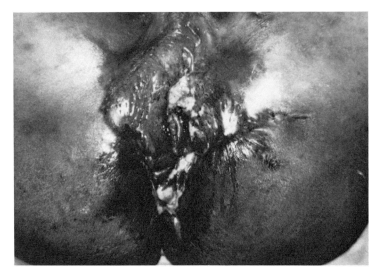

A

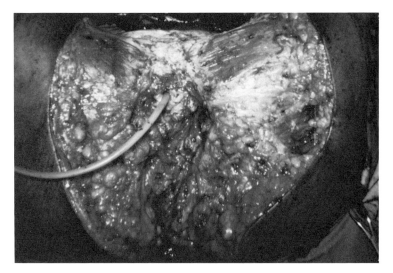

B

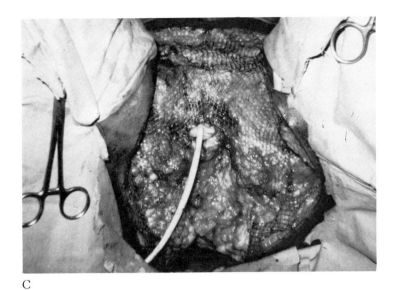

C

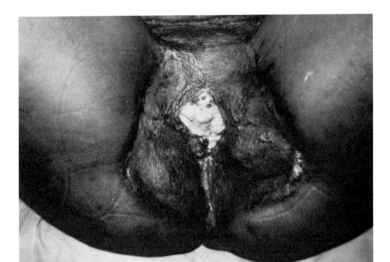

D

FIG. 55-1. A. Highly advanced lymphogranuloma venereum with recurrent perirectal and perineal abscesses. This case required 22 previous admissions to the hospital. B. Wide excision was
performed. C. Mesh graft was used. D. Postoperative appearance 1 year after surgery. The
patient is healed, employed, and has a normal sex life. Extensive disease involving the majority of
the perineal tissues must always be excised in a radical fashion, and resurfacing of the area completed as described in the text. (From *Plast. Reconstr. Surg.* 51:217, 1973. Copyright © 1973, The
Williams & Wilkins Co., Baltimore.)

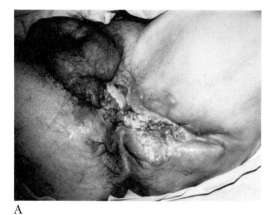

A

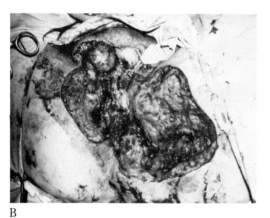

B

FIG. 55-2. A and B.   Lymphogranuloma venereum in a male patient, requiring extensive resection and grafting.

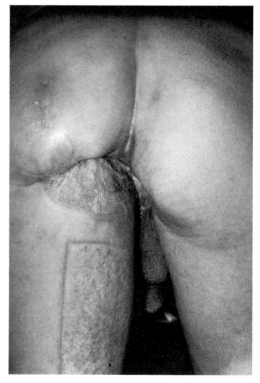

FIG. 55-3.   Postoperative healing after grafting. (Note donor site on thigh.) The patient had been confined to bed for months prior to surgery. He is now healed after excision and grafting.

Cavernous Hemangioma of the Penis

DAVID N. MATTHEWS

An infant with this disorder was referred to our hospital for assessment and treatment (Fig. 55-4) The immense hemangioma involved the scrotum and pubis as well as the penis. Since there had been transient hematuria, it was decided that it would be necessary to pass a cystoscope to see if the bladder was also involved. The child was anaesthetized, and, as a preliminary to cystoscopy, a soft rubber catheter was passed. When it had traversed only half the length of the penis, a little bright red blood appeared through the catheter and within a few seconds the child died of ventricular fibrillation. Post-mortem examination revealed an air embolus.

The case is presented to draw attention to the fact that air embolus is the major hazard in the surgery of giant hemangiomas in infants and young children. With only a minute quantity of air, ventricular fibrillation is instantaneous and lethal. Venous channels connecting the hemangioma with the systemic circulation are often the diameter of an adult thumb. Whenever excising such a lesion, the surgeon should always have a bowl of sterile saline on hand so the wound can at once be flooded by an assistant if the diathermy needle opens any cavernous space. In a total of over 100 such cases, the author once lost a child with a giant cavernous hemangioma of the calf muscles at operation from the same cause.

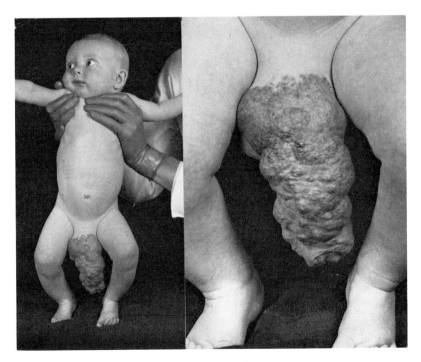

FIG. 55-4.   Cavernous hemangioma of the penis in an infant.

Snake Bite of the Penis

CLIFFORD C. SNYDER

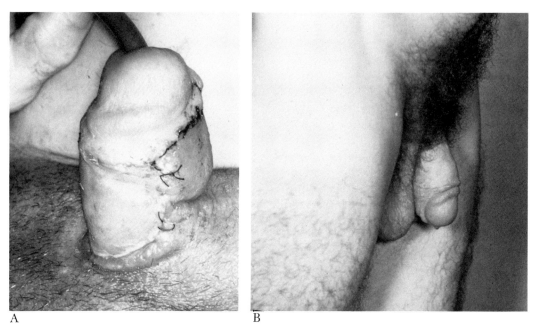

A   B

FIG. 55-5. Snake bite of the penis causing dorsal skin slough. A. Skin graft to the dorsum of the penis. B. Postoperative appearance. This patient was bitten by a rattlesnake carried in a cloth bag, as the bag brushed against the patient. The skin loss was reconstructed by a split skin graft.

Washer on Penis

CHARLES E. HORTON
ROBERT HARRELL

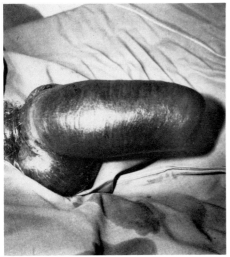

A

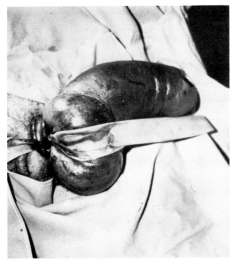

B

FIG. 55-6. A and B. Steel washer around the base of the penis. (Note distal edema and discoloration.) Special drills were necessary to remove the washer. The skin circulation returned uneventfully.

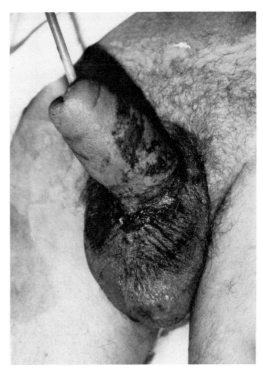

FIG. 55-7. Appearance after removal of the washer from the penis and recovery of skin viability. Many patients place strings or rubber bands around the base of the penis. Fibrous tissue reaction under the area of pressure may be so severe that surgical release of the *subcutaneous* fibrous tissue band is required.

Silastic Implants to the Buttocks

JOSEPH E. O'MALLEY

ROGER J. BARTELS ET AL.

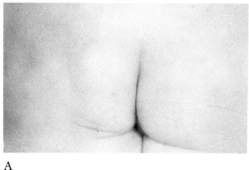
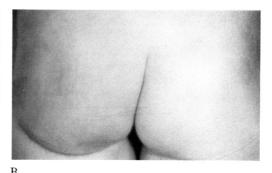

A   B

FIG. 55-8. A and B. Cronin Silastic breast implants to the buttocks. This patient had thin, sagging buttocks and desired augmentation. Breast prostheses were inserted with pleasing results to the patient. (From R. J. Bartels, J. E. O'Malley, W. Douglas, and R. G. Wilson, *Plast. Reconstr. Surg.* 44:500, 1969. Copyright © 1969, The Williams & Wilkins Co., Baltimore.)

Punitive Ablation of the Male Genitalia

DAVID MATTHEWS

Reconstruction of the penis in a single operation was performed on a boy of 16 years of age who had been mutilated at the age of four by punitive genital ablation. The genitalia had evidently been held up and cut off with a downward stroke; the penile shaft was thus cut obliquely, with the urethra severed in the perineum and a part of the corpora remaining. The scrotum was largely missing; the left testis was absent and a small part of the right testis and its duct remained. There was suprapubic scarring and scarring in the groin with much scarring of the remnants of the scrotum. The residual part of the corpora was completely buried in the abdominal skin.

Figure 55-9 depicts the initial condition, but it is not completely accurate in that it shows much more of the penile shaft than was in fact present and does not show the scrotal mutilation.

The first stage of the operation was to raise two small flaps on the ventral surface of the penis with which to restore the urethra by the Denis Browne fistula procedure (Figs. 55-10 and 55-11). Two abdominal flaps were then raised and sutured around the shaft of the penis after dissecting this from the abdominal wall. (Figs. 55-12 and 55-13). The abdominal defect was then closed with rotation flaps (Fig. 55-14). The urinary stream was diverted by a perineal catheter for 3 weeks after the operation, and intermittent urethral dilatation was necessary for a few months. The operation was carried out more than 20 years ago, and the restored organ has remained satisfactory urologically and sexually. The restoration is shown in Figure 55-15.

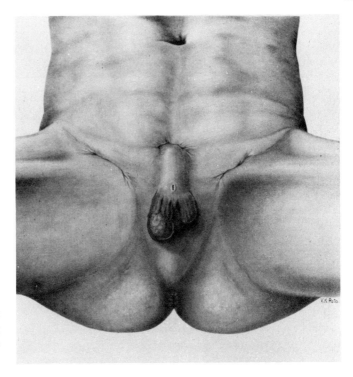

FIG. 55-9. Penile ablation: preoperative state. (Drawing is not entirely accurate—see text.)

FIG. 55-10. Flaps were raised on the ventral surface of the penis.

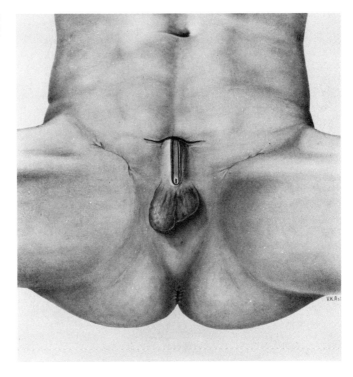

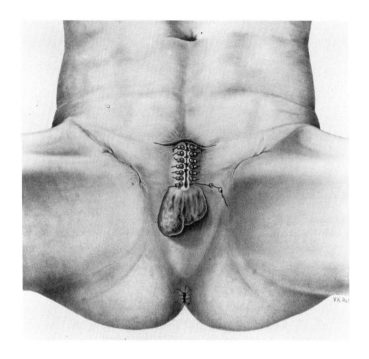

FIG. 55-11.   Restoration of the urethra.

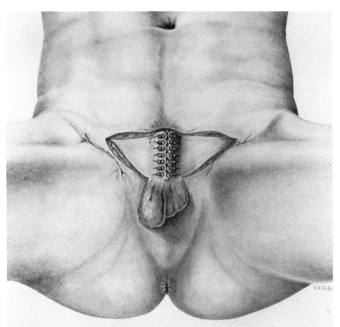

FIG. 55-12.   Abdominal flaps were raised.

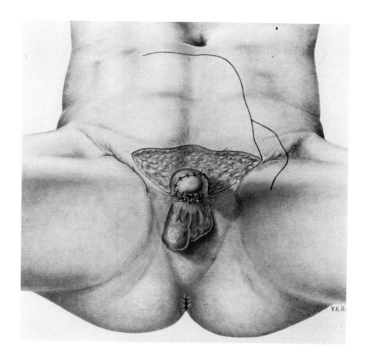

FIG. 55-13. Abdominal flaps were sutured around the penile shaft.

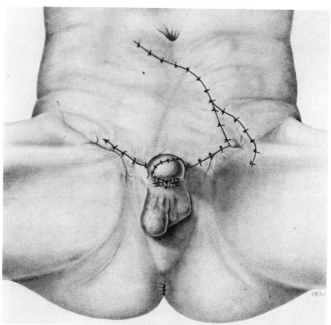

FIG. 55-14. Closure of the abdominal defect with rotation flaps.

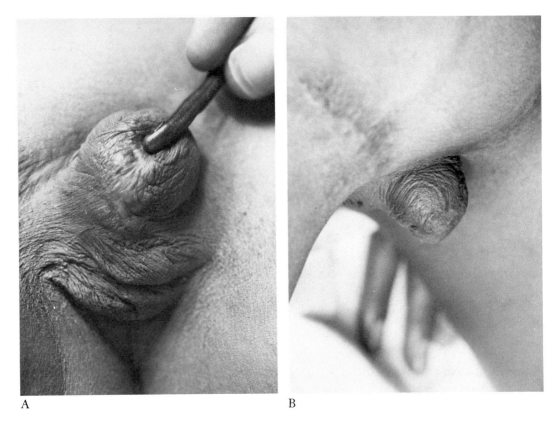

A   B

FIG. 55-15.   A and B.   Postoperative appearance.

Congenital Perineal Webbing

CHARLES E. HORTON

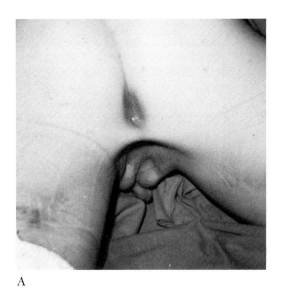

A   B

FIG. 55-16. A. Congenital perineal webbing. B. Condition was corrected with two Z-plasties.

Fournier's Disease of the Scrotum

CHARLES E. HORTON

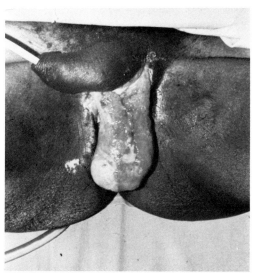

FIG. 55-17. Fournier's idiopathic gangrene of the scrotum requiring skin grafts for coverage.

Gangrene of the Skin of the Penis

CHARLES E. HORTON

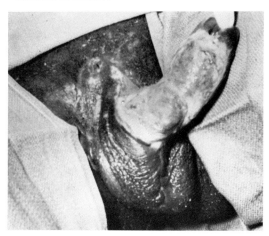

FIG. 55-18. Gangrene of the skin of the penis in a paraplegic. A tight, condom-type drainage bag was tied around the base of the penis to treat urinary incontinence. Skin grafting was required.

Radionecrosis of the Vulval Region: Tubed Pedicle Repair

IAN MCGREGOR

A 78-year-old woman was referred for treatment of an area of radionecrosis in the vulval region. Nine years previously, a vulvectomy had been performed for leukoplakia. Seven years later, a well-differentiated squamous cell carcinoma on the left side of the introitus and encroaching on the urinary meatus was treated with a radium implant. A dose of 6000 rads at 0.5 cm was recorded. One year later, the introitus was contracted and she had an ulcerated lesion around the urethral meatus. A biopsy examination was performed on the area, which showed considerable radiation effects but no evidence of tumor. The introitus was enlarged, but it contracted again within the year. The ulcer was still present.

An abdominal tubed pedicle was raised, 4½ by 9 inches in size. This was based on the left superficial epigastric vessels and crossed the midline. The upper end was delayed 6 weeks later (Fig. 55-19) and detached after 19 days. An area of skin and subcutaneous tissue 6 cm in diameter surrounding the meatus and introitus was removed, and the tubed pedicle was inset (Fig. 55-20). After 3 weeks, the pedicle was divided and completely inset. Excess tube was then excised. A biopsy specimen showed that the recurrent carcinoma had been completely excised, and there was no sign of further growth 1 year later (Fig. 55-21).

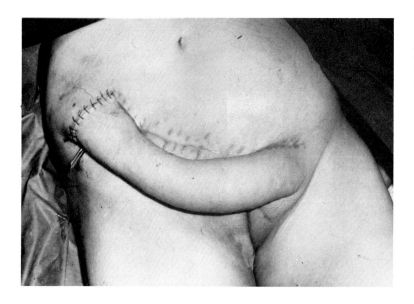

FIG. 55-19. Tubed pedicle was based on the left superficial epigastric vessels and the upper end was delayed.

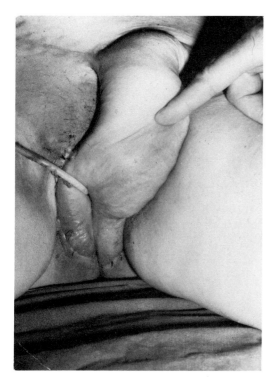

FIG. 55-20. Vulval region was excised and the upper end of the tube inset.

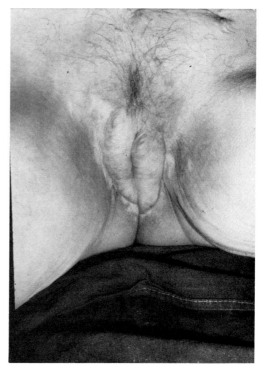

FIG. 55-21. Completed repair.

Attempt to Enlarge Normal Penis

WILLIAM DOUGLAS

A 41-year-old white male stated that about 3 years prior to treatment, he awoke in an alcoholic stupor to find his penis swollen and painful. He was told that his companion (whom he described as an "ex-intern who was a narcotic addict and who was later imprisoned on narcotic charges convictions") had injected his penis with petrolatum jelly in an attempt to make his normal penis larger.

Physical examination of the genitalia revealed that the skin of the entire shaft of the penis and the adjacent 1 inch of the scrotum was replaced by fibrotic tissue with deep craters (Fig. 55-22A and B). There was general induration of the entire area, but no inguinal lymphadenopathy. A single indurated area about 8 mm in diameter was also present on the glans. A wide excision was performed (Fig. 55-22C). Closure of the defect with a split-thickness skin graft was successful (Fig. 55-22D and E). The pathological diagnosis of the excised specimen was fat necrosis, fibrosis, and chronic inflammation of the penis.

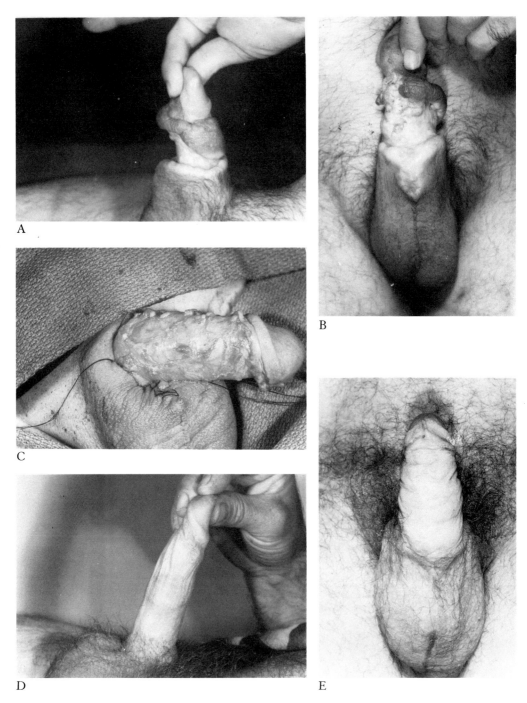

FIG. 55-22. A and B. Preoperative view. C. View at operation. D and E. Skin graft.

Circumcision Burn

LORENZO ADAMS

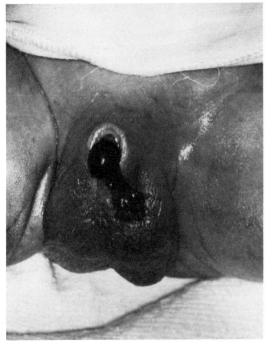 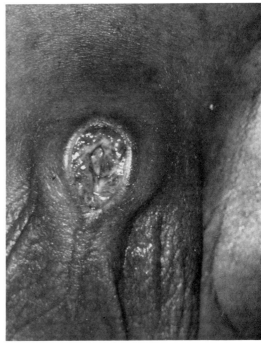

FIG. 55-23. Necrosis of penis due to malfunction of electrical current at time of circumcision.

Spider Bite

FRANK MASTERS

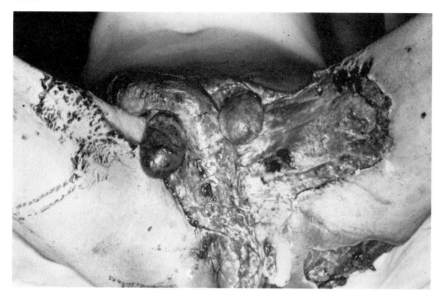

FIG. 55-24.   Brown spider bite of genital area causing massive necrosis. These spiders are seen frequently in outhouses. The bite typically causes extensive tissue necrosis. (From F. Masters and D. W. Robinson. *J. Trauma* 8:430, 1968. Copyright © 1968, The Williams & Wilkins Co., Baltimore.)

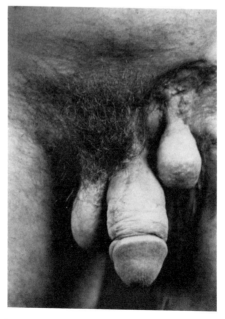

FIG. 55-25.   Reconstruction after split-thickness grafting.

Index

Index